ARTHROPLASTY - UPDATE

Edited by **Plamen Kinov**

Arthroplasty - Update
http://dx.doi.org/10.5772/56149
Edited by Plamen Kinov

Contributors

Hiran Amarasekera, Ricardo Becerro De Bengoa Vallejo, Marta Elena Losa Iglesias, Miguel Fuentes Rodriguez, Tsutomu Gomi, Hiroshi Hirano, Masahiro Nakajima, Kalman Tóth, Pietro Melloni, Maite Veintemillas, Anna Marin, Rafael Valls, Michael Soudry, Jean Yves Lazennec, Ali Sina Shahi, Hamid Reza Seyyed Hossein Zadeh Ardebili, Samih Tarabichi, Usama Hassan, Mehrnoush Hassas Yeganeh, Aidin Masoudi, Gholam Hossein Kazemian, Pablo Renovell, Antonio Silvestre, Oscar Vaamonde, Manuel Villanueva, Antonio Ríos-Luna, Francisco Chana-Rodriguez, Antonio J Pérez Caballer, Jose-Antonio De Pedro, Hamid Reza Seyyed Hosseinzadeh, Mohammad Emami, Farivar Abdollahzadeh Lahiji, Sina Emami, Andrew Gordon, Mark Wilkinson, Hosam E Matar, Michelle Maree Dowsey, Trisha Peel, Peter Choong, Kirsty Buising, Plamen Kinov, Peter Tivchev, Francisco Argüelles, Fernando Almeida, Raúl Lopez, Nahum Rosenberg, Maruan Haddad, Doron Norman, Asim Rajpura, Timothy Board, Alper Gokce, Vladan Stevanovic, Zoran Stanisa Vukasinovic, Dusko Spasovski, Branislav Starcevic, Dragana Matanovic, Zoran Bascarevic, Moby Parsons, Eun Kyoo Song, Jong-Keun Seon, Ji-Hyeon Yim, Nadr M. Jomha, M. Elizabeth Pedersen, Angela Scharfenberger, Gordon Goplen, Adrian J Cassar Gheiti, Kevin J Mulhall, Takedani, Rubin, Scott Ritterman, Timothy McTighe

Published by InTech

Janeza Trdine 9, 51000 Rijeka, Croatia

Publishing Process Manager Danijela Duric
Technical Editor InTech DTP team
Cover InTech Design team

Additional hard copies can be obtained from orders@intechopen.com

Arthroplasty - Update, Edited by Plamen Kinov
p. cm.
ISBN 978-953-51-0995-2

For EU product safety concerns:
IN TECH d.o.o., Prolaz Marije Krucifikse Kozulić 3, 51000 Rijeka, Croatia,
info@intechopen.com or visit our website at intechopen.com.

Meet the editor

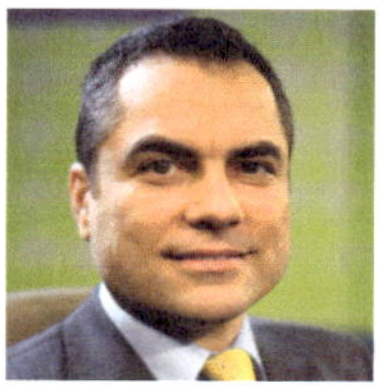

Assoc. Professor Plamen Kinov, MD, PhD, is a Head of Joint Replacement Unit at Department of Orthopedics, Medical University of Sofia, Bulgaria, with his scientific interests focused on hip and knee replacement. He graduated medicine with honors in 1995 at the Medical University of Pleven, Bulgaria and completed his training in orthopedics at Medical University of Sofia, Bulgaria. He was a research fellow at the Department of Orthopedics, University of Graz, Austria and a visiting fellow in Graz, Austria, Munich, Germany, and Bologna, Italy. He was awarded International Society of Orthopedic Surgery and Traumatology (SICOT) Abdel Hay Mashhour Award and Bulgarian Orthopedics and Traumatology Association (BOTA) Award. He is an author of over 120 scientific publications. He is a Treasurer of the Bulgarian Orthopedics and Traumatology Association (BOTA) and was a Secretary of BOTA and an Editorial Secretary of Bulgarian Journal of Orthopedics and Traumatology. Plamen Kinov is a member of European Federation of National Associations of Orthopedics and Traumatology (EFORT), American Academy of Orthopedic Surgeons (AAOS), European Hip Society (EHS), among other scientific societies.

Contents

Preface

Arthroplasty is one of the most dynamic and rapidly expanding spheres of orthopedics and medical science. The successive stages of development of the technique of joint replacement include introduction of uncemented implants, emergence of biomaterials and ceramics, and evolution of bearing surfaces. Last but not least, credit to the success of arthroplasty is attributed to continuous improvements in surgical technique and introduction of mini-invasive techniques during the last decade. All these contribute to the tremendous success and unusual popularity of the intervention. As a result, it is not a surprise that the number of arthroplasties increases steadily every year and nowadays more than one million patients undergo the procedure annually worldwide. Moreover, based on the global aging of the population and higher arthritis prevalence, the demand for the procedure is expected to increase steadily.

The purpose of this book is to provide an overview of the up-to-date developments in orthopedic surgery. It is a sequel of a successful series dedicated to one of the fastest growing fields in orthopedics - arthroplasty. Aiming at dissemination of scientific research this book provides a profound overview of the recent evolution of technology and surgical techniques. The process of improving care for patients and standards of treatment requires straightforward access to up-to-date research and knowledge. The format of the publication allows easy and quick reference to shared ideas and concepts. We hope, that the current book will add significant contribution to the success of this endeavor.

New technologies, improvements in implant design and advances in surgical technique have yielded favorable outcomes after joint replacement and decreased rate of complications. In short-term perspective mini-invasive surgery may offer certain advantages. However, successful clinical outcome after arthroplasty is a function of stable and long-lasting fixation of the implant. This in addition to a pain-free joint with a functional range of motion defines the arthroplasty as successful.

New developments of implant design have been extensively reviewed and current treatment approaches have been critically discussed in the light of clinical outcome by the contributing authors. Consideration of new technologies in implant design and advances in surgical technique is an integral part to preoperative planning and decision making. Such approach helps expand the armamentarium for solving difficult problems such as osteolysis in primary and revision setting. Valuable contribution of this book is the detailed and exhaustive review of predictors of clinical outcome following total joint replacement. Special attention was given to various complications after arthroplasty. Despite the great success of joint replacement surgery, infection of the prosthesis is still a concern. Increased morbidity, necessity for further operations, prolonged hospital stay, and finally, higher costs are inevitable consequences of this devastating complication. Due to these facts, periprosthetic infections were widely discussed in a separate book section. Prophylaxis, diagnostics and treatment of this serious complication were viewed from different perspectives. Special attention was attributed to the role of various microorganisms and biofilm in the pathogenesis of prosthetic joint infections, specific characteristics of particular microorganisms and to providing optimal treatment strategy. As the book chapters were written by different authors, some topics had been discussed in repetition. In such a project this is inevitable. However, the analyses of the problems from different standpoints only increased the value of the book.

The book could be used as a reference manual in studying of joint replacement, and as for analysis of the occurred questions, related to endoprosthetics. I acquired - upon the editing - a new and detailed view on the process of writing a medical book. Besides, the editing of this book allowed me to extend my horizon of knowledge and led to appearance of new questions as well, related to my scientific researches in the field of joint replacement. I also used the possibility of quick review of a given theme and of obtaining the essence of presentation. It became possible through an analysis of the thesis and aim of the author, review of the examples for illustrating of the thesis and searching for a practical application of the presented ideas. This is an approach, which would also help the reader in a brief review of the problem in our increasingly busy daily life.

I would like to thank the contributing authors for their commitment to the project and providing of up-to-date review of joint replacement. I thank them for sparing time and resources, sharing their knowledge and experience. Without their enthusiasm, accuracy and responsibility, the book would hardly be realizable. I would like to thank Silvia Vlase and Danijela Duric, the Publishing Process Managers, for their kind assistance. Last but not least, I thank our readers to whom this book is addressed and without whom it would be fruitless.

Plamen Kinov, MD, PhD
Assoc. Professor and Head,
Joint Replacement Unit, Dept. of Orthopedic Surgery,
University Hospital Queen Giovanna
ISUL, Sofia, Bulgaria

Section 1

Decision Making for Arthroplasty

Chapter 1

Surgical Approaches to the Hip Joint and the It's Clinical Implications in Adult Hip Arthroplasty

Hiran Amarasekera

Additional information is available at the end of the chapter

http://dx.doi.org/10.5772/55212

1. Introduction

The Hip joint can be approached in many ways and therefore many different exposures have been described. The choice of which approach to use depend on the type of surgery, what part of the hip needs to be exposed, age of the patient and surgeon's preference and expertise.

When approaching the hip it is also important to consider whether the surgery is done for trauma or elective surgery, whether the patient is an adult or a child whether it is conservative hip surgery or replacement surgery and what part needs to be accessed for the specific surgery such as the acetabulum, femoral head or whether both need equal access as in total hip arthroplasty.

The main aim of this chapter is to discuss the available surgical approaches in the adult hip when elective reconstructive surgery is done such as total hip resurfacing and revision hip arthroplasty.

The advantages and dis-advantages and the clinical relevance of these approaches to each surgery and basic surgical steps are discussed including the traditional approach and the modification of these approaches.

For completion of the chapter most approaches and classifications are mentioned but the emphasis is mainly on the common approaches used in hip arthroplasty. A good approach to the hip should have good access to both femoral head and acetabulum, should have minimal dissection of soft tissues, leading to reduced operative time and blood loss, less post operative pain and early mobilisation, least risk of damage to neurovascular bundles muscles and tendons with minimal risk of infection thrombosis and dislocation. However in practice there is no one ideal approach hence many approaches have been described and used among orthopaedic surgeons over the years.

2. Classification of different surgical approaches

Surgical approaches to the hip joint can be classified in many ways. One simple classification is based on the direction of approach. (Fig 1) The common approaches used based on this classification are the anterior, antero-lateral and posterior. Some of the different ways of classifying surgical approaches to the hip is given below. [1]

a. **Based on the direction**

1. Anterior type
2. Lateral and antero lateral type
3. Posterior type
4. Medial type
5. Combined e.g. anterior and posterior

b. **Based on incision and invasiveness**

1. Standard incision e.g. Posterior
2. Mini incision posterior (MIS)

c. **Based on type od surgery**

1. Open surgical e.g. anterior
2. Arthroscopic

It is also important to know that certain new approaches described are essentially a modification of an existing approach. E.g. Trochanteric flip approach is a modification of an anterior type approach. [2]

3. Surgical approaches to the hip joint

Before performing any surgical approach it is important understand the anatomical principles that lie behind the surgical dissection.

Like in all orthopaedic surgeries positioning the patient, draping and preparing the area, identification of landmarks and making the incision along skin creases, are important to remember. It is also important to note that all incisions should be made along the identified line of incision but the initial incision is best made within the middle half of the incision line so that if needed this can be extended in either direction. Previous concept of "Big surgeons make big incisions" does not hold true in modern day practice as the demand is for mini incisions and key hole surgery as they give a better cosmetic outcome.

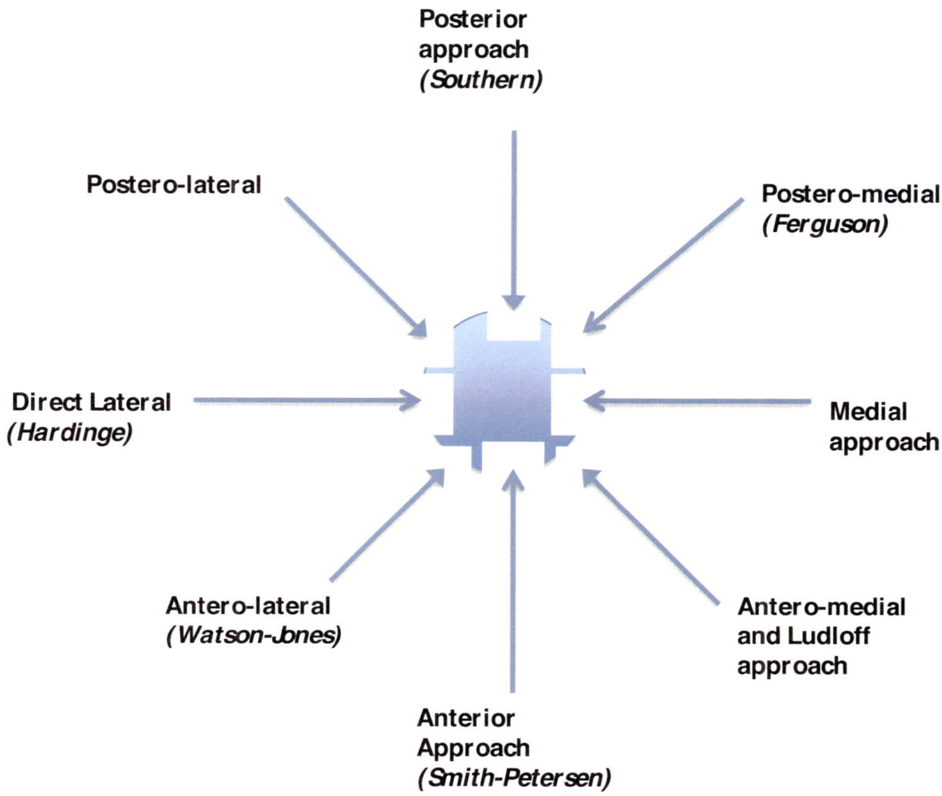

Figure 1. All directions the hip can be approached.

Another principle in operative orthopaedic surgery is the attempt to go directly to the operative area whether it is a bone or a joint. This minimises the lateral dissection thus avoiding damage to soft tissues such as nerves and vessels.

The concept of "*internervous plane*" is important to understand before any surgical approach is done. This means that all deep dissection should be done by dissecting and separating the muscles between two nervous planes so that all muscles supplied by one nerve and it's branches are retracted towards one side to avoid damage and denervating the muscles. (Fig 2)

It is not always possible to dissect along the internervous plane. Sometimes dissection planes are developed by splitting the muscles. (Fig 3) The principles of muscle splitting incision are

1. Always muscles are split longitudinally along the line of the fibres.
2. Splitting is done away from the neuromuscular junction to avoid denervation.
3. Bulk of the muscle is retracted along with the nerve-so that most of the muscle will retain the nerve supply.

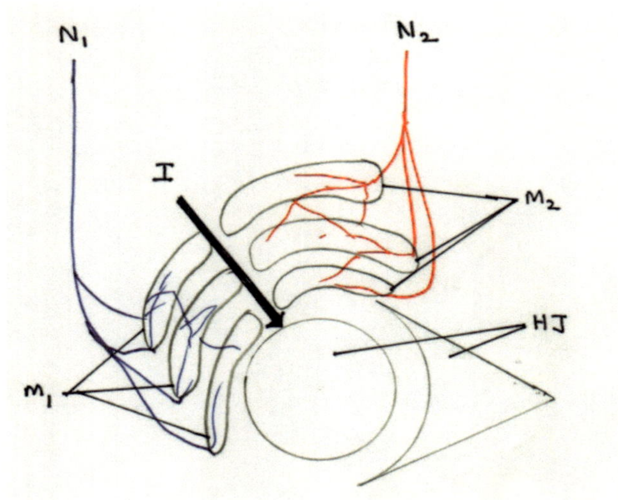

Figure 2. Concept internervous plane, (HJ, Hip Joint; N1Nerve supplying the muscle group M1; N2 nerve supplying the muscle groupM2; I internervous plane)

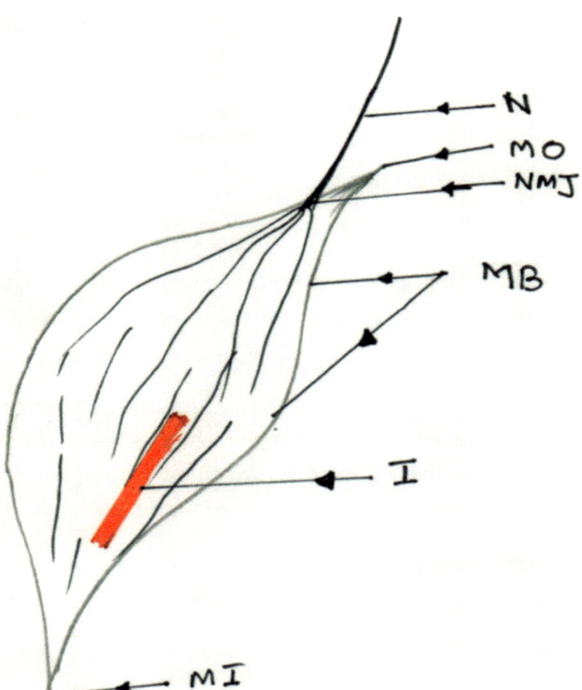

Figure 3. Muscle splitting incisions *(I)* are made along the line of the fibres, away from the Neuro-muscular junction *(NMJ) MO: Muscle Origin, MB: muscle Belly, MI: Muscle Insertion, N: Nerve*

http://dx.doi.org/10.5772/55212

In the next few paragraphs the following approaches are described in relation to the clinical implications.

1. **Anterior approaches**

a. Anterior type approach is Smith Peterson approach

b. Mini incision anterior approach

2. **Lateral approaches**

a. Direct Lateral /Hardinge

b. Antero-Lateral /Watson Jones

3. **Posterior approach**

a. Southern Approach [3]

4. **Medial approaches**

a. Antero medial

b. Postero-medial (Ferguson Approach)

c. Ludloff's approach

5. **Modern**

a. Arthroscopic

b. Minimally invasive

6. **Modified and combined approaches**

a. Trochanteric Flip Ganz [2]

b. Antero –lateral minimally invasive [4]

c. Mini incision posterior approach [5]

d. Modified antero-lateral [6]

e. Combined approaches [7]

Out of these approaches it is important understand that the medial approaches are rarely used in hip arthroplasty due to poor access to acetabulum and femoral head.

Even though a detailed description of each surgical approach is beyond the scope of this chapter all the salient features of above approaches are discussed with regard to their key steps, key advantages, key limitations, specific complications, common surgical procedures done through the approach, modifications of the traditional approach and other key issues.

The approaches described in depth below are the surgical approaches used commonly in hip arthroplasty.

4. The anterior approach *(Smith-Petersen)*

a. Key steps

This approach initially described by Smith-Peterson [8] is one of the approaches but not a very popular approach used by arthroplasty surgeons as the femoral exposure is limited. It is mainly used for arthrotomies to drain the hip in presence of infection. The key steps and the details are given below.

Position: Supine with a pillow under the pelvis on the operating side

Incision: Longitudinal incision lies between anterior iliac crest towards upper thigh curving over anterior superior iliac spine.

Soft tissue dissection: This is between sartorius and the tensor fasciae lata and rectus femoris and gluteus medius.

Internervous plane: Lies between the sartorius (Femoral nerve) and the tensor fasciae latae (Superior gluteal nerve)

Arthrotomy: Adduct and externally rotate the leg and incise the capsule longitudinally or with W or T shape incision.

Dislocation: by external rotation

Closure: In layers capsule rarely closed. Fascial planes are closed and skin

b. Key advantages

The advantages of this approach include preservation of the vascularity, stability following the procedure with less chance of dislocation. Limited morbidity, high stability and with good access to the acetabulum are key advantages of this approach. [9] The approach limits muscle cutting and separation, reduce chance of dislocations, and makes it easier to take intra-operative radiographs as the patient is supine in position. Key muscle groups the extensors and the abductors are kept intact the along with the medial circumflex femoral artery and it's branches. [10], [11]

c. Key Limitations

The key limitation of this approach is the limited access making it technically demanding to place components in arthroplasty. Even though the approach to the acetabulum is good approach to proximal femur is limited through this approach. Some encourage to use a fracture table to get a better approach to the femur [12] while others use the standard operating table. [13]

Even though many total hip arthroplasties and even resurfacing hip replacements are done using this approach [10] due to limited access and technical demanding nature [14] this may not be a popular approach among arthroplasty surgeons.

d. Specific complications, [15]

Damage to lateral cutaneous nerve and the anterior cutaneous nerve should be kept in mind. [16]

e. Common surgical procedures

Even though hip arthroplasty is not commonly done some surgeons still prefer to do total hip arthroplasty [17] and hip resurfacing [10] through an anterior approach.

f. Modifications to the approach

The modification of this approach includes two incision direct anterior approach and minimally invasive direct anterior approaches. [18], [19] Low blood loss, early recovery, early mobilisation reduced operating time are the advantages of the minimally invasive anterior approach. [20]

5. Antero-lateral approach *(Watson-Jones)*

Described initially by Watson-Jones [21] approaches the hip between tensor fascia lata and the gluteus medius muscle planes.

a. Key Steps:

Position: The patient can be positioned supine or laterally on the table

In the supine position a sand bag may be placed under the pelvis on the operating side.

Incision: Longitudinal incision is made while flexing the hip slightly extending over the centre of the greater trochanter running posteriorly along the shaft of the femur.

Soft tissue dissection: This is done by identifying the plane between the tensor fasciae latae and the gluteus medius taking care not to damage the inferior branch of the superior gluteal nerve as it supplies the former muscle.

Vastus lateralis is identified and the muscle is detached from the origin and the capsule identified.

Internervous plane: Since the superior gluteal nerve supply both gluteus medius and tensor fasciae latae it is difficult to define a true internervous plane for this approach. However as long as the plane between these muscles are not dissected superiorly up to the origin the nerve will remain intact.

Arthrotomy: The capsule is divided longitudinally over the anterior superior femoral neck.

Dislocation: This is done by applying external rotation, traction and adduction to dislocate the hip.

Closure: The wound is closed in layers starting with the capsule. If a trochanteric osteotomy is performed it has to be re attached.

b. Key advantages

The key advantages of the approach include stability, less chance of posterior dislocation, less risk to sciatic nerve damage unless during dislocation where traction can stretch the nerve. Precautions should also be taken not to damage the superior gluteal nerve.

c. Key limitations

One of the key limitations is that possibility of abductors getting weak during dissection or by denervation of the nerve supply. [22]

d. Specific complications

Damage to superior gluteal nerve and lateral circumflex femoral artery (LCFA) should be kept in mind.

Damage to the femoral nerve and vessels are a relatively rare complication.

e. Modifications

Mueller modified the approach to avoid trochanteric osteotomy.

Another recent modification for this approach is the minimally invasive approach.[4] Antero lateral minimally invasive approach (ALM) has been described as a good alternative [23] to traditional approaches as it reduces hospital stay, surgical time, blood loss, morbidity, and encourages early mobilisations, and recovery. Even though some report high complication rates [24] with this approach over all this is an approach with many advantages in the modern day practice. However this is a technically demanding procedure that needs expertise.

Trochanteric flip approach developed by Ganz et al is can be considered as a modification or combined type approach where steps of posterior approach is used but the hip is dislocated anteriorly by performing a trochanteric flip osteotomy.[2]

f. Advantages

The key advantage of this approach is the protection of medial circumflex femoral artery thus preserving the main blood supply to the hip. Therefore this becomes an important approach to use in conservative hip surgery and the surface replacement of the hip joint as this can protect the femoral head and neck from developing avascular necrosis (AVN). [25] The key step of this approach is the trochanteric flip osteotomy where a bony flip of around 1.5cm made over the greater trochanter and reflected anteriorly along with vastus lateralis, gluteus medius and minimus and the hip is dislocated anteriorly thus avoiding and dissection of short external rotators.

g. Key limitations

The key limitations include the patient need to be non-weight bearing for six weeks or until the trochanteric osteotomy is healed. Non-union and separation of the osteotomy are other potential complications. [6] (Fig 4)

6. Direct lateral approach

Direct lateral approach also called as the trans-gluteal approach initially described by Kocher in 1903 [26] popularised by Hardinge in the modern age [27] gives good exposure to the hip

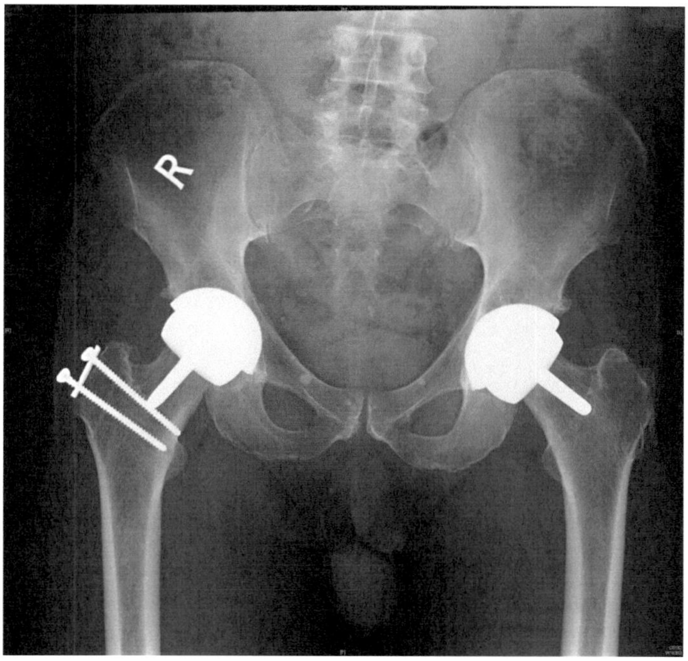

Figure 4. Post-operative X ray of patient showing Hip resurfacing done through Posterior approach (Left Hip) and Trochanteric flip approach (Right hip), note the re-attachment of the osteotomy with screws and loosening of the lower screw.

joint preserving most of gluteus medius minimus and vastus lateralis, and the vascularity. It exposes the femur well with good access to the joint.

a. Key steps

Position: This can either be done on lateral or supine position

Incision: from mid point of greater trochanter longitudinally along the femoral shaft extending around 8-10 cm with proximal extension up to anterior superior iliac spine. [27]

Incision: Usually it is made about 7-10 cm below the tip of the greater trochanter along the anterior border of the femur.

Soft tissue dissection: Gluteal fascia and illio tibial band divided and plane between tensor facia late and gluteus maximus is identified. Gluteus medius incised and approach via gluteus medius and vastus muscles.

Internervous plane: As the gluteus medius tendon and muscle fibres and the vastus lateralis muscles are split there is no true internervous plane. However it is important are split protect the superior gluteal nerve by making the incision distal to the point which it enters the muscle.

Dislocation: Leg can be externally rotated and abducted for dislocation [27].

Closure: Illio tibial ligament initially re attached followed by gluteus medius suturing.

b. Key advantages

This approach gives good access to the hip and yet preserves vascularity and minimise risk of damage to sciatic nerve as compared to the posterior approach.

c. Key limitations

Damage to gluteal muscle mainly medius can increase recovery time,

d. Specific complications

Complications are relatively rare with low dislocation rates. Heterotopic ossification may be a problem in selected cases. [28]

e. Common surgical procedures

Total hip replacements, hip resurfacing, [29] trauma, and many procedures can be done via this.

f. Modifications

Modifications include the trans gluteal approach. [30] This has been compared with Watson Jones approach and appear to be a good alternative to the traditional approach. [31] According to some authors the surgical exposure can be improved by modifying the way muscle fibres are split, fascia is cut retractors are placed and closing the wound. [32]

Lateral trans trochanteric approach was initially described in 1881 by Ollier and popularised by Sir John Charnley provide a good exposure hip joint is mainly used in revision arthroplasties. [33]

7. Posterior approach

Also called, as the Southern approach is one of the commonest approaches used by the orthopaedic surgeons at present.

a. Key Steps

Position: Mostly done in lateral position

Incision: standard incision is 10-15 cm long curve-linear extending from posterior superior iliac spine to greater trochanter and extending down in a variable distance along the shaft of the femur. The modern incisions are shorter than the standard. As this can be extended if needed it is sensible to initially make a smaller incision and extend if needed.

Soft tissue dissection: Initially fascia lata and vastus lateralis is cut. The gluteus maximus fibres are split. Then the hip is internally rotated and short external rotators are cut after holding them with stay sutures.

Obturator internus and piriformis is detached and reflected backwards to protect the sciatic nerve.

Internervous plane: As we split through the fibres of gluteus maximus rather than between muscle planes it is difficult to find a true internervous plane. How ever as the nerve enters the muscle medial to the split the muscle denervation is unlikely.

Arthrotomy: Capsule is incised with a T shaped incision

Closure: Capsular closure is described but the practicality is an issue mainly following hip arthroplasty procedures.

It is important re-attached the external rotators and obturator internus and piriformis.

b. Key advantages

This is a good approach that provides excellent exposure to both acetabulum and the femoral head and neck equally making it easier to surgical procedures well.

c. Key Limitations

Due to the possibility that blood supply may get damaged resulting in AVN has limited it's used in conservative hip surgery such as open hip debridement, open surgery for hip impingement and use of this in paediatric population is not recommended.

d. Specific Complications

The posterior approach has specific complications these are

1. Damage to sciatic nerve, which could be either stretching which recover usually, or permanent damage, which will result in a foot drop.

2. Damage to inferior gluteal vessels, branches of profunda femoris vessels and rarely femoral vessels.

3. Invariably branches of medial circumflex femoral artery are cut during this approach, which can theoretically give rise to AVN of femoral head and neck. This does not matter in total hip replacement as the head and neck is removed but in conservative procedures including hip resurfacing arthroplasty. Many authors have challenged however the clinical implications of this blood flow drop. [34]- [37] Some argue the blood supply drop is transient which may recover during post-operative period. [38]

e. Common surgical procedures

This is in an approach commonly used to do Primary and revision total hip replacements, hip resurfacings, and other procedures such as open reduction of hip dislocations and fixation of acetabular fractures.

f. Modifications

Minimally invasive (MIS) posterior approach is a modification. This approach when compared with standard lateral approach has similar outcomes during early post-operative period such as surgical duration, blood loss and hospital stay but long term results such as Harris Hip score is higher in the MIS. [39] Similar results have been achieved when compared with postero-lateral approaches. [40] When compared with the standard posterior approach it was found to be less blood loss, less post-operative pain and early recovery. [41] Gibson approach [42] is another modification and can be considered a poster-lateral type of approach.

8. Postero-lateral approach

Initially described by Langenback in 1874 [43] is another approach that can be used in hip arthroplasty surgery. Compared with trans trochanteric approach it is believed that this has less blood loss and shorter hospital stay. [44]

6.Medial approaches are mainly used developmental dysplasia of the hip, in young patients and children as it protects most soft tissues and blood supply to the hip joint.

The medial approaches can be further sub classified to antero-medial, postero-medial (Ferguson) and Ludloff's approach

a. Antero-medial approach,

b. Postero-medial approach

c. Ludloff's approach

These approaches are mainly used in children to treat DDH and open reduction of CDH and other conservative procedures. [45], [46]

The minimally invasive approaches to the hip joint used in hip arthroplasty.

Due to ion crease blood loss, slow recovery increase intra operative time, and delay in discharge more and more orthopaedic surgeons have been keen to develop minimally invasive approaches. These are usually modifications of existing approaches so that a surgeon preferring a certain standard approach can try the minimally approaches. The commonest minimally invasive approaches are minimally invasive antero lateral, minimally invasive direct lateral [24] minimally invasive posterior, minimally invasive anterior

The principles include shorter skin incision either single or multiple, minimal soft tissue dissection, without compromising the access or the quality of the surgery.

Optimal incision is around 8-9 cm either used as single or two separate incisions. [47] [48]

The results suggests better immediate outcomes and similar long term out comes in total hip arthroplasty for antero lateral MIS [23], postero-lateral MIS [49]

The reasons for developing Modified and modern approaches to the hip joint was mainly driven by the concept of minimal invasive surgeries being developed through out the surgical fields as they are supposed to be less invasive with low intra-operative complications such as low blood loss, less tissue dissection and less operative time, with early recovery, early mobilisation and early discharge from hospital. With development of smaller implants better instrumentation, better pre-operative planning, use of navigation, and better intra-operative imaging it has been possible to develop and use minimally invasive approaches to major surgeries like total hip arthroplasty or revision hip surgery. How ever at present there is debate over the long term out comes quality of surgery including implant positioning and learning curve for minimally invasive approaches over standard surgical approach. The answers to these questions will come from the research done comparing minimally invasive approaches versus the standard surgical approaches.

9. Conclusion

In conclusion it is important note that there are multiple surgical approaches to the hip joint and some better suited for arthroplasty and some for more conservative hip surgery. A checklist of factors one should consider before an approach is selected is,

1. What type of surgery? Is it conservative or hip arthroplasty?
2. If is arthroplasty, is it Total hip replacement, Hip resurfacing or a Revision hip replacement?
3. Age of patient? Adult young adult or a child
4. What part of the hip do you need the best exposure to? Acetabular socket, Femoral head and neck or both
5. Surgeon's preference and competence in doing the approach.
6. Whether the surgery is elective or trauma/emergency.

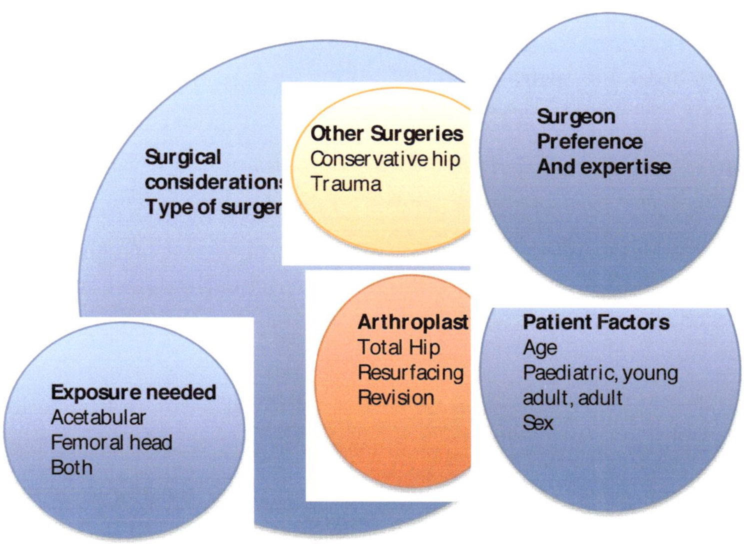

Figure 5. Show different factors that has to be taken to consideration when selecting

The relationship between the outcome of surgery and the surgical approach is still less understood, even though many comparison studies have been done. [50] [51] The final decision on what surgical approach to use is a clinical decision that has to be made by the operating surgeon.

Author details

Hiran Amarasekera

Orthopaedic Research Fellow/ PhD Student, Warwick Medical School, University of Warwick, And University Hospital of Coventry and Warwickshire, UK

References

[1] Gerdesmeyer, L, Gollwitzer, H, Bader, R, & Rudert, M. Surgical approaches in hip resurfacing]. *Orthopade* (2008).

[2] Ganz, R, Gill, T. J, Gautier, E, Ganz, K, Krugel, N, & Berlemann, U. Surgical dislocation of the adult hip: A TECHNIQUE WITH FULL ACCESS TO THE FEMORAL HEAD AND ACETABULUM WITHOUT THE RISK OF AVASCULAR NECROSIS. *J Bone Joint Surg Br* (2001). B-, 8, 1119-24.

[3] Hunter, S. C. Southern hip exposure. *Orthopedics* (1986).

[4] Jerosch, J, Theising, C, & Fadel, M. E. Antero-lateral minimal invasive (ALMI) approach for total hip arthroplasty technique and early results. *Arch Orthop Trauma Surg* (2006).

[5] Mcminn, D. J, Daniel, J, Pynsent, P. B, & Pradhan, C. Mini-incision resurfacing arthroplasty of hip through the posterior approach. *Clin Orthop Relat Res* (2005). *441*, 91-8.

[6] Khan, R. M, Cooper, G, & Hull, J. B. Hip resurfacing through a modified anterolateral approach, as compared with the Ganz trochanteric flip osteotomy: a two year follow-up study. *Hip Int* (2009).

[7] Lusskin, R, Goldman, A, & Absatz, M. Combined anterior and posterior approach to the hip joint in reconstructive and complex arthroplasty. *J Arthroplasty* (1988).

[8] Smith-petersen, M. N. Approach to and exposure of the hip joint for mold arthroplasty. *J Bone Joint Surg Am* (1949). A-, 1, 40-6.

[9] Light, T. R, & Keggi, K. J. Anterior approach to hip arthroplasty. *Clin Orthop Relat Res* (1980).

[10] Kreuzer, S, Leffers, K, & Kumar, S. Direct anterior approach for hip resurfacing: surgical technique and complications. *Clin Orthop Relat Res* (2011).

[11] Judet, J, & Judet, H. Anterior approach in total hip arthroplasty]. *Presse Med* (1985).

[12] Horne, P. H, & Olson, S. A. Direct anterior approach for total hip arthroplasty using the fracture table. *Curr Rev Musculoskelet Med* (2011).

[13] Lovell, T. P. Single-incision direct anterior approach for total hip arthroplasty using a standard operating table. *J Arthroplasty* (2008). Suppl:64-8., 23-7.

[14] Goytia, R. N, Jones, L. C, & Hungerford, M. W. Learning curve for the anterior approach total hip arthroplasty. *J Surg Orthop Adv* (2012).

[15] Barton, C, & Kim, P. R. Complications of the direct anterior approach for total hip arthroplasty. *Orthop Clin North Am* (2009).

[16] Bhargava, T, Goytia, R. N, Jones, L. C, & Hungerford, M. W. Lateral femoral cutaneous nerve impairment after direct anterior approach for total hip arthroplasty. *Orthopedics* (2010).

[17] Bender, B, Nogler, M, & Hozack, W. J. Direct anterior approach for total hip arthroplasty. *Orthop Clin North Am* (2009).

[18] Oinuma, K, Eingartner, C, Saito, Y, & Shiratsuchi, H. Total hip arthroplasty by a minimally invasive, direct anterior approach. *Oper Orthop Traumatol* (2007).

[19] Rachbauer, F. Minimally invasive total hip arthroplasty. Anterior approach]. *Orthopade* (2006).

[20] Hallert, O, Li, Y, Brismar, H, & Lindgren, U. The direct anterior approach: initial experience of a minimally invasive technique for total hip arthroplasty. *J Orthop Surg Res* (2012).

[21] Watson-JonesFractures of the neck of femur. *British Journal of surgery* (1936). *23*, 787-808.

[22] Pawlowski, Z, Bohatyrewicz, A, Czajkowski, A. A, Kominiak, P, & Gusta, A. Early abductor muscle strength after total hip replacement performed by antero-lateral approach]. *Chir Narzadow Ruchu Ortop Pol* (2002).

[23] Walde, T. A, Blattgerste, D, Sehmisch, S, Kuttler, W, Walde, H. J, & Koster, G. Early results and patient satisfaction after total hip arthroplasty using a minimally invasive anterolateral approach. *Hip Int* (2009).

[24] Spaans, A. J. van den Hout JA, Bolder SB. High complication rate in the early experience of minimally invasive total hip arthroplasty by the direct anterior approach. *Acta Orthop* (2012).

[25] Amarasekera Surface Replacement of the Hip Joint. In: K.Fokter S, ed. *Recent Advances in Hip and Knee Arthroplasty*, 1 ed. Croatia: Intech, (2012). , 2012, 181-90.

[26] Kocher, T. In: *Text book of operative surgery*. London: Adams and Charles Blac, (1903).

[27] Hardinge, K. The direct lateral approach to the hip. *J Bone Joint Surg Br* (1982).

[28] Foster, D. E, & Hunter, J. R. The direct lateral approach to the hip for arthroplasty. Advantages and complications. *Orthopedics* (1987).

[29] Gerdesmeyer, L, Gollwitzer, H, Diehl, P, Buttgereit, B, & Rudert, M. The minimally invasive anterolateral approach combined with hip onlay resurfacing. *Oper Orthop Traumatol* (2009).

[30] Bauer, R, Kerschbaumer, F, Poisel, S, & Oberthaler, W. The transgluteal approach to the hip joint. *Arch Orthop Trauma Surg* (1979).

[31] Eyb, R. Clinical results following the transgluteal and anterolateral (Watson-Jones) approach to hip prosthesis implantation]. *Z Orthop Ihre Grenzgeb* (1985).

[32] Warren, P. J, Jennings, G. J, & Fletcher, M. D. Improvement in surgical exposure of the hip using the direct lateral approach. *Ann R Coll Surg Engl* (2002).

[33] Mulliken, B. D, Rorabeck, C. H, Bourne, R. B, & Nayak, N. The surgical approach to total hip arthroplasty: complications and utility of a modified direct lateral approach. *Iowa Orthop J* (1995). *15*, 48-61.

[34] Amarasekera, H. W, Costa, M. L, Foguet, P, Krikler, S. J, Prakash, U, & Griffin, D. R. The blood flow to the femoral head/neck junction during resurfacing arthroplasty: A COMPARISON OF TWO APPROACHES USING LASER DOPPLER FLOWMETRY. *J Bone Joint Surg Br* (2008).

[35] Amarasekera, H. W, Costa, M. L, Parsons, N, Achten, J, Griffin, D. R, Manktelow, S, & Williams, N. R. SPECT/CT bone imaging after hip resurfacing arthroplasty: is it feasible to use CT attenuation correction in the presence of metal implants? *Nucl Med Commun* (2011).

[36] Campbell, P, Mirra, J, & Amstutz, H. C. Viability of femoral heads treated with resurfacing arthroplasty. *J Arthroplasty* (2000).

[37] Amarasekera, H, Costa, M, Prakash, U, Krikler, S, Foguet, P, & Griffin, D. FEMORAL BLOOD FLOW DURING HIP RESURFACING: A COMPARISON OF TWO APPROACHES USING LASER DOPPLER FLOW MEASUREMENT. *Journal of Bone & Joint Surgery, British 2012*B-SUPP III:148.

[38] Amarasekera, H, Roberts, P, Costa, M, Parsons, N, Achten, J, Griffin, D, & Williams, N. Scintigraphic assessment of bone status at one year following hip resurfacing: comparison of two surgical approaches using SPECT-CT scan. *Bone and Joint Research* (2012).

[39] Schleicher, I, Haas, H, Adams, T. S, Szalay, G, Klein, H, & Kordelle, J. Minimal-invasive posterior approach for total hip arthroplasty versus standard lateral approach. *Acta Orthop Belg* (2011).

[40] Fink, B, & Mittelstaedt, A. Minimally invasive posterior approach for total hip arthroplasty]. *Orthopade* (2012).

[41] Fink, B, Mittelstaedt, A, Schulz, M. S, Sebena, P, & Singer, J. Comparison of a minimally invasive posterior approach and the standard posterior approach for total hip arthroplasty A prospective and comparative study. *J Orthop Surg Res* (2010).

[42] Gibson, A. Posterior exposure of the hip joint. *J Bone Joint Surg Br* (1950). B-, 2, 183-6.

[43] Pellegrini VJaECM. Surgical approaches to the hip. In: Evarts C, ed. *Surgery of the Musculoskeletal system*. NewYork: Churchil Livingstone, (1990).

[44] Aglietti, P, & Salvati, E. The postero-lateral approach for total hip prosthesis. *Ital J Orthop Traumatol* (1981).

[45] Di Mascio LCarey-Smith R, Tucker K. Open reduction of developmental hip dysplasia using a medial approach: a review of 24 hips. *Acta Orthop Belg* (2008).

[46] Broughton, N. S, Graham, H. K, Nattrass, G. R, Torode, I. P, Marshall, P. D, Sullivan, O, & Ludloff, M. s medial approach for open reduction of congenital dislocation of the hip. *J Bone Joint Surg Br* (1997).

[47] Noble, P. C, Pfluger, G, Junk-jantsch, S, Thompson, M. T, Alexander, J. W, & Mathis, K. B. The optimal skin incision for minimally invasive total hip arthroplasty performed via the anterolateral approach. *J Arthroplasty* (2012).

[48] Wetzel, R, & Dorsch, M. Minimally invasive approach to implantation of a hip endoprosthesis]. *Orthopade* (2006).

[49] Varela Egocheaga JRSuarez-Suarez MA, Fernandez-Villan M, Gonzalez-Sastre V, Varela-Gomez JR, Murcia-Mazon A. [Minimally invasive posterior approach in total hip arthroplasty. Prospective randomised trial]. *An Sist Sanit Navar* (2010).

[50] Barber, T. C, Roger, D. J, Goodman, S. B, & Schurman, D. J. Early outcome of total hip arthroplasty using the direct lateral vs the posterior surgical approach. *Orthopedics* (1996).

[51] Jolles, B. M, & Bogoch, E. R. Posterior versus lateral surgical approach for total hip arthroplasty in adults with osteoarthritis. *Cochrane Database Syst Rev* (2006). CD003828.

Chapter 2

Preoperative Planning of Total Knee Replacement

A.O. Erdogan, N.S. Gokay and A. Gokce

Additional information is available at the end of the chapter

http://dx.doi.org/10.5772/55023

1. Introduction

Total knee replacement (TKR) surgery is the gold standard method in the treatment of end stage knee arthritis with a high success. Relieving pain effectively, restoring range of motion and improving function are the major goals of arthroplasy. Patient satisfaction rates were reported as 90% to 95% after TKR. [1-3] Better clinical results were gained in younger population than the older patients. Unfortunately, primary osteoarthritis is seen mainly in the elderly. However, inflamatory arthritis, trauma, avascular necrosis and hemophilia are some of the secondary causes leading osteoarthritis in younger population.. Nearly 1 million TKR surgeries are performed on earth per year and this number is increasing day by day, with the novel designed surface technologies. Despite the fact that new implant technologies secure better results, a revision procedure may be required in some of the patients. Ofcourse the amount of revision surgeries is also increasing in parallel with primary TKR surgeries. Unfortunately, the clinical result of revision total knee arthroplasty isn't succesfull enough as primary total knee arthroplasty.

Polyethylene (PE) wear, aseptic loosening, instability and infections are counted among the factors leading revision surgery [4,5]. The incidence of PE wear is decreased nowadays by the development of ultra high cross-linked polyethilens (UHMWPE). PE wear is a serious problem leading to aseptic loosening. Malalingment, malrotation and soft tissue imbalance after TKR surgery are the other factors which may cause in aseptic loosening. Instability and problems related with patella are among the other situations in which revision surgery may be requiredIt is very clear that surgical technique of primary TKR is the main risk factor for early failures [6, 7]. Extensive preoperative planning is very important considering aforementioned particulars to achieve accurate prosthetic seating with proper axial alignment. In this chapter, the preoperative planning issues including pre-operative preparations of patient and surgeon will be discussed.

2. Pre-operative clinical evaluation

Pre-operative clinical evaluation is very substantial in assessing the current medical status and determining the relative risk profile of the patient. It is very important for the orthopaedic surgeon to understand the basic principles and nuances involved. Preoperative planning initiates with selection of an apropriate candidate for TKR procedure. The patient's expectations and general risk factors plays an import role in this decision. Questioning of the patient's complaints and life quality, assesment of the medical condition and detailed physical examination are the essentials of preoperative clinical evaluation.

3. Indication of TKR

Total knee replacement was found to be quite effective in terms of improvement in health-related quality of life dimensions, with the occasional exception of the social dimension. The underlying disease is not a life threatening one. The primary indications for total knee arthroplasty are pain and loss of function. Clinical evaluation of the patient has to be initiated by questioning of the complaints and disabilities.

There must be a significant and disabling pain which is resistant to the medical treatment. Spinal disease, ipsilateral hip pathologies, peripheral vascular disease, meniscal pathologies, and bursitis of the knee should be considered in differential diagnosis. The real source of the knee pain must be displayed.

The patient's quality of life should be questioned and significant reduction might be taken into consideration It should be remembered that the patients, which are less satisfied following TKR, are the ones with mild pre-operative complaints. All conservative treatment modalities should be exhausted before surgery. The frequent indications for TKR surgery are given on table 1.

Osteoarthritis
Inflammatory arthritis
Rheumatoid arthritis
Osteochondromatosis
Villonodular synovitis
Metabolic arthritis
Osteonecrosis
Gout, pseudogout
Posttraumatic arthritis
Intraarticular fractures
Malaligned ankylosis
Failed high tibial osteotomies

Table 1. The major indications for total knee arthroplasty

4. Contrendications of TKR

Contraindications must be well known and considered before the surgery decision. Absolute contraindications for total knee arthroplasty include knee sepsis, chronic infection, extansor mechanism dysfunction, severe vascular disease, recurvatum deformity secondary to muscular weakness, presence of well functioning knee arthrodesis. There are also relative and contraversial contraindications. These include medical conditions that preclude safe anesthesia, inadequate soft tissue coverage, morbid obesity, neuropathic arthropathy, and history of osteomyelitis around knee joint. A preoperative condition that can adversly affect the patient's outcome can be considered as a relative contraindication.

5. Medical condition of the patient

A comprehensive medical history and physical examination are the cornerstones of the preoperative assessment. Patient's medical comorbidities should be optimized preoperatively. Cardiovascular diseases, cerebrovascular diseases, pulmonary diseases, neurologic conditions, rheumatoid arthritis, uropathy, morbid obesity, haematologic and endocrine diseases are the important situations which may affect the intraoperative and postoperative morbidity and mortality.. Drug history of the patient must be questioned too. Sources of infection such as dental, dermatological, urological or respiratory tract infections must be ruled out. Age alone was not found to be an obstacle for an effective surgery, however age related comorbidities should be considered. Additional risks for infection, previous surgeries should be adressed before surgery. Every patient must have a general medical evaluation including laboratory tests, electrocardiogram and chest graphy. The type of the procedure also may enhance the medical risks. For example, simultaneously performed bilateral TKR may be associated with an increased risk of cardiac, respiratory or neurological complications. Low preoperative mental health has also an influence on outcome after TKR [10].

The detailed physical examination should include the range of motion, ligament status, circulation and skin condition evaluation. Furthermore alignment of lower extremities, patellar instability and gait analysis should to be assessed. Additional knowledge and scientific dissemination of surgery outcomes should help to ensure better management of the patients after total knee arthroplasty and to optimize the procedure [12].

Underlying or predisposing orthopaedic diseases, which may interact the outcome of TKR should be reviewed previously. Examples of such common musculoskeletal conditions are as follows: 1) Nerve entrapments affecting motor functions of lower extremity, 2) Adjacent joint degenerative arthritis 3) Presence of any inflamatory arthritis, which may flare after surgery 4) Any musculoskletal disability affecting postoperative mobility 5) Thromboembolic history or predispositions.

6. Radiographic assesment

An apropriate musculoskeletal radiologic study is essential in planning of TKR. The presence of bone defects might be detected and pre-operative decision whether to use a primary or revision implant should be given. Determination of the joint line is also important in determining the flexion/extension space and balance of the ligaments.

Tracking of the quadriceps mechanism and rotational deformites are other important issues for patellar stability, however may not be assessed on direct radiographs especially in deformed knees with fixed valgus position.

Conventional radiographs are usually adequate for initial radiographic evaluation to confirm the diagnosis or assess the severity of the disease. Preoperative radiographic planning for total knee arthroplasty begins by obtaining a high quality standing antero-posterior (AP) and lateral 52-inch casette graphies. Additional views such as Merchant, tunnel, patella sunrise, orthoroentgenogram or advanced imaging modalities such as CT, MRI may be necessary in extraordinary conditions such as congenital dislocation of the patella, post traumatic deformities, severe deformities, tumors and congenital anomalies.

6.1. AP view

The AP view should be obtained with the patient in a standing position. The joint space on the weight bearing AP film should be more than 3 mm or within 50% of the joint space of the contralateral knee. Normally, the lateral joint space is wider than the medial space. Articular surfaces of the medial and lateral joint compartments may be best assessed on this view. The presence of associated osteophytes and subcondral bone changes are some of the findings which may be seen on AP graphies.

6.2. Lateral view

The lateral aspect of the knee is leaned against the x ray film cassette and flexed 30°. The excessive glide in flexion may be an indicator of posterior cruciate ligament tightness and therefore PCL sacrifiying prosthesis must be considered before the surgery. Patellar height should be assessed on this view using Insall-Salvati ratio. The Insall-Salvati is the ratio of the patellar tendon length (LT) to the length of the patella (LP) (Figure 1). The values above 1,2 is considered as "Patella Alta", while the values below 0,8 is considered as "Patella İnfera". Suprapatellar and posterior regions must be evaluated in terms of detecting the loose bodies.

Posterior of the knee joint is easily observed on this view and overhanging bone structure or osteophytes should be determined. If left unresected, this overhanging bone can impinge on tibial PE and result with flexion limitation and early wear of the PE.

The lateral view may also allow size selection of the femoral component (Figure 2). Oversizing will create tightness in fexion and increased tension in quadriceps mechanism and undersizing will create looseness in flexion and anterior cortical notching of the femur is also inevitable. Careful preoperative planning with using templates aims to achieve the correct AP dimension for restoring normal kinematics and quadriceps muscle function.

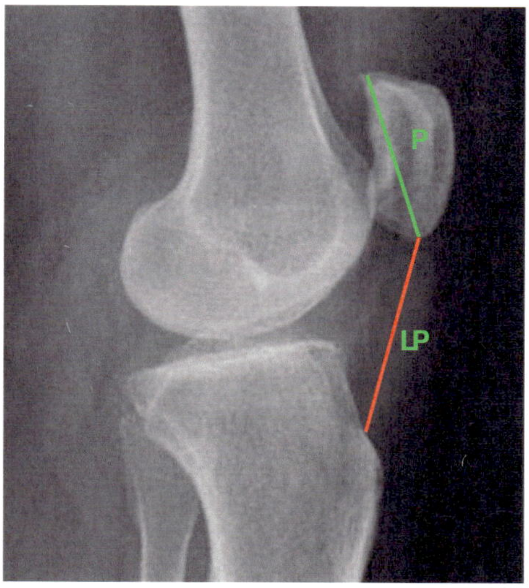

Figure 1. Patella height is assessed via measuring Insall-Salvati ratio (LP/P) on lateral graphies

6.3. Standing orthorontgenogram (52-inch casette three joint view)

Standing ap view of the lower extremities from hips to ankles is helpful preoperatively for assessing overall alignment (mechanical axis) of the lower extremity. The knee is normally in 7 degree of valgus alignment on AP view.

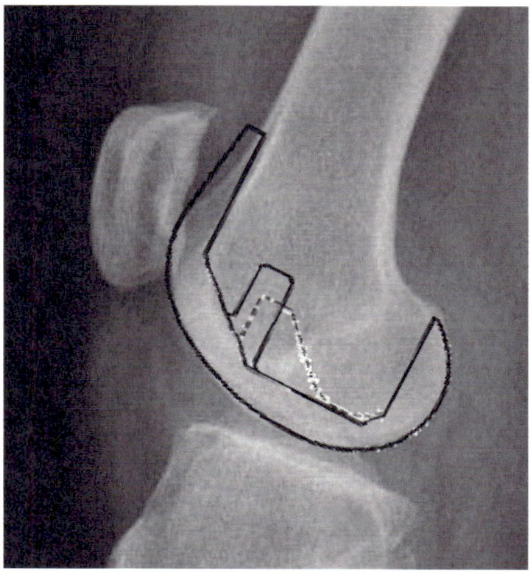

Figure 2. Proper size of the femoral component is assessed via evaluation of the pre-operative lateral radiographs.

The orthorontgenogram allows the surgeon to determine the varus or valgus alignment of the knees, leg length discrepancy and the presence of extraarticular deformities.

It is essential to ensure to take this radiograph in neutral rotation of the legs to obtain the most accurate measurements. It should be confirmed via inspecting the relationship between the tibia and the fibula, distally and proximally.

6.4. Merchant view

Merchant view helps to assess the patellofemoral alignment, trochlear grove and articular surfaces. Preoperatively patellar subluxation seen on this view should alert the surgeon for lateral release of the patella during TKR. Merchant view demonstrates both the patellar and trochlear surfaces. Subluxation can be assessed by measuring the congruence angle (Figure 3). Congruence angle demonstrates the relationship of apex of patella with the trochlear grove's bisector. Two lines are drawn to measure the congruence angle. First line is the bisector line of femoral sulcus angle and it establishes a zero reference line. Second line is drawn from the apex of the sulcus angle to the lowest point of the patellar articular ridge.

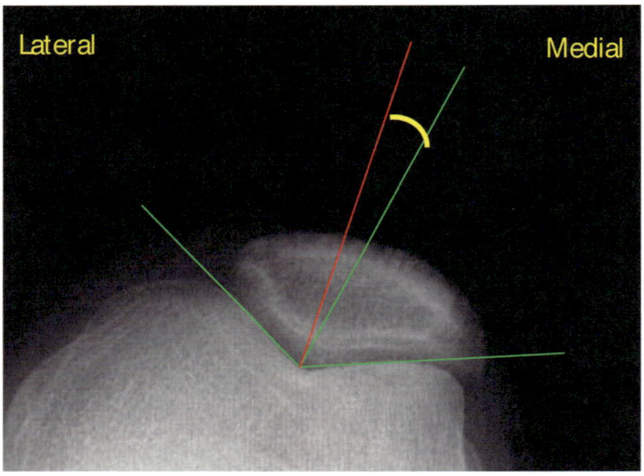

Figure 3. The congruence angle (α) lower than 16° to lateral or medial direction is considered as normal.

If congruence angle is lateral to the reference line this means the angle is positive while angles medial to the reference lines are considered as negative. The angles lower than 16 degree are considered as normal.

6.5. Tunnel view

Tunnel view shows the posterior aspect of the intercondylar notch and it is useful to evaluate osteocondritis dissecans or intraarticular loose bodies in young patients.

6.6. Patella sunrise view

This is called the sunrise view because the patella appears to be rising over the horizon. The sunrise view also helps to identify the patellar malalignment.

7. Surgeon's preperation

Preoperative planning is essential component for surgeon in TKR to obtain desired clinical outcome and radiographic result. Correct implant selection with proper size is one of the important stage in preoperative planning. Patient's and surgeon's expectations should be taken into consideration pre-operatively to improve the outcomes and increase the satisfaction after operation [12]. Pre-operative planning of the bone cuts may simplify the surgery. Positioning of the components is very important in acquiring the accurate alignment. Mechanical axis measurement and alignment evaluation on AP and lateral planes may performed on standing X-rays. Also entry points for intramedullary guide pins should be determined for the correct component position.

During the process of planning of TKR, the surgeon aims to obtain the optimal fitting of the implant and the optimal extremity alignment. This is possible for the surgeon by thinking three-dimensionally. The prediction of the surgery pre-operatively should improve the precision of the process and shorten the length of the operation. It should also reduce the complication rate.

8. Templating

Most of the knee replacement systems provide a large number of options for treating conditions that are encountered during surgery. The different systems serve the surgeons different sizes of implants in a wide range. Intra-operative determination of the implant sizes was found more accurate than the pre-operative templating. However pre-operative templating is useful in obtaining proper implant positioning. Working with templates is widely accepted approach, which can help determine component sizes, predict amounts of bony resection, and anticipate surgical steps. Acetate templating was found accurate and reliabile [13]. However, with widespread use of digital radiographs the use of digital templating has recently grown due to advances in reducing errors associated with manipulating films and templates (Figure 4).

Combining digital templating with picture archiving and communication system PACS brings advantages include saving health care costs, quick and reproducible planning, remote access, and the ability to keep a permanent digital record of the surgical plan.

Templating should also work in preparing the surgeon to some extreme scenarios which may be encountered during surgery. For example; Standart cruciate retaining or sacrifiying implant systems are usually enough to solve the problem in large majority of cases. Constrained or even more complicated sytems with extension stems or wedges may be necessiated in small number of primary cases (Figure 5). Modular systems should be required due to intraoperative complications such as fractures or ligament tears.

Constrained condylar knee prosthesis (CCK) is commonly used in total knee replacement to overcome the severe ligamentous imbalance problem. CCK may also be preferred if the lateral

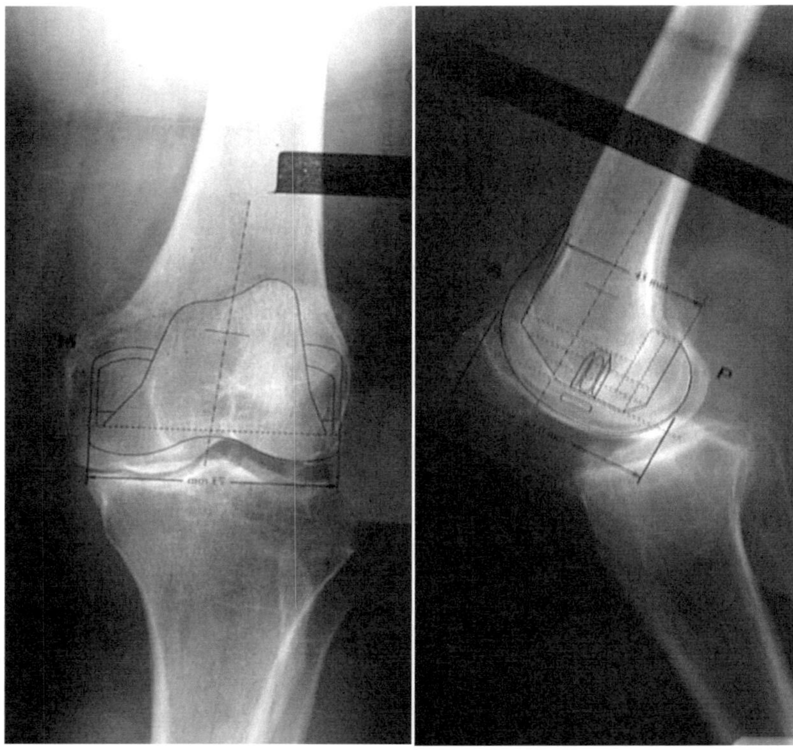

Figure 4. Templating

collateral ligament laxity more than 2 mm persists, even after adequate medial soft tissue release in patients with varus deformity of greater than 20°.

Although women have greater functional limitations than men, at the time of the surgery, they recover faster in early post-operative period. Women also have a greater improvement in WOMAC scores than men after primary surgery. Specific anatomic differences are blamed to be responsible for gender-specific differences after TKR. However, there are conflicting data in the literature regarding these gender-specific outcomes [14].

There are also efforts in reducing costs and improving quality of care, which may planned in preoperative period. Template-directed instrumentation was proposed for simplifying the surgical instruments and saving sterilization costs of unnecessary implant trays as saving measurement. In this novel approach, surgical planning combines digital templating with prepared instruments and components used intraoperatively [15].

Computer based navigation should be prefered in complex cases to overcome the heavily distorded anatomy or malalignment. There are also several quite recent technologies, like patient specific surgical cutting guide systems or robotic assisted implantations in cases of surgeon's special interest. Beside the medical aspects surgeons have to deal with cost considerations and even discuss with the patient in preoperative planning period [16].

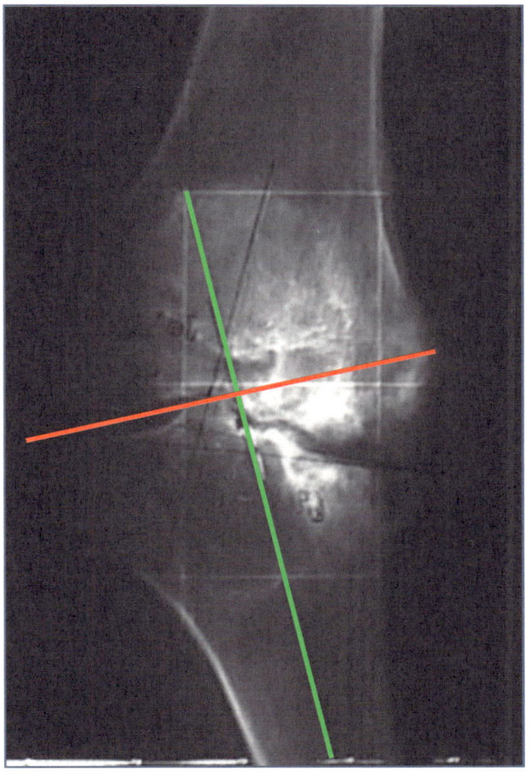

Figure 5. Wedge and modular extension stems should be considered in patients which present with a such pre-operative radiograph.

Author details

A.O. Erdogan, N.S. Gokay and A. Gokce

Namik Kemal University School of Medicine, Department of Orthopaedics and Traumatology, Tekirdag, Turkey

References

[1] Colizza, W. A, & Insall, J. N. Scuderi GR: The posteriorstabilized knee prosthesis: Assessment of polyethylene damage and osteolysis after a ten-year minimum follow-up. J Bone Joint Surg 77A:(1995). , 1713-1720.

[2] Emmerson, K. P, & Moran, C. G. Pinder IM: Survivorship analysis of the kinematic stabilizer total knee replacement: A year follow-up. J Bone Joint Surg 78B:441-445, (1996). , 10-14.

[3] Ranawat, C. S, & Luessenhop, C. P. Rodriquez JA: The press-fit condylar modular total knee system: Four to six year results with a posterior-cruciate-substituting design. J Bone Joint Surg 79A:(1997). , 342-348.

[4] Robertsson, O, & Lidgren, L. Annual Report- The Swedish Knee Arthroplasty Register. *Annual Report SKAR* (2008). , 1-37.

[5] Mulhall, K. J, Ghomrawi, H. M, Scully, S, Callaghan, J. J, & Saleh, K. J. Current etiologies and modes of failure in total knee arthroplasty revision. *Clin Orthop Relat Res* (2006). , 446, 45-50.

[6] Manley, M, Ong, K, Lau, E, & Kurtz, S. M. Total Knee Arthroplasty Survivorship in the United States Medicare Population Effect of Hospital and Surgeon Procedure Volume. *J Arthroplasty* (2008).

[7] Schroer, W. C, Calvert, G. T, Diesfeld, P. J, & Reedy, M. E. LeMarr AR. Effects of increased surgical volume on total knee arthroplasty complications. *J Arthroplasty* (2008). Suppl 1):61-67.

[8] Crekarell, J. R, & Guyton, J. L. Arthroplasty of ankle and knee. Canale ST (ed). Campbell's operative orthopaedics. 10th edition, St Louis: Mosby, (2003).

[9] Aydogdu, S. ve ark. Diz artroplastisinde genel ilkeler endikasyonlar. Ege R. Diz sorunları. Ankara, bizim büro basımevi, (1998). , 439-459.

[10] Vissers, M. M, Bussmann, J. B, Verhaar, J. A, Busschbach, J. J, Bierma-zeinstra, S. M, & Reijman, M. Psychological factors affecting the outcome of total hip and knee arthroplasty: a systematic review. Semin Arthritis Rheum. (2012). , 41(4), 576-88.

[11] Ethgen, O, Bruyère, O, Richy, F, Dardennes, C, & Reginster, J. Y. Health-related quality of life in total hip and total knee arthroplasty. A qualitative and systematic review of the literature. J Bone Joint Surg Am. (2004). A(5):963-74., 86.

[12] Ghomrawi, H. M, Mancuso, C. A, Westrich, G. H, & Marx, R. G. Mushlin AI Discordance in TKR Expectations Between Patients and Surgeons; Expectations Discordance Study Group.Clin Orthop Relat Res. (2012). Jul 21.

[13] Peek, A. C, Bloch, B, & Auld, J. How useful is templating for total knee replacement component sizing? Knee. (2012). Aug;doi:j.knee.2011.03.010. Epub 2011 May 10., 19(4), 266-9.

[14] Liebs, T. R, Herzberg, W, Roth-kroeger, A. M, Rüther, W, & Hassenpflug, J. Women recover faster than men after standard knee arthroplasty. Clin Orthop Relat Res. (2011). , 469(10), 2855-65.

[15] Hsu, A. R, Gross, C. E, Bhatia, S, & Levine, B. R. Template-directed Instrumentation in Total Knee Arthroplasty: Cost Savings Analysis. Orthopedics. (2012). Nov 1;35(11):edoi:, 1596-600.

[16] S.David Stulberg Chapter 3 Preoperative Planning and Prosthetic Selectin in book Knee Arthroplasty edited Thomas P. Sculco and Ermanno A. Martucci, New York: Springer Wien; 2002. 250.

Chapter 3

Special Considerations in Asian Knee Arthroplasty

Hamid Reza Seyyed Hosseinzadeh, Samih Tarabichi,
Ali Sina Shahi, Mehrnoush Hassas Yeganeh,
Usama Hassan Saleh, Gholam Reza Kazemian and
Aidin Masoudi

Additional information is available at the end of the chapter

http://dx.doi.org/10.5772/53595

1. Introduction

Human body is a unique correlation between anatomy and physiology. It is mandatory to have adequate knowledge on this issue former to perform any kind of surgery. As in all parts of human body, there are several variations in human knee concerning middle-eastern and Asian ethnicity, which should be considered for performing total knee arthroplasty among these races. These differences involve both in anatomical and physiological features, causing variations in a wide spectrum from metabolic syndromes to morphology of knee components.

During total knee replacement, the accurate bone cutting, adequate balancing of the soft tissues and proper coverage of the resected surface were important factors for achieving a successful outcome. In recent years, many studies have identified shape differences in the knee within the Caucasian population. Total knee replacement is a precise procedure, requiring accurate soft tissue balancing and resection of bone thickness equal to the thickness of the implanted prosthetic component. Proper bone cuts for rotational alignment of the femur and tibia in the axial plane represents the key for a balanced flexion gap and proper patella tracking. Both represent important parameters for high flexion. [1] A properly shaped prosthesis can provide the best coverage and avoid soft tissue impingement. Thus, it becomes important to obtain the anthropometric data to achieve the best stability and longevity for implant. Total knee prostheses based on the accurately morphologic data of knee, gender morphologic difference, and the morphologic correlations between tibia and femur may be expected to give better results.

Differences among males and females have been widely reported, with females having a smaller mediolateral to anteroposterior ratio and more narrow distal femurs and different proximal tibia geometry. [2, 3] However, ethnic differences have not received much focus given that most existing TKA implant designs are based on the Caucasian population. But, many studies have determined that the prostheses designed for Caucasian patients are not suitable for Asian patients. Anatomic differences have been identified between both sex and ethnicity, with Caucasian subjects having a higher tibial torsion angle and lower varus alignment than Japanese.

As mentioned above, accurate sizing and proper placement of prosthetic components plays a major role in the success and long term survival of total knee arthroplasty (TKA). The femoral component sizing is an important determinant for achieving a well-balanced flexion-extension gap in a TKA. Mediolateral sizing of the femoral component is necessary for proper patellofemoral tracking and uniform stress distribution over the resected distal femoral surface; this contributes to the long term stability of the prosthesis. [1] Most of the total knee prostheses currently available have been developed using measurements from Caucasians. Caucasian knees have been shown to be generally larger than Asian knees. [4] It follows that these discrepancies may give rise to implant size mismatch with the resected bony surface of Asian patients. Several studies have found that the femoral aspect ratio (mediolateral [fML]/ anteroposterior [fAP]) of the prostheses used in Asia were not suitable for Asian patients. For instance, Ho et al reported that 3 of 5 TKA systems used in China tended to cause mediolateral overhang of the component across the width of the resected femurs of Chinese patients. The authors also found a larger femoral aspect ratio in small knees and a proportionally smaller ratio in large knees, but all the 5 sets of implant systems examined in the study showed little changes in the aspect ratio with AP length. [2]

Iorio et al showed that the Japanese patients had a significantly less postoperative range of motion than white patients. Furthermore, 4.1% Japanese patients required revision after primary posterior cruciate-retaining TKA within an average follow-up of 6.6 years, whereas only 2.6% of their American cohort needed revision within an average follow-up of 9 years. The authors suggested that the racial morphologic differences might be a factor causing the differences in outcome. [5]

Systematic differences have also been observed. ACL laxity among Japanese is higher than Caucasians. [4] It has also been proven that the ACL laxity is significantly different between Malaysians and Caucasians. [6] This could be the result of different life style. The systematic differences are explained further through the chapter.

Some rare complications accompanied by TKA are more common among the ethnicity, such as insufficiency fracture. This could be as a result of having greater rates of risk factors like: osteoporosis, overweight and gross varus deformity. Insufficiency fracture would be presented by no history of trauma, sudden unset pain, knee instability and deformity. The patient surprisingly is unable to walk. Unfortunately it is common to be misdiagnosed as MCL insufficiency.

That's why it is very important to have special consideration while performing total knee arthroplasty among Asian or middle-eastern ethnicity.

These findings on TKA mismatching have led some researchers to suggest that Asia Pacific people should have special designs of TKA prosthesis system.

2. Three-dimensional morphology of the knee reveals ethnic differences

In recent years, many studies have identified shape differences in the knee within the Caucasian population. [7, 8, 9] Shape analyses have identified sex differences in the femoral midshaft, distal femur, and patella. [10] Ethnic differences have not received much focus given that most existing TKA implant designs are based on the Caucasian population. Many studies have reported the anatomy and comparison of East Asian populations (Japanese, Chinese, Indian) to existing implant systems. Mahfouz et al in a comprehensive, 3D analysis of the knee morphology identified shape differences in the distal femur and proximal tibia among the ethnic groups. [11]

They found AMs (East Asian Male) had a smaller ML/AP (mediolateral/anteroposterior) ratio than CMs (Caucasian Male) (1.33 ± 0.12 versus 1.4 ± 0.06), contrary to Yue et al. The mean and SD values of the ML for CMs (79 ± 4.6 mm) and CFs (Caucasian Female) (68.6 ± 4.8 mm) were comparable to those published by Yue et al. The normalized ratios and nonlinear shape analysis in this research supported differences between East Asians and Caucasians independent of any scale factor. They also found differences in the ratio between AAF/CF (African American Female/Caucasian Female) and AAM/CM (African American Male/ Caucasian Male), with the mean ratio being larger in CMs compared to AAMs and CFs compared to AAFs. [11, 12, 13]

This finding conflicts with Gillespie et al. who reported a larger ML/AP ratio in African Americans than in Caucasians; however, their African American population was from the early 20th century, which could account for differing anatomic features from the current population. [3, 13] The radii of curvature analysis on both the medial and lateral condyles revealed AMs and AFs (American Female) tend to have more curved condyles (ie, smaller radius of curvature) than Caucasians, implying a larger ROM. This finding agrees with Leszko et al. who found an increased ROM of 153° for AF and 151° for AM compared to 146° for CM. [14] Women from all ethnic groups had smaller, narrower knees with a smaller ML/AP ratio.

This study by Mahfouz et al. shows that AAMs and AAFs have larger AP dimensions than their Asian and Caucasian counterparts and AMs and AFs have smaller AP dimensions than CMs and CFs. When compared to CFs with similar AP dimensions, AMs have larger ML dimensions. In analyzing ethnic differences in tibial anatomy, AAMs have larger LAPs (lateral anteroposterior diameter) and smaller MAPs (medial anteroposterior diameter) (Figure 1-B) than CMs, while also having larger ML and AP dimensions than AMs. AMs and AFs have smaller ML and AP dimensions than CMs and CFs. This study also identifies shape differences in the distal femur and proximal tibia between sexes in each ethnic population. Males across all ethnicities have average 9-mm larger ML and 5-mm larger AP dimensions than their female counterparts. AAMs and CFs have shallower patellar grooves than AAFs and CMs. Females have more curved femurs in all ethnicities. Males have larger tibial AP dimensions than females. AAMs and CMs have larger ML dimensions than AAFs and CFs, respectively. Differences in femoral and tibial shapes are also identified in comparing shapes across populations based on differences in ML/AP, AML/PML (anterior mediolateral length/posterior mediolateral length), and MAP/LAP ratios. [11] (Figure 1-A)

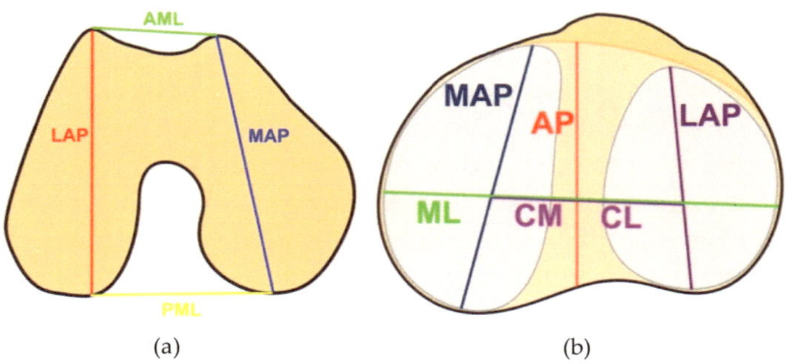

Figure 1. A) Diagram illustrating measurements on the distal femur. AML = Anterior mediolateral length, PML = Posterior mediolateral length, LAP = Lateral anteroposterior diameter, MAP = Medial anteroposterior diameter. B) Diagram illustrating measurements on the proximal tibia. ML = Mediolateral width, AP = Anteroposterior length, MAP = Medial anteroposterior length, LAP = Lateral anteroposterior length.

3. Normal development of the knee angle

Development of the knee angle from bowlegs (varus) in the infant to knock knees (valgus) in early childhood is a part of normal and physiological development. Several researchers have studied knee angle variation in various parts of the world and many of them have tried to set standards for certain ethnic/social groups. [15, 16, 17]

The TFA has been described as the angle defined by the mechanical axis of the femur intersecting the mechanical axis of the tibia.

There are studies available regarding normal development of the knee angle in whites, Chinese, Nigerians, Koreans, and Turkish children. Saini UC et al. have found that none of the subjects had a varus knee alignment in the more than 3 years age groups. Also, even for the children in the 2 years age group, the mean TFA was positive, indicating a mean valgus alignment in Indian children, even at the age of 2 years. [18] This was contrary to the findings of the largest study carried to date by Cheng et al. in the Chinese population, which showed a mean varus TFA at the age of 2 years. After 3 years, the authors noted a rapid decrease in the mean IMD in the Chinese children, reaching 0 cm at the age of 8 years, with a normal range of ±3 cm. [19] In Turkish children, Arazi et al noted a significantly higher degree of valgus angle than that in previous reports. The maximal mean valgus angle was 9.6° at 7 years of age for boys and 9.8° at 6 years of age for girls. These differences were considered to be racial differences between Turkish children and those of other races. Turkish children aged between 3 and 17 years were found to exhibit up to 11° physiologic valgus. The authors concluded that a measurable varus angle or a valgus higher than 11° during this period should be considered as abnormal. [20] In a study conducted by Heath and Staheli in white children, using clinical measurements of the TFA and the ICD and IMD, children were maximally bow-legged at the age of 6 months and progressed toward approximately neutral knee angles (0.0°) by the age of 18 months. They found the greatest mean knock knee of 8° at the age of 4 years, which was followed by a gradual decrease to a mean of 6° at 11 years of age. Normal children aged 2–11 years had knock knee up to 12° and IMD up to 8 cm. The existence of bowlegs after the age of 2 years was found to be abnormal. [21] Yoo et al. carried out a study on normal healthy Korean children, with full-length anteroposterior view standing radiographs. They found that the overall patterns of the chronological changes in the knee angle were similar to those described previously in western or Asian children, but the knee angle development was delayed, i.e., genu varum before 1 year, neutral at 1.5 years, increasing genu valgum with a maximum value of 7.8° at 4 years, followed by a gradual decrease to approximately 5–6° of genu valgum of the adult level at 7–8 years of age. Although the use of different techniques to estimate the knee angles might be responsible for variations in observations in different studies, it is more likely that these variations are possibly due to the ethnical and racial differences that might exist in different population groups. [22] Arazi et al found the weight of children at a specific age to have a negative correlation with the ICD of the subject. However, this correlation was found to be weak and although statistically significant, it might not be of any clinical significance. The only possible explanation to this might be the relatively thick thighs of the heavier children, which is expected to subjectively decrease the ICD. However, considering the fact that fixed body landmarks on the body should not change even in obese children, this result is hard to explain. [20]

Oginni et al. who measured the knee angles of 2,036 normal Nigerian children up to an age of 12 years. In their study, they found the majority of the knees to be bowed (varus) in the first 6 months. At 21–23 months of age, the distribution of angles became strongly bimodal: about half being varus and half being valgus (knock-kneed). After this, the knee angle was found to be valgus in most of the children. They concluded that the change from varus to valgus in individual infants might be sudden (a few weeks), although the changeover of the whole population appeared smooth and gradual. The authors also concluded that varus knee alignment was uncommon after 2 years in Nigerian children and large knee angles between 2 and 5 years suggested rickets. However, in their study, the children became maximally and uniformly knock-kneed (-7.1° ± 1.4°) between 3 and 3.5 years, with little change thereafter. [23] This is contrary to the findings in Indian children, in whom the maximum valgus has been found to occur at an age of 5–6 years. [18] As the literature shows, there is a wide variation in the normal development of the knee angle, which might be physiological.

3.1. Development of tibiofemoral angle in Indian children

Saini et al. observed the highest mean IMD of 4.5 cm in children aged 5 years, with a minimum mean of 1 cm at the age of 9 years. They also found that the maximum mean valgus was seen at the age of 6 years in Indian children. Thereafter, the valgus alignment decreased in Indian children and the mean TFA stabilized to lie between 4 and 5° in most of the children after the age of 10 years. Indian girls overall showed more valgus at the knees than boys and the results were statistically significant, especially at the age of 6 years, when peak valgus was achieved in Indian children. The maximum TFA of 11° was seen in a 6-year-old perfectly healthy girl. They also found a boy with a valgus knee angle of 10.5° at the age of 5 years. [18]

In India, there are statistically significant differences between the mean TFA of boys and girls in the age groups of 3, 5, and 6 years (Table 2). The mean TFA is significantly higher in Indian girls of age groups 3 and 6 years, while Indian boys of age group 5 years showed a significantly higher mean TFA. After the age of 6 years, there are no statistically significant differences between the mean TFA of Indian boys and girls.

Neither height nor body mass of a child at a specific age group have statistically significant correlation with the mean TFA or the ICD or IMD. [18]

Age in years	Mean TFA of males (±SD)	Mean TFA of females (±SD)
2	1.0 ± 3.1	1.0 ± 3.6
3	1.6 ± 3.6	3.4 ± 1.5
4	3.9 ± 1.4	4.8 ± 1.3
5	7.5 ± 2.2	5.9 ± 1.8
6	7.2 ± 2.6	9.0 ± 1.9
7	5.8 ± 1.5	6.4 ± 2.0
8	5.7 ± 2.5	6.7 ± 1.8
9	5.3 ± 2.2	5.9 ± 1.0
10	5.3 ± 2.3	5.6 ± 1.9
11	4.58 ± 2.35	5.30 ± 2.49
12	4.70 ± 2.15	5.16 ± 0.98
13	4.68 ± 1.95	5.10 ± 0.87
14	4.56 ± 1.45	5.00 ± 0.63
15	4.55 ± 2.13	5.00 ± 0.81
Total	4.61 ± 2.96	5.39 ± 2.45

Table 1. Mean TFA ± SD distribution amongst male and female children at different ages

3.2. Development of tibiofemoral angle in Korean children

Yoo JH et al found that in Korean children, knee alignment or aTFA was in varus alignment in infancy, and became neutral at an average age of 1.5 yr. Development into valgus alignment continued until age 4 yr when it peaked at 7.8°. It then decreased slowly to plateau at 5-6° at age 7 to 8 yr, and remained at this level thereafter. This pattern of knee alignment change is similar to that found previously in other ethnic groups, except that the valgus peak occurred later. [22]

3.3. Axial alignment of the lower extremity in Chinese adults

Achieving normal axial alignment of the lower extremity is important to surgeons who perform reconstructive surgery of the knee. The normal alignment of the lower extremity in Caucasians has been documented by Moreland et al. with use of radiographs of the lower extremity. [24]

Tang WM et al. showed that the extremities of the Chinese women had a mean of 2.2 ± 2.5 degrees of varus alignment, and those of the Chinese men had a mean of 2.2 ± 2.7 degrees of varus alignment. The knees of Chinese female subjects, therefore, were in more varus alignment than were those in the white female subjects in the study by Hsu et al. [17, 25]

The inferolateral angle (Angle A in figure 2) between the knee joint surface and the mechanical axis of the tibia is an index of knee joint obliquity. If this angle is 90 degrees, the knee-joint surface is perpendicular to the mechanical axis. The knee-joint surface is inclined toward the medial side if this angle is larger than 90 degrees. This angle was a mean (and standard deviation) of 95.4 ± 2.5 degrees (range, 89.0 to 100.0 degrees) in the women and 94.9 ± 2.3 deegrees (range, 90.5 to 102.0 degrees) in the men in this study. The mean medial inclination (Angle B in figure 2) of the knee joint surfaces in Chinese female and male subjects therefore was 5.4 ± 2.5 degrees and 4.9 ± 2.3 degrees, respectively, which is significantly more oblique than the commonly reported 3 degrees. The inferolateral angle in both the right and the left extremity in Chinese male subjects was significantly larger than that in the white subjects in the study by Moreland et al. In the study by Hsu et al., this angle was a mean of 91.0 ± 1.4 degrees in thirty white men (sixty lower extremities) who ranged in age from twenty-five to forty years and a mean of 90.1 ± 1.9 degrees in thirty white women who ranged in age from twenty-five to forty years. [24, 25]

As noted by Insall, one should be cautious in describing what is "normal" because of the substantial individual variations. Currently, designers of most total knee arthroplasty systems recommend placement of the components in such a way that the transverse axis of the artificial knee joint is perpendicular to the mechanical axes of the tibia and the femur. The resulting alignment of the lower extremity, therefore, is in close proximity to the alignment documented by Moreland et al. and Hsu et al. The mechanical axes of the femur and the tibia did not form a straight line in either Chinese males or females. This finding is in contrast to the general consensus that has been described previously. The Chinese females had more varus alignment of the knee than did the white female subjects in the study by Hsu et al. The authors did not find the same difference between the Chinese male subjects and the white male subjects described by Moreland et al. and Hsu et al. Insall and Hungerford et al. described a 3-degree varus alignment of the knee-joint surface with reference to the mechanical axis of the tibia. Although Moreland et al. confirmed this 3-degree varus in white men, the finding was not reproduced in the study by Hsu et al. In this study of Chinese subjects, the surface of the knee joint had a medial inclination with respect to the tibia that was a mean of 5.4 degrees in the women and 4.9 degrees in the men. The values were found to be significantly different from those of the white subjects in the studies of Moreland et al. and Hsu et al. Therefore, if the tibial cut in a total knee arthroplasty is placed perpendicular to the mechanical axis of the tibia, 5 degrees of external rotation of the femoral component instead of the commonly reported 3 degrees might be necessary to produce a rectangular flexion gap in Chinese patients. [24, 25]

Fang et al. showed that femora in Chinese individuals are more bowed. In such patients, a short intramedullary rod entering the femur at the apex of the inter-condylar notch (femoral anatomical axis I) with a 4-degree distal cutting block is more likely to produce a distal femoral cut that is perpendicular to the mechanical axis of the femur. However, the choice of the cutting block should be individualized according to the preoperative planning on weight-bearing radiographs of the whole lower extremity. It is also interesting to note that the designers of some instrumentation systems have recommended use of a distal femoral cutting block with a smaller angle in taller individuals on the basis of the assumption that taller patients have a smaller physiological valgus angle of the femur. [26]

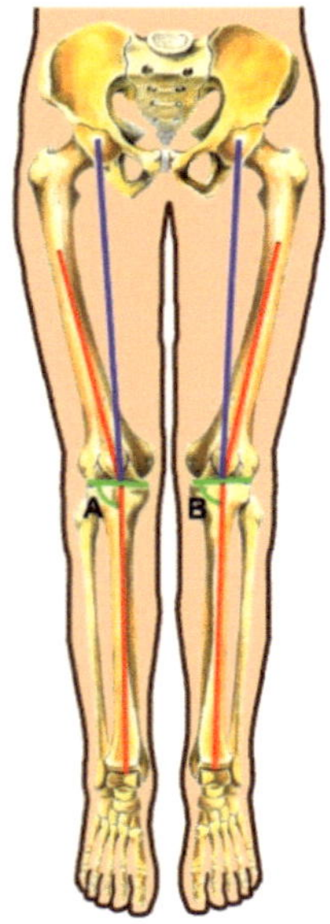

Figure 2. Diagram showing the anatomic (red) and mechanical (green) axes of the lower limb and the angles between them.

3.4. Axial alignment of the lower extremity in healthy Indian adults

Mullaji et al showed that the mean HKTA angle in healthy indian adults was 1.3° ± 0.8° of varus,mean distal femoral axis-femoral mechanical axis angle was 5.5° ± 0.8°, mean femoral condylarmechanical axis angle was 93.1° ± 1.6°, and mean femoral bow was 0.4° ± 1.2°. [27]

3.5. Variances in sagittal femoral shaft bowing

Tang WM et al have confirmed in Chinese patients distal sagittal bowing is a constant and important feature, and it affects the positioning of the femoral component on the sagittal plane. There is a dilemma of implanting the femoral component either according to the anatomy of the distal femur ignoring the bowing, or according the longitudinal axis of the femur on the sagittal plane. On one hand, following the distal anatomy might sufficiently flex the femoral component that it results in an undesirable impingement of the anterior aspect of the polyethylene post on knee extension if posterior-stabilized implants are used and thus become a source of osteolysis-inducing polyethylene particles. However, following the longitudinal axis of the femur might result in an extended femoral component that could compromise the anterior cortex of the distal femur. In Chinese patients who have undergone TKA, distal sagittal bowing of the femur is common but the common pattern is posteromedial osteoarthritis. This apparent inconsistency could be the result of differences in tibial slope and the joint line obliquity in Chinese patients. [28]

4. Three dimensional morphometry of the Chinese knees

4.1. Proximal tibial morphology

The average tibial mediolateral (tML) and tibial anteroposterior (tAP) measurement for Chinese knees are 73.0±4.6 mm and 48.8±3.4 mm, respectively. Males have larger values for tML and tAP compared with females. The male subject have larger values than female subject in the mediolateral dimension under a given anteroposterior dimension. [29] To evaluate possible differences between the medial and lateral plateau, Bo Cheng et al measured the tMAP and tLAP, and found that the tMAP was larger than the tLAP by an average of 5.6±3.2 mm in males and 5.1±2.2 in females, the CL had larger values than CM (Figure 1, B) by an average of 4.9±2.2 mm in males and 4.3±1.7 mm in females. They also calculated the aspect ratio of the tibia (tML/tAP%). The average aspect ratio of the tibia was 149.7±5.2. (Table 2) The aspect ratio showed a definitely negative correlation with tAP. From the relationship between the aspect ratio (tML/tAP %) and tAP, the authors found that there were large values in the aspect ratio with the smaller tAP, and that males have larger values in the aspect ratio than females having the same values for anteroposterior dimension. Compared with the five tibial components, only one of the prostheses had a declining change in the aspect ratio parallel with the increasing tAP. Even so, but the rate of change did not match that of the Chinese population. [29]

4.2. Distal femoral morphology

The femoral mediolateral (fML) and femoral anteroposterior (fAP) measurements are 71.0±3.0 mm and 64.1±2.7 mm, respectively. The male have larger values in fML and fAP compared with female. Comparing the morphological data with similar values for five conventional femoral components currently used in China, Bo Cheng et al found that two of the prostheses had large values in fML dimension with all range of the fAP. This was more evident with reference to female. They found that males have larger values in mediolateral dimension than females under the same value in the anteroposterior dimension. They also found that the fMAP had larger values than fLAP by an average of 0.8±0.3 mm in males and 0.5±0.2 mm in females. The average aspect ratio was 111.1±2.7 (Table 3) and had a negative correlation with the fAP. The femoral aspect ratio was higher for smaller knees and proportionally lower for larger knees. Female subjects had a smaller aspect ratio with the same anteroposterior dimension. Only one of the five femoral components showed a similar negative correlation with the fAP. Even so, the rate of change was not the same as that of the Chinese population. [29]

4.2.1. Morphologic relationships between the tibia and femur

Bo Cheng et al also analyzed the correlation between the tibial mediolateral (tML) and femoral mediolateral (fML) dimension, and between the tibial mediolateral (tML) and femoral anteroposterior (fAP)measurement. The results showed that the fML and fAP were strongly correlated with the tML. As the tML increasing, the fML and fAP also increased. [29]

Parameters	Male	Female	Combined
Tibial mediolateral (tML)	76.4±2.8	68.8±4.6	73.0±4.6
Tibial middle anteroposterior(tAP)	51.3±2.0	45.7±1.9	48.8±3.4
Tibial medial anteroposterior (tMAP)	53.3±2.5	47.5±2.4	50.7±2.4
Tibial lateral anteroposterior (tLAP)	47.7±2.7	42.4±2.3	45.3±2.5
Medial to central distance (CM)	13.2±2.6	11.9±2.0	12.7±2.1
Lateral to central distance (CL)	18.1±2.4	16.2±2.3	17.3±2.3
Aspect ratio (tML/tAP)	149.0±5.7	150.7±6.1	149.7±5.2
tMAP–tLAP	5.6±3.2	5.1±2.2	5.4±2.8

Table 2. Average values of the tibia morphology measurement (mm).

http://dx.doi.org/10.5772/53595

Parameters	Male	Female	Combined
Femoral anteroposterior (fAP)	66.6±2.4	61.0±2.7	64.1±2.7
Femoral mediolateral (fML)	74.4±2.9	66.8±3.1	71.0±3.0
Femoral medial anteroposterior (fMAP)	52.6±2.4	49.8±3.2	51.3±3.3
Femoral lateral anteroposterior (fLAP)	51.8±3.7	49.3±4.1	50.7±4.0
Aspect ratio (fML/fAP %)	111.7±3.3	109.6±3.6	111.1±2.7
fMAP–fLAP	0.8±0.3	0.5±0.2	0.6±0.3

Table 3. Average values of the femur morphology measurement (mm).

4.2.2. Utility

Quantification of the tML and tAP revealed that the female has a smaller tibial surface than the male, and both have smaller values than the Caucasian population. In the tibia of the Chinese population, the morphologic data showed a decreasing aspect ratio (tML/tAP %) as the tAP dimension increased, which is similar in many studies. In contrast, a majority of the implants had a relatively constant aspect ratio. Comparing five major conventional prostheses, it is evident that tML is undersized with the smaller tAP, and overhang with the larger tAP. This is more evident in male knee. In the morphology of the femur, females have a smaller aspect ratio with the same femoral anteroposterior dimension, which suggest that women have generally narrower femora than men when the femoral anteroposterior dimension is adequate. These results suggest that the prostheses which are suitable for Caucasian patients may be larger than ideal for Chinese patients. Bo Cheng et al also found that the femoral condyles in the Chinese population are asymmetric. These results may imply that asymmetric femoral component could prevent soft tissue irritation.

Since the tML is strongly correlated with the fML and fAP, it is important to consider the tibia and femur as a whole. Therefore, the tML and fAP should be considered as the criteria to design gender-specific proper prostheses suitable for most of Chinese population.

4.3. Distal rotational alignment of the chinese femur

Yip et al showed a statistically significant difference in Whiteside-epicondylar angle when using the mechanical (2.3°) compared with the anatomic (1.1°) axes in Chinese population. The posterior condylar angle in this study was shown to be 5.1° (for men) and 5.8° (for women). [30] (Figure 3)

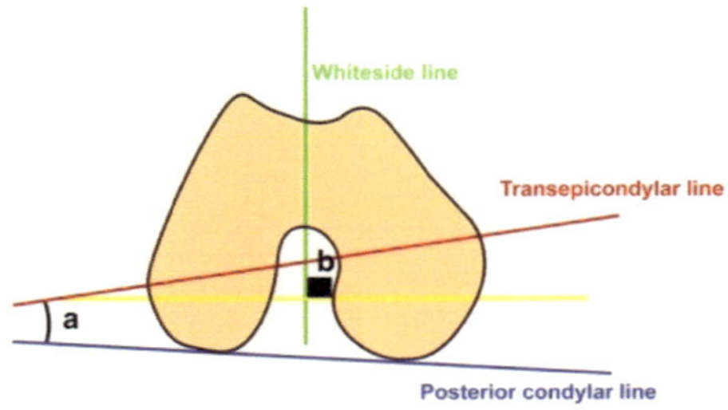

Figure 3. The whiteside-epicondylar (a) and Posterior condylar (b) angles.

4.3.1. The offset of the tibial shaft from the tibial plateau in Chinese people

Tang et al conducted a study to identify the location of the tibial shaft axis on the tibial plateau with the use of magnetic resonance imaging scans in a Chinese population. All of the measurements were made at three resection levels. The first resection level was just distal to the subchondral bone of the medial tibial plateau, which represented the clinical situation of the level of a bone cut in a proximal tibial segment with mild bone loss. The second resection level was 5mm distal to the subchondral bone of the medial tibial plateau, which represented the level of a bone cut in a proximal tibial segment with moderate bone loss. The third resection level was 10 mm distal to the subchondral bone of the medial tibial plateau, which represented the level of a bone cut in a proximal tibial segment with severe bone loss. They showed that the mean offset (and standard deviation) of the tibial shaft from the tibial plateau was 7.23 ± 2.44 mm (range, 1.62 to 12.26 mm), 6.33 ± 2.26 mm (range, 1.31 to 11.36 mm), and 4.75 ± 2.07 mm (range, 0.46 to 9.36 mm) at the first, second, and third resection levels, respectively. In almost all the knees that were examined, the tibial shaft axis was located anterolateral to the center of the tibial plateau at all resection levels. The anteroposterior and mediolateral offsets and the anteroposterior and mediolateral dimensions of the tibial plateau in the male group were significantly larger than those in the female group at each resection level. [31]

4.3.2. Utility

Several studies have revealed that the axis of the tibial shaft is, on the average, located anteromedial to the center of the tibial plateau in the Western population, for whom a medially offset stem seems more suitable. [32-34]

But, these results confirm that the axis of the tibial shaft does not overlap the center of the tibial plateau in Chinese people. Abraham et al. performed total knee arthroplasty in twenty cadaver tibiae and found that the average distance between the center of the tibial diaphysis and the center of the tibial metaphysis was 4.1 mm at the resection level of the fibular head. In view of the findings of Abraham et al. [35] as well as this study, it would appear that an offset stem would be more suitable for Chinese patients who need a long-stemmed tibial component. These authors also noted that there was a large variation in the offset of the tibial shaft from the tibial plateau, ranging from0.46 to 12.26 mm, so it would be desirable to have a wide range of offset stems available—for example, from 0 to 16 mm, in 2-mm or 4-mm increments. [35]

In a study on Iranian normal adult knees, we assessed the tibial plateau shift angle (TPSA) in order to assess our hypothesis that the proximal tibia of Iranian knee is not the same as the western knees. Our TPSA findings demonstrate that tibial plateau was not symmetrical and the Cp passes medial to Cs. This shows that the tibial plateaus in Iranian knees have a medial offset in regard to tibial shaft. So we consider that the center of the tibial plateau should not be used as a landmark of the tibial component.

Yoo et al. studied the placement of the tibial stem in close relation to the medial tibial cortex when using total knee replacements (TKRs) with medially-offset tibial stems in Korean patients. They found that the midline of the tibial stem was located medial to the tibial shaft axis in 79.7% of knees. In 6.5% of knees there was radiological contact between the tibial stem or cement mantle and the medial tibial cortex. This study has shown that the medially-offset stem in the tibial component may not be a good option for knees undergoing replacement Korean patients. (Figure 4) These researches show that some tibial base-plates specifically designed for Caucasians may not be suitable for Asian people and it remains a necessity to design a special tibial base-plate for these ethnic groups. [36] (Figure 5)

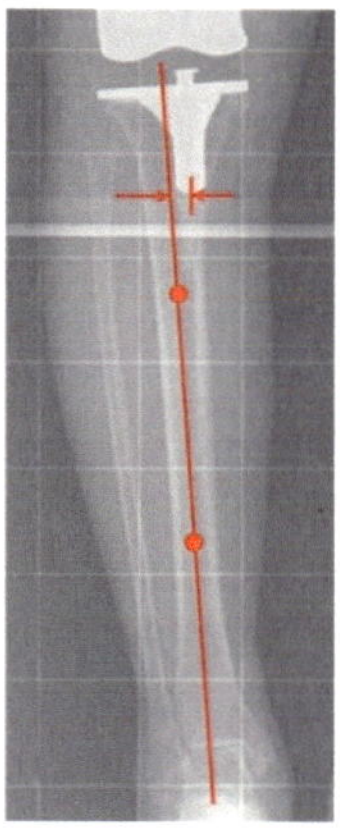

Figure 4. Anteroposterior postoperative radiograph showing the distance between the tip of the stem and the tibial shaft axis (between arrows)

4.4. Posterior slope of tibial plateau in Chinese

Kapandji found that the tibial plateau was inclined posteriorly for 5 ° to 6 ° with the horizontal and called this *retroversion* in the sagittal plane of the tibia. Insall and Kelly quoted that the posterior slope was approximately 10 ° with respect to the shaft of the tibia in western population. [38] Chiu et al. studied the posterior tibial slope in Chinese population. On visual inspection, they found that the posterior slope of the medial tibial plateau was 14.8 °

(SD, 4.2°; range, 5°-25°), and that of the lateral tibial plateau was 11.8 ° (SD, 3.8°; range, 4°-23°). The association between the posterior slopes of the medial and lateral tibial plateau was not strong.

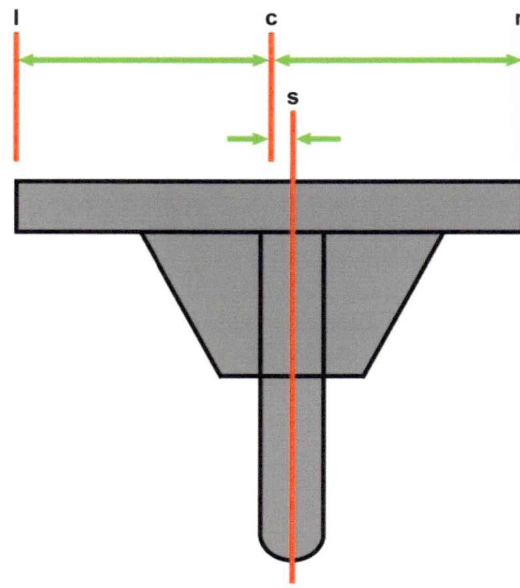

Figure 5. Diagram showing a right tibial component with a medially-offset stem. The tip of the stem (s) is located medial to the center of the tibial tray (c) which is equidistant from the medial (m) and lateral (l) borders of the tibial component. The distance between c and s corresponds to the amount of medial offset.

The difference between the posterior slopes of the medial and lateral tibial plateau was statistically significant. On radiographic assessment, they showed that the posterior slope was 14.7 ° (SD, 3.7°; range, 5°-22 °) with the extramedullary alignment line and 11.5 ° (SD, 3.6°; range, 2°-18.5 °) with the intramedullary alignment line. The association between the posterior slopes with the 2 alignment lines was strong. The difference between the posterior slopes with the 2 alignment lines was statistically significant. The posterior slope of the medial tibial plateau on visual inspection showed stronger correlation to the posterior slopes determined by radiographs. The posterior slope of the lateral tibial plateau on visual inspection had weaker correlation to the posterior slopes with the intramedullary alignment line and extramedullary alignment line in the radiographs. [38]

4.5. Ethnical differences of knee anthropometry

4.5.1. Between Chinese and white men and women

Recent anthropometric studies have suggested that current design of total knee arthroplasty (TKA) does not cater to racial anthropometric differences. Most of the commercially available TKA prostheses are designed according to the anthropometric data of white knees, which has been suspected as the cause of the component mismatch in Asian people. Several studies have compared the morphology of Asian knees to that of TKA prostheses currently used in Asia and found that the femoral aspect ratio (mediolateral [fML]/anteroposterior [fAP]) of these prostheses were not suitable for Asian patients. Iorio et al showed that the Japanese patients had a significantly less postoperative range of motion than white patients. Furthermore, 4.1% Japanese patients required revision after primary posterior cruciate-retaining TKA within an average follow-up of 6.6 years, whereas only 2.6% of their American cohort needed revision within an average follow-up of 9 years. The authors suggested that the racial morphologic differences might be a factor causing the differences in outcome. [5]

Yue B et al showed that the fML dimension of Chinese females (72.8 ± 2.6 mm; range, 70.0-79.1 mm) was significantly smaller than that of white females (76.4 ± 4.0 mm; range, 70.3-82 mm) (P =.002). The fAP dimension was 58.8 ± 2.5 mm (range, 53.2-63 mm) for Chinese females and 59.7 ± 2.6 mm (range, 54.6-64.1 mm) for white females. The difference in fAP dimension was not statistically significant. A statistically significant difference was noted between the fML/fAP ratios of Chinese females (1.24 ± 0.04; range, 1.17-1.32) and white females (1.28 ± 0.06; range, 1.16-1.39). The morphological data showed a progressive decline in the fML/fAP ratio with increasing fAP dimension for both races. However, there was a distinct offset between the fML/fAP ratio of Chinese and white females, indicating that the Chinese females had a smaller fML/fAP ratio than white females for the same fAP dimension.(Table 5) Measurements of tibia showed that the tibial size of Chinese females was generally smaller than that of white females. However, the tibial aspect ratio did not show any significant difference between Chinese (1.78 ± 0.1; range, 1.56-1.96) and white females (1.76 ± 0.08; range, 1.58-1.89). The medial/lateral posterior tibial slopes showed no difference between the 2 groups. The average medial slope was 5.4° ± 2.3° (range, 1.4°-10.1°) for Chinese females and 6.5° ± 2.9° (range, 0.6°-10.7°) for white females. The average lateral slope was 4.8° ± 2.8° (range, 0.3°-10.6°) for Chinese females and 5.8° ± 2.7° (range, 0.8°-10.4°) for white females. Chinese males had an average fML dimension of 82.6 ± 3.6 mm (range, 72.6-87.1 mm), which was significantly smaller than that of white males (86.0 ± 5.6 mm; range, 74.9-100.2 mm). The fAP size averaged 65.0 ± 2.8 mm (range, 59.4-70.3 mm) for Chinese males and 67.5 ± 3.6 mm (range, 62.4-75.3 mm) for white males. The difference was statistically significant between fAP size of Chinese and white males. The femoral aspect ratio (fML/fAP) of Chinese males averaged 1.27 ± 0.03 (range, 1.22-1.33) and white males 1.28 ± 0.07 (range, 1.12-1.37), and there was no statistically significant difference. The tibial dimension of Chinese males was generally smaller than that of white males. A significant difference was noted for the tibial aspect ratio, with Chinese males averaging 1.82 ± 0.07 (range, 1.70-1.95) and white males averaging 1.75 ± 0.11 (range, 1.58-1.87). The morphological data showed a progressive decline in the tibial aspect ratio with increasing average tAP dimension for both races. The lines representing change in tibial aspect ratio with increasing average tAP dimension for Chinese and white males were nearly coincident. Therefore, the differences in tibial aspect ratios between the 2 groups may be caused by the average tAP dimensions of Chinese males that were generally smaller than those of white males. The medial/lateral plateau posterior slope showed no significant difference between the 2 groups.

The average medial slope was 6.0° ± 2.5° (range, 2.7°- 12.0°) for Chinese males and 5.1° ± 3.3° (range, −3.0° to 11.1°) for white males. The average lateral slope was 5.2° ± 3.6° (range, −1.8° to 14.0°) for Chinese males and 5.6° ± 2.7° (range, 2.5°-15.1°) for white males. [39] (Table 5)

	fML (mm)	fAP (mm)	fML/fAP
Chinese female	72.8 ± 2.6 (70.0-79.1)	58.8 ± 2.5 (53.2-63)	1.24 ± 0.04 (1.17-1.32)
White female	76.4 ± 4.0 (70.3-82)	59.7 ± 2.6 (54.6-64.1)	1.28 ± 0.06 (1.16-1.39)
Chinese male	82.6 ± 3.6 (72.6-87.1)	65.0 ± 2.8 (59.4-70.3)	1.27 ± 0.03 (1.22-1.33)
White male	86.0 ± 5.6 (74.9-100.2)	67.5 ± 3.6 (62.4-75.3)	1.28 ± 0.07 (1.12-1.37)

Table 4. Femoral Measurements Categorized by Race and Sex.

	Tibial Plateau Dimensions					Posterior Tibial Slope (deg)		
	MPAP (mm)	LPAP (mm)	Average AP (mm)	tML (mm)	tML/Avg. tAP	MPPS	LPPS	Average Posterior Slope
Chinese female	41.5 ± 3.0 (37.6-48.6)	33.2 ± 3.2 (28.7-40.2)	37.3 ± 2.8 (34.5-44.1)	66.2 ± 2.1 (63.1-69.5)	1.78 ± 0.10 (1.56-1.96)	5.4 ± 2.3 (1.4-10.1)	4.8 ± 2.8 (0.3-10.6)	5.1 ± 2.3 (1.4-9.9)
White female	43.4 ± 1.9 (39.2-46.5)	35.2 ± 3.8 (26.5-40.0)	39.3 ± 2.6 (34.1-43.3)	69.0 ± 4.2 (61.3-74.4)	1.76 ± 0.08 (1.58-1.89)	6.5 ± 2.9 (0.6-10.7)	5.8 ± 2.7 (0.8-10.4)	6.1 ± 2.5 (0.7-9.8)
Chinese male	46.1 ± 2.4 (42.0-49.5)	36.8 ± 2.1 (34.1-40.7)	41.5 ± 2.1 (38.0-45.1)	75.2 ± 3.6 (67.6-81.5)	1.82 ± 0.07 (1.70-1.95)	6.0 ± 2.5 (2.7-12.0)	5.2 ± 3.6 (-1.8-14.0)	5.6 ± 2.8 (0.4-11.9)
White male	49.3 ± 3.1 (42.5-53.5)	40.7 ± 2.9 (35.6-48.4)	45.0 ± 2.8 (39.9-50.2)	78.7 ± 5.4 (67.1-89.1)	1.75 ± 0.11 (1.58-1.97)	5.1 ± 3.3 (-3.0-11.1)	5.6 ± 2.7 (2.5-15.1)	5.3 ± 2.5 (0.8-12.7)

Table 5. Tibial Measurements Categorized by Race and Sex

The present study showed that the dimensions of Chinese knees were generally smaller than white knees. In addition, Chinese females had a significantly narrower distal femur than white females, whereas Chinese males had a wider proximal tibia than their white counterparts. These results proved the hypothesis that there is a distinct difference in size and shape between the Chinese and white knees. [39] Harvey et al also showed that there are more valgus alignment of the distal femur in Chinese. [40]

A proper design of femoral aspect ratio of femoral TKA components is critical to obtain an ideal coverage of the resected bone surface. It must be noted that the differences in average values of femoral aspect ratio between Chinese and white females cannot be explained by differences in knee size alone, and this may point to a distinct variation in femoral shape between the 2 races. Given this, it is possible that the components designed based on white knee data may produce a mediolateral component overhang in Chinese females. [41]

The geometry of tibial plateau has a direct influence on the biomechanics of tibiofemoral joint and is considered as an important factor in TKA design and implantation. [9, 42]

The study by Yue et al. showed that Chinese subjects generally had a smaller size of proximal tibia than white subjects in both sexes. Interestingly, the tibial aspect ratio of Chinese males was significantly larger than that of white males (1.82 ± 0.07 vs 1.75 ± 0.11). However, the present study also found a larger tibial aspect ratio in small knees and a proportionally smaller ratio in large knees. Therefore, the differences of the tibial aspect ratios between the 2 groups may be caused by the average tAP dimensions of Chinese males that were generally smaller than those of white males. This study showed that there was no difference in medial/lateral posterior slope between Chinese and white subjects in either sex. [39]

4.5.2. Anthropometry of the Japanese proximal tibia

Uehara et al, in a comparative study between CT and intraoperative measurements of tibial dimensions, showed that the average ML length on the CT scan was significantly larger (74.3 ± 6.6 mm [mean ± SD]) compared with the intraoperative measurement (71.4 ± 5.0 mm). In contrast, the average AP length on the CT scan was significantly smaller (48.3 ± 5.4 mm) compared with the intraoperative measurement (50.3 ± 3.6 mm). [43]

4.5.3. Variations between Japanese and Caucasian populations in the healthy young adult knee joint

Hovinga et al showed that there was a significant difference in alignment between Caucasian and Japanese groups. The mechanical alignment in Caucasians was slightly varus (0.55 ± 0.338, 57%varus), while78% of Japanese subjects exhibited a varus alignment (1.64 ± 0.438). A significant difference also existed between male and female subjects, with women exhibiting a higher percentage of valgus alignment (50%) than men (36%). The average torsion angle was 37.58 for all subjects. Tibial torsion measurements showed significant differences with ethnicity; Caucasians demonstrated a higher torsion angle than Japanese. No difference based on gender was observed. The tibial width for all subjects was 74.1 ± 0.77 mm. The lateral width was 39.4 ± 0.52 mm, while the medial width was 34.6 ± 0.42 mm. Medial and lateral widths were greater in males than in females, but no ethnic differences were found. The laxity measurement for Caucasian females was 6.4 ± 0.36 mm, and for males was 4.9 ± 0.35 mm. For Japanese females, the laxity was 8.1 ± 0.65 mm, and for males 6.9 ± 0.56 mm. Significant differences were found for both gender and ethnicity. [4]

Based on this study, a higher varus alignment, lower tibial torsion, and higher ACL laxity were found in Japanese compared to Caucasian populations. Males demonstrated a higher varus alignment, larger tibial width, and lower ACL laxity compared to females. [4]

Tamari et al performed a clinical study aimed to investigate whether or not there were ethnic, gender, and age-related differences in FTA and torsion of the lower limb among healthy Japanese and Australian Caucasian populations. They found that the Japanese had significantly greater FTA than the Australian Caucasians. Moreover, there was gender difference in this variable, that is, the female subjects had significantly smaller FTA than the males. The femoral antetorsion was significantly smaller in middle and older age groups compared to the younger age group in the Japanese subjects. Femoral antetorsion of the Japanese was significantly greater than that of the Australian subjects. Further, the females had greater femoral antetorsion than the male subjects. They also found that the tibiofibular torsion was significantly larger in the younger and middle age groups compared to the older age group of the females, whereas there were no significant age-related differences in the male subjects. But, there was no ethnic difference in tibiofibular torsion. Tibiofibular torsion of the females was significantly smaller than that of the male subjects. [7]

4.5.4. Morphometry of the Korean proximal tibia

Kwak et al assessed the morphometry of the proximal tibia of Korean ethnicity. Their results are as follows. (Table 6)

4.5.4.1. ML and AP dimensions

The average mediolateral (ML) and middle anteroposterior (AP) dimensions for the Korean population were 73.5±5.6 mm and 47.3±3.8 mm, respectively. The males were found to have larger values for the AP and ML dimensions when compared to the females. Comparison of the AP and ML dimensions to the height of the person showed a statistically significant, positive correlation with the height of the person. [44]

4.5.4.2. Medial and lateral anteroposterior dimensions of the tibial condyle

The medial tibial plateau is larger than the lateral tibial plateau anteroposteriorly by an average of 3.9±2.9 mm in the males and 3.7±2.7 mm in the females. This result favors the need for asymmetry in the tibial component for the Korean population.

Accordingly, the gross size of the proximal tibia (ML and AP) in the females was found to be smaller than that in the males. Both the AP and ML lengths were found to be smaller than the Caucasian population. This research shows that the ML dimension is more strongly correlated to the height of the person when compared to the AP dimension. They also found that the MAP was located closer to the centre of the tibial plateau (C) as compared to the LAP, which further confirmed the asymmetry of the proximal tibia. [44]

This study revealed a higher aspect ratio for the smaller AP dimensions of the proximal tibia and a lower aspect ratio for the larger AP dimensions of the proximal tibia. In other words, this means that with every increase in the AP dimension of the proximal tibia, the shape of the anticipated tibial component becomes less oval (mediolaterally) for use in the Korean population. In the Japanese study, the aspect ratio in women varied from 138 to 142.86, however, they found that as the ML dimensions increased the aspect ratio increased. In contrast, to the pattern of the study population, the majority of the symmetric conventional implants showed a relatively constant aspect ratio or an increase in the aspect ratio (NexGen) with the increase of the AP dimension of the proximal cut. Thus, a tibial component that would be suitable for the Korean population would be one whose aspect ratio decreased with increase in the anteroposterior dimension. [44]

4.5.5. Anthropometric measurements of knee joints in Thai population

Chaichankul et al assessed the knee morphology in Thai population and found that the femoral aspect ratio and the tibial aspect ratio were significantly different between males and females. This study also demonstrated that when the tibial AP dimension increased, there was a decreasing tibial AP/ML aspect ratio, while most implants had a relatively constant aspect ratio. [45] (Table 7 and 8)

Parameter	Male	Female	Combined
Mediolateral length (ML)	76.1±4.0	67.64±3.12	71.9±5.6
Middle anteroposterior length (AP)	48.2±3.3	43.2±2.3	45.7±3.8
Medial anteroposterior (MAP)	48.5±3.7	43.5±2.9	45.9±4.2
Lateral anteroposterior (LAP)	44.6±3.2	39.8±2.5	42.2±3.7
Medial to centre distance (CM)	14.4±5.1	12.9±3.5	13.7±4.4
Lateral to centre distance (CL)	19.7±3.5	15.9±5.6	17.8±5.1
Aspect ratio	158	156	157
Height (cm)	165.9±4.8	156.4±5.0	161.2±6.8
MAP–LAP difference	3.9±2.9	3.7±2.7	3.8±2.8

Table 6. Average values (in mm) of the measured data from the cadavers

Parameters	Total	Male	Female
	Mean±SD (range)	**Mean±SD (range)**	**Mean±SD (range)**
Resected AP length (mm)	45.43±4.5 (35–56.9)	48.55±3.73 (40–56.9)	43.32±3.69 (35–55)
Resected ML width (mm)	64.06±6.31 (52–78.9)	70.15±3.87 (61.4–78.9)	59.91±3.75 (52–76.3)
Aspect ratio (ML width/AP length)×100	141±12 (111–177)	145±11 (124–177)	139±12 (111–177)

Table 7. The distal femoral condyle dimensions.

Parameters	Total	Male	Female
	Mean±SD (range)	**Mean±SD (range)**	**Mean±SD (range)**
Resected AP length (mm)	46.04±4.4 (37.6–56.6)	50.15±3.09 (44–56.6)	43.23±2.57 (37.6–52)
Resected ML width (mm)	68.8±5.8 (57.8–86)	74.44±3.44 (65.6–86)	64.95±3.45 (57.8–78.6)
Aspect ratio (ML width/AP length)×100	67±3 (59–77)	67±3 (61–75)	67±3 (59–77)

Table 8. The proximal tibial dimensions.

4.5.6. Anthropometric measurements of the Indian population

Vaidya et al examined the anthropometric characteristics of Indian normal knees by CT scan and dry bone measurement. They found that the mean anteroposterior diameter of the femur in men was 61.09 mm and in women was 55.58 mm. Most men (27 of 38) had a range of anteroposterior diameter between 55 and 65 mm, whereas most women (40 of 48) had a range between 49 and 59 mm. In the cadaveric study, the mean anteroposterior diameter was 55.26 mm, and most (19 of 25) had a range between 52 and 60 mm. [46]

Assuming the lowest cut-off value of the anteroposterior diameter of the lower end of the femur in the study population to be 55 mm (55 mm being the smallest size of commercially available prosthetic femoral component), it was observed that a statistically significant number of Indian population (approximately 40%) had measurements lower than this value. This percentage was more significant in women (60.4%), in whom the mean anteroposterior diameter was 52.01 mm, than in men. The clinical implication of this statistical analysis is that there is a substantial number of Indians in whom the problem of component oversizing is likely to occur. [46]

4.5.7. Morphology of proximal tibia in Iranian

4.5.7.1. Lateral offset of tibial shaft in relation to tibial plateau

In a study on Iranian normal adult knees, we assessed the tibial plateau shift angle (TPSA) in order to assess our hypothesis that the proximal tibia of Iranian knee is not the same as the western knees. TPSA is the angle formed between central line (Cs)of the tibial shaft and the mechanical axis of the tibia which goes through the central point (Cp) of the tibial articular surface and the center of ankle. Our results are shown in Table 9.

	Our study			Japanese			Americans			France
Parameter	**Mean**	**SD**	**Range**	**Mean**	**SD**	**Range**	**Mean**	**SD**	**Range**	**Mean**
TA	93.8	1.54	90.3-98	97.2	3.8	89-106	93	1.6	90-96.5	93
TPSA	2.11	3.64	-3.4-7.4	2.21	1.5	-3.0-7.0	-	-	-	-

Table 9. Representation of the amount of tibial shaft offset in Iranian and its comparison with other studies.

Our TPSA findings demonstrate that tibial plateau was not symmetrical and the Cp passes medial to Cs. This shows that the tibial plateaus in Iranian knees have a medial offset in regard to tibial shaft. So we consider that the center of the tibial plateau should not be used as a landmark of the tibial component.

4.5.7.2. Posterior tibial slope

We assessed the tibial slope in normal adults in Iran. The mean slope angle was 9.4±1.8 degrees. We found no statistical relationship between age and gender and posterior tibial slope. The normal posterior tibial slope angle in this Iranian population was different from other ethnic groups (Table 10). It may be necessary to consider these differences in designing tibial components for knee arthroplasty. [47]

Study	Ethnic group	Number	Range of slope (degrees)	Mean ± (SD)
Moore et al (1974)	American	50	7 – 22	14 ± 3.7
Jiang et al (1994)	Thai	50	0 – 20	10 ± 4
Matsuda et al (1999)	Japanese	30	5 – 15.5	10.7
Chiou et al (2000)	Chinese	25	5 – 22	14.7 ± 3.7
Our study (2009)	Iranian	108	2 – 18	9.4 ± 1.8

Table 10. Comparison of posterior tibial slope between Iranians and other ethnic groups

5. Patella

Patella-related problems are among the issues of concern during and after TKA. Information regarding anthropometric patellar dimensions can play an important role during the design of patellar prostheses and the development of surgical techniques. [48] Thickness, height/width ratio, and relative position of the median ridge all have implications relating to the selection of patellar components, patellofemoral contact stress, and patellar tracking in the trochlear groove. [49]

Patellar thickness is a challenging consideration during patellar resurfacing for TKA. A thin patella can reduce patellofemoral contact force but also poses the potential risk of stress fracture and anteroposterior instability. Increasing patellar thickness might be expected to increase effective quadriceps moment arm at low flexion angles of the knee but potentially reduces range of motion and predisposes to patellar subluxation. It commonly is assumed that it is desirable for a resurfaced patella to be equal to its original thickness, and a bony patellar thickness of at least 15 mm should be maintained. However, it is not uncommon to find, intraoperatively, the patella is too thin to simultaneously satisfy these criteria. Three surgical options should be considered with a thin patella: (1) leave the patella unresurfaced; (2) restore the original patellar thickness by removing bone to account for the thickness of the prosthesis, while accepting thin residual bone; and (3) leave residual bone of adequate thickness, while accepting an increase in overall patellar thickness. To solve this problem, the only versatile option is to use a specifically designed patellar prosthesis with less thickness. [9, 50]

Patellar height/width ratios and the position of the median patellar ridge have clinical implications for TKA with patellar resurfacing. Because the mediolateral width of a patella typically is larger than its height, a dome-shaped patella component chosen by the height does not cover the entire resected surface of the patella. It has been recommended the patella be placed at the medial margin of a resected patella to help patellofemoral tracking by decreasing the Q angle. In addition, the position of the median ridge is another factor to consider when selecting the size of a patellar component. The median ridge can act as a fulcrum for patellofemoral tracking and thus can influence restoration of normal kinematics after TKA with patellar resurfacing. If an orthopaedic surgeon attempts to restore the original position of the median ridge, he or she may have to select a smaller component, which reduces patellofemoral articulation contact area. [9]

The only article in the literature that we could find on this subject was by Kyun Kim et al. They performed an anthropometric assessment of patella on Korean knees (Figure 6) and its comparison to the western knees. They found that Koreans had thinner and smaller patellae than Westerners. The mean central ridge thickness was 21.2 mm in women and 23.1 mm in men, whereas corresponding reported mean thicknesses in Western patients are 21.8 to 22.5 mm and 23.9 to 26.1 mm. In Koreans, mean heights and widths were 33.1 mm and 41.0 mm in women and 36.2 mm and 45.6 mm in men, whereas corresponding values in Western patients are 35.0 mm and 42.7 mm in women and 39.4 mm and 49.5 mm in men. However, despite these differences in thicknesses, widths, and heights, the width/height ratios and ridge positions were similar in Koreans and Westerners. [50] (Table 11)

Some studies have advocated reestablishment of original thickness and adequate residual bony thickness as key surgical guidelines. However, in Korean patients, these two guidelines often cannot be satisfied. In such cases, the surgeon is forced to choose between restoring the original thickness while accepting a low residual bony thickness and retaining sufficient residual bony thickness while accepting an increased overall thickness. But if Koreans can have a specifically designed patellar prosthesis with less thickness, this problem will be better resolved. [51]

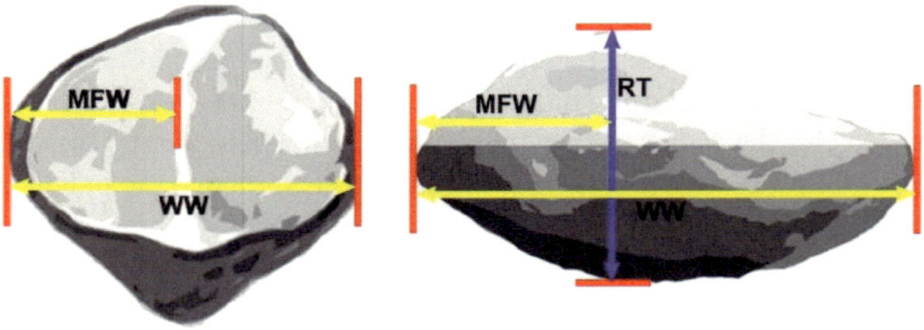

Figure 6. The schematic drawings show anthropometric dimensions before bone resection, including medial facet width (MFW), whole patella width (WW), and thickness at the median ridge (RT).

Study	Thickness at central ridge (mm)	Ridge position	Mediolateral width (mm)	Superoinferior height (mm)	Width/height Ratio	Residual bony thickness after bone resection (mm)	Overall thickness after implantation (mm)
This study							
Female (n = 713)	21.2 (17–26)	0.45 (0.23–0.67)	41.0 (25–51)	33.1 (23–43)	1.24 (0.72–1.78)	12.5 (10–15)	21.2 (17–25)
Male (n = 39)	23.1 (20–26)	0.44 (0.23–0.52)	45.6 (36–52)	36.2 (31–52)	1.27 (0.81–1.50)	13.5 (12–16)	22.7 (20–26)
Baldwin and House (2005)							
Female (n = 57)	21.8 (18–27)	0.43	42.7 (32–50)	35.0 (28–43)	1.22 (1.06–1.56)		
Male (n = 35)	23.9 (20–30)	0.42	49.5 (44–64)	39.4 (34–45)	1.26 (1.05–1.51)		
Chmell et al.(1996)							
Female (n = 123)	22.6 (17.5–28)						
Male (n = 75)	26.1 (20–33)						
Hitt et al.(2003)							
Female (n = 209)	22.5						
Male (n = 128)	25.3						

Table 11. Comparisons of the anthropometric dimensions of the patellae of Korean and Western patients (based on published values)

6. Is ethnicity influencing in vivo normal knee kinematics?

Current TKA reduces pain, restores mobility, and provides satisfactory longevity. Surgery is sometimes refused in non-Western cultures due to the anticipated limited postoperative ROM. [52]

Therefore, improvements to facilitate deep flexion activities are required in the present TKA designs to be accepted by Asian people. To make design changes, it is important to understand which factors influence deep flexion capabilities. Since Asian populations can achieve more flexion than Caucasians (156.9°, 157.3°, 159.6°, 160°, 162° or even 165° for Asian populations and 143.8°, 145° for Caucasian), ethnicity might reveal certain factors leading to higher knee flexion. [53 - 55]

Physiologic and anatomic characteristics can vary considerably between individuals. Research data originating from different regions of the world suggest ROM may be a function of ethnicity or a lifestyle. Caucasians can flex to about 140°, while in societies where daily activities require full kneeling or squatting as in Japan, India, or the Middle East, subjects achieve up to 165°, providing an energy-saving flexed posture. Saudi Arabian men flex their knees, on average, to 159.6°, 15° more than Scandinavians. Muslims maintain the flexion of 157.3° in their prayer position. [54, 55]

Leszko et al. assessed the knee kinematics in Asian and Caucasian population. They found that Caucasian women achieved similar maximum flexion as the Japanese women and Japanese men. These three groups also outnumbered the Caucasian males capable of achieving knee flexion greater than 150°. Consequently, the average maximum flexion was lower for Caucasian men than for Caucasian women or Japanese men. These differences were also apparent when comparing the flexion ROM; the highest was attained by Japanese women, followed by Japanese men, Caucasian women, and Caucasian men. The maximum axial rotation was lower for Caucasian men compared to Caucasian women. Caucasian women and both Japanese groups achieved similar average maximum axial rotation. The absolute range of axial rotation revealed a similar trend; it was lower for Caucasian men than for the three other groups, and there was no difference among the three other groups. When compared at each flexion increment, the femur rotated externally with increasing flexion, in a similar pattern for all four groups. [9]

However, in deep flexion, Caucasian men had the least amount of external rotation. For all groups, the femur was slightly abducted at the beginning of the activity but adducted with increasing knee flexion. Above 120° of flexion, the femur remained about 4° adducted for Caucasian women and both Japanese groups, while for Caucasian men, the adduction reduced and the femur became slightly abducted at 150° of flexion. The lateral tibio-femoral contact point translated posteriorly in virtually the same pattern for all four groups and there was no difference at any flexion increment or in the absolute range of translation between any of the groups. The AP translation of the medial tibio-femoral contact point was also similar for all groups, except at maximum flexion where it was more posterior for Caucasian men than for Caucasian women. Similarly, the AP translation of the lateral femoral flexion facet center was similar between the groups at any flexion as was the medial femoral flexion facet center translation at each flexion increment. However, the posterior translation of the femoral flexion facet center from full extension to maximum flexion was higher for Caucasian men than for any other group. The medial and lateral condyles moved in different modes. The lateral condyle was spinning and rolling posteriorly throughout the ROM. However, the medial condyle counter-translated in the early flexion and then was spinning until 120°. Above 120°, the motion changed to more of a rolling type for both condyles, which may justify the use of the term "posterior femoral rollback." There were no differences in the type of motion of the lateral condyle between the analyzed groups at any flexion increment. However, above 120° of flexion, the medial condyle revealed more rolling for Caucasian men compared to Caucasian women and both Japanese groups. [9]

This study suggested higher axial rotation is not related to the lateral condyle, as its motion was almost identical for all three groups (the lateral femoral condyle was spinning and rolling in the same manner for all four groups). The differences were observed on the medial condyle.

From full extension to maximum flexion, for Caucasian men, the medial tibio-femoral contact point and flexion facet center translated more posteriorly than for any other group. The medial condyle was also rolling more for the Caucasian men than for any other group above 120°. In fact, for the three other groups, the medial condyle remained more stationary, spinning close to the center of the tibial plateau, possibly allowing the lateral condyle to pivot about it and to rotate more externally. The ability to achieve more external rotation may also be related to ACL laxity, as it was higher for Japanese than for Caucasians. [9]

7. Conclusion

Almost all prosthetic implants have been designed and manufactured to accommodate the knee anatomy of Western Caucasians, and there is some doubt about the application of these systems to Asians, as the size of Asians differs from that of Caucasians. Moreover, even if the smallest size from each Western prosthesis company is used, it may be too big for some Asian subjects.

However, all the problems with matching a conventional knee prosthesis with Asian knees is not the mere size. It is important not to consider Asian knees as a smaller western Caucasian knees. As we reviewed in above paragraphs, there are many differences in various anatomic parameters between Asian and Caucasian knees. In Chinese, Korean and Iranian knees, it has been shown that the tibial anatomic axis does not pass through the same point of plateau as the western Caucasian knees. It is a noteworthy point to consider while marking the tibial entry point, otherwise, in Asian knees, the tibial component would be inserted in varus or the tibial medial cortex would be fractured.

Besides, the relationship between these parameters in Asian knees are far different from western Caucasian knees. As it was described in multiple studies in Chinese, Japanese, Korean and Indian population, the mediolateral diameter of the distal femur is smaller than their counterpart in western population with the same AP diameter. There is also a more important aspect of difference between these two groups of knees, which is great disparity among changes in these parameters. In other words, in contrast to western Caucasian knees, there are some parameters in the Asian knees which decrease upon increasing the other parameters and the size of the knee. As it has been shown in Chinese knees, the femoral aspect ratio was higher for smaller knees and proportionally lower for larger knees and female subjects had a smaller aspect ratio with the same anteroposterior dimension. On the tibial side, the aspect ratio (tML/tAP %) showed a definitely negative correlation with tAP, which means that there were large values in the aspect ratio with the smaller tAP, and that males have larger values in the aspect ratio than females having the same values for anteroposterior dimension. Although, there are some prostheses that consider this negative correlation between tibial aspect ratio and tAP, however, the rate of change did not match that of the Asian population.

There is also a huge number of differences in the angular parameters between Asian and western Caucasian knees. Distal femoral coronal angle, posterior femoral condylar angle, proximal tibial varus angle and posterior tibial slope have all been shown to be different in Asian from western Caucasian knees. It means that standard considerations while preparing and cutting distal femur and proximal tibia may not be appropriate for Asian knees, otherwise, soft tissue tension, ligament balancing and ROM of the joint may be disturbed.

Patellar dimensions are also different between these two ethnic groups, so although specific considerations in patellar resurfacing techniques for Asians are necessary, a specifically designed patellar prosthesis with less thickness is imperative to accommodate thinner patella of Asian ethnicity.

Aside from technical considerations for Asian knees which of course must be different from western knees, there seems to be necessary to have some specifically designed knee prostheses for Asian population. These prostheses must take into account not only the differences in size, but also the variations in aspect ratios in size parameters and their specific changes with changes in other parameters. Another consideration in Asian knee prostheses is their need for more flexion than their western counterparts. For achieving deep flexion after TKA, prosthesis design, although not as important as the technical consideration, is an significant point.

8. Summary

As you've read through the chapter it is clear that knees are different in different ethnic population.

These differences vary in a wide spectrum. For example, three-dimensional morphology of the Knee represents that the shape of the distal femur and proximal tibia is different among the ethnic groups. The normalized ratios and nonlinear shape analysis of the studies supported differences between East Asians and Caucasians independent of any scale factor.

There is a strong correlation between the femoral mediolateral (fML) and femoral anteroposterior (fAP) dimensions with the tibial mediolateral (tML) measurements, and as the latter increases, there is an increase in the formers.

Quantification of the tML and tAP (tibial anteroposterior) revealed that among Chinese population females have a smaller tibial surface than males, and both have smaller values than the Caucasian population. The morphologic data of the tibia showed a decreasing aspect ratio (tML/tAP %) as the tAP dimension increased, which is similar in many studies. In contrast, a majority of the implants had a relatively constant aspect ratio. Comparing five major conventional prostheses, it is evident that tML is undersized with the smaller tAP, and overhang with the larger tAP. This is more evident in male knees. In the morphology of the femur, females have a smaller aspect ratio with the same femoral anteroposterior dimension, which suggest that women have generally narrower femora than men when the femoral anteroposterior dimension is adequate. These results suggest that the prostheses which are suitable for Caucasian patients may be larger than ideal for Chinese patients. Since the tML is strongly correlated with the fML and fAP, it is important to consider the tibia and femur as a whole. Therefore, the tML and fAP should be considered as the criteria to design gender-specific proper prostheses suitable for most of Chinese population.

Dimensions of Chinese knees were generally smaller than white knees. In addition, Chinese females had a significantly narrower distal femur than white females, whereas Chinese males had a wider proximal tibia than their white counterparts. These prove the hypothesis that there is a distinct difference in size and shape between the Chinese and white knees. Another point is that the femoral condyles are asymmetric among Chinese population.

Anatomical differences could be observed even during childhood developments. Arazi et al found a negative correlation between the weight of children at a specific age with the ICD of the subject. However, this correlation was found to be weak and although statistically significant, it might not be of any clinical significance. The only possible explanation to this might be the relatively thick thighs of the heavier children, which is expected to subjectively decrease the ICD. Literature shows that there is a wide variation in the normal development of the knee angle, which might be physiological.

Axial alignment of the lower extremity has also seemed to be different among different races. Achieving normal axial alignment of the lower extremity is important to surgeons who perform reconstructive surgery of the knee.

In the study by Tang et al, the extremities of Chinese women had a mean of 2.2 ± 2.5 degrees of varus alignment, demonstrating that the knees of Chinese female is in more varus alignment than those in the white females.

Several studies have revealed that the axis of the tibial shaft is, on the average, located anteromedial to the center of the tibial plateau in the Western population, for whom a medially offset stem seems more suitable. But, some studies confirm that the axis of the tibial shaft does not overlap the center of the tibial plateau in Chinese people. It seems that an offset stem would be more suitable for Chinese patients who need a long-stemmed tibial component. Among Asian population, there is a large variation in the offset of the tibial shaft from the tibial plateau, ranging from 0.46 to 12.26 mm.

In a study on Iranian normal adult knees, we assessed the tibial plateau shift angle (TPSA) in order to assess our hypothesis that the proximal tibia of Iranian knee is not the same as the western knees. Our TPSA findings demonstrate that tibial plateau was not symmetrical and the central point (Cp) passes medial to central shaft line (Cs). This shows that the tibial plateaus in Iranian knees have a medial offset in regard to tibial shaft. So we suggest that the center of the tibial plateau should not be used as a landmark of the tibial component. Therefore, some tibial base-plates specifically designed for Caucasians may not be suitable for Asian people and it remains a necessity to design a special tibial base-plate for these ethnic groups.

Some variances have also been observed in sagittal femoral shaft bowing. In Chinese patients distal sagittal bowing is a constant and important feature, and it affects the positioning of the femoral component on the sagittal plane. There is a dilemma of implanting the femoral component either according to the anatomy of the distal femur ignoring the bowing, or according the longitudinal axis of the femur on the sagittal plane. On one hand, following the distal anatomy might sufficiently flex the femoral component that it results in an undesirable impingement of the anterior aspect of the polyethylene post on knee extension if posterior-stabilized implants are used and thus become a source of osteolysis-inducing polyethylene particles. However, following the longitudinal axis of the femur might result in an extended femoral component that could compromise the anterior cortex of the distal femur. In Chinese patients who have undergone TKA, distal sagittal bowing of the femur is common but the common pattern is posteromedial osteoarthritis. This apparent inconsistency could be the result of differences in tibial slope and the joint line obliquity in Chinese patients.

The posterior tibial slope has also a unique feature in Asians. Kapandji found that the tibial plateau was inclined posteriorly for 5 ° to 6 ° according to the horizontal plane and called this *retroversion* in the sagittal plane of the tibia. We assessed the tibial slope in normal adults in Iran. The mean slope angle was 9.4±1.8 degrees. We found no statistical relationship between age and gender and posterior tibial slope. The normal posterior tibial slope angle in this Iranian population was different from other ethnic groups. It may be necessary to consider these differences in designing tibial components for knee arthroplasty.

Special considerations in total knee arthroplasty for Asians: Recent anthropometric studies have suggested that current design of total knee arthroplasty (TKA) does not cater to racial anthropometric differences. Most of the commercially available TKA prostheses are designed according to the anthropometric data of white knees, which has been suspected as the cause of the component mismatch in Asian people. Several studies have compared the morphology of Asian knees to that of TKA prostheses currently used in Asia and found that the femoral aspect ratio (medio-lateral [fML]/antero-posterior [fAP]) of these prostheses were not suitable for Asian patients.

Patella-related problems are among the issues of concern during and after TKA. Information regarding anthropometric patellar dimensions can play an important role during the design of patellar prostheses and the development of surgical techniques. Thickness, height/width ratio, and relative position of the median ridge all have implications relating to the selection of patellar components, patella-femoral contact stress, and patellar tracking in the trochlear groove. The only article in the literature that we could find on this subject was by Kyun Kim et al. They found that Koreans had thinner and smaller patellae than Westerners. Patellar thickness is a challenging consideration during patellar resurfacing for TKA. A thin patella can reduce patella-femoral contact force but also poses the potential risk of stress fracture and anteroposterior instability. It commonly is assumed that it is desirable for a resurfaced patella to be equal to its original thickness, and a bony patellar thickness of at least 15 mm should be maintained. However, it is not uncommon to find, intra-operatively, the patella is too thin to simultaneously satisfy these criteria. To solve this problem, the only versatile option is to use exclusively designed patellar prosthesis with less thickness.

Yet the importance of these issues is more distinguished when one considers the geographical variation in the epidemiology of osteoarthritis, which has been well documented. The ratio of knee osteoarthritis to hip osteoarthritis is 9:1 for Chinese individuals in Hong Kong,

3:1 for white individuals in the United States, and 1:2 for Swedish individuals. The racial differences in the axial alignment of the lower extremity may contribute to the variation in this ratio. The authors suspect that the larger knee-joint-obliquity angle in Chinese individuals may contribute to the higher ratio of knee osteoarthritis to hip osteoarthritis among Chinese adults.

One should be cautious in describing what is "normal" because of the substantial individual variations. Currently, designers of most total knee arthroplasty systems recommend placement of the components in such a way that the transverse axis of the artificial knee joint is perpendicular to the mechanical axes of the tibia and the femur. The resulting alignment of the lower extremity, therefore, is in close proximity to the alignment documented by Moreland et al. and Hsu et al. The mechanical axes of the femur and the tibia did not form a straight line in either Chinese males or females. This finding is in contrast to the general consensus that has been described previously.

And ultimately, the answer to this question: "Are in vivo normal knee kinematics influenced by ethnicity?" is, **YES**.

Author details

Hamid Reza Seyyed Hosseinzadeh[1*], Samih Tarabichi[2], Ali Sina Shahi[1], Mehrnoush Hassas Yeganeh[1], Usama Hassan Saleh[2], Gholam Reza Kazemian[1] and Aidin Masoudi[1]

*Address all correspondence to: hhosseinzadehmd@yahoo.com

1 Shahid Beheshti Unversity of Medical Sciences, Tehran, Iran

2 American Hospital, Dubai, United Arab Emirates

References

[1] Hofmann S, et al. Bone Cuts and Implant Positioning to Achieve High Flexion. Techniques in Knee Surgery, 2011; 10(2): 77-86.

[2] Bellemans J et al. Both Morphotype and Gender Influence the Shape of the Knee in Patients Undergoing TKA. Clin Orthop Relat Res (2010) 468:29–36

[3] Gillespie RJ, et al. Gender differences in the anatomy of the distal femur. J Bone Joint Surg Br. 201;93(3):357-63.

[4] Hovinga KR, et al. (2009). Anatomic variations between Japanese and Caucasian populations in the healthy young adult knee joint. J Orthop Res. 2009;27(9):1191-6.

[5] Iorio R, et al. Primary posterior cruciate-retaining total knee arthroplasty: a comparison of American and Japanese cohorts. J Surg Orthop Adv. 2007 Winter;16(4):164-70.

[6] Kamarul T, et al. Normal Anterior Cruciate ligament Laxity in the Malaysian Population. J Malaysian Orthopaedic. 2007; Vol 1: No 2.

[7] Tamari K, et al. Ethnic-, Gender-, and Age-Related Differences in Femorotibial Angle, Femoral Antetorsion, and Tibiofibular Torsion. Clinical Anatomy 19:59–67 (2006)

[8] Henry D, et al. Restoration of Femoral Anatomy in TKA With Unisex and Gender-specific Components. Clin Orthop Relat Res (2008) 466:2711–2716

[9] Hitt K, et al. Anthropometric Measurements of the Human Knee: Correlation to the Sizing of Current Knee Arthroplasty Systems. J Bone Joint Surg Am. 85-A; Supplement 4: 2003

[10] Conley S, et al. The Female Knee: Anatomic Variations. J Am Acad Orthop Surg 2007;15 (suppl 1):S31-S36

[11] Mahfouz M, et al. Three-dimensional morphology of the knee reveals ethnic differences. Clin Orthop Relat Res. 2012;470(1):172-85.

[12] Nelson AE, et al. Static knee alignment measurements among Caucasians and African-Americans: The Johnston County Osteoarthritis Project. J Rheumatol 2009;36(9): 1987–1990

[13] Yue B, et al. Gender differences in the knees of Chinese population. Knee Surg Sports Traumatol Arthrosc. 2011;19(1):80-8.

[14] Leszko F, et al. Comparison of in vivo patellofemoral kinematics for subjects having high-flexion total knee arthroplasty implant with patients having normal knees. J Arthroplasty. 2010;25(3):398-404.

[15] Espandar R, et al. Angular Deformities of the Lower Limb in Children. Asian Journal of Sports Medicine, 2010;Vol 1 (No 1): 46-53

[16] Sabharwal S, Zhao C. The Hip-Knee-Ankle Angle in Children: Reference Values Based on a Full-Length Standing Radiograph. J Bone Joint Surg Am. 2009;91:2461-8

[17] Tang WM, Zhu YH, Chiu KY. Axial alignment of the lower extremity in Chinese adults. J Bone Joint Surg Am. 2000; 82-A(11):1603-8.

[18] Saini UC, et al. Normal development of the knee angle in healthy Indian children: a clinical study of 215 children. J Child Orthop. 2010;4(6):579-86.

[19] Cheng N, Shi QY. Rehabilitation exercises after single total knee replacement: a report of 38 cases. Zhongguo Gu Shang. 2010; 23(3): 220-1.(Abstract)

[20] Arazi M, et al. Normal development of the tibiofemoral angle in children: a clinical study of 590 normal subjects from 3 to 17 years of age. J Pediatr Orthop. 2001; 21(2): 264-7.

[21] Heath CH, Staheli LT. Normal limits of knee angle in white children—genu varum and genu valgum. J Pediatr Orthop. 1993; 13(2): 259-62.

[22] Yoo JH, et al. Development of tibiofemoral angle in Korean children. J Korean Med Sci. 2008; 23(4): 714-7.

[23] Oginni LM, et al. Knee angles and rickets in nigerian children. J Pediatr Orthop. 2004; 24(4): 403-7.

[24] Moreland JR, et al. Radiographic analysis of the axial alignment of the lower extremity. J Bone Joint Surg Am. 1987; 69(5): 745-9.

[25] Hsu RW, et al. Normal axial alignment of the lower extremity and load-bearing distribution at the knee. Clin Orthop Relat Res. 1990; (255): 215-27.

[26] Fang Y, et al. The biomechanical study of rotating-arm self-locking intramedullary nails in comminuted femoral shaft fractures. Sheng Wu Yi Xue Gong Cheng Xue Za Zhi. 2006 Oct;23(5):1041-4.(Abstract)

[27] Mullaji AB, et al. Distal femoral rotational axes in Indian knees. J Orthop Surg (Hong Kong). 2009; 17(2): 166-9.

[28] Tang WM, et al. Sagittal bowing of the distal femur in Chinese patients who require total knee arthroplasty. J Orthop Res. 2005; 23(1): 41-5.

[29] Cheng FB, et al. Three dimensional morphometry of the knee to design the total knee arthroplasty for Chinese population. Knee. 2009; 16(5): 341-7..

[30] Yip DK, et al. Distal rotational alignment of the Chinese femur and its relevance in total knee arthroplasty. J Arthroplasty 2004; 19: 613.

[31] Tang Q, et al. The offset of the tibial shaft from the tibial plateau in Chinese people. J Bone Joint Surg Am. 2010. 18; 92(10): 1981-7.

[32] Hicks CA, et al. The anatomy of the tibial intramedullary canal. Clin Orthop Relat Res. 1995; 321: 111-16.

[33] Westrich GH, et al. Resection specimen analysis of proximal tibial anatomy based on 100 total knee arthroplasty specimens. J Arthroplasty. 1995; 10: 47-51.

[34] Wevers HW, et al. Improved fit by asymmetric tibial prosthesis for total knee arthroplasty. Med Eng Phys. 1994;16: 297-300.

[35] Abraham R, et al. An anatomical study of tibial metaphyseal/diaphyseal mismatch during revision total knee arthroplasty. J Arthroplasty. 2007 Feb; 22(2): 241-4.

[36] Yoo JH, et al. The relationship of the medially-offset stem of the tibial component to the medial tibial cortex in total knee replacements in Korean patients,. J Bone Joint Surg [Br] 2008; 90-B: 31-6

[37] Kapandji IA. The knee ligaments as determinants of trochleo-condylar profile. Med Biol Illus. 1967; 17(1): 26-32.(Abstract)

[38] Chiu KY, et al. Posterior slope of tibial plateau in Chinese. J Arthroplasty. 2000; 15(2): 224-7.

[39] Yue B, et al. Differences of Knee Anthropometry Between Chinese and White Men and Women. J Arthroplasty. 2011; Vol. 26: No. 1

[40] Harvey WF, et al. Knee alignment differences between Chinese and Caucasian subjects without osteoarthritis. Ann Rheum Dis. 2008; 67(11): 1524-8.

[41] Hosaka K, et al. Asian-Specific total knee system: 5-14 year follow-up study. Musculoskeletal Disorders 2011, 12:251

[42] Hashemi J, et al. The Geometry of the Tibial Plateau and Its Influence on the Biomechanics of the Tibiofemoral Joint. J Bone Joint Surg Am. 2008; 90-A: 12.

[43] Uehara K, et al. Anthropometry of the proximal tibia to design a total knee prosthesis for the Japanese population. J Arthroplasty. 2002; 17(8): 1028-32.

[44] Kwak DS, et al. Morphometry of the proximal tibia to design the tibial component of total knee arthroplasty for the Korean population. Knee. 2007; 14(4): 295-300.

[45] Chaichankul C, et al. Anthropometric measurements of knee joints in Thai population: correlation to the sizing of current knee prostheses. Knee. 2011; 18(1): 5-10.

[46] Vaidya SV,et al. Anthropometric measurements to design total knee prostheses for the Indian population. J Arthroplasty. 2000; 15(1): 79-85.

[47] Hosseinzadeh HR, et al. Measurment of Posterior Tibial Slope. Iranian Journal of Orthopaedic Surgery Vol 9, No 2, Spring 2010:121-5

[48] Hsu HC, et al. Influence of patellar thickness on patellar tracking and patellofemoral contact characteristics after total knee arthroplasty. J Arthroplasty. 1996; 11: 69–80.

[49] Baldwin JL, House CK. Anatomic dimensions of the patella measured during total knee arthroplasty. J Arthroplasty. 2005; 20: 250–257.

[50] Kim TK, et al. Clinical implications of anthropometric patellar dimensions for TKA in Asians. Clin Orthop Relat Res. 2009; 467(4): 1007-14.

[51] Koh JS, et al. Influence of patellar thickness on results of total knee arthroplasty: does a residual bony patellar thickness of 12 mm lead to poorer clinical outcome and increased complication rates? J Arthroplasty. 2002; 17: 56–61.

[52] Noble PC, et al. Does total knee replacement restore normal knee function? Clin Orthop Relat Res. 2005; 431: 157–165.

[53] Hemmerich A, et al. Hip, knee, and ankle kinematics of high range of motion activities of daily living, J Orthop Res. 2006; 24: 770–781.

[54] Freeman MA, Pinskerova V. The movement of the knee studied by magnetic resonance imaging. Clin Orthop Relat Res. 2003; 410: 35–43.

[55] Freeman MA, Pinskerova V. The movement of the normal tibiofemoral joint. J Biomech. 2005; 38: 197–208.

Chapter 4

Predictors of Pain and Function Following Total Joint Replacement

Michelle M. Dowsey and Peter F. M. Choong

Additional information is available at the end of the chapter

http://dx.doi.org/10.5772/53245

1. Introduction

Osteoarthritis (OA) is one of the most disabling diseases in developed countries and is responsible for significant disability in over 43 million people worldwide, 27 million of whom are 60 years of age or older [1]. Age is the strongest predictor of the development and progression of osteoarthritis, as such the number of people suffering with OA is expected to continue to increase over the coming years due to the ageing population [2]. Other predictors associated with OA include; gender, obesity, physical inactivity, smoking, excess alcohol and injuries [2].

Total joint replacement is the treatment of choice (among suitably 'fit' candidates) for end-stage OA [3]. It is a high-cost and high-volume procedure, which dominates surgical waiting lists and this is expected to become critical with the rapidly ageing population [4]. The number of hip and knee replacement being performed each year has risen markedly over the past decade in most OECD countries [2]. On average, the rate of hip replacement has increased by over 25% and the rate of knee replacement has nearly doubled. While joint replacement surgery is mainly carried out in people aged 60 and over, the rate of surgery is also increasing in younger people due to the increasing prevalence of obesity, advances in surgery and greater patient demand.

Many studies have confirmed the beneficial impact of TJR on pain, disability and quality of life [5, 6]. However, surgery is not without risk. In the immediate post-operative period, there is a small but important risk of severe complications [7-9] and in the longer term there is the risk of prosthesis failure, primarily through loosening, resulting in the need for complex revision surgery [10]. While the majority can expect improvements in pain and function in the intermediate period, there is a minority who remain dissatisfied after TJR and this is despite procedurally excellent outcomes. There are a number of risk factors for continuing pain and disability after surgery and given the increasing demand for TJR, understanding more about the determinants of good and bad outcomes has become an imperative.

This chapter provides an overview of baseline patient characteristics and predictors associated with pain and function following total joint replacement.

2. Incidence

The incidence of dissatisfaction or suboptimal outcome following total joint replacement varies in the literature. Quantifying the influence of a single patient factor on the functional and quality of life outcomes in joint replacement is a complex process. Variations in reporting may in part be due to the range of instruments used to measure patient centred outcomes and the lack of consensus and consistency amongst health professionals in how these tools are used [11-14]. Furthermore, to understand the complexities of what contributes to a suboptimal outcome, large data sets with samples representative of the total study population and extensive follow-up are essential, however this is a labour intensive and challenging process.

In 1998 our institution established a joint replacement registry to respond to this issue and to contribute to our understanding of what constitutes and predicts a good versus poor outcome following TJR. The St Vincent's Total Joint Replacement Registry (SVHM JRR) currently contains over 8000 procedures undertaken in over 7000 consecutive patients, and grows by approximately 800 procedures each year. Data include patient demographics, diagnoses, and type of surgery, prostheses, co-morbidities and peri-operative interventions, and an extensive range of outcomes including death, re-hospitalisation and complications. The registry includes marginalised and disadvantaged groups and is characterised by i) cultural and linguistic diversity (15% from a non-English speaking background representing over 20 languages); ii) 15% rural representation; and iii) socio-economic diversity (20% are ranked as living in the most "disadvantaged" socio-economic areas (Australian Bureau of Statistics [15]). Since 2006, we have obtained near complete (> 99%) 12 month follow-up of our cohort. Pain and functional outcomes as well as quality of life (QoL) are measured using validated surveys including; the Harris Hip Score [13, 16], the International Knee Society Score[17, 18] and Short Form Health Survey[12, 13, 19].

From our registry and that of the literature, dissatisfaction (variously measured) is as high as 50% among patients undergoing total joint replacement [20-25]. The level of dissatisfaction amongst recipients of hip and knee replacement is considerably different with a much higher rate of satisfaction reported amongst patients undergoing hip than knee replacement.

2.1. Pain

Chronic pain is a major global health care problem reported in 1 in 5 adults. The major causes of non-cancer chronic pain are; arthritis (40%) and surgery or injury (25%). For many, chronic pain substantially impairs daily physical activities, social activities and ability to enjoy life [26]. It carries a major economic burden with estimated costs running into billions in many OECD countries; US$635 billion in America [27], EUR$32 billion in Sweden [28] and AU$34 billion in Australia [29].

Chronic disabling pain is the primary indicator for recommending TJR in those with radiographic evidence of arthritis. For those that present with early disease, conservative treatment modalities including physical and pharmacological therapies are the first line of treatment [30, 31] however arthritis is a progressive disease and non-surgical modalities can effectively delay but not negate the need for eventual surgical intervention. Surgical interventions such as arthroscopy, bone marrow stimulation or osteotomy, may be recommended in carefully selected patients, however TJR remains the most effective and cost effective intervention for relieving pain and restoring function in suitably fit patients [32, 33]

Total joint replacement is a major surgical procedure that requires multidisciplinary input prior to and after surgery to ensure the best possible outcome. Recovery from surgery is optimized with the inclusion of rehabilitation programs which are tailored to restore mobility and independence [34]. Time to recovery can vary following TJR and most patients will report substantial gains between 3 to 6 months after surgery. Patients undergoing THR report faster recovery in terms of both pain and function, with significant improvements occurring within the first 3 months of surgery [35]. In comparison patients undergoing TKR are more likely to report improvement between 3 to 6 months [36, 37]. Overall a continuing pattern of improvement can be observed up to 12 months following surgery [5, 38].

While on average a majority of patients report an improvement in pain following total joint replacement [39, 40] for a substantial number of individuals the level of improvement is sub-optimal or does not meet expectation at 12 months or more after surgery. In total knee replacement ongoing pain has been reported in as many as 53% of patients and for hip replacement the incidence is as high as 38% (Table 1).

The causes of ongoing pain following TJR are not clearly understood. Recent literature reports a high prevalence of features of pain sensitisation in knee OA patients. Wylde et al (2011) identified 70% of patients as having various somatosensory abnormalities in a study of 117 knee OA patients [44]. Hochman et al (2011) reported neuropathic symptoms in 28% of older adults with chronic symptomatic knee OA [52]. Ohtori et al (2012) reported similar findings with neuropathic symptoms in as many as 20.6% of patients with radiographically confirmed knee OA [53]. These mechanisms of pain are not necessarily addressed by undergoing joint replacement.

Recent trials of the use of second-generation antiepileptic drugs (AED's), which are commonly used to treat neuropathic pain however, report mixed results in TJR studies. Both Gabapentin and Pregalbin use are associated with a reduction in post-operative opioid consumption following knee replacement [54, 55]. A randomized controlled trial comparing pre-operative Pregalbin to placebo has also reported a significant reduction in neuropathic pain at 6 months post TKR [54]. In contrast, Gabapentin had no effect on post-operative opioid consumption or pain scores at 6 months following total hip replacement [56]. While pre-operative Pregalbin has shown to reduce post-operative opioid consumption following THR, the longer term effects on post surgery pain have not been reported.

Overall higher rates of persistent pain are reported after knee replacement as compared to hip replacement (Table 1). Features of pain sensitisation and neuropathic type symptoms are also predominately reported in knee OA patients. This may explain the differences in response to AED's between hip and knee replacement recipients and is an indication that the underlying mechanisms of persistent pain following surgery differ according to the surgical site.

Author	Cohort	Follow-up	Pain Measure	Incidence of Ongoing Pain
Liu et al 2012 [41]	TJR = 1030	Minimum 1 year 32% response rate	McGill Pain Questionnaire [42]	Persistent pain THR = 38.0% TKR = 53.0%
Dowsey et al 2012 [40]	TKR = 478	99.4% at 1 year 93.5% at 2 years	IKSS [43] pain	Moderate to severe pain 29.5% at 12 months 30.6% at 2 years
Wylde et al 2011 [44]	THR = 909 TKR = 860	3 to 4 years 73.0% hip and knee	WOMAC [45] pain	Persistent pain THR = 27.0% TKR = 44.0%
Singh & Lewallen 2010 [46]	THR = 9,154 (2yrs) 6,243 (5yrs)	62.3% at 2 years 52.7 at 5 years	Mayo [47] Hip Score	Moderate to severe pain 8.1% at 2 years 10.6% at 5 years
Czurda et al 2010 [5, 48]	TKR = 411	18 to 42 months 80.3%	WOMAC [45] pain	Knee pain 13.9%
Wylde et al 2009 [49]	THR = 1,534 TKR = 857	5 to 8 years 72.5% hip 71.5% knee	Oxford [50] pain	Moderate to severe pain THR = 13.0% TKR = 26.0%
Baker et al 2007 [51]	TKR = 9417	87.4% at 1 year	Oxford [50] pain	Persistent pain 19.8% at 1 year

(IKSS – International Knee Society Score, WOMAC – Western Ontario and McMaster Universities Arthritis Index)

Table 1. Incidence of self reported pain > 12 months following TJR

2.2. Function

While arthritis accounts for 40% of non-cancer chronic pain it is the leading cause of disability in most developed countries. [57-59]. For many sufferers of arthritis even the most basic daily activities such as dressing, walking and stair climbing are substantially restricted. Pain and deformity associated with the progression of arthritis are the main contributors to impeding function and activity. As such joint replacement surgery that results in amelioration of pain and correction of deformity should lead to improved function and activity participation. However poor function and difficulty with daily activities have been reported up to 51% of TJR recipients, (Table 2).

A decrease in activity participation outside those required for basic daily functioning has also been noted in a proportion of patients who have undergone TJR. Wylde et.al interviewed 56 hip and 60 knee replacement patients about their leisure activities [60]. They reported that THR patients participated in 209 leisure activities but rated 82% of these activities as difficult to perform prior to surgery and TKR patients participated in 171 leisure activities 86% of which were rated as difficult to perform prior to surgery due to joint problems. At 1 year post surgery THR patients still rated 25% of leisure activities as difficult to perform and TKR patients rate 32% of leisure activities difficult to perform. In a larger study Groen et.al measured adherence to an activity regimen recommended to maintain health in patients who underwent total knee replacement and found that 42% of patients were not active enough to maintain their health and fitness [61].

Author	Cohort	Follow-up	Functional Measure	Incidence of Functional Impairment
Dowsey et al 2012 [40]	TKR = 478	99.4% at 1 year 93.5% at 2 years	IKSS [43] function	Poor function 48.9% at 12 months 50.7% at 2 years
Wylde et al 2009 [49]	THR = 1,534 TKR = 857	5 to 8 years 72.5% hip 71.5% knee	Oxford [50] function	Extreme difficulty with individual activities THR = 5% to 17% TKR = 7% to 24%
Franklin et al 2008 [175]	TKJR = 17270	46.6% at 1 year	SF12 PCS [12] function	Function score worse than baseline = 19.0%
Lubbeke et al 2007 [62]	THR = 435	4 to 6 years 80.2%	HHS [16] function	Fair or poor function 9.0%
Nilsdotter et al 2003 [25]	THR = 211	26 to 65 months 94%	OARSI Criteria [63]	No improvement in function = 8.7%
Singh & Lewallen 2010 [64]	THR = 9,154 (2yrs) 6,243 (5yrs)	62.3% at 2 years 52.7% at 5 years	Mayo [47] Hip Score	Moderate to severe activity limitation 30% at 2 years 35% at 5 years
Singh et al (2010) [126]	TKR = 10,957 (2 yrs) 7,404 (5yrs)	65.0% at 2 years 57.0% at 5 years	IKSS [43] function	Moderate to severe activity limitation 20.7% at 2 years 27.1% at 5 years

(SF-12 PCS – Short Form 12 Physical Component Summary, HHS – Harris Hip Score, OARSI – Osteoarthritis Research Society International

Table 2. Incidence of self reported functional impairment > 12 months following TJR

As function and activity levels depends on all other joints and systems, not just the joint being replaced, improvements may not be achieved as a result of joint replacement alone in patients who have multiple joint arthropathy or systemic health issues. Functional outcomes also seem to be dependent on the site of joint replacement (Table 2). Consistent with pain outcomes, a higher proportion of patients undergoing TKR report poor function or difficulty with activities than do patients undergoing THR. Demographic and patient characteristics are of predictive value in determining barriers to functional gain and activity participation following TJR recipients.

3. Predictors of pain and function

Intuitively, those who present with the "worst" symptoms might be those who should be prioritized for TJR. However, the literature reports a mismatch between patient reported symptom severity and response to surgery and it is becoming clearer that TJR outcomes are influenced by a multitude of factors. Recent work has identified a number of baseline risk factors for continuing pain and disability after TJR and these can be stratified into those which are modifiable and non-modifiable. Non-modifiable risk factors include; age, gender, socio-economic status, aetiology and culture and ethnicity. Modifiable risk factors include; psychological state, co-morbidities, obesity, baseline symptom severity and patient expectation.

Importantly, our work to date has demonstrated that a majority of baseline patient characteristics (obesity, mental health, co-morbidities, radiographic OA severity, baseline pain and function) associated with sub-optimal outcome following TJR are those that could be "modified" with appropriate intervention [8, 39, 40, 65]; hence there is opportunity to alter patient outcomes. Appreciating the nature of patient pre-operative risk factors and the impact of different outcomes is critical for improving response rates to surgery.

3.1. Patient demographics

3.1.1. Age

As age is the strongest predictor of the development and progression of osteoarthritis the ageing population has no doubt contributed to the world wide increase in TJR numbers. However, TJR in younger patients is also on the rise particularly for knee replacement [66], and this is likely due in part to the rising incidence of obesity in patients presenting for surgery [8, 39]. The median age at presentation for joint replacement demonstrates a downward trend over the past 10 years at our institution (Figure 1)

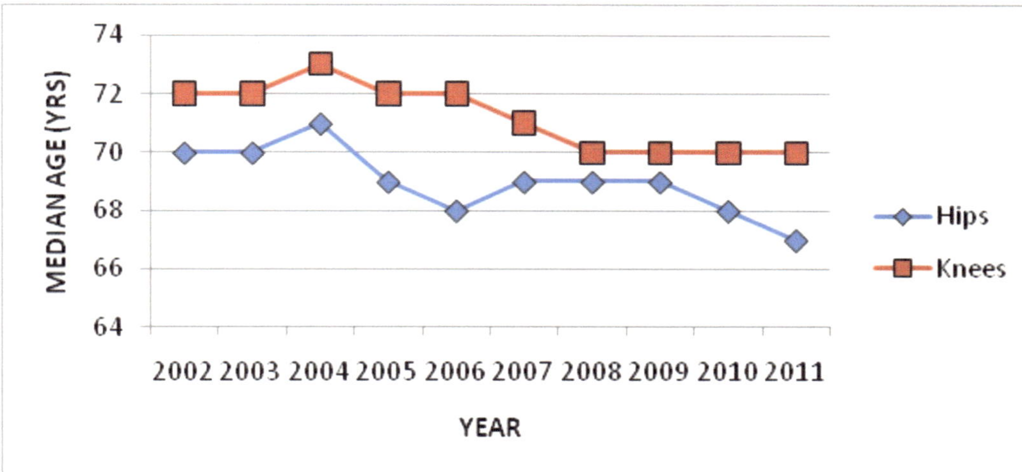

Figure 1. Median age at presentation for primary elective TJR (SVHM JRR)

Total joint replacement in the elderly carries a higher risk of peri-operative complication, requires a longer recovery time and is associated with a significant mortality rate in the longer term [67, 68]. However advancing age is not a barrier to pain and functional improvements after TJR surgery [67, 68] and excellent pain relief has been reported in individuals in their 80's and 90's [69-71]. While advancing age is associated with poorer function and activity levels following TJR [40] higher satisfaction with activity levels have been reported in those older than 70 years when compared to their younger counterparts [72].

3.1.2. Gender

Worldwide more females than males undergo joint replacement each year, with the greatest difference being for knee replacement. Various National Joint Replacement Registries report the ratio of females to males undergoing knee replacement as high as 2:1 and this concurs with gender patterns at our institution (Figure 2), [73-76]. Despite these figures inequities in referral patterns and reluctance in women to undergo joint replacement, resulting in late presentation have been reported [77, 78]. A gender bias in physician referral for knee replacement was identified in one study, with family physicians twice as likely and orthopaedic surgeons 22 times more likely to recommend knee replacement to male patients [79]. However it has also been identified that women delay seeking joint replacement until a later point in their functional decline [77].

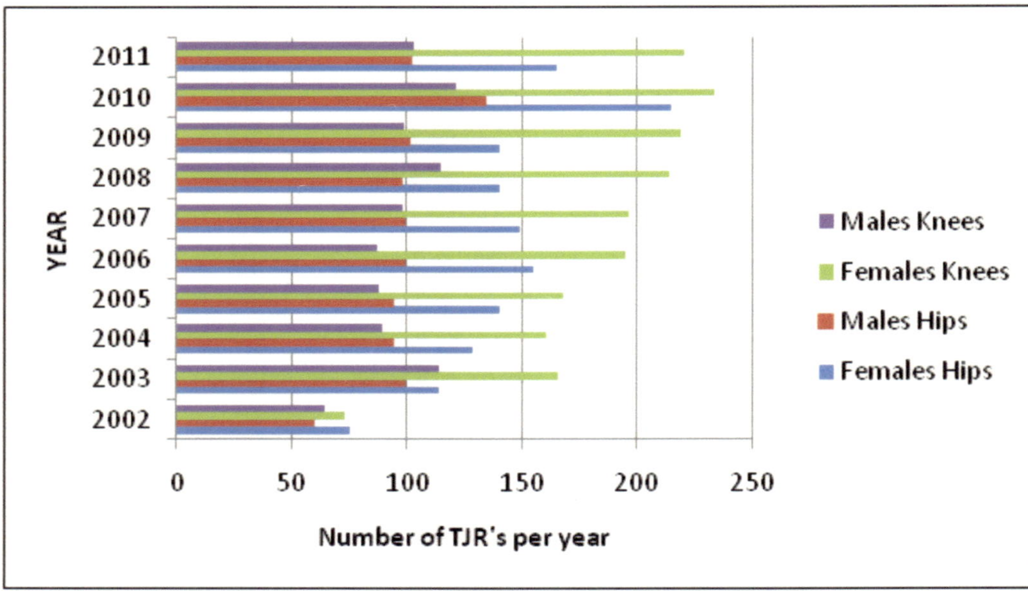

Figure 2. Gender breakdowns at presentation for primary elective TJR (SVHM JRR)

Females generally present with worse self-reported pain and functional impairment compared to males at the time hip and knee replacement [80-83], as such females do not tend to achieve the same level of physical function after surgery as males [84, 85]. However when taking into account baseline pain and function, women generally demonstrate greater improvements in pain and function scores after surgery than men [84-86]. Faster recoveries in terms of pain and function have also been reported in females undergoing total knee replacement when compared to males [87]. Despite this a significantly higher odds of poor function at 12 months (OR 1.81; 95% CI 1.08-3.03) and 2 years (OR 2.06; 95% CI 1.20 – 3.53) post knee replacement have been reported by women undergoing TKJR [40]. Impairment with specific activities such as stair climbing, despite achieving greater improvements in knee flexion, have also been reported in females compared to males [86]. These data suggest women may benefit from tailored rehabilitation programs following joint replacement surgery.

3.1.3. Socio-economic status

Differences among nations in their socio-economic fabric, ethnic composition, health care systems and cultural expectations, may confound studies examining the importance of socioeconomic status as a predictor of outcome following TJR. Variations in classifications of socio-economic status also require that caution should be exercised in making direct comparisons between studies. To date studies have largely focused on socio-economic status in patients undergoing total hip replacement, with most data derived from cohorts in Western countries.

A large UK study by Jenkins et.al (2009) reported significant differences in SF-36 physical improvement between the least and most "deprived groups" 18 months post THR [88]. A study based in Scotland by Clement et.al (2011) reported similar findings. In a cohort of 1312 patients who underwent primary THR a significant improvement in Oxford scores across all socioeconomic categories was noted, however social deprivation predicted a poorer functional outcome [89]. In a smaller study based in the US, Allen-Butler et.al (2011) conducted a secondary analysis of a prospective randomised study originally comparing 2 different hip stems. They also concluded that individual socioeconomic parameters such as education level, household income, as well as being African American were associated with lower Harris Hips Scores up to 2 years post THR [90]. Finally a German based study by Schafer et.al (2010) also concluded that socioeconomic parameters independently predicted response to THR as measured using the WOMAC [91]. An increased risk for "non-response" to surgery at 6 months was demonstrated in widowed patients, those who lived alone, those on a disability pension and those who had a shorter duration of school education.

Only one study reported outcomes according to socioeconomic status in patients undergoing total knee replacement. In a multicentre study conducted in several countries (USA, UK, AU, Canada) socio-economic status did not appear to affect the outcome of knee replacement [92]. Socioeconomic data were derived from a pre-operative questionnaire regarding education, income, working status and living arrangements, to allow for direct comparison between countries. Despite reporting a correlation between lower income and worse pre-operative pain and function, there were no differences in post-operative pain and function at 24 months.

Despite variations in definitions and study designs, patient reported outcomes following THR are consistently poorer for disadvantaged groups. In contrast there is a dearth of literature on TKR with only one study that reported no differences in patient reported outcomes. Poorer outcomes in socioeconomically disadvantaged groups may occur as a result underutilization of health services [93] and this has important implications in relation to preparing disadvantaged patients for joint replacement surgery.

3.1.4. Culture and ethnicity

Racial and ethnic TJR utilization disparities exist and are likely due to a lower willingness to undergo surgery amongst ethnic minorities rather than lower disease prevalence [78, 94, 95]. Poor health literacy, financial constraints, cultural influences and concerns about possible outcomes are amongst reported reasons for a lower willingness to undergo surgery and delayed presentation [96-100]. As such self-reported baseline pain and function are worse amongst ethnic minorities presenting for total joint replacement surgery [100-103].

Substantial improvements in pain and function have been reported following primary total joint replacement irrespective of race and ethnicity however ethnic minorities do report worse outcomes following both hip and knee replacement surgery. Lavernia et al (2011) studied patient reported outcomes in a large cohort of hip and knee replacements (739 hips and 1010 knees) and found that ethnic minorities had worse pain, function and well-being scores 2 years after surgery compared to Whites and worse outcomes was most pronounced for African Americans [103]. Kamath et al (2010) reported similar findings for African-Americans undergoing TKJR [100]. In an Australian study of 237 TKR's, 41 were non-English speaking patients, Dowsey et al (2009) reported poorer International Knee Society pain and function scores at 12 months after surgery in those who required Interpreters compared to their English speaking counterparts[104]. A Swedish study analysed 1216 patients' pre and 1 year after THR, comparing those who were born inside and outside the country. Krupic et al (2012) reported lower self care and activity scores and more pain amongst those born abroad [102].

Promoting greater dialogue with health care providers and understanding the health literacy needs of ethnic minorities may help to address willingness to undergo joint replacement surgery and lead to better patient reported outcomes [105, 106].

3.2. Patient characteristics

3.2.1. Aetiology

Osteoarthritis is the principle diagnosis for a majority of total joint replacements performed each year [73-76]. In Australia it accounted for 88% of primary elective total hip replacement and 97% of primary elective knee replacement in 2010 [73]. The remaining diagnoses for elective THR included avascular necrosis (3.7%), dysplasia (1.3%) and rheumatoid arthritis (1.3%) and for TKR; rheumatoid arthritis (1.7%), inflammatory arthritis (0.5%) and necrosis (0.4%) [73].

Despite the worldwide increase in TJR numbers in recent years, the rate of joint replacement surgery in patients with rheumatoid arthritis has remained relatively stable and for some countries a decrease in numbers has been noted [107-110]. Contemporary treatment of rheumatoid arthritis now includes disease modifying medications or biologics, anti-tumour necrosis factor drugs and corticosteroids are proving to be more effective in the management of this immune disease when taken in combination as opposed to mono-therapy [111]. Despite advances in conservative management of rheumatoid arthritis, joint replacement remains a viable treatment option for those with significant joint pain and stiffness although joint destruction, osteoporosis and severe deformity make surgery technically challenging in this group [110]. Nevertheless rheumatoid patients demonstrate substantial improvements in pain, function and quality of life following TJR [112-115]. Although functional outcomes after surgery are inferior, rheumatoid patients report equivalent pain relief from TJR when compared to OA patients[110].

Aside from rheumatoid arthritis total hip replacement in young adults is generally reserved for those with developmental dysplasia (DDH) and slipped upper femoral epiphysis (SUFE). Anatomical abnormalities including acetabular or femoral deformity, leg length discrepancy and the age at which joint replacement is performed can contribute to higher failure rates observed in these patient compared to patients with osteoarthritis [73, 116, 117]. Setting aside the higher likelihood of revision surgery for patients who have hip replacement for DDH or SUFE in the longer term, post-operative outcome scores for these patients are comparable to patients with OA in the short term. No significant differences in Oxford hips scores at 6 months have been observed in THR patients with either DDH or SUFE when compared OA patients [118, 119]. Excellent functional outcomes have also been reported in patients with DDH under the age of 30 years with an average Harris Hips score of 90.6 at 9 [3-14] years follow-up [117]. Similar Harris Hip Scores (average 93) have been reported in THR for SUFE at 15 years follow-up [120].

3.2.2. Co-morbidities

Individual comorbidities such as diabetes, cardiovascular and respiratory disease are commonly reported in patients undergoing TJR and many patients carry multiple comorbidities [7, 8, 39, 40, 121]. When reported as a composite, self-reported functional outcomes are poorer in patients with multiple comorbidities for both hip and knee replacement. Lingard et al (2004) reported an association with higher comorbidity and poorer SF-36 physical function scores at 1 year after knee replacement [122] and Gandhi et al (2010) reported similar findings at 3 [1–8] years [123]. In total hip replacement Young et al (2008) reported better functional outcomes following hip replacement in those had no comorbid disease [124].

Deyo-Charlson comorbidity index, a validated clinical comorbidity index [125] is an independent predictor of functional outcome in TJR. Singh & Lewallen (2010) studied activity limitation and dependence on walking aids in both hip and knee replacement patients 2 and 5 years after surgery. Deyo-Charlson comorbidity index independently predicted a greater reliance on walking aids at 2 and 5 years after both total hip and knee replacement and higher odds of moderate to severe activity limitation at 2 years after knee replacement [64, 126]. We have reported similar findings in patients undergoing TKR using an Age-Adjusted Charlson Comorbidity Index [127], demonstrating higher odds of reporting poor function at 2 years in those with a higher comorbidity index [40].

Very little is known about the effect of individual comorbidities on patient reported outcomes in TJR. A recent study of 677 consecutive primary knee and 547 consecutive primary hip replacements, demonstrated an association between metabolic syndrome risk factor and 1 year WOMAC scores [128]. Metabolic syndrome risk factors were self-reported and defined as body mass index >30kg/m^2, hypercholesterolemia, hypertension and diabetes. While increasing number of metabolic risk factors were associated with higher (worse) WOMAC scores, individual risk factors were found to better predict outcome. Obesity predicted higher WOMAC scores in both total hip and total knee replacement and hypertension also predicted higher WOMAC scores in total hip replacement only.

3.2.3. Obesity

Obesity features prominently in the patho-physiological mechanisms underpinning OA especially end-stage OA requiring TJR [129]. Obesity affects 1 in 4 members of the community, but our data indicate a 2-3 fold over-representation of obesity in patients presenting for TJR (Figure 3). The economic impact of obesity-related OA in Australia was estimated to be $221.3 million in 2005 [130]. While the real costs of treating obese patients with TJR remain unknown, we have demonstrated higher episode of care costs for TKR in the first 12 months

(+$1,821[95% CI $245, $3,398]; p=0.024) in a comparative cohort of 520 patients [131]. The cost of THR is also estimated to be higher for obese ($523) and morbidly obese patients, ($1,432) patients [132]. In addition to the increasing overrepresentation of obese patients presenting for TJR (Figure 3) our data demonstrates that the severity of obesity is also increasing over time (Figure 4), as such developing strategies to reduce the burden of obesity-related joint disease should be an imperative [133].

Weight loss in obese patients awaiting TJR is a problem because the symptoms of disabling arthritis may limit an individual's ability to exercise. Patients often identify this as the reason for the inability to lose weight, and believe that joint replacement would be critical for weight loss. However, numerous studies have confirmed that undergoing total joint replacement does not result in clinically significant weight loss and as many as one-third of patients gain weight at 12 months after surgery [8, 39, 134-140]. It has also been demonstrated that weight gain continues to increase over time after joint replacement [141].

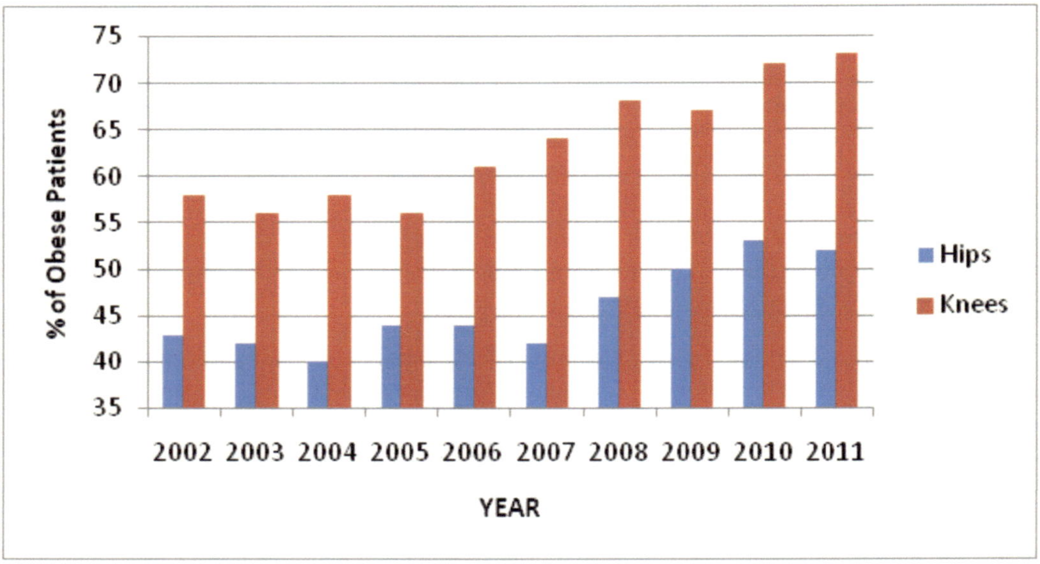

Figure 3. Obesity rates in OA patients at presentation for primary elective TJR (SVHM JRR)

Data from our registry demonstrates that both the number of obese patients presenting for joint replacement (Figure 3) and the average BMI of patients is increasing over time, particularly in the past 5 years. Of note there are higher rates of obesity and a more rapid rise in average BMI demonstrated amongst recipients of knee replacement compared to recipients of hip replacement, with females undergoing knee replacement recording the highest BMI average.

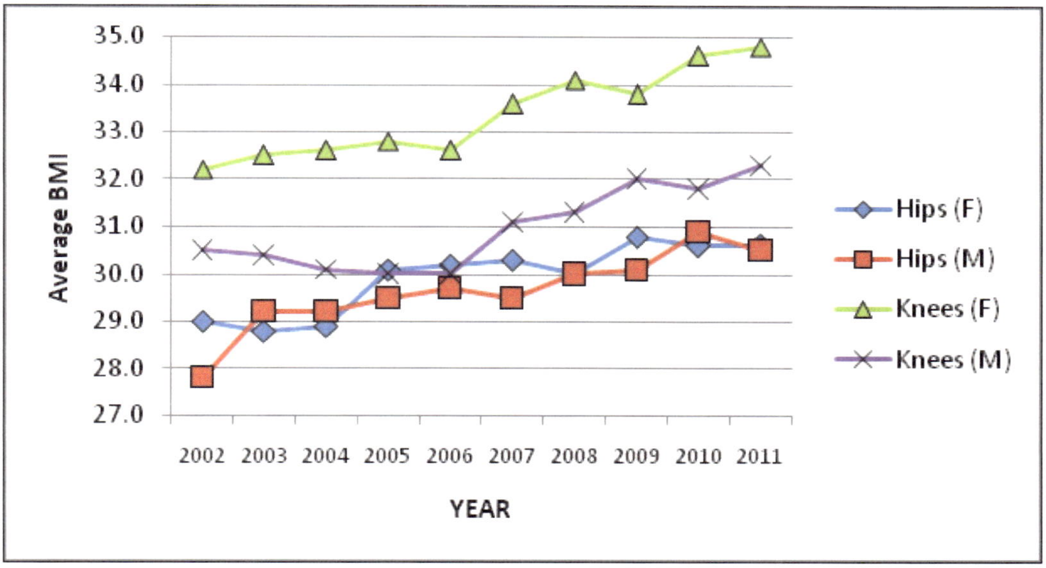

Figure 4. Mean BMI of OA patients at presentation for primary elective TJR (SVHM JRR)

Although widely reported there remains disagreement in the literature as to the impact of obesity on patient reported outcomes following TJR. Numerous reviews confirm that obese patients report substantial improvements in pain and function following joint replacement surgery [142-145]. However when limited to level 1 studies [146], the evidence does suggests that obese and particularly morbidly obese patients may not achieve the same level of functional improvement after TJR when compared to non-obese patients in both the short and longer term.

3.2.3.1. Outcomes for primary THR

Obesity and advancing BMI have been shown to have a negative impact on pain and more so function after primary elective total hip replacement in both the short and longer term. Functional gains and activity levels after THR remain poorer for obese when compared to non-obese individuals. Obese groups also report worse pain and higher usage of pain medication after THR. A review of level 1 large cohort studies is presented.

Moran et al (2005) compared functional and QoL outcomes using the Harris Hip Score (HHS) and Short-Form-36 (SF-36) in 800 patients undergoing total hip replacement, pre surgery (100% follow-up) and at 6 (97% follow-up) and 18 months (86% follow-up) [147]. BMI was found to be a significant predictor of poorer function at both 6 and 18 months. The authors concluded that the difference between obese and non-obese scores were small and therefore not clinically significant, however this was based on comparing post-operative scores only and the change in scores between groups was not provided.

Gandhi et al (2010) investigated the influence of self-reported metabolic syndrome risk factors defined as obesity, hypertension, hypercholesterolemia and diabetes on patient function in a consecutive cohort of 547 primary hip replacements [128]. As measured using the WOMAC obesity was associated with higher odds (2.4; 95% CI 1.4 – 4.2) of less functional improvement at 12 months after surgery.

Dowsey et al (2010) compared pain, function (HHS) and quality of life (SF-12) in a consecutive cohort of 471 primary THR's with 98.5% follow-up. Function and physical health scores were worse at baseline and 12 months after surgery for obese and morbidly obese patients. Baseline mental health scores were also worse in obese and morbidly obese patients, however were comparable at 12 months with obese patients demonstrating a significantly greater improvement in scores compared to non-obese patients [39].

Lubbeke et.al (2007) reported significantly poorer functional outcomes in obese patients (n=182), who underwent primary THR compared to non-obese patients (n=635), at 5 years follow-up, as measured using the Harris Hip Score [148]. Eighty-one percent of hips in the non obese group and 70% in the obese group had a good to excellent results according to their HHS. When broken down by gender it was obese females who demonstrated significantly poorer outcomes compared to non-obese females with very little differences in outcomes demonstrated between obese and non obese males.

Singh & Lewallen (2010) measured activity limitation and dependence on walking aids in 5,707 patients at 2 years and 3,289 patients at 5 years after primary total hip replacement [64]. Predictors of moderate to severe activity limitation (defined as limitation in 3 or more activities), included BMI > 30kg/m^2 at both time intervals. Obese (BMI > 30kg/m^2) patients had higher odds of complete dependence on a walking aid at 2 years and severely obese (BMI >35kg/m^2) had a higher odds of complete dependence on a waking aid at 5 years.

Singh & Lewallen (2010) also examined pain as measured by the Mayo Hip Score and the use of pain medications at 2 and 5 years following primary total hip replacement in the same cohort of patients [46]. The odds of reporting ongoing moderate to severe pain at 2 years after surgery were higher in those with a BMI 35-39.9kg/m^2 (OR 1.8; 95% CI 1.2 – 2.4) and BMI > 40kg/m^2 (1.7; 95% CI 1.0 – 2.9) compared to those with a BMI < 25kg/m^2. At 5 years the odds of reporting ongoing moderate to severe pain was higher for all weight groups compared to the baseline group; BMI 25 – 29.9kg/m^2, (OR 1.5; 95% CI 1.1 – 2.1); BMI 30-34.9kg/m^2, (OR 1.8; 95% CI 1.2 – 2.6); BMI 35-39.9kg/m^2, (OR 1.9; 95% CI 1.2 – 3.1); and BMI > 40kg/m^2, (OR 3.1 95% CI 1.7 – 5.7). BMI 35-39kg/m^2 was also a predictor of non-steroidal anti-inflammatory use at 2 years and BMI 30-34.9kg/m^2 predicted use of opioid medication at 5 years after THR.

3.2.3.2. Outcomes for primary TKR

Obesity and advancing BMI have been shown to have a negative impact on function after primary elective total knee replacement in both the short and longer term. Functional gains and activity levels after TKR are poorer for obese when compared to non-obese individuals.

Obese groups however do report comparable pain outcomes compared to non-obese patients after surgery. A review of level 1 large cohort studies is presented.

Gandhi et al (2010) investigated the influence of self-reported metabolic syndrome risk factors defined as obesity, hypertension, hypercholesterolemia and diabetes on patient function in a consecutive cohort of 677 primary knee replacements with 83% follow-up [128]. As measured using the WOMAC, obesity (BMI > 30kg/m^2) was associated with higher odds (3.6; 95% CI 0.02 – 7.2) of less functional improvement at 12 months after surgery.

Rajgopal et al (2008) compared functional outcomes between morbidly obese (BMI > 40kg/m^2) and non-morbidly obese (BMI < 40kg/m^2) patients 12 months after total knee replacement in a series of 550 patients; of which 69 patients were classified as morbidly obese [149]. BMI ≥ 40 predicted 12 month WOMAC scores (coefficient −5.188, 95% CI −9.771 −0.606), however no differences in the change in WOMAC or SF-12 scores were demonstrated when comparing morbidly obese to non-morbidly obese patients.

We also measured improvement in pain, function and quality of life from baseline to 12 months following elective primary knee replacement in consecutive series of 529 patients with 98% follow-up [8]. The change in IKSS function scores were 10 points lower for both obese (BMI > 30kg/m^2) and morbidly obese (BMI > 40kg/m2) patients compared to non-obese (BMI <30kg/m^2), (p=0.002). No significant difference in IKSS pain scores was noted between the 3 groups at baseline or 12 months and there was no significant difference in SF-12 scores between the 3 groups at baseline or 12 months.

Singh et al (2010) measured activity limitation in 4,701 patients at 2 years and 2,395 patients at 5 years after primary knee replacement [126]. Predictors of moderate to severe activity limitation (defined as limitation in 3 or more activities), included all BMI groups > 30 compared to BMI < 25kg/m^2 at 2 years after surgery; BMI 30-34.9kg/m^2, (OR 1.5; 95% CI 1.0 – 2.0); BMI 35-39.9kg/m^2, (OR 1.8; 95% CI 1.3 – 2.7); and BMI > 40kg/m^2, (OR 3.0 95% CI 2.0 – 4.5). Higher BMI also predicted moderate to severe activity limitation at 5 years; BMI 35-39.9kg/m^2, (OR 2.1; 95% CI 1.4 – 3.3); and BMI > 40kg/m^2, (OR 3.9 95% CI, 2.3 – 6.5).

Sing et al (2011) also examined whether BMI was associated with pain as measured using the IKSS after primary knee replacement at 2 and 5 years after surgery [150]. Patients were classified into BMI groups as above for comparison. In contrast to their study on activity limitation, there was no association demonstrated between BMI and ongoing moderate to severe pain at either 2 or 5 years after TKR.

Our findings mirror that of Singh et al (2010 & 2011). We reported pain and function outcomes in a cohort of 478 consecutive primary elective total knee replacements at 1 and 2 years post surgery with 99% and 94% follow-up respectively [40]. Each incremental increase in BMI significantly increased the odds of poor function as measured using the IKSS at 12 months (OR 1.07, 95% CI 1.03 – 1.12) and at 2 years (OR 1.09, 95% CI 1.05 – 1.14). However we found no association between advancing BMI and ongoing moderate to severe pain at either time point.

3.2.4. *Psychosocial state*

Psychological distress leading to patient dissatisfaction after TJR is an important cause for TJR failure. Pre-operative psychological distress is associated with excessive analgesic intake and higher rates of hospital readmission and long term mortality [151]. Our research has also drawn a link between poorer pre-operative mental health and weight gain after TJR [39]. Published results from the SVHM TJR cohort and that of others have i) identified a high rate (30-60%) of self-reported psychological distress in TJR patients [152-154] and ii) determined that pre-operative psychological distress is an independent risk factor for poorer post-operative outcomes after surgery [8, 65]. A number of recent comprehensive literature reviews have found pre-operative psychological distress to be an independent predictor of pain and function after TKR in a majority of published studies [155, 156].

Psychological co-morbidities and traits reported in TJR patients include; anxiety, depression, neuroticism, catastrophising and poor self-esteem. These individual traits and poorer pre-operative mental health scores in general are associated with poorer function and/or greater pain after TJR in the short and longer term.

In general pre-operative psychological distress is associated with poorer pain and worst function 1 year after total joint replacement. We have reported an association between lower SF-12 MCS scores and risk for ongoing moderate to severe pain and poor function at 12 months and 2 years following TKR. Lingard et al (2004) also reported an association between lower SF-36 MCS scores and worse WOMAC pains scores at 1 and 2 years after TKR [122]. An analysis of pre-operative and one-year post-operative data in 6,158 patients from the Swedish Hip Arthroplasty Register, also demonstrated that anxiety/depression measured on the EQ-5D [157] was a strong predictor of pain after THR [158].

Anxiety is a psychological and physiological state characterized by somatic, emotional, cognitive, and behavioural components [159]. Anxiety can occur as a result of transient negative stimuli such as in a threatening situation and this is referred to as state anxiety. In contrast trait anxiety is referred to as a general tendency to experience anxiety [160]. In patients undergoing total hip replacement trait anxiety has shown to correlate with impaired health related quality of life 3 to 6 months after surgery [161, 162]. In contrast state anxiety had no effect on outcome suggesting pre-existing anxiety disorder rather than anxiety induced by fear of surgery predicts poorer outcomes form joint replacement.

Pre-existing depression has been shown to predict greater pain and poorer function in patients undergoing total knee replacement at 1 year and it has also been demonstrated that worse outcomes persist at 5 years [20, 163]. However this finding is not consistent, with some studies suggesting that there is no association between depression measured prior to surgery and pain and function outcomes following TJR. Of note Riddles et al (2010) measured the association between a range of psychological comorbidities including depression, anxiety and panic disorders, self efficacy and fear of movement and found that only pain catastrophising predicted poorer pain outcomes after total knee replacement [164],

Pain catastrophising has been described as a tendency to magnify or exaggerate the threat value or seriousness of pain sensations [165]. Pre-operative pain catastrophising is a predictor of worse post-surgical pain following TKR in the short (6 weeks and 6 months) term, but does not correlate with function [164, 166]. The correlation between catastrophising and poorer post-operative pain has also been shown to persist at 24 months following TKR [167]. To date the link between pain catastrophising and post operative pain after TJR seems to be unique to knee replacement, with no evidence of pain catastrophising in total hip replacement patients.

Neuroticism is a personality trait described as an enduring tendency to experience negative emotional states [168]. There is a dearth of literature examining the association between neuroticism and TJR, however one study on total hip replacement did report that neuroticism was amongst a number of psychological traits that predicted poorer quality of life outcomes at 6 months after surgery [162].

3.3. Baseline symptom severity

Total joint replacement is most often performed for the management of "end-stage' arthritis characterised by retractable pain, loss of function and deformity [30]. According to the NIH statements for both hip and knee replacement, candidates for elective TJR should have radiographic evidence of joint damage, moderate-to-severe persistent pain that is not adequately relieved by an extended course of nonsurgical management, and clinically significant functional limitation resulting in diminished quality of life [32, 33]. However there is discordance between radiographic changes and patient reported symptom severity at presentation for surgery, with some people receiving joint replacement reporting severe preoperative symptoms of pain and disability and mild radiographic changes [80, 83].

3.3.1. Baseline clinical symptoms

Baseline symptom severity is a predictor of outcome for both total hip and knee replacement. Several studies have concluded that those with worse pain and poor function at the time of surgery also report comparatively worse pain and function after surgery, suggesting that surgery could be prioritized based on clinical symptom severity [169].

In a multicentre study involving more than 200 hip and knee replacements Fortin et al (1999] reported that lower preoperative physical function scores predicted worse WOMAC pain and function at 6 months compared to those with higher baseline function scores [170]. Fortin et al (2002) continued to follow the cohort up at 2 years post surgery and confirmed that their initial findings at 6 months persisted [169], concluding that undergoing surgery earlier in the course of functional decline may be associated with better outcome.

In a larger study involving 860 recipients of primary TKR from 3 different countries, Lingard et al (2004) reported that worse baseline WOMAC pain scores were a strong determinant of worse pain at 1 and 2 years after surgery. Pre-operative WOMAC function was also the strongest predictor of worse function at both 1 and 2 years after surgery [122].

3.3.2. Baseline radiographic characteristics

In contrast to clinical symptoms emerging literature suggests that those with the worst radiographic OA symptoms report better outcomes after total joint replacement.

We recently evaluated the association between pre-operative radiographic changes and outcomes after primary total knee replacement for osteoarthritis. We reported that pain relief was unsatisfactory in about 30% and functional improvement suboptimal in about 50% of patients [40]. In this study radiographic OA severity was measured using a modified version of the Kellgren-Lawrence Classification system [80]. We noted that radiographic OA severity was an independent predictor of pain and function at 12 months following TKR. Patients with evidence of mild radiographic OA changes were 5 times more likely (OR 5.39, 95% CI 1.23 – 15.69) to report moderate to severe pain at 12 months post TKR than those with severe radiographic changes.

Merle-Vincent et al (2011) examined predictors of satisfaction in 299 patients undergoing primary TKR and reported an association between radiographic OA severity and outcome 2 years after surgery [171]. Those with severe pre-operative joint space narrowing were nearly 4 times more likely to report satisfaction with surgery at 2 years compared to those with mild to moderate narrowing, (OR 3.9, 95% CI 1.1 – 14.3).

Valdes et al (2012) examined predictors of chronic pain using the WOMAC in 860 patients who had undergone TKR and 928 patients who had undergone THR with an average of 3.2 years follow-up [172]. They reported an OR 1.56 (95% CI 1.04 – 2.36) of ongoing pain in TKR patients with a Kellgren-Lawrence grade <3 and in THR patients with minimal joint space narrowing (>2mm width).

Cushnaghan et al (2007) reported on long term (approximately 8 years) functional outcomes following THR in a series of 282 patients matched with 295 community controls [173]. Radiographic OA severity defined as Croft grade 5 OA[174] was a predictor of greater functional improvement in cases as measured using the SF-36 physical function scores (19.4, 95% CI 7.7 – 31.2), when compared to cases with Croft grade < 3.

These findings suggest an inverse relationship between baseline radiographic OA and outcome up to 8 years following total joint replacement. More severe radiographic changes predict worse pain and to a lesser degree suboptimal function after surgery, providing important implications for timing of joint replacement.

4. Conclusion

Total joint replacement is the most effective and cost effective treatment for end-stage osteoarthritis. Most patients derive substantial benefits from joint replacement surgery; however those that don't are subject to chronic pain and disability and a higher risk for revision surgery. The causes of poor outcomes of surgery are multifactorial but almost certainly patient selection is a key determinant. While those who present with the "worst" symptoms might

http://dx.doi.org/10.5772/53245

be those who should be prioritized for TJR, the literature reports a mismatch between patient reported symptom severity and response to surgery. Although many risk factors are recognised, their individual or combined contributions to the *absolute risk* of suboptimal outcome after TJR remains poorly quantified. Importantly a majority of baseline patient characteristics (obesity, mental health, co-morbidities, radiographic OA severity, baseline pain and function) associated with sub-optimal outcome following TJR are those that could be "modified" with appropriate intervention. However baseline risk factors tend to remain unidentified or identified and managed at the point of surgery, which is too late. Hence there remains a need for exploring early interventions where there is opportunity to alter patient outcomes.

Acknowledgements

Dr Dowsey holds an NHMRC Early Career Australian Clinical Fellowship (APP1035810)

Author details

Michelle M. Dowsey[1] and Peter F. M. Choong[2]

1 University of Melbourne, Department of Surgery, St. Vincent's Hospital Melbourne, Australia

2 Department of Orthopaedics, St. Vincent's Hospital Melbourne, Australia

References

[1] World Health Organization. World Report on Disability. Malta: WHO; 2011 [cited 06/08/2012. Available from: http://www.who.int/disabilities/world_report/2011/en/index.html.

[2] Organization for Economic Co-operation and Development. Health at a Glance 2011: OECD Indicators. Heatlh Care Activities: 47 Hip and Knee Replacement [serial on the Internet]. 2011 06/08/2012]: Available from: http://www.oecd-ilibrary.org.

[3] Wang Y, Simpson JA, Wluka AE, Teichtahl AJ, English DR, Giles GG, et al. Relationship between body adiposity measures and isk of primary knee and hip replacement for osteoarthritis: a prospective cohort study. Arthritis Res Ther. 2009;11(2):R31.

[4] Productivity Commission. Economic implications of an aging Australia. Austrtalian Government Research Report (Canberra, 2005).

[5] Nilsdotter AK, Toksvig-Larsen S, Roos EM. A 5 year prospective study of patient-relevant outcomes after total knee replacement. Osteoarthritis Cartilage. 2009 May; 17(5):601-6.

[6] Santaguida PL, Hawker GA, Hudak PL, Glazier R, Mahomed NN, Kreder HJ, et al. Patient characteristics affecting the prognosis of total hip and knee joint arthroplasty: a systematic review. Can J Surg. 2008 Dec;51(6):428-36.

[7] Dowsey MM, Choong PF. Obese diabetic patients are at substantial risk for deep infection after primary TKA. Clin Orthop Relat Res. 2009 Jun;467(6):1577-81.

[8] Dowsey MM, Liew D, Stoney JD, Choong PF. The impact of pre-operative obesity on weight change and outcome in total knee replacement: a prospective study of 529 consecutive patients. J Bone Joint Surg Br. 2010 Apr;92(4):513-20.

[9] Malviya A, Martin K, Harper I, Muller SD, Emmerson KP, Partington PF, et al. Enhanced recovery program for hip and knee replacement reduces death rate. Acta Orthop. 2011 Oct;82(5):577-81.

[10] Australian Orthopaedic Association. National Joint Replacement Registry. Annual Report. Adelaide:AOA. 2010; Available from: www.dmac.adelaide.edu.au/aoanjrr/publications.jsp..

[11] Ashby E, Grocott MP, Haddad FS. Outcome measures for orthopaedic interventions on the hip. J Bone Joint Surg Br. 2008 May;90(5):545-9.

[12] Dunbar MJ, Robertsson O, Ryd L, Lidgren L. Appropriate questionnaires for knee arthroplasty. Results of a survey of 3600 patients from The Swedish Knee Arthroplasty Registry. J Bone Joint Surg Br. 2001 Apr;83(3):339-44.

[13] Ostendorf M, van Stel HF, Buskens E, Schrijvers AJ, Marting LN, Verbout AJ, et al. Patient-reported outcome in total hip replacement. A comparison of five instruments of health status. J Bone Joint Surg Br. 2004 Aug;86(6):801-8.

[14] Pollard B, Johnston M, Dieppe P. What do osteoarthritis health outcome instruments measure? Impairment, activity limitation, or participation restriction? J Rheumatol. 2006 Apr;33(4):757-63.

[15] Australian Bureau of Statistics. Postal Area (POA) Index of Relative Socio-economic Advantage and Disadvantage. Canberra: Commonwealth of Australia; 2008 [Accessed 1/2/2011]; Available from: www.abs.gov.au.

[16] Harris WH. Traumatic arthritis of the hip after dislocation and acetabular fractures: treatment by mold arthroplasty. An end-result study using a new method of result evaluation. J Bone Joint Surg Am. 1969 Jun;51(4):737-55.

[17] Bach CM, Nogler M, Steingruber IE, Ogon M, Wimmer C, Gobel G, et al. Scoring systems in total knee arthroplasty. Clin Orthop Relat Res. 2002 Jun(399):184-96.

[18] Davies AP. Rating systems for total knee replacement. Knee. 2002 Dec;9(4):261-6.

[19] Sanderson K, Andrews G. The SF-12 in the Australian population: cross-validation of item selection. Aust N Z J Public Health. 2002 Aug;26(4):343-5.

[20] Brander VA, Stulberg SD, Adams AD, Harden RN, Bruehl S, Stanos SP, et al. Predicting total knee replacement pain: a prospective, observational study. Clin Orthop Relat Res. 2003 Nov(416):27-36.

[21] Dickstein R, Heffes Y, Shabtai EI, Markowitz E. Total knee arthroplasty in the elderly: patients' self-appraisal 6 and 12 months postoperatively. Gerontology. 1998;44(4): 204-10.

[22] Jones CA, Beaupre LA, Johnston DW, Suarez-Almazor ME. Total joint arthroplasties: current concepts of patient outcomes after surgery. Rheum Dis Clin North Am. 2007 Feb;33(1):71-86.

[23] Jones CA, Voaklander DC, Johnston DW, Suarez-Almazor ME. Health related quality of life outcomes after total hip and knee arthroplasties in a community based population. J Rheumatol. 2000 Jul;27(7):1745-52.

[24] Mancuso CA, Salvati EA, Johanson NA, Peterson MG, Charlson ME. Patients' expectations and satisfaction with total hip arthroplasty. J Arthroplasty. 1997 Jun;12(4): 387-96.

[25] Nilsdotter AK, Petersson IF, Roos EM, Lohmander LS. Predictors of patient relevant outcome after total hip replacement for osteoarthritis: a prospective study. Ann Rheum Dis. 2003 Oct;62(10):923-30.

[26] European Federation of ISAP chapters. EFICF's declaration on pain as a major health problem, a disease in its own right: Available from: http://www.iasp-pain.org/AM/Template.cfm?Section=Press_Release&Template=/CM/ContentDisplay.cfm&ContentID=2908.

[27] (IOM) Institute of Medicine. Relieving pain in America: A Blueprint for Transforming Prevention, Care, Education and Research. Washington DC, 2011.

[28] Gustavsson A, Bjorkman J, Ljungcrantz C, Rhodin A, Rivano-Fischer M, Sjolund KF, et al. Socio-economic burden of patients with a diagnosis related to chronic pain--register data of 840,000 Swedish patients. Eur J Pain. 2012 Feb;16(2):289-99.

[29] Access Economics. The high price of pain: the economic impact of persistent pain in Australia: MBF Foundation in conjunction with the University of Sydney, 2007.

[30] Choong PF, Dowsey MM. Update in surgery for osteoarthritis of the knee. Int J Rheum Dis. 2011 May;14(2):167-74.

[31] Sinusas K. Osteoarthritis: diagnosis and treatment. Am Fam Physician. 2012 Jan 1;85(1):49-56.

[32] NIH consensus conference: Total hip replacement. NIH Consensus Development Panel on Total Hip Replacement. JAMA. 1995 Jun 28;273(24):1950-6.

[33] NIH Consensus Statement on total knee replacement December 8-10, 2003. J Bone Joint Surg Am. 2004 Jun;86-A(6):1328-35.

[34] Jones CA, Beaupre LA, Johnston DW, Suarez-Almazor ME. Total joint arthroplasties: current concepts of patient outcomes after surgery. Clin Geriatr Med. 2005 Aug;21(3): 527-41, vi.

[35] Laupacis A, Bourne R, Rorabeck C, Feeny D, Wong C, Tugwell P, et al. The effect of elective total hip replacement on health-related quality of life. J Bone Joint Surg Am. 1993 Nov;75(11):1619-26.

[36] Shields RK, Enloe LJ, Leo KC. Health related quality of life in patients with total hip or knee replacement. Arch Phys Med Rehabil. 1999 May;80(5):572-9.

[37] Rissanen P, Aro S, Sintonen H, Slatis P, Paavolainen P. Quality of life and functional ability in hip and knee replacements: a prospective study. Qual Life Res. 1996 Feb; 5(1):56-64.

[38] Huang NF, Dowsey MM, Ee E, Stoney JD, Babazadeh S, Choong PF. Coronal Alignment Correlates With Outcome After Total Knee Arthroplasty: Five-Year Follow-Up of a Randomized Controlled Trial. J Arthroplasty. 2012 Aug 3.

[39] Dowsey MM, Liew D, Stoney JD, Choong PF. The impact of obesity on weight change and outcomes at 12 months in patients undergoing total hip arthroplasty. Med J Aust. 2010 Jul 5;193(1):17-21.

[40] Dowsey MM, Nikpour M, Dieppe P, Choong PF. Associations between pre-operative radiographic changes and outcomes after total knee joint replacement for osteoarthritis. Osteoarthritis Cartilage. 2012 Jul 16.

[41] Liu SS, Buvanendran A, Rathmell JP, Sawhney M, Bae JJ, Moric M, et al. A Cross-Sectional Survey on Prevalence and Risk Factors for Persistent Postsurgical Pain 1 Year After Total Hip and Knee Replacement. Reg Anesth Pain Med. 2012 Jul;37(4):415-22.

[42] Melzack R. The McGill Pain Questionnaire: major properties and scoring methods. Pain. 1975 Sep;1(3):277-99.

[43] Insall JN, Dorr LD, Scott RD, Scott WN. Rationale of the Knee Society clinical rating system. Clin Orthop Relat Res. 1989 Nov(248):13-4.

[44] Wylde V, Hewlett S, Learmonth ID, Dieppe P. Persistent pain after joint replacement: prevalence, sensory qualities, and postoperative determinants. Pain. 2011 Mar;152(3): 566-72.

[45] Bellamy N, Buchanan WW, Goldsmith CH, Campbell J, Stitt LW. Validation study of WOMAC: a health status instrument for measuring clinically important patient relevant outcomes to antirheumatic drug therapy in patients with osteoarthritis of the hip or knee. J Rheumatol. 1988 Dec;15(12):1833-40.

[46] Singh JA, Lewallen D. Predictors of pain and use of pain medications following primary Total Hip Arthroplasty (THA): 5,707 THAs at 2-years and 3,289 THAs at 5-years. BMC Musculoskelet Disord. 2010;11:90.

[47] Kavanagh BF, Fitzgerald RH, Jr. Clinical and roentgenographic assessment of total hip arthroplasty. A new hip score. Clin Orthop Relat Res. 1985 Mar(193):133-40.

[48] Czurda T, Fennema P, Baumgartner M, Ritschl P. The association between component malalignment and post-operative pain following navigation-assisted total knee arthroplasty: results of a cohort/nested case-control study. Knee Surg Sports Traumatol Arthrosc. 2010 Jul;18(7):863-9.

[49] Wylde V, Blom AW, Whitehouse SL, Taylor AH, Pattison GT, Bannister GC. Patient-reported outcomes after total hip and knee arthroplasty: comparison of midterm results. J Arthroplasty. 2009 Feb;24(2):210-6.

[50] Dawson J, Fitzpatrick R, Murray D, Carr A. Questionnaire on the perceptions of patients about total knee replacement. J Bone Joint Surg Br. 1998 Jan;80(1):63-9.

[51] Baker PN, van der Meulen JH, Lewsey J, Gregg PJ. The role of pain and function in determining patient satisfaction after total knee replacement. Data from the National Joint Registry for England and Wales. J Bone Joint Surg Br. 2007 Jul;89(7):893-900.

[52] Hochman JR, Gagliese L, Davis AM, Hawker GA. Neuropathic pain symptoms in a community knee OA cohort. Osteoarthritis Cartilage. 2011 Jun;19(6):647-54.

[53] Ohtori S, Orita S, Yamashita M, Ishikawa T, Ito T, Shigemura T, et al. Existence of a neuropathic pain component in patients with osteoarthritis of the knee. Yonsei Med J. 2012 Jul 1;53(4):801-5.

[54] Buvanendran A, Kroin JS, Della Valle CJ, Kari M, Moric M, Tuman KJ. Perioperative oral pregabalin reduces chronic pain after total knee arthroplasty: a prospective, randomized, controlled trial. Anesth Analg. 2010 Jan 1;110(1):199-207.

[55] Clarke H, Pereira S, Kennedy D, Gilron I, Katz J, Gollish J, et al. Gabapentin decreases morphine consumption and improves functional recovery following total knee arthroplasty. Pain Res Manag. 2009 May-Jun;14(3):217-22.

[56] Clarke H, Pereira S, Kennedy D, Andrion J, Mitsakakis N, Gollish J, et al. Adding gabapentin to a multimodal regimen does not reduce acute pain, opioid consumption or chronic pain after total hip arthroplasty. Acta Anaesthesiol Scand. 2009 Sep;53(8): 1073-83.

[57] Dunlop DD, Manheim LM, Yelin EH, Song J, Chang RW. The costs of arthritis. Arthritis Rheum. 2003 Feb 15;49(1):101-13.

[58] Mathers CD, Vos ET, Stevenson CE, Begg SJ. The Australian Burden of Disease Study: measuring the loss of health from diseases, injuries and risk factors. Med J Aust. 2000 Jun 19;172(12):592-6.

[59] Yelin E, Murphy L, Cisternas MG, Foreman AJ, Pasta DJ, Helmick CG. Medical care expenditures and earnings losses among persons with arthritis and other rheumatic conditions in 2003, and comparisons with 1997. Arthritis Rheum. 2007 May;56(5): 1397-407.

[60] Wylde V, Livesey C, Blom AW. Restriction in participation in leisure activities after joint replacement: an exploratory study. Age Ageing. 2012 Mar;41(2):246-9.

[61] Groen JW, Stevens M, Kersten RF, Reininga IH, van den Akker-Scheek I. After total knee arthroplasty, many people are not active enough to maintain their health and fitness: an observational study. J Physiother. 2012;58(2):113-6.

[62] Lubbeke A, Katz JN, Perneger TV, Hoffmeyer P. Primary and revision hip arthroplasty: 5-year outcomes and influence of age and comorbidity. J Rheumatol. 2007 Feb;34(2):394-400.

[63] Escobar A, Gonzalez M, Quintana JM, Vrotsou K, Bilbao A, Herrera-Espineira C, et al. Patient acceptable symptom state and OMERACT-OARSI set of responder criteria in joint replacement. Identification of cut-off values. Osteoarthritis Cartilage. 2012 Feb;20(2):87-92.

[64] Singh JA, Lewallen DG. Predictors of activity limitation and dependence on walking aids after primary total hip arthroplasty. J Am Geriatr Soc. 2010 Dec;58(12):2387-93.

[65] Paulsen MG, Dowsey MM, Castle D, Choong PF. Preoperative psychological distress and functional outcome after knee replacement. ANZ J Surg. 2011 Oct;81(10):681-7.

[66] A WD, Robertsson O, Lidgren L. Surgery for knee osteoarthritis in younger patients. Acta Orthop. 2010 Apr;81(2):161-4.

[67] Hamel MB, Toth M, Legedza A, Rosen MP. Joint replacement surgery in elderly patients with severe osteoarthritis of the hip or knee: decision making, postoperative recovery, and clinical outcomes. Arch Intern Med. 2008 Jul 14;168(13):1430-40.

[68] Stroh DA, Delanois R, Naziri O, Johnson A, Mont M. Total knee arthroplasty in patients over 80 years of age. J Knee Surg. 2011 Dec;24(4):279-83.

[69] Joshi AB, Gill G. Total knee arthroplasty in nonagenarians. J Arthroplasty. 2002 Sep; 17(6):681-4.

[70] Joshi AB, Markovic L, Gill G. Knee arthroplasty in octogenarians: results at 10 years. J Arthroplasty. 2003 Apr;18(3):295-8.

[71] Pagnano MW, McLamb LA, Trousdale RT. Primary and revision total hip arthroplasty for patients 90 years of age and older. Mayo Clin Proc. 2003 Mar;78(3):285-8.

[72] Dahm DL, Barnes SA, Harrington JR, Sayeed SA, Berry DJ. Patient-reported activity level after total knee arthroplasty. J Arthroplasty. 2008 Apr;23(3):401-7.

[73] Australian Orthopaedic Association. National Joint Replacement Registry Annual Report. Adelaide2011.

[74] Swedish Hip Arthroplasty Register. Annual Report 2010 Göteborg, 2011: Available from: http://www.shpr.se/en/default.aspx.

[75] The Swedish Knee Arthroplasty Register Annual Report 2010 Lund, 2011: Available from: http://www.knee.nko.se/english/online/thePages/contact.php.

[76] National Joint Replacement Registry for England and Wales. 8th Annual Report 2011 Hertfordshire, 2011: Available from: www.njrcentre.org.uk.

[77] Karlson EW, Daltroy LH, Liang MH, Eaton HE, Katz JN. Gender differences in patient preferences may underlie differential utilization of elective surgery. Am J Med. 1997 Jun;102(6):524-30.

[78] Mujica-Mota RE, Tarricone R, Ciani O, Bridges JF, Drummond M. Determinants of demand for total hip and knee arthroplasty: a systematic literature review. BMC Health Serv Res. 2012 Jul 30;12(1):225.

[79] Borkhoff CM, Hawker GA, Kreder HJ, Glazier RH, Mahomed NN, Wright JG. The effect of patients' sex on physicians' recommendations for total knee arthroplasty. CMAJ. 2008 Mar 11;178(6):681-7.

[80] Dieppe P, Judge A, Williams S, Ikwueke I, Guenther KP, Floeren M, et al. Variations in the pre-operative status of patients coming to primary hip replacement for osteoarthritis in European orthopaedic centres. BMC Musculoskelet Disord. 2009;10:19.

[81] Ackerman IN, Graves SE, Wicks IP, Bennell KL, Osborne RH. Severely compromised quality of life in women and those of lower socioeconomic status waiting for joint replacement surgery. Arthritis Rheum. 2005 Oct 15;53(5):653-8.

[82] Hoogeboom TJ, van den Ende CH, van der Sluis G, Elings J, Dronkers JJ, Aiken AB, et al. The impact of waiting for total joint replacement on pain and functional status: a systematic review. Osteoarthritis Cartilage. 2009 Nov;17(11):1420-7.

[83] Dowsey MM, Dieppe P, Lohmander S, Castle D, Liew D, Choong PF. The association between radiographic severity and pre-operative function in patients undergoing primary knee replacement for osteoarthritis. Knee. 2012 Mar 23.

[84] Lavernia CJ, Alcerro JC, Contreras JS, Rossi MD. Patient perceived outcomes after primary hip arthroplasty: does gender matter? Clin Orthop Relat Res. 2011 Feb; 469(2):348-54.

[85] O'Connor MI. Implant survival, knee function, and pain relief after TKA: are there differences between men and women? Clin Orthop Relat Res. 2011 Jul;469(7):1846-51.

[86] Ritter MA, Wing JT, Berend ME, Davis KE, Meding JB. The clinical effect of gender on outcome of total knee arthroplasty. J Arthroplasty. 2008 Apr;23(3):331-6.

[87] Liebs TR, Herzberg W, Roth-Kroeger AM, Ruther W, Hassenpflug J. Women recover faster than men after standard knee arthroplasty. Clin Orthop Relat Res. 2011 Oct; 469(10):2855-65.

[88] Jenkins PJ, Perry PR, Yew Ng C, Ballantyne JA. Deprivation influences the functional outcome from total hip arthroplasty. Surgeon. 2009 Dec;7(6):351-6.

[89] Clement ND, Muzammil A, Macdonald D, Howie CR, Biant LC. Socioeconomic status affects the early outcome of total hip replacement. J Bone Joint Surg Br. 2011 Apr; 93(4):464-9.

[90] Allen Butler R, Rosenzweig S, Myers L, Barrack RL. The Frank Stinchfield Award: the impact of socioeconomic factors on outcome after THA: a prospective, randomized study. Clin Orthop Relat Res. 2011 Feb;469(2):339-47.

[91] Schafer T, Krummenauer F, Mettelsiefen J, Kirschner S, Gunther KP. Social, educational, and occupational predictors of total hip replacement outcome. Osteoarthritis Cartilage. 2010 Aug;18(8):1036-42.

[92] Davis ET, Lingard EA, Schemitsch EH, Waddell JP. Effects of socioeconomic status on patients' outcome after total knee arthroplasty. Int J Qual Health Care. 2008 Feb; 20(1):40-6.

[93] Dixon A, Le Grand J, Henderson J, Murray R, Poteliakhoff E. Is the British National Health Service equitable? The evidence on socioeconomic differences in utilization. J Health Serv Res Policy. 2007 Apr;12(2):104-9.

[94] Irgit K, Nelson CL. Defining racial and ethnic disparities in THA and TKA. Clin Orthop Relat Res. 2011 Jul;469(7):1817-23.

[95] Ang DC, James G, Stump TE. Clinical appropriateness and not race predicted referral for joint arthroplasty. Arthritis Rheum. 2009 Dec 15;61(12):1677-85.

[96] Dunlop DD, Song J, Manheim LM, Chang RW. Racial disparities in joint replacement use among older adults. Med Care. 2003 Feb;41(2):288-98.

[97] Hanchate AD, Zhang Y, Felson DT, Ash AS. Exploring the determinants of racial and ethnic disparities in total knee arthroplasty: health insurance, income, and assets. Med Care. 2008 May;46(5):481-8.

[98] Ibrahim SA. Racial and ethnic disparities in hip and knee joint replacement: a review of research in the Veterans Affairs Health Care System. J Am Acad Orthop Surg. 2007;15 Suppl 1:S87-94.

[99] Dunlop DD, Manheim LM, Song J, Sohn MW, Feinglass JM, Chang HJ, et al. Age and racial/ethnic disparities in arthritis-related hip and knee surgeries. Med Care. 2008 Feb;46(2):200-8.

[100] Kamath AF, Horneff JG, Gaffney V, Israelite CL, Nelson CL. Ethnic and gender differences in the functional disparities after primary total knee arthroplasty. Clin Orthop Relat Res. 2010 Dec;468(12):3355-61.

[101] Joshy S, Datta A, Perera A, Thomas B, Gogi N, Kumar Singh B. Ethnic differences in preoperative function of patients undergoing total knee arthroplasty. Int Orthop. 2006 Oct;30(5):426-8.

[102] Krupic F, Eisler T, Garellick G, Karrholm J. Influence of ethnicity and socioeconomic factors on outcome after total hip replacement. Scand J Caring Sci. 2012 May 23.

[103] Lavernia CJ, Alcerro JC, Contreras JS, Rossi MD. Ethnic and racial factors influencing well-being, perceived pain, and physical function after primary total joint arthroplasty. Clin Orthop Relat Res. 2011 Jul;469(7):1838-45.

[104] Dowsey MM, Broadhead ML, Stoney JD, Choong PF. Outcomes of total knee arthroplasty in English- versus non-English-speaking patients. J Orthop Surg (Hong Kong). 2009 Dec;17(3):305-9.

[105] Schonberg MA, Marcantonio ER, Hamel MB. Perceptions of physician recommendations for joint replacement surgery in older patients with severe hip or knee osteoarthritis. J Am Geriatr Soc. 2009 Jan;57(1):82-8.

[106] Suarez-Almazor ME, Souchek J, Kelly PA, O'Malley K, Byrne M, Richardson M, et al. Ethnic variation in knee replacement: patient preferences or uninformed disparity? Arch Intern Med. 2005 May 23;165(10):1117-24.

[107] Hekmat K, Jacobsson L, Nilsson JA, Petersson IF, Robertsson O, Garellick G, et al. Decrease in the incidence of total hip arthroplasties in patients with rheumatoid arthritis--results from a well defined population in south Sweden. Arthritis Res Ther. 2011;13(2):R67.

[108] Skytta E, Honkanen P, Eskelinen A, Huhtala H, Remes V. Fewer and older patients with rheumatoid arthritis need total knee replacement. Scand J Rheumatol. 2012 Jul 24.

[109] Sokka T, Kautiainen H, Hannonen P. Stable occurrence of knee and hip total joint replacement in Central Finland between 1986 and 2003: an indication of improved long-term outcomes of rheumatoid arthritis. Ann Rheum Dis. 2007 Mar;66(3):341-4.

[110] Clement ND, Breusch SJ, Biant LC. Lower limb joint replacement in rheumatoid arthritis. J Orthop Surg Res. 2012;7:27.

[111] Donahue KE, Gartlehner G, Jonas DE, Lux LJ, Thieda P, Jonas BL, et al. Systematic review: comparative effectiveness and harms of disease-modifying medications for rheumatoid arthritis. Ann Intern Med. 2008 Jan 15;148(2):124-34.

[112] Borstlap M, Zant JL, Van Soesbergen M, Van der Korst JK. Effects of total hip replacement on quality of life in patients with osteoarthritis and in patients with rheumatoid arthritis. Clin Rheumatol. 1994 Mar;13(1):45-50.

[113] Kageyama Y, Miyamoto S, Ozeki T, Hiyoshi M, Kushida K, Inoue T. Outcomes for patients undergoing one or more total hip and knee arthroplasties. Clin Rheumatol. 1998;17(2):130-4.

[114] Kirwan JR, Currey HL, Freeman MA, Snow S, Young PJ. Overall long-term impact of total hip and knee joint replacement surgery on patients with osteoarthritis and rheumatoid arthritis. Br J Rheumatol. 1994 Apr;33(4):357-60.

[115] March LM, Barcenilla AL, Cross MJ, Lapsley HM, Parker D, Brooks PM. Costs and outcomes of total hip and knee joint replacement for rheumatoid arthritis. Clin Rheumatol. 2008 Oct;27(10):1235-42.

[116] Tabutin J, Cambas PM. Hip arthroplasty up to the age of 30 and considerations in relation to subsequent revision. Hip Int. 2009 Jul-Sep;19(3):201-5.

[117] Dudkiewicz I, Salai M, Ganel A, Blankstein A, Chechik A. Total hip arthroplasty in patients younger than 30 years of age following developmental dysplasia of hip (DDH) in infancy. Arch Orthop Trauma Surg. 2002 Apr;122(3):139-42.

[118] Boyle MJ, Frampton CM, Crawford HA. Early results of total hip arthroplasty in patients with slipped upper femoral epiphysis compared with patients with osteoarthritis. J Arthroplasty. 2012 Jun;27(6):1003-7.

[119] Boyle MJ, Frampton CM, Crawford HA. Early results of total hip arthroplasty in patients with developmental dysplasia of the hip compared with patients with osteoarthritis. J Arthroplasty. 2012 Mar;27(3):386-90.

[120] Pietrzak K, Strzyzewski W, Pucher A, Kaczmarek W. [Total hip replacement after Legg-Calve-Perthes disease]. Chir Narzadow Ruchu Ortop Pol. 2011 May-Jun;76(3): 129-33.

[121] Dowsey MM, Choong PF. Obesity is a major risk factor for prosthetic infection after primary hip arthroplasty. Clin Orthop Relat Res. 2008 Jan;466(1):153-8.

[122] Lingard EA, Katz JN, Wright EA, Sledge CB. Predicting the outcome of total knee arthroplasty. J Bone Joint Surg Am. 2004 Oct;86-A(10):2179-86.

[123] Gandhi R, Dhotar H, Razak F, Tso P, Davey JR, Mahomed NN. Predicting the longer term outcomes of total knee arthroplasty. Knee. 2010 Jan;17(1):15-8.

[124] Young NL, Cheah D, Waddell JP, Wright JG. Patient characteristics that affect the outcome of total hip arthroplasty: a review. Can J Surg. 1998 Jun;41(3):188-95.

[125] Deyo RA, Cherkin DC, Ciol MA. Adapting a clinical comorbidity index for use with ICD-9-CM administrative databases. J Clin Epidemiol. 1992 Jun;45(6):613-9.

[126] Singh JA, O'Byrne M, Harmsen S, Lewallen D. Predictors of moderate-severe functional limitation after primary Total Knee Arthroplasty (TKA): 4701 TKAs at 2-years and 2935 TKAs at 5-years. Osteoarthritis Cartilage. 2010 Apr; 18(4):515-21.

[127] Hall WH, Ramachandran R, Narayan S, Jani AB, Vijayakumar S. An electronic application for rapidly calculating Charlson comorbidity score. BMC Cancer. 2004 Dec 20;4:94.

[128] Gandhi R, Razak F, Davey JR, Mahomed NN. Metabolic syndrome and the functional outcomes of hip and knee arthroplasty. J Rheumatol. 2010 Sep;37(9):1917-22.

[129] Lementowski PW, Zelicof SB. Obesity and osteoarthritis. Am J Orthop (Belle Mead NJ). 2008 Mar;37(3):148-51.

[130] Access-Economics. The economic costs of obesity. (Commissioned by Diabetes Australia, 2006).

[131] Leung A, Liew D, Lim J, Page C, Boukris-Sayag V, Mundae M, et al. The effect of joint aspiration and corticosteroid injections in osteoarthritis of the knee. Int J Rheum Dis. 2011 Oct;14(4):384-9.

[132] Kim SH. Morbid obesity and excessive hospital resource consumption for unilateral primary hip and knee arthroplasty. J Arthroplasty. 2010 Dec;25(8):1258-66.

[133] Kouris-Blazos A, Wahiqvist M. Health economics of weight management: evidence and cost. Asia Pac J Clin Nutri. 2007;16 (Suppl.1):329-38.

[134] Aderinto J, Brenkel IJ, Chan P. Weight change following total hip replacement: a comparison of obese and non-obese patients. Surgeon. 2005 Aug;3(4):269-72, 305.

[135] Donovan J, Dingwall I, McChesney S. Weight change 1 year following total knee or hip arthroplasty. ANZ J Surg. 2006 Apr;76(4):222-5.

[136] Heisel C, Silva M, dela Rosa MA, Schmalzried TP. The effects of lower-extremity total joint replacement for arthritis on obesity. Orthopedics. 2005 Feb;28(2):157-9.

[137] Jain SA, Roach RT, Travlos J. Changes in body mass index following primary elective total hip arthroplasty. Correlation with outcome at 2 years. Acta Orthop Belg. 2003 Oct;69(5):421-5.

[138] Lachiewicz AM, Lachiewicz PF. Weight and activity change in overweight and obese patients after primary total knee arthroplasty. J Arthroplasty. 2008 Jan;23(1):33-40.

[139] Middleton FR, Boardman DR. Total hip arthroplasty does not aid weight loss. Ann R Coll Surg Engl. 2007 Apr;89(3):288-91.

[140] Woodruff MJ, Stone MH. Comparison of weight changes after total hip or knee arthroplasty. J Arthroplasty. 2001 Jan;16(1):22-4.

[141] Zeni JA, Jr., Snyder-Mackler L. Most patients gain weight in the 2 years after total knee arthroplasty: comparison to a healthy control group. Osteoarthritis Cartilage. 2010 Apr;18(4):510-4.

[142] Vincent HK, Horodyski M, Gearen P, Vlasak R, Seay AN, Conrad BP, et al. Obesity and long term functional outcomes following elective total hip replacement. J Orthop Surg Res. 2012 Apr 25;7(1):16.

[143] Gillespie GN, Porteous AJ. Obesity and knee arthroplasty. Knee. 2007 Mar;14(2):81-6.

[144] Samson AJ, Mercer GE, Campbell DG. Total knee replacement in the morbidly obese: a literature review. ANZ J Surg. 2010 Sep;80(9):595-9.

[145] Dowsey MM, Choong PF. Early outcomes and complications following joint arthroplasty in obese patients: a review of the published reports. ANZ J Surg. 2008 Jun; 78(6):439-44.

[146] Wright JG, Swiontkowski MF, Heckman JD. Introducing levels of evidence to the journal. J Bone Joint Surg Am. 2003 Jan;85-A(1):1-3.

[147] Moran M, Walmsley P, Gray A, Brenkel IJ. Does body mass index affect the early outcome of primary total hip arthroplasty? J Arthroplasty. 2005 Oct;20(7):866-9.

[148] Lubbeke A, Stern R, Garavaglia G, Zurcher L, Hoffmeyer P. Differences in outcomes of obese women and men undergoing primary total hip arthroplasty. Arthritis Rheum. 2007 Mar 15;57(2):327-34.

[149] Rajgopal V, Bourne RB, Chesworth BM, MacDonald SJ, McCalden RW, Rorabeck CH. The impact of morbid obesity on patient outcomes after total knee arthroplasty. J Arthroplasty. 2008 Sep;23(6):795-800.

[150] Singh JA, Gabriel SE, Lewallen DG. Higher body mass index is not associated with worse pain outcomes after primary or revision total knee arthroplasty. J Arthroplasty. 2011 Apr;26(3):366-74 e1.

[151] Burg MM, Benedetto MC, Soufer R. Depressive symptoms and mortality two years after coronary artery bypass graft surgery (CABG) in men. Psychosom Med. 2003 Jul-Aug;65(4):508-10.

[152] Lingard EA, Riddle DL. Impact of psychological distress on pain and function following knee arthroplasty. J Bone Joint Surg Am. 2007 Jun;89(6):1161-9.

[153] Walton MJ, Newman JH. Pre-operative mental wellbeing and the outcome of knee replacement. Knee. 2008 Aug;15(4):277-80.

[154] Caracciolo B, Giaquinto S. Self-perceived distress and self-perceived functional recovery after recent total hip and knee arthroplasty. Arch Gerontol Geriatr. 2005 Sep-Oct;41(2):177-81.

[155] Paulsen M, Dowsey M, Castle D, Choong P. Pre-Operative Psychological Distress and Functional Outcome after Knee Replacement. ANZ J of Surg. 2010;[E-pub ahead of print] 20/1/2011.

[156] Vissers MM, Bussmann JB, Verhaar JA, Busschbach JJ, Bierma-Zeinstra SM, Reijman M. Psychological factors affecting the outcome of total hip and knee arthroplasty: a systematic review. Semin Arthritis Rheum. 2012 Feb;41(4):576-88.

[157] Rabin R, de Charro F. EQ-5D: a measure of health status from the EuroQol Group. Ann Med. 2001 Jul;33(5):337-43.

[158] Rolfson O, Dahlberg LE, Nilsson JA, Malchau H, Garellick G. Variables determining outcome in total hip replacement surgery. J Bone Joint Surg Br. 2009 Feb;91(2):157-61.

[159] Seligman MEP, Walker, E.F. & Rosenhan, D.L.,. Abnormal psychology, (4th ed.). New York: W.W. Norton & Company, Inc.; 2001.

[160] Quigley L, Nelson AL, Carriere J, Smilek D, Purdon C. The effects of trait and state anxiety on attention to emotional images: An eye-tracking study. Cogn Emot. 2012 May 30.

[161] Montin L, Leino-Kilpi H, Katajisto J, Lepisto J, Kettunen J, Suominen T. Anxiety and health-related quality of life of patients undergoing total hip arthroplasty for osteoarthritis. Chronic Illn. 2007 Sep;3(3):219-27.

[162] Badura-Brzoza K, Zajac P, Brzoza Z, Kasperska-Zajac A, Matysiakiewicz J, Piegza M, et al. Psychological and psychiatric factors related to health-related quality of life after total hip replacement - preliminary report. Eur Psychiatry. 2009 Mar;24(2):119-24.

[163] Brander V, Gondek S, Martin E, Stulberg SD. Pain and depression influence outcome 5 years after knee replacement surgery. Clin Orthop Relat Res. 2007 Nov;464:21-6.

[164] Riddle DL, Wade JB, Jiranek WA, Kong X. Preoperative pain catastrophizing predicts pain outcome after knee arthroplasty. Clin Orthop Relat Res. 2010 Mar;468(3): 798-806.

[165] Chaves JF, Brown JM. Spontaneous cognitive strategies for the control of clinical pain and stress. J Behav Med. 1987 Jun;10(3):263-76.

[166] Sullivan M, Tanzer M, Stanish W, Fallaha M, Keefe FJ, Simmonds M, et al. Psychological determinants of problematic outcomes following Total Knee Arthroplasty. Pain. 2009 May;143(1-2):123-9.

[167] Forsythe ME, Dunbar MJ, Hennigar AW, Sullivan MJ, Gross M. Prospective relation between catastrophizing and residual pain following knee arthroplasty: two-year follow-up. Pain Res Manag. 2008 Jul-Aug;13(4):335-41.

[168] Matthews G, and Ian J. Deary, I.J.,. Personality traits. Cambridge, UK: Cambridge University Press.; 1998.

[169] Fortin PR, Penrod JR, Clarke AE, St-Pierre Y, Joseph L, Belisle P, et al. Timing of total joint replacement affects clinical outcomes among patients with osteoarthritis of the hip or knee. Arthritis Rheum. 2002 Dec;46(12):3327-30.

[170] Fortin PR, Clarke AE, Joseph L, Liang MH, Tanzer M, Ferland D, et al. Outcomes of total hip and knee replacement: preoperative functional status predicts outcomes at six months after surgery. Arthritis Rheum. 1999 Aug;42(8):1722-8.

[171] Merle-Vincent F, Couris CM, Schott AM, Conrozier T, Piperno M, Mathieu P, et al. Factors predicting patient satisfaction 2 years after total knee arthroplasty for osteoarthritis. Joint Bone Spine. 2011 Jul;78(4):383-6.

[172] Valdes AM, Doherty SA, Zhang W, Muir KR, Maciewicz RA, Doherty M. Inverse relationship between preoperative radiographic severity and postoperative pain in patients with osteoarthritis who have undergone total joint arthroplasty. Semin Arthritis Rheum. 2012 Feb;41(4):568-75.

[173] Cushnaghan J, Coggon D, Reading I, Croft P, Byng P, Cox K, et al. Long-term outcome following total hip arthroplasty: a controlled longitudinal study. Arthritis Rheum. 2007 Dec 15;57(8):1375-80.

[174] Croft P, Cooper C, Wickham C, Coggon D. Defining osteoarthritis of the hip for epidemiologic studies. Am J Epidemiol. 1990 Sep;132(3):514-22.

[175] Franklin PD, Li W, Ayers DC. The Chitranjan Ranawat Award: functional outcome after total knee replacement varies with patient attributes. Clin Orthop Relat Res. 2008 Nov; 466(11):2597-604.

Section 2

Surgical Techniques and Technologies

Chapter 5

The Acrylic Bone Cement in Arthroplasty

Hamid Reza Seyyed Hosseinzadeh,
Mohammad Emami, Farivarabdollahzadeh Lahiji,
Ali Sina Shahi, Aidin Masoudi and Sina Emami

Additional information is available at the end of the chapter

http://dx.doi.org/10.5772/53252

1. Introduction

1.1. The genesis and evolution of acrylic bone cement

1.1.1. History

Otto Röhm is known as the developer of polymethylmethacrylate (PMMA) in 1901. Industrial-size chemical synthesis of MMA was achieved in the 1920s in the laboratories of Rohm and Haas, and the first biomedical applications of PMMA was the fabrication of dentures. In the 1930s it was discovered that the mixing of MMA monomer and benzoyl peroxide initiator with prepolymerized PMMA powder resulted in the formation of a dough-like material which could slowly harden into a glassy polymer. This two-component polymer (cement) was initially used to close cranial defects. Because of the transparency, strength, and stability of polymethylmethacrylate, the commercial production of cast sheets of it in the early 1930s led to its utilization as a denture base and prosthetic material. Originally pieces of the material were molded under heat and pressure.[1, 2, 3] In 1935, an injection molding technique was introduced by ICI for dentures in which the melted PMMA was injected into dried plaster molds under hydraulic pressure. These techniques proved to be too cumbersome. In 1936, as was mentioned above, it was discovered that mixing of methyl methacrylate monomer with the ground polymer produced a dough that could be shaped in plaster molds and could be polymerized into a solid mass by using benzoyl peroxide as a polymerization initiator. In the next few years, it was found that improved molding characteristics could be obtained using a powder that was a mixture of ground and spherical (bead) polymer particles.[1, 2]

The discovery of the dough molding technique led to the near universal use of these acrylic resins for dentures and prostheses for cranioplasties in the 1940s.[4] In 1943, German chemists discovered that if a tertiary amine such as dimethyl-pare-toluidine was added along with the benzoyl peroxide, the dough could be polymerized at room temperature. Based on this development, Kulzer and Degussa companies refined a dough-like, workable form of PMMA in 1943. Their developments led to the introduction of cold-cured PMMA, which hardens at room temperature. In the 1940s, with the advent of acrylic femoral hemiarthroplasties by Jean and Robert Judet, PMMA attracted interest in the field of orthopaedics. Kiaer and Haboush separately reported using PMMA to affix femoral implants in the early 1950s. The success with and the popularity of PMMA in orthopaedics is attributable to Sir John Charnley, whose work was affected by his exposure to the field of dentistry (because his father was a dentist) and his inherent interest in biomaterials. Charnley's early clinical accomplishments established a foundation for the continued use of PMMA in orthopaedics. Charnley had a long experience in producing his own instruments and gadgets. Charnley was interested in the work on thin sectioning of bones and rocks embedded in cast acrylic resin. He also performed a research into Judet prostheses and acrylic joints cast in alginate molds. He performed some arthroplasties with acrylic bone cement and reported the preliminary results of six cases in the British Journal of Bone and Joint Surgery in 1960. It is important to appreciate that this advance was not simply the use of acrylic cement but rather a conscious recognition of its ability to fill completely the medullary canal and adapt to the bone interface, so facilitating stress transfer, minimizing local stresses, and thereby stabilizing and anchoring the prosthesis. It was a new technique and provided the basis for the development of Charnley's concept of low friction arthroplasty during the next decade.[1, 2]

For over 40 years, poly(methylmethacrylate) (PMMA)-based bone cement, commonly known as acrylic bone cement, has been used for fixation of total joint replacement prostheses to periprosthetic bone. Today, most acrylic bone cements on the market consist of two components: a liquid and a powder one, which are mixed in the operating room until they become dough-like and are then applied to the bone prior to insertion of the component of the joint replacement prosthesis. The primary function of cements is to fix the joint replacement prosthesis to the periprosthetic bone tissue.[5] The basic component of acrylic bone cements is methylmethacrylate (MMA), which is an ester of methacrylic acid. In 1951, Kaier and Jansen in Copenhagen were the first to use PMMA bone cement for the fixation of acrylic cups to the subchondral bone of the femoral head. In 1953, Haboush used bone cement as a seating material for femoral head replacements without inserting it into the medullary canal. In 1958, Sir John Charnley used acrylic bone cement to fix femoral prostheses in the femur, as is done in modern-day joint arthroplasty these days. Charnley used a self-curing PMMA cement called Nu-Life, which was a pink-colored denture repair material. These early total hip replacements had a high incidence of failure, and it was not because of the cement or stems but because of the use of polytetrafluoroethylene (PTFE) acetabular cups. In 1966, CMW began to supply the first sterilized bone cement, formulated specifically for fixation of total joint replacement prostheses.[5] Nowadays, uncemented total hip replacement prostheses designs have largely been introduced in the orthopedic market, but acrylic cements continue to be one of the best primary methods of fixation of joint replacement prostheses, especially for knee replacement prostheses. In addition, injectable formulations of acrylic bone cements have been used for applications in vertebroplasty.

Several factors such as their chemical composition, viscosity, porosity, radiopacifiers and antibiotic additives, mixing methods, sterilization, temperature during handling, mechanical properties, and biocompatibility, affect the clinical performance of bone cements.

2. Composition and chemistry

The methylmethacrylate monomer consists of two carbon atoms that are covalently bound, with one of the carbon atoms covalently bonded to two hydrogen atoms and the other attached via a covalent bond to a methyl and acrylic group. Polymerization of MMA monomer produces PMMA, which is a polymer or a macromolecule. Hardened acrylic bone cement consists of linear, uncross-linked PMMA macromolecules of various lengths ranging from a few tens of thousands to a few million grams per mole. Acrylic bone cements comprise two components, often supplied in a 2:1 ratio: (a) a powder component, usually in a 40 g package, and (b) a liquid component, in a 20 mL ampoule.[2, 6](Table 1) There are several reasons for using a two-component bone cement instead of simply polymerizing pure MMA monomer:

The polymerization of MMA monomer is too slow and can take several hours or days, depending on the type and amount of reaction initiator used.

Pure MMA monomer has a very low viscosity and can easily diffuse into the blood stream, which can lead to cardiorespiratory and vascular complications.

The heat of polymerization can easily increase the temperature of the cement to over 100°C (boiling point for MMA = 100.3°C), which could lead to boiling of the volatile MMA monomer. The use of less amount of monomer and the presence of prepolymerized PMMA beads in the powder decreases the number of polymerization reaction and hence, the amount of released heat and assists in heat dissipation, decreasing the overall temperature.

After polymerization of pure MMA into PMMA, there would be a volumetric shrinkage of 21% due to differences in the density of the MMA monomer and the PMMA polymer. This amount of shrinkage is unacceptable and would lead to a large gap at the cement-bone and cement-prosthesis interface, compromising the fixation of the prosthesis.

The powder is the variable part in composition of bone cements among different brands, which contributes to differences in properties. (Figure 1) The powder component primarily consists of prepolymerized PMMA beads of 10 to 150 μm diameter, contributing to 83% to 99% of the powder. The prepolymerized beads of different bone cements include copolymers of MMA with styrene, methyl acrylate, or butyl methacrylate comonomers. The remaining components include a radiopacifier, either barium sulfate (BaSO4) or zirconium dioxide (ZrO2) (8% to 15% by weight), as well as an initiator, benzoyl peroxide (0.75% to 2.6%). The MMA monomer can self-polymerize under exposure to heat and light, but, this reaction is very slow. Therefore, dibenzoyl peroxide (BPO) reaction initiator in powder form is included in the powder component. Other variations include the initiator tri-n-butylborane and accelerator 2,5-dimethylhexane- 2,5-hydroperoxide(in Bonemite, chlorophyll dye and ethanol and ascorbic acid. The initiator, radiopacifier, and antibiotic powders all consist of particles of approximately 1 μm in diameter. [7]

Constituent	Role
Powder components	
Polymer	Polymethylmethacrylate
Co-polymer (e.g. MA-MMA)	Alter physical properties of the cement
Barium sulphate or Zirconium dioxide	Radio-opacifiers
Antibiotics*	Antimicrobial prophylaxis
Dye (e.g. chlorophyll)	Distinguish cement from bone
Liquid components	
Monomer	Methylmethacrylate monomer
N,N-dimethyl-p-toluidine (DMPT)	Initiates cold curing of polymer
Benzoyl peroxide	Reacts with DMPT to catalyze polymerization
Hydroquinone	Stabilizer preventing premature polymerization
Dye (e.g. chlorophyll)	Distinguish cement from bone
*Plain bone cements do not contain antibiotics	

Table 1. Commercial constituents of bone cement

The monomer, a colorless liquid with a characteristic odor, is packaged in ampules. The liquid components remain relatively constant among commercially available cements. 97% to 99% of this liquid consists of methylmethacrylate. N,N-dimethyl-para-toluidine (DMPT) makes up 0.4% to 2.8% by weight and acts as an accelerator to speed up the polymerization and setting of the cement. Since MMA can spontaneously polymerize during storage, addition of trace amounts of a stabilizer, usually hydroquinone (15 to 75 ppm), stabilizes and prevents premature polymerization of monomers.

MMA polymerizes by the mechanism of free radical polymerization, which consists of three steps: initiation, propagation, and termination. The initiation step involves decomposition of BPO monomer into radicals at room temperature.[7] (Figure 2)

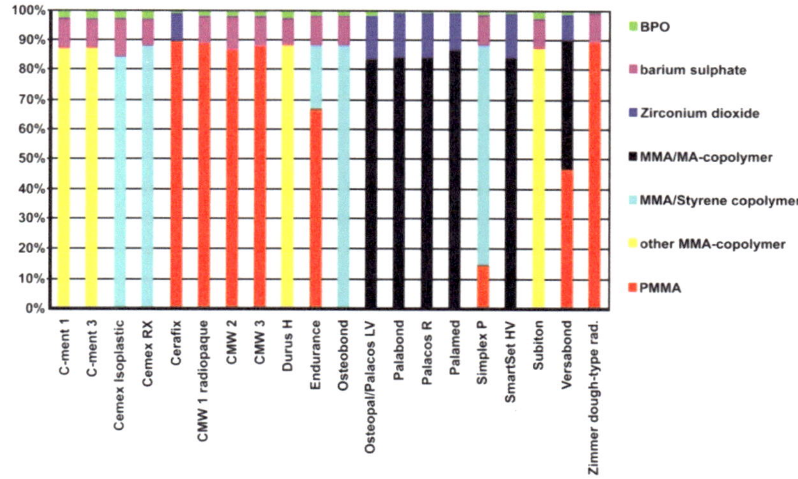

Figure 1. The composition of the powder of several PMMA bone cements on the market.

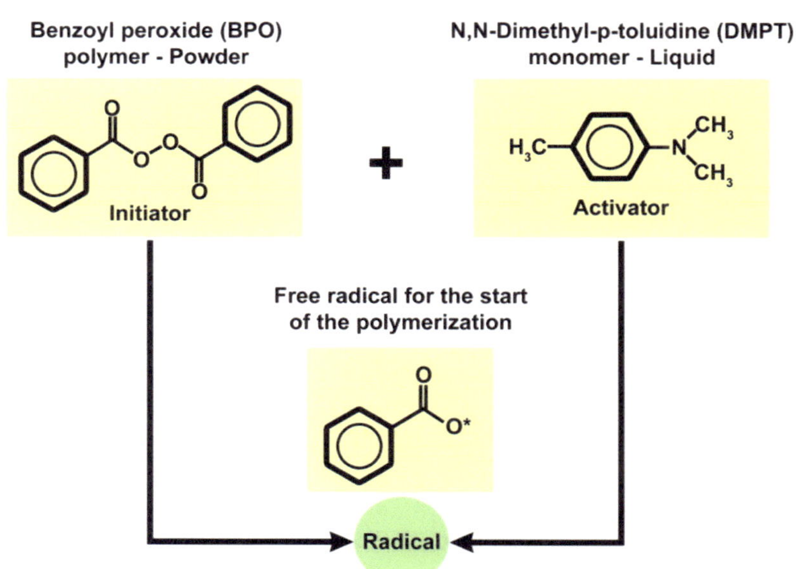

Figure 2. The initiation of the polymerization of MMA: BPO from the powder and DMPT from the liquid react to form radicals, starting the curing of bone cements.

Upon mixing of the two components, the DMPT in the liquid component decomposes BPO into a benzoyl radical and a benzoate anion as follows:

$$(C_6H_5COO)_2 + CH_3C_6H_4N(CH_3)_2 \longrightarrow C_6H_5COO^* + C_6H_5COO- + CH_3C_6H_4N(CH_3)_2^+ \longrightarrow CH_3C_6H_4NCH_3CH_2{}^* + H^+ \quad (1)$$

where BPO = $(C_6H_5COO)_2$, DMPT= $CH_3C_6H_4N(CH_3)_2$, benzoyl radical = $C_6H_5COO^*$, and benzoate anion = C_6H_5COO-.

The second step of the free radical polymerization is chain propagation in which the benzoyl radical reacts with the MMA monomer as follows:

$$C_6H_5COO^* + CH_2{=}CCH_3COOCH_3 \longrightarrow C_6H_5COO\text{-}CH_2\text{-}CCH_3COOCH_3 + CH_2{=}CCH_3COOCH_3 \longrightarrow C_6H_5COO\text{-}CH_2CCH_3COOCH_3\text{-}CH_2CCH_3COOCH_3 \quad (2)$$

The free radical attacks one of the double bonds of the MMA monomer. One electron of the double bond pairs up with the electron of the free radical to form a bond between the oxygen of the benzoyl free radical and one of the carbon atoms of the MMA monomer while the second electron of the double bond shifts to the other carbon atom, which then turns into a free radical. This free radical then attacks another MMA monomer and the chain propagates until a PMMA of relatively high molecular weight, on the order of 100,000 to 1,000,000 g/mol, is achieved. Finally, chain termination can be achieved by chain coupling as follows:

$$\text{-}CH_2CXCH_3{}^* + {}^*CXCH_3CH_2\text{-} \longrightarrow \text{-}CH_2CXCH_3\text{-}CXCH_3CH_2\text{-} \quad (3)$$

or, to a lesser extent, by disproportionation via transfer of a hydrogen atom as follows:

$$\text{-}CH_2CXCH_3{}^* + {}^*CXCH_3CH_2\text{-} \longrightarrow \text{-}CH_2C_XCH_2 + CXH{=}CH\text{-}^{\cdot\cdot} \quad (4)$$

where X refers to the substituent $COOCH_3$.

The glass transition temperature of PMMA is about 105°C, but the glass transition temperature of hardened PMMA-based bone cement can be lower due to plasticization effects of residual monomer and water. With proceeding of polymerization, the growing polymer chains slowly turn into a hard, glassy material, and it becomes difficult for the monomer to diffuse through the hardened PMMA matrix to continue chain propagation. [8]

The hardened acrylic bone cement consists primarily of linear, uncross-linked PMMA macromolecules of various lengths, but their length (or molecular weight) can vary widely. The molecular weight of the hardened cement depends on several factors, such as (a) the molecular weight of the monomer used (usually MMA), (b) the molecular weight of the prepolymerized beads, (c) the ratio of the initiator and the accelerator, (d) the presence of stabilizers, (e) the ambient temperature during polymerization, and (f) the sterilization method.[7, 8]

3. Properties

3.1. Heat production during polymerization

Combining powder and liquid monomer initiates an exothermic reaction. In vitro, the peak temperatures reach 113°C. In vivo temperatures are reported to be between 40° and 56°C. Methylmethacrylate monomer, the basic building block of PMMA, contains carbon-carbon double bonds, which react with the free radical produced by the activator and initiator. The monomer free radical interacts with other monomer molecules, creating a growing polymer chain. During the polymerization, the powder changes to a workable dough. [7]

This reaction releases 52 KJ/mole of monomer, equating to heat production of 1.4 to 1.7×10^8 J/m^3 of cement. The production of heat by the curing cement has been studied *in vitro* and *in vivo* and modeled using finite element analysis. *In vitro* studies have shown that the thicker cement mantles, the higher ambient temperatures and the greater ratio of monomer to polymer the more heat is produced. Recorded temperatures range between 70°C and 120°C. Collagen denatures with prolonged exposure to temperatures in excess of 56°C, and the risk of causing thermal damage to bone has been emphasized by several authors. However, *in vivo* studies have recorded lower peaks of temperature. In 1977, Reckling and Dillon measured the temperature at the bone cement interface in 20 THRs. The maximum temperature was 48°C.[9] The reasons for the lower in vivo temperature are:

1. The thin layer of the bone cement
2. Blood circulation
3. The large surface area of the interface
4. Poor thermal conductivity of the cement
5. Heat dissipation to the prosthesis and to the vital tissue.

So, the temperature increase greater than the coagulation temperature of proteins is avoided.

Harving, Soballe and Bunger recorded temperatures above 56°C but only for two to three minutes. Even though, such temperatures may sometimes be reached, animal studies have shown no adverse effects. Nevertheless, concerns regarding thermal and chemical injury persisted.[3]

3.2. Curing of a bone cement

By mixing the powder and liquid, two different processes are started. First, the polymer powder takes up the monomer liquid, forming a more or less viscous fluid or a dough. This phenomenon is because of the swelling and dissolution processes of monomer and polymer powder. Swelling and dissolution processes are physical processes and they are important for the working characteristics of a bone cement. Second, a chemical process is initiated, which is responsible for the final hardening of the bone cement. The initiator BPO from the polymer powder and the activator DMPT from the liquid interact to produce free radicals in the so-called ''initiation reaction''. These radicals are able to start the polymerization of MMA by adding to the polymerizable double-bond of the monomer molecule. This results in a growing polymer chain that builds up macromolecules. Because of the high number of radicals generated, many rapidly growing polymer chains are formed and, therefore, there is a fast conversion of MMA to PMMA. If two growing polymer chains meet, the chains are terminated by combining both, resulting in an unreactive polymer molecule. The polymerization of MMA is an exothermic reaction, resulting in a temperature increase in the curing bone cement.[7] This temperature maximum can be influenced by:

1. The chemical composition of the cement
2. By the powder to liquid ratio
3. By the radiopacifier.

3.3. Volume shrinkage

Because a polymerization means a conversion of a large number of monomer molecules to a much smaller number of polymer molecules, there is a volume shrinkage during curing of the bone cement. The reason for this shrinkage is the decreasing molecular distance between free monomer molecules before the polymerization and the molecular distance of the molecules bonded in the polymer chain. The volume shrinkage of pure MMA is approximately 21%. By using prepolymerized powder, the content of MMA in commercially available bone cements is reduced to approximately one third of the whole mass. The theoretic volume shrinkage of bone cements is therefore approximately 6%–7%. The real shrinkage is lower, however, because of the air inclusions in the cement dough. So, the real volume shrinkage of hand-mixed bone cement thus might be lower than the shrinkage of vacuum-mixed bone cement, because vacuum-mixed cement has hardly any air inclusions. Because acrylic bone cement absorbs water, its volume shrinkage is compensated by the expansion caused by the water-uptake.[8]

4. Processing and handling of bone cement

The handling characteristics and setting times of acrylic cements are of great importance for orthopedic surgeons. The handling of bone cements can be described by four different phases with their corresponding viscosities:

1. The mixing phase (up to 1 minute) is the period during which the powder and the liquid are homogenized thoroughly. The powder and the liquid can be mixed manually by using a bowl and a spatula or by a special mixing system, applying vacuum to avoid the formation of voids.
2. The waiting phase (up to several minutes, according to the type of cement and the handling temperature) is the period to reach a non-sticky state of the cement.

3. The working phase (2–4 minutes, according to the type of cement and the handling temperature) is the period during which the surgeon can inject the cement and insert the prosthesis. The viscosity of the cement has to be high enough to withstand the bleeding pressure. Blood pervasion of the cement results in a reduction of the strength of the cement. A late application at a too high viscosity level may result in poor interfaces between the prosthesis, the cement, and the bone.

4. The hardening phase (1–2 minutes) is the period of the final setting process and the development of the polymerization heat.

The effect of the temperature on the length of the phases is clearly visible. The information given by the temperature versus time curves of different cements is not always comparable, because manufacturers use different determination methods resulting in variant lengths of the working phases. This disagreement is caused by the lack of a universal detection method. A wide experience and knowledge by the surgeon is therefore helpful to find the optimal range of time to inject the cement and to fix the prosthesis. The method described in ISO 5833 and ASTM F 451 to determine a viscosity-like parameter is the intrusion test. This is not really a test method for the determination of the true viscosity. To perform this test, the mixed cement is placed in a plastic mold and is loaded with a force of 49 N for 1 minute. The depth of the intrusion of the cement into four drill holes is measured. This method is only available for high viscosity bone cements. In the standard ASTM F 451, there is another extrusion viscosity test described with a capillary rheometer for low viscosity bone cements. [7]

In the Standards, there are two further time parameters defined: the doughing time and the setting time. The doughing time end by the beginning of the working phase and it is determined by recording from the start time of mixing until the mixture is able to separate cleanly from a gloved finger. The second time parameter is the setting time, which is defined as the time to reach a temperature midway between ambient and maximum. The end of setting time marks the final hardening of the bone cement. [8]

During the waiting period swelling of the beads occurs and allows the polymerization to proceed, leading to an increase in viscosity. At this stage, the cement turns into a sticky dough. The working period begins when the cement is no longer sticky but of sufficiently low viscosity to permit the surgeon to easily apply the cement into the prepared place. During this period, the chain propagation continues, along with an increase in viscosity. The viscosity of the cement must be carefully assessed before inserting the cement because with a very low viscosity the cement would not be able to withstand the bleeding pressure. This would result in blood lamination in the cement, which can weaken the cement. The heat produced during this period, results in thermal expansion of the cement. On the other hand, there is a volumetric shrinkage of the cement as the MMA monomer converts into the denser PMMA polymer.

The final stage is the hardening period, when the polymerization terminates and leads to a hardened cement. The temperature of the cement continues to elevate during this period and then slowly decreases to body temperatures. During this period, the cement undergos volumetric shrinkage along with thermal shrinkage as the cement cools down to body temperature. While the manufacturer can determine the hardening period length using in vitro measurements at a controlled temperature and humidity in a laboratory environment, it is difficult to predict the hardening period in vivo, with accuracy due to variations in the ambient environment in the operating room, the body temperature, and thickness of the cement mantle, all of which can alter the setting times of the cement. Several factors, such as the type of mixing method used, the viscosity of the cement, the precooling of the monomer and/or powder, the preheating of the powder component, and the preheating of the prosthesis, can also significantly alter the times of some of the handling phases. Thus it is important for the surgeon to know each of the factors that can alter the duration of each phase. [7]

4.1. Viscosity and handling properties

The dynamic viscosity (η) of fluids is denoted by shear stress (F)/shear rate (S) [$\eta = F/S$]. Fluids are designated as Newtonian if shear stress is linearly related to shear rate. Cement in its liquid phase of curing behaves as a non-Newtonian fluid with viscosity decreasing as shear rate is increased. This is called pseudoplastic or shear thinning behaviour. However, the viscosity of all cements increases during polymerisation as the polymer chains lengthen.[10]

The mixed cement begins as a viscous liquid, then turns into a viscoelastic material, and finally hardens into a predominantly elastic solid. Thus, it is important to monitor both the dynamic viscosity as well as the viscoelastic parameters, such as storage modulus (G'), loss modulus (G"), and tanδ (their ratio). A high storage modulus indicates that the material is more solid-like whereas a high loss modulus shows that the material is more viscous.[7]

The viscosity of bone cements at the dough stage is determined mainly by the chemical composition and the powder to monomer ratio. These aspects should never be modified in the operating theater to modify the viscosity. There are some methods to modify the viscosity without changing other characteristics of the cement, however. One of them is the prechilling of the cement. The velocity of the reaction, and with it the viscosity, depends on the temperature. Prechilling of cements, especially of high viscosity cements, has been introduced with the introduction of mixing systems to make mixing of cement in these systems more convenient and to improve the quality of the mixture, especially with respect to porosity. [8]

Another method for applying this change is preheating the cement, to accelerate the polymerization and thus, reducing the operation time. But it has been shown that by this heat application to the cement powder, various characteristics of the cement itself or the cemented construct are either enhanced, degraded, or marginally affected, which depends on the structure of the cement powder and its stability against the heat. Specifically, these properties are significantly decreased when the principal constituent in the powder has a low resistance to degradation by the preheat temperature (as is the case of the PMMA polymer in Cemex XL and CMW 1 cements) but are not when the resistance is high (as in the case of a mixture of PMMA + MMA styrene copolymer in Surgical Simplex P cement).[11]

Manufacturers can also change the viscosity of cement by changing the molecular weight, by using co-polymers, and by varying the methods of sterilization. In addition, the curing process itself can be controlled by altering the proportions of the initiator (Toluidine) and the monomer, and this can change the working properties.

The cement must be liquid enough during the working phase to be forced through a delivery device and then flow under pressure to penetrate the interstices of cancellous bone, achieving micro-interlock. Bone cements are usually divided into three categories: high, medium and low viscosity:

Low. These have a long waiting phase of three minutes, also known as a sticky phase. The viscosity rapidly increases during the working phase and the hardening phase is one to two minutes long.

Medium. There is a long waiting phase of three minutes, but during the working phase, the viscosity only increases slowly. Hardening takes between one minute 30 seconds, and two minutes 30 seconds.

High. A short waiting/sticky phase is followed by a long working phase. The viscosity remains constant until the end of the working phase. The hardening phase lasts between one minute 30 seconds and two minutes. High viscosity cements are therefore forgiving for the surgeon and are in predominant use in orthopaedics. [3]

However, the rates of curing are very sensitive to environmental factors. Low ambient temperatures during storing and mixing, and high humidity both prolong setting time. Typical representatives of high viscosity cements are Palacos R (Biomet Inc.; Warsaw/USA; Schering-Plough; Heist-op-den-Berg/Belgium; Heraeus Kulzer; Wehrheim/Germany), Palamed (Biomet Merck; Ried/Switzerland; Heraeus Kulzer), CMW 1 (DePuy; Blackpool/England), Simplex P (Stryker; Limerick/Ireland), and Cemfix 1 (Teknimed; Vic en Bigorre/France), whereas Osteopal (Biomet Merck; Heraeus Kulzer), Palacos LV (Schering-Plough; Heraeus Kulzer), Osteobond (Zimmer; Warsaw/USA), Versabond (Smith & Nephew; Memphis/USA), Cemfix 3 (Teknimed), Sulcem 3 (Zimmer; Baar/Switzerland), and CMW 3 (DePuy) are examples of low viscosity cements. [7]

The high viscosity during mixing might be a disadvantage, because this supports the entrapping of air. The viscosity is the most important handling property for the surgeon and determines the working properties of the cement.

4.2. Residual monomer and monomer release

Radical polymerization of the MMA in bone cement generally does not proceed to completion, because the mobility of remaining monomer molecules is inhibited at high conversion rates. There will remain, therefore, some residual monomer. Directly after curing, the content of residual monomer is approximately 2%–6%. In the following 3 weeks this content decreases to approximately 0.5%. The main part (approximately 80%) of the total residual monomer is post-polymerized slowly. A smaller part of the residual monomer is released from the cement and metabolized to carbon dioxide and water in the citric acid cycle.(Figure 3) In earlier times, released MMA was considered the main reason for perioperative respiration and circulation upset. However, these effects are definitely the result of the increase in the intramedullary pressure and fat embolism. They are not caused by the residual monomer. [7]

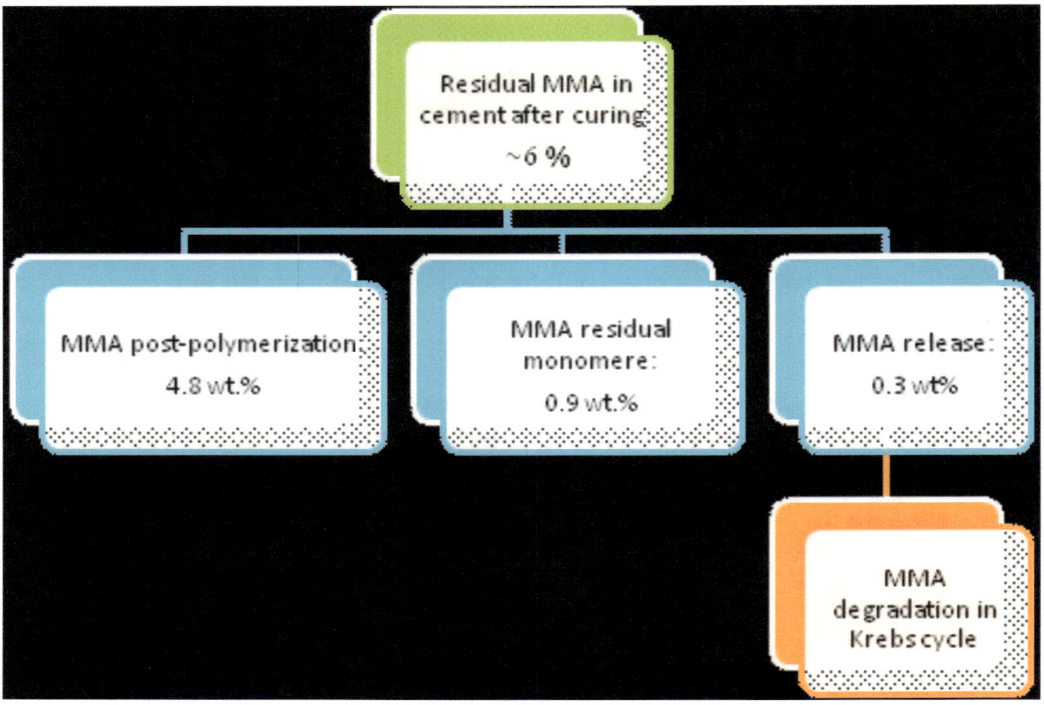

Figure 3. Residual monomer in acrylic bone cement: post-polymerization and release with subsequent degradation.

4.3. Radiopacity

After a total joint replacement, if the cement does not have a distinct opacity, the surgeon cannot monitor the healing process clearly. This is the reason why radiopaque materials are added to bone cements, so the hardened cement is radiopaque. Barium sulfate or zirconium dioxide is used as opacifiers in all available bone cements.(Figure 4) The radiopacifier does not contribute to the polymer chain. It is dispersed uniformly in the polymer powder and in the resulting solid bone cement. Animal experiments and in vivo studies with different cell cultures showed more osteolytic changes by using barium sulfate than by using zirconium dioxide. Despite the low solubility of barium sulfate, toxic barium ions can be released. On the other hand, the abrasive properties of zirconium dioxide seem to be a disadvantage. All bone cements examined contain 8.0%–15.0% opacifier within the polymer. Zirconium dioxide provides higher opacity to bone cements compared to barium sulfate. Bone cements with more than 15.0% zirconium dioxide in the polymer have the most distinct opacity.[2, 3, 7]

4.4. Molecular weight and sterilization

The molecular weight of the polymer powder particles is affected strongly by the sterilization procedure used. Sterilization by γ-irradiation or β-irradiation significantly lowers the molecular weight, whereas sterilization by ethylene oxide has no influence on the molecular weight of the polymer. The molecular weight influences the swelling properties and the mechanical properties of the bone cement; therefore, low molecular weights have a few disadvantages. Sterilization by ethylene oxide is the preferred method for bone cements, because there is no change in material properties during sterilization. [12]

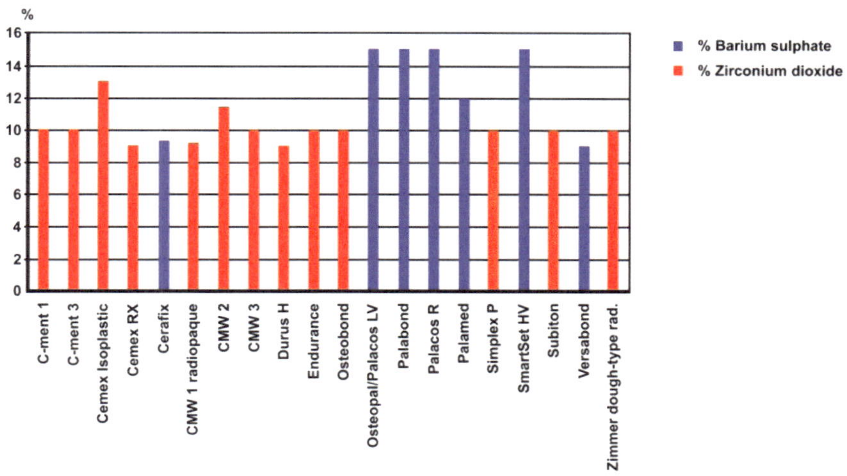

Figure 4. Content of radiopaquer in the powder of several acrylic bone cements; two radiopaquer agents are used in commercial products: Barium sulfate and Zirconium dioxide.

5. Cement morphology

The composition of hardened cement consists of prepolymerized beads of PMMA or their copolymers fused with the polymerized MMA monomer, in addition to radiopacifiers and additives, such as powders of antibiotics, as well as pores or voids and residual initiator. These parts of a cement composition act as flaws. These flaws can be due to: (a) air dissolved within the powder particles; (b) air entrapment during mixing of powder and liquid monomer; (c) incomplete fusion of prepolymerized PMMA beads with the setting MMA; (d) evaporation of the volatile monomer due to the heat of reaction during setting; (e) air entrapment during transfer of the dough to the gun; and (f) air entrapment during introduction of cement into the medullary canal. The major problem associated with the presence of flaws is that when a critical flaw size is achieved, the flaws act as sites of stress concentration, leading to weakening of the cement. But if the critical flaw size is not reached, they act as crack blunting part of the cement upon its fracture. In other words, the cracks deviate from their path when they encounter flaws in their path associated with pores and radiopacifier particles. The Griffith crack criterion assumes that there exists a critical flaw size unique to each material above which its fracture strength is compromised. For PMMA, the critical flaw size is 70 μm. Thus, if the pores are smaller than the critical flaw size for PMMA, the porosity will not compromise the fracture strength of bone cement. It is generally well known that hardened bone cement contain macropores (pore diameter greater than 1 mm) and micropores (pore diameter 0.01-1.0 mm). Based on the Griffith theory, elimination of the macropores would be more important than elimination of the micropores, especially the pores much smaller than 70 μm in diameter. The most common method of eliminating pores is to use centrifugation and vacuum mixing methods. Another source of flaws that can be potential sites of high stress concentration is radiopacifier powder particles. A radiopacifier powder, usually barium sulfate or zirconium oxide, consists of particles with a broad range of sizes, from approximately 0.2 to 2 μm in diameter. Zirconium oxide is a harder material than barium sulfate. Thus, if there is loosening, there could be concerns with regards to third body abrasive wear in the bearing surface of the joint replacement. Barium sulfate is generally insoluble, but there are concerns about toxicity of barium ions. Poor spread of radiopacifier particles in the region between the prepolymerized cement beads can affect both crack initiation and crack propagation, especially if they are larger than the critical flaw size for PMMA. The radiopacifier particles do not bond with PMMA and instead reside within pores, which are larger than these particles due to cement shrinkage. [13, 8]

6. Mixing techniques and its effect on porosity

Mixing techniques are of great importance in determining the content and size of flaws that can affect the cement toughness. Historically, three methods of mixing of cement have been employed: (a) hand mixing in air; (b) hand mixing followed by centrifugation; and (c) hand mixing in an evacuated mixing device, commonly known as "vacuum mixing." [8, 14]

Hand mixing involves mixing of the liquid and powder components in an open bowl using a spatula at a speed of 1 to 2 Hz for a period of duration of approximately 2 minutes. The hand-mixing method can introduce a porosity of 7% or higher. It is confirmed that excessive mixing can lead to increased porosity. By decreasing the number of beats and waiting for a short duration after wetting the powder component with the monomer the porosity of cement can be reduced to approximately 5%. Centrifugation was later introduced as a method to eliminate pores. In this method, the liquid and powder components are initially hand mixed and then placed in a tube and subjected to centrifugation at a speed of 2300 to 4000 rpm for a duration of 0.5 to 3 minutes. With this method the total porosity decreases to 1% or less, which is significantly lower than the porosity observed in hand mixing. It is obvious that for centrifugation to be effective, the viscosity of the cement must be relatively low, allowing the air bubbles to flow to the surface of the cement under the centrifugal force. One way to assist centrifugation is to chill the MMA monomer prior to mixing. One potential disadvantage of the centrifugation mixing technique is that it can lead to an inhomogeneous distribution of radiopacifier particles in the centrifuged cement, due to the difference in density of radiopacifier particles and PMMA and MMA monomer. The third type of mixing technique is vacuum mixing, in which the two components of bone cements are placed in a mixing bowl and are mixed after subjecting the bowl to vacuum conditions. The vacuum-mixing devices have proven to substantially decrease porosity in cements to less than 1% and consequently to increase their fatigue properties. Another major reason for using vacuum mixing is that MMA monomer is contained within the mixing bowl, which limits exposure to its vapors. Toxicology information obtained from materials safety data sheets (MSDSs) show that MMA monomer is harmful if inhaled, swallowed, or absorbed through the skin. [8, 14]

It must be noted that this reduction in the porosity of cement mantle with vacuum-mixing, is not always the case. Messick et al found that vacuum-mixed cement does not result in overall lower porosity of the cement, but the distribution of porosity may be different when compared with that of hand-mixed cement.(Figure 5) It has also been demonstrated that very high vacuum levels can be associated with the presence of cracks in the cement.[15]

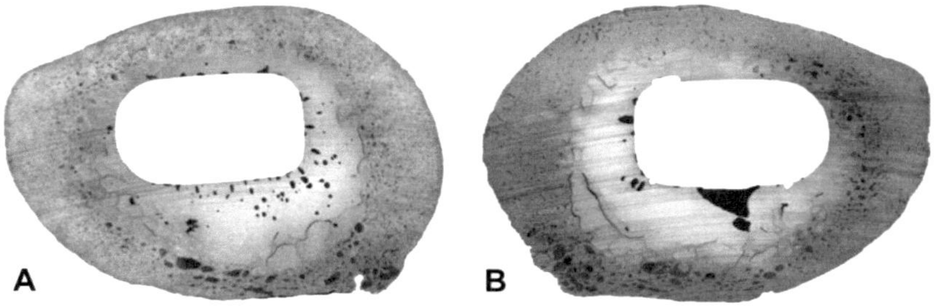

Figure 5. Representative sections illustrating the distribution of porosity for A) hand- and B) vacuum-mixed cement.

7. Mechanical and physical properties

7.1. Static mechanical properties (Table 2)

The main function of acrylic bone cement is the stable fixation of endoprostheses. The cement must endure considerable stresses, thus, sufficient strength is one of the most important demands to achieve a stable fixation and to guarantee long-term stability of the implant. The cement layer has the effect of an elastic buffer between prosthesis and bone. Because of its close adaptation to bone and its viscoelastic properties, it can reduce the stress concentrations at the interface with the bone. In the end, transferring load from the prosthesis to the bone as efficiently as possible also is decisive for the long-term stability of the implant. The mechanism of loading is especially complex for hip arthroplasty; therefore, it is difficult to define what sufficient strength actually means. The total load affecting bone cement is a mixture of compressive loading combined with bending, tension, shear, and torsion. It has been extremely difficult to simulate this complex situation in the laboratory. Two mechanical tests have been introduced into ISO 5833, the relevant standard for testing acrylic bone cements. These tests are the compression and the four-point bending test for the determination of the compressive strength, the bending strength and the bending modulus (modulus of elasticity or Young's modulus), respectively. The standard ASTM F 451 includes the compression test only. Generally there are two different fundamental measuring principles to determine mechanical properties of bone cements: applying static (also called quasistatic) stresses and dynamic stresses. Static tests are destructive tests with a uniaxial single loading, increasing until failure, in contrast to dynamic tests that involve a cyclic loading.[16]

The compression test according to the standards ISO 5833 and ASTM F 451 is a static method in which the compressive strength is defined as the maximum stress that a material can withstand before failure in compression. The test is executed with a universal testing machine equipped to record load versus crosshead displacement. The minimum requirement for the compressive strength is 70 MPa according to the standards. All commercial antibiotic and plain bone cements meet this requirement. Between both cement types, no significant differences in compressive strength are observable.[10]

The second mechanical test according to ISO 5833 is the four-point bending test, also performed with a universal testing machine. According to ISO 5833 the minimum requirement for the bending strength is 50 MPa and for the bending modulus it is 1800 MPa, respectively. Again, all commercial cements clearly fulfill the requirements. The addition of antibiotics reduces the bending strength, but the differences between antibiotic and plain cement are not always statistically significant. The bending modulus represents the ratio of stress to corresponding strain of the material within the elastic range characterizing the relative stiffness of the material. Stiff materials have a high modulus, eg, glass and ceramics; ductile materials like rubber have a low modulus. Within the elastic range the stress and strain are directly proportional following Hooke's Law, and if the load is released, the material regains its initial dimensions. The elastic range is limited by a stress limit, the so-called "proportional limit" at which the physical properties of the material actually change and the material might not recover its initial shape after releasing load. As already mentioned the cement acts as a mechanical buffer. For this purpose the modulus of elasticity of bone cement has to be lower than the moduli of the metallic prosthesis and the bone. The modulus must not decrease to below a minimum value, however; therefore, a lower limit for the modulus is established in ISO 5833. The modulus varies with temperature, which means the higher the temperature, the lower the modulus. Testing bone cement at 23°C is not a really convenient way to get meaningful results for the application in the human body. The mechanical performance of bone cements is influenced by various parameters, such as composition of the cement, porosity, and preparation of the cement. The addition of radiopacifier and antibiotics to a bone cement slightly decreases the mechanical strength. These additives are necessary to get radiograph opacity and antibiotic protection of the implant, which are important attributes of bone cements. Despite these additives, the resulting cements easily meet the requirements. [16,17]

Although bone cement has a high compressive strength, it is susceptible to fracture that might result from tensile loading. Tensile tests therefore are performed according to ISO 527-1 or ASTM D 638. These standards describe a static test method applicable for all polymer materials. The uniaxial tensile test is executed with flat tapered specimens. The ultimate tensile strength is defined as the maximum stress that a material can withstand before failure in tension. The tensile strength is approximately 50 –60 MPa and there are no significant differences between the tested materials. Again, the addition of antibiotics seems to reduce the tensile strength, but the differences between antibiotic and plain cement are not statistically significant. [18]

The compressive strength of bone cement is higher than the flexural strength and that is higher than the tensile strength. This descending order is found in all polymer materials. That means tensile loading may be a higher risk factor for failure than compressive loading. In vivo, simple tensile loading, however, does not play an important part in reality; complex combinations of different loading types are more relevant. From a physical point of view, bending is a mixture of compressive and tensile loading; therefore, the bending test actually is a realistic test. [17]

One further static test applied with bone cements is the shear strength test according to ASTM D732. This mechanical parameter is important because debonding of the stem–cement interface has been implicated in the initiation of failure of cemented femoral stems. The interface static shear strength is influenced by surface roughness, cement type, and porosity. Surface finish has the greatest effect on the interface strength. Increasing the surface roughness increases the interface shear strength. Increasing the surface roughness to greater than a certain value, however, has no additional affect. Cement type and porosity have a minor influence on the static interface strength. [19]

Furthermore, there are methods to determine fracture properties, such as fracture toughness (ASTM E399 and ISO 13,586) and impact strength (ISO 179/ISO 180/DIN 53,435). There is a correlation between the two methods. For a given specimen configuration, g-irradiation produced a statistically significant decrease in fracture toughness because of the concomitant depreciation in molecular weight. Impact strength is a measure of the energy required to cause a material to fracture when struck by a sudden blow. The addition of radiopacifier and antibiotics together with pores in the cement might have a negative effect on the impact strength. [20]

7.2. Water uptake and glass transition

When considering the mechanical tests described previously, one fact should be taken into account: most of the tests are executed with dry specimens at room temperature. The cement has to perform its task in the human body, however, in contact with body fluid and at a temperature of 37°C. Mechanical properties of polymers vary relative to their temperature and water uptake. The absorption of water results in a lower modulus of elasticity and in a less stiff material. The decreasing stiffness may even be advantageous for fracture resistance and long-term stability of the implant. The water uptake of commercial bone cements is approximately 1%–2% for plain bone cements and slightly higher for antibiotic bone cements. There is high initial water uptake during the first days of incubation at 37°C. The bone cements are completely water-saturated 4–8 weeks after incubation. The glass transition temperature is a physical parameter defining the softening range of a material. Softening means a transition from a hard and rigid glassy state with a high modulus to a soft rubbery state with a low modulus by heating the polymer. If the material for anchoring endoprosthesis is in the rubbery state, there would be a high risk for subsidence of the femoral stem and no stable fixation of the implant would be possible. Bone cements therefore can be used only for fixation of endoprostheses at temperatures less than their glass transition temperature in the glassy state. The glass transition temperatures of acrylic bone cements in a dry state range from 80°–100°C. These are high temperatures compared with the temperature of the human body. The water absorption of the cement, however, results in a reduction in glass transition temperature of approximately 20°–30°C after 8 weeks of incubation in water. The glass transition temperatures of water-saturated bone cements are approximately 60°–70°C. The addition of antibiotics does not lower the glass transition significantly. Considering the pronounced difference between the glass transition temperature and the temperature of the human body, the risk for sinking of the implant caused by creep seems to be very low.[16]

Property	Value range (MPa)
Ultimate tensile strength	36 to 47
Ultimate compressive strength	80 to 94
Bending strength (4 point configuration)	67 to 72
Shear strength	50 to 69
Mean fracture toughness (K_{ic})**	1.52 to 2.02 (MPa$\sqrt{m}$)

*Simplex P, Palacos R, CMW1

**K_{ic}, mean fracture toughness of brittle materials

Table 2. Mechanical properties of three cement brands*

7.3. Creep behavior

Polymers such as PMMA bone cements exhibit a combination of elastic and viscous behavior called viscoelasticity. When a polymer is subjected to a constant load, the resulting deformation can be divided into two parts: the immediate elastic deformation and the time-dependent, continuous deformation. The immediate elastic deformation happens instantaneously by applying load. It is a recoverable deformation essentially independent of time. Following this rapid deformation there is a delayed continuous deformation resulting from stress. One part of this deformation is recoverable in time after releasing load. This part is called delayed elastic deformation or primary creep. The second part of this continuous deformation is a non-recoverable permanent deformation called secondary creep.[21]

Different test methods are described in the standard ASTM D 2990 to measure creep. The specimen is loaded by tensile, compressive, or flexural stress. In each method the change in length of the specimen is measured and divided by the original length for the calculation of creep. All plastic materials including acrylic bone cement creep to a certain extent. The degree of creep depends on several factors, such as composition of the material, temperature, load, and load duration. Delayed injection time of acrylic bone cement increased creep compared with bone cement prepared according to standard injection procedures. Creep therefore depends not only on the material properties, but also on the cement handling by the surgeon.[22] It has been proposed that creep of acrylic bone cement may contribute to loosening of cemented total joint replacements. The long-term prosthetic subsidence rates caused by creep of acrylic cement, however, are small. On the other hand, cement creep relaxes cement stresses and creates a more favorable stress distribution at the interfaces. [3, 16]

7.4. Fatigue behavior

To ensure survival of the cement in the human body, the bone cement must be able to withstand the varying loads it endures. The fatigue properties of the cement thus are of particular significance, and they may determine when a correctly used cement will fail or not. Many studies have dealt with this topic, measuring fatigue properties in different ways. Today three different standard testing procedures are used to characterize the fatigue behavior:

- Four-point bending arrangement recommended by ISO 5833 standard
- Uniaxial pure tensile test with flat tapered specimens according to ISO 527
- Uniaxial compression–tension test with cylindrical tapered specimens according to ASTM F2118
- The first method is equivalent to the bending test method according to ISO 5833.

7.5. Fatigue testing

Fatigue testing is a dynamic test and is executed with a sinusoidal cyclic loading under stress control. The tests are continued until failure or until run-out. The run-out limit is a predetermined number of cycles at which the testing on a specimen is stopped, eg, 5 million or 10 million cycles. The second method is equivalent to tensile testing according to ISO 527. Again, the test run is performed with a sinusoidal cyclic loading under stress control until failure or until run-out. The third method is according to ASTM F2118. The specimens are subjected to fully reversed compressive and tensile loading in a sinusoidal cyclic manner. Again, the tests are continued until failure or until the run-out limit is reached. Most fatigue tests run at a specified frequency, eg, 5 Hz, in buffered saline solutions at 37°C.[16]

For tension–compression, the preliminary results exhibit a steeper decrease that might be caused by a possibly stronger deterioration from the additional compressive loading. The materials behave in a similar way under bending and uniaxial tension. The simplest test configuration is the standardized four-point bending test according to ISO 5833. Additionally the preparation of the specimens for the tension–compression is much more complex than the preparation of specimens for the bending test. For these two reasons the four-point bending is the preferred method for fatigue testing. The environmental conditions in which these experiments are conducted have a considerable influence on the fatigue life. Bone cements have different fatigue behavior if tested dry or in aqueous solution. The tests in air at room temperature result in a stress-number of cycles-curve (S-N-curve) of considerably higher slope. To simulate the body environment, tests should be performed in an appropriate liquid, such as simulated body fluid or Ringer's solution. The results of tests in air at laboratory temperature should be rated carefully.

Furthermore, the sterilization process of the polymer powder has an influence on fatigue behavior of acrylic bone cements. Sterilization by γ-irradiation or b-irradiation significantly lowers the molecular weight of the polymer powder and the resulting cured bone cement, whereas sterilization by ethylene oxide has no influence on the molecular weight of the polymer. Bone cement with high molecular weight has a better fatigue performance than a cement with low molecular weight.[17]

Porosity is a major cause of reduced fatigue life of bone cement. Pores or other inclusions serve to concentrate stress in the material and often initiate fatigue cracks within the bone cement. These cracks ultimately lead to failure. The sources of porosity are air initially surrounding the powder, which is trapped during wetting of the powder, air trapping in the cement during mixing, and air trapping in the cement during transfer from mixing container to application device. Hand-mixed bone cement in an open bowl has a significantly higher number of pores than bone cement mixed in a vacuum mixing system. Modern cement mixing systems reduce cement porosity and enhance cement strength by eliminating the chances of air entrapment in the cement.[23]

8. Antibiotics

Buchholz and Engelbrecht were the first to add gentamicin antibiotic to a bone cement.[3] Initially the antibiotic was added by hand, and subsequently during manufacture, making antibiotic-loaded acrylic cement widely available as part of antimicrobial prophylaxis in primary arthroplasty. It was shown later, that oxacillin, cefazolin, and gentamicin are all stable in PMMA bone cement and were released in active form. The largest release of antibiotics occurred in the first 24 hours, but high bactericidal concentrations of the antibiotics were measured in the periprosthetic bone for up to 21 days after implantation. A small amount of antibiotic elution is observed even after 5 years. Bone cement without any antibiotics had no bacteriostatic effect on *Staphylococcus aureus, Escherichia coli,* and *Pseudomonas aeruginosa* organisms. [24]

Bone cements can function as a matrix for the local application of antibiotics. Because of the high local concentration of an antibiotic in the surroundings of the implant, the use of bone cements has great advantages compared with a systemic antibiotic therapy. The artificial implant is especially sensitive to bacterial contamination on its surface, because the microorganisms may proliferate there almost unhampered by the immune defense of the body. As the bacteria rapidly generate a protective mucus layer and go to an inactive state with low sensitivity to antibiotics, a local antibiotic treatment is important. The pharmacokinetics of the antibiotic release from the matrix is of clinical importance. The local antibiotic concentrations reached must be clearly greater than the minimal inhibitory concentration and the minimal bactericidal concentration for the organisms. Not all antibiotics are suitable for use in bone cements. To avoid the development of resistant strains, a high initial level with a subsequent controlled release for days or weeks is important. The following bacteriologic and physical and chemical factors should be considered in the choice of an antibiotic:

1. Broad antibacterial spectra, including gram-positive and gram-negative organisms
2. Good bactericidal effect in low concentrations
3. Low incidence of primary resistant germs
4. Low rate of development of resistances
5. Low protein bonding
6. Low allergic potential
7. Little effect on bone cement mechanics
8. Chemical and thermal stability
9. Good solubility in water
10. Good release from bone cement

Based on these requirements and release tests, gentamicin has become the favorite antibiotic for bone cements since the early 1970s. Gentamicin is the most common additive because it has, amongst other features, a good spectrum of concentration-dependent bactericidal activity, thermal stability and high water solubility. [7]

Antibiotics are added in the form of powder, which is unable to diffuse through a hard, glassy polymer. So the mechanism of elution of the antibiotics is believed to be closely related to water-absorbing properties of the cement with respect to time and distance from the surface of the cement. The diffusion rate of the antibiotics depends on several factors, such as the chemical composition of the cement, the surface area at the cement-bone interface, and cement handling. For example, Palacos cement containing prepolymerized beads of P(MMA-co-MA) were shown to elute gentamicin at more rapidly than Simplex containing prepolymerized beads of P(MMA-co-S). In addition, vacuum mixing, which decreases the porosity in bone cement, can also alter the kinetics of the elution of antibiotics and was shown to decrease their rate of elution by 50%.[25]

Penner et al investigated the release of vancomycin and tobramycin from bone cement separately or combined in nonvacuum preparations. They observed that the combined use of the 2 antibiotics led to an increased elution of both from cement. Baleani et al also showed that the presence of meropenem broadened the antibacterial spectrum and enhanced the elution of vancomycin from cement. [26]

Since powder gentamicin is a costly antibiotic and is not available for hand-mixing with bone cement in operating rooms, many researchers have tried to add liquid gentamicin to bone cements. The liquid gentamicin, a much less costly antibiotic (1/20 the price of tobramycin) with a broad antimicrobial spectrum, is widely available throughout the world, but there is always a fear of deteriorating the mechanical properties of the bone cement by adding liquid gentamicin. Hsieh PH et al investigated the use of liquid gentamicin, alone and in combination with vancomycin, incorporated into acrylic bone cement as a potential treatment of complex orthopedic infections. They assessed the cement specimens loaded with

480 mg of liquid gentamicin, 4 g of powdered vancomycin, or both antibiotics for elution characteristics, bioactivity, compressive strength, and porosity. Vancomycin elution was enhanced by 146% with the addition of gentamicin liquid, and gentamicin elution was enhanced by 45% when combined with vancomycin. Bioassay confirmed the bactericidal activity of the released antibiotics. Adding liquid gentamicin increased porosity, whereas adding vancomycin did not. Compressive strength decreased by 13%, 37%, and 45% in specimens containing vancomycin, liquid gentamicin, and both antibiotics, respectively.(Table 3) Despite inferior mechanical properties, the temporary nature of cement beads and spacers makes the liquid gentamicin–vancomycin mixture a potentially more cost-effective regimen in bone cement to treat musculoskeletal infections. [27]

	Vancomycin	Gentamicin	Both antibiotics
Porosity* (%)	5.8 ± 2.6	16.8 ± 1.9	22.4 ± 3.4
Compressive strength (MPa)	79.69 ± 6.2	57.99 ± 1.5	50.32 ± 4.9

*Porosity as a percentage of the total area.

Table 3. Porosity and ultimate compressive strength of the specimens

Other antibiotics with suitable spectra against orthopaedic infecting organisms, such as cefazolin, ciprofloxacin, linezolid, levofloxacin and rifampin, have been tested according to their elution and bactericidal activities and have been shown that all these antibiotics may be suitable for incorporation into polymethylmethacrylate for management of orthopaedic infections.[28] (Table 4)

But it worth noting that all antibiotics are not suitable for adding to bone cements. Goss et al have shown that amphotericin B does not elute from polymethylmethacrylate bone cement. However, addition of this antifungal increases the mechanical strength by forming covalent crosslinks in the PMMA matrix, imparting better mechanical properties. [29]

Antibiotics premixed into the cement by the manufacturer can be advantageous since the addition of antibiotic powder manually can lead to agglomeration and a decrease in the mechanical strength of the cement. Antibiotics are added to cement in the powdered form since it was demonstrated that the addition of liquid antibiotics resulted in a decrease in mechanical strength due to interference with the early stages of polymerization of the MMA monomer. The amount of antibiotic powder required for a therapeutic level of elution is approximately 0.5 to 2 g in a standard 40-g package of prepolymerized PMMA powder. Note that antibiotic powder, like radiopacifiers and pores, also results in defects or flaws in bone cement. The flexural strength of antibiotic-containing cement was shown to be lower than that of cement without antibiotics, and the toughness of antibiotic-containing cement decreased further with excessive amounts of antibiotics. A likely reason for this is that excess amounts of undissolved antibiotics agglomerate into aggregates exceeding the critical flaw size for PMMA. However, doses of 2 g of well-dispersed antibiotic powder may not have any adverse effect on the mechanical properties of bone cement if the size of the inclusions remains below the critical flaw size for PMMA.

Antimicrobial	Amount (%)	AUC (μg/mL/h)	Peak concentration (μg/mL)	Time no longer detectable (h)	Percent in the bead before elution
Cefazolin	2.5	18 ± 3	15 ± 2	2 ± 0	56 ± 2
	7.5	162 ± 33	62 ± 23	10 ± 1	42 ± 4
	15	792 ± 47	147 ± 22	26 ± 1	54 ± 5
Ciprofloxacin	2.5	23 ± 5	5 ± 0	45 ± 3	36 ± 3
	7.5	112 ± 3	15 ± 1	45 ± 5	36 ± 7
	15	307 ± 10	54 ± 3	48 ± 0	31 ± 3
Gatifloxacin	2.5	157 ± 34	15 ± 2	48 ± 0	45 ± 2
	7.5	190 ± 65	19 ± 1	48 ± 0	47 ± 4
	15	499 ± 51	51 ± 3	48 ± 0	50 ± 3
Levofloxacin	2.5	33 ± 4	7 ± 1	48 ± 0	28 ± 3
	7.5	123 ± 7	26 ± 3	48 ± 0	23 ± 3
	15	291 ± 59	52 ± 10	48 ± 0	24 ± 3
Linezolid	2.5	Not detected	<5	0 ± 0	96 ± 5
	7.5	213 ± 53	43 ± 4	12 ± 4	88 ±4
	15	224 ± 155	64 ± 47	22 ± 2	84 ± 4
Rifampin	2.5	5 ± 2	4 ± 1	2 ± 1	21 ± 1
	7.5	147 ± 15	15 ± 2	37 ± 1	27 ± 4
	15	409 ± 46	31 ± 11	48 ± 0	24 ±1

AUC: area under the curve

Table 4. Parameters of release from PMMA for studied antimicrobials

8.1. Costs of antibiotic-loaded bone cement

Currently the increased acquisition cost of commercially available antibiotic-loaded bone-cement products is considerable. Compared with the cost of plain bone-cement products, the cost of equivalent antibiotic-loaded bone-cement products is increased anywhere from $284 to $349 (United States dollars) per 40-g packet. If the historical 11% usage of antibiotic-loaded bone cement increased to 50% of the estimated 500,000 primary total joint arthroplasties performed annually in the United States, and if two packets of cement (at a $300 increased cost per packet) were used for each joint replacement, the increase in overall health-care costs would be $117,000,000 for the 195,000 additional cases. This estimated increased health-care cost must be balanced with the potential cost savings associated with a realized reduction in the rate of infection associated with routine use of antibiotic-loaded bone cement for prophylaxis in primary total joint replacement. At an approximately $50,000 cost for the treatment of an infection at the site of a total joint replacement, there would have to be 2340 fewer infected patients among the additional 195,000 patients for the routine use of antibiotic-loaded bone cement to be fiscally neutral. With a rather high estimated infection rate of 1.5%, a deep postoperative infection could be expected to develop in 2925 of 195,000 patients. In other words, the rate of deep periprosthetic infection would need to be reduced from this 1.5% to 0.3% to recover the costs associated with the routine use of commercially available low-dose antibiotic-loaded bone cement in primary total joint arthroplasty. Moreover, while the estimated costs for the treatment of an infection at the site of a total joint arthroplasty do not account for morbidity and mortality associated with the treatment required, the increased costs associated with the treatment of more drug-resistant organisms are unknown. [30]

8.2. Choice of antibiotic in antibiotic-loaded bone cement used prophylactically

The aminoglycoside antibiotics were originally selected for use in antibiotic-loaded bone cement because of their broad bacterial coverage and their low allergy profile. Because the level of gentamicin or tobramycin in the joint is often ten times greater than safe blood levels, the efficacy of those drugs is excellent unless the organism has a specific resistance to them. Gentamicin and tobramycin are also the only antibiotics currently available in commercially premixed low-dose antibiotic-loaded bone-cement preparations. As mentioned above, however, low doses of other types of antibiotics, including several of the cephalosporins, have been hand-mixed into bone-cement preparations, and those preparations have had good success in prophylactic applications. Allergic reactions have not been reported, to our knowledge, but it is prudent for the surgeon to consider the individual patient's allergy history before selecting the antibiotic for antibiotic-loaded bone cement. There has been considerable research on the primary bacterial contaminants in total joint surgery.

Al-Maiyah et al. took 627 blood-agar impressions of the gloved hands of surgical personnel during the performance of fifty total hip arthroplasties in England. Bacteria grew on culture of fifty-seven impressions (9%); 69% were coagulase-negative staphylococci, 12% were Micrococcus, 9% were diphtheroids, and 6% were *Staphylococcus aureus*. Of the coagulase-negative staphylococci, only 52% were sensitive to cefuroxime. In contrast, Ridgeway et al. found *Staphylococcus aureus* in 50% of the surgical site infections (both superficial and deep) in their multiple-hospital study in England. More than half of the *Staphylococcus aureus* isolates were methicillin-resistant. Thus, it appears that staphylococcal species are the primary bacteria toward which antibiotic-loaded bone cement would be directed. The currently available commercial gentamicin or tobramycin-loaded bone cements provide sufficient elution concentrations to be bactericidal even against methicillin-resistant organisms. Vancomycin may also be added to bone cement, but it has a lower efficacy than gentamicin or tobramycin at these concentrations. The use of vancomycin should be considered in revisions following primary arthroplasties in which gentamicin or tobramycin-loaded bone cement had been used because of the prevalence of gentamicin resistance in association with such revisions. Cephalosporins may also be considered for antibiotic-loaded bone cement that is to be used prophylactically but may not be effective against methicillin-resistant organisms.[30]

9. Adverse effects of bone cement

9.1. Cardiopulmonary complications

Cardiopulmonary complications associated with PMMA have been reported in conjunction with hip arthroplasty and VA. Prior studies have postulated that PMMA-associated hypoxia, hypotension, and death may occur as a result of the toxic effects of monomer or anaphylaxis. Other literature indicates that the application of PMMA may lead to embolization of marrow debris and neurogenic reflex, thus adversely affecting cardiopulmonary function. Pulmonary infarction and death have been reported as a result of embolization of PMMA that was injected in liquid state following VA. [2]

9.2. Hypersensitivity to components of methylmethacrylate, especially benzoyl peroxide

A small but significant proportion of cemented total knee arthroplasties develop early aseptic loosening. Polyethylene debris is unlikely to be the cause in the small subgroup that experiences early loosening. Allergy to polymethylmethacrylate bone cement or its constituents has been reported in dentistry, dermatology, and joint arthroplasty. Although allergy to polymethylmethacrylate bone cement or its constituents is unusual, the possibility of a systemic inflammatory response and consequent pain and loosening must be considered. Benzoyl peroxide is an essential component of bone cement. Direct evidence for allergic reactions to benzoyl peroxide has been reported in dental and dermatological literature. The currently accepted model for this delayed hypersensitivity is that a hapten such as benzoyl peroxide conjugates with a body protein, which creates a neoantigen capable of stimulating an immune response. This hypersensitivity places the patient at risk of developing insidious pain, a systemic inflammatory response, and possibly aseptic loosening. After revision to uncemented femoral and tibial components, the patient's symptoms vastly improved.[31]

9.3. Presence of components of methylmethacrylate in serum and breast milk

Singh et al. reported dose-related teratogenic and fetal toxic effects of methacrylic acid administered via the intraperitoneal route in rats. McLaughlin et al. exposed pregnant mice to very high vapor concentrations of methacrylic acid of 1330 parts per million for two consecutive hours, twice daily. The mice demonstrated no evidence of fetal toxicity or teratogenic effects; in fact, there was a slight increase in fetal weight with methacrylic acid exposure. The only published study that has addressed methacrylic acid exposure during lactation involved a patient undergoing arthroplasty, not operating room personnel who were exposed to methacrylic acid vapors. In that study, Hersh et al. found undetectable levels of polymethylmethacrylate in breast milk that was collected thirty-six hours after hybrid total hip arthroplasty in a twenty-nine-year-old woman who was five months postpartum. Linehan et al. showed undetectable levels of methacrylic acid (at the 0.5-part-per-million level) in the serum and breast milk of two lactating surgeons who had been exposed to typical operating room conditions without the use of personal exhaust systems. [32]

10. Composite bone cements

PMMA-based bone cement has a high modulus but low toughness compared with ductile polymers. In order to address the lack of fracture toughness and fatigue strength, many investigators who have developed new composite PMMA cements use the concept of fiber reinforcement and incorporate a low-volume fraction of chopped fibers of approximately 1% to 2%.[33] Several types of fibers, such as fibers made of carbon, polyethylene terephthalate, oriented PMMA, ultra high molecular weight polyethylene, titanium, aramid, Kevlar, graphite, steel, and zirconia fibers with and without acrylic coating have been used to reinforce PMMA-based bone cement.[33-6] While these composites have displayed improved fatigue failure properties, biocompatibility concerns and complications of processing have prevented their implementation in the manufacture of PMMA bone cement.

Author details

Hamid Reza Seyyed Hosseinzadeh, Mohammad Emami, Farivarabdollahzadeh Lahiji, Ali Sina Shahi, Aidin Masoudi and Sina Emami

Akhtar Orthopaedic Hospital, Shahid Beheshti University of Medical Sciences, Iran

References

[1] Dennis, C., et al. (2005). The genesis and evolution of acrylic bone cement Orthop Clin N Am , 36(2005), 1-10.

[2] Todd, J., et al. (2010). DO Polymethylmethacrylate: Properties and Contemporary Uses in Orthopaedics, J Am Acad Orthop Surg 2010; , 18, 297-305.

[3] Webb, J. C. J., et al. (2007). The role of polymethylmethacrylate bone cement in modern orthopaedic surgery J Bone Joint Surg [Br] 2007;B:851-7., 89.

[4] Kuehn KD, et al. Acrylic bone cements: Composition and properties. Orthop Clin North Am (2005). , 36, 17-28.

[5] Charnley, J., et al. (1964). The bonding of prostheses to bone by cement. J Bone Joint Surg Br 1964; , 46, 518-529.

[6] Webb JC, et al. (2007). The role of polymethylmethacrylate bone cement in modern orthopaedic surgery. J Bone Joint Surg Br 2007; , 89, 851-857.

[7] Klaus-Dieter, K., et al. (2005). Acrylic bone cements: composition and properties Orthop Clin N Am , 36(2005), 17-28.

[8] Anuj Bellare, et al. (2007). orthopaedic bone cement, the adult hip, second edition, 2007, LWW, , 144-155.

[9] Reckling FW, et al. (1977). The bone- cement interface temperature during total joint replacement. J Bone Joint Surg 1977;59A: , 80-2.

[10] Lewis, G., et al. (1997). Properties of acrylic bone cement: state of the art review. J Biomed Mater Res 1997; , 38, 155-82.

[11] Gladius Lewis, et al. (2007). Preheating Acrylic Bone Cement Powder Is Not Recommended for All Brands. *The Journal of Arthroplasty*, 22(3).

[12] Lewis, G., et al. (1998). Effect of sterilization method on properties of Palacos R acrylic bone cement. *Biomaterials*, 117 EOF-24 EOF.

[13] Bridgens, J., et al. (2008). Stockley Orthopaedic bone cement DO WE KNOW WHAT WE ARE USING? J Bone Joint Surg [Br] 2008;B:643-7., 90.

[14] Macaulay, W., et al. (2002). Differences in bone-cement porosity by vacuum mixing, centrifugation, and hand mixing. J Arthroplasty 2002; , 17, 569-75.

[15] Messik, K. J., et al. (2007). Vacuum-mixing cement does not decrease overall porosity in cemented femoral stems. J Bone Joint Surg [Br]2007;B:1115-21., 89.

[16] Klaus-Dieter Kuehn, et al. (2005). Acrylic bone cements: mechanical and physical properties Orthop Clin N Am , 36(2005), 29-39.

[17] Demian HW, et al. (1998). Regulatory perspective on characterization and testing of orthopedic bone cements. *Biomaterials*, 19, 1607-18.

[18] Harper EJ, et al. (2000). Tensile characteristics of ten commercial acrylic bone cements. J Biomed Mater Res 2000; , 53(5), 605-16.

[19] Wang JS, et al. (2003). Factors affecting the static shear strength of the prosthetic stem-bone cement interface. J Mater Sci Mater Med 2003; , 14, 55-61.

[20] Lewis, G., et al. (2000). Correlation between impact strength and fracture toughness of PMMA-based bone cements. *Biomaterials*, 21(8), 775-81.

[21] Verdonschot, N., et al. (2000). Creep properties of three low temperature-curing bone cements: a preclinical assessment. J Biomed Mater Res 2000; , 53, 498-504.

[22] Lee AJ, et al. (2002). Factors affecting the mechanical and viscoelastic properties of acrylic bone cement. J Mater Sci Mater Med 2002; , 13, 723-33.

[23] Lewis, G., et al. (1999). Effect of two variables on the fatigue performance of acrylic bone cement: mixing method and viscosity. Biomed Mater Eng 1999; , 9, 197-207.

[24] Armstrong, M., et al. (2002). Antibiotic elution from bone cement: a study of common cement-antibiotic combinations. *Hip International*, 12, 23-7.

[25] Perry AC, et al. (2002). Antimicrobial release kinetics from polymethylmethacrylate in a novel continuous flow chamber. Clin Orthop Relat Res. 2002; , 403, 49-53.

[26] Baleani, M., et al. (2008). Biological and biomechanical effects of vancomycin and meropenem in acrylic bone cement. J Arthroplasty. 2008 Dec; Epub 2008 Apr 14., 23(8), 1232-8.

[27] Hsieh PH, et al. (2009). Liquid gentamicin and vancomycin in bone cement: a potentially more cost-effective regimen. J Arthroplasty. 2009 Jan; Epub 2008 Feb 14., 24(1), 125-30.

[28] Anguita-Alonso, P., et al. (2006). Comparative study of antimicrobial release kinetics from polymethylmethacrylate. Clin Orthop Relat Res. 2006 Apr; , 445, 239-44.

[29] Goss, B., et al. (2007). Elution and mechanical properties of antifungal bone cement. J Arthroplasty. 2007 Sep; Epub 2007 Jul 25., 22(6), 902-8.

[30] Jiranek WA, Hanssen AD, Greenwald AS. ((2006).)Antibiotic-loaded bone cement for infection prophylaxis in total joint replacement. J Bone Joint Surg Am. 2006 Nov; Review., 88(11), 2487-500.

[31] Edwards SA, et al. (2007). Hypersensitivity to benzoyl peroxide in a cemented total knee arthroplasty: cement allergy. J Arthroplasty. 2007 Dec; Epub 2007 Jan 18., 22(8), 1226-8.

[32] Linehan CM, et al. (2006). Serum and breast milk levels of methylmethacrylate following surgeon exposure during arthroplasty. J Bone Joint Surg Am. 2006 Sep; , 88(9), 1957-61.

[33] Kotha, S., et al. (2009). Reinforcement of bone cement using zirconia fibers with and without acrylic coating. J Biomed Mater Res A. 2009 Mar 15; , 88(4), 898-906.

[34] Kotha SP, et al. (2006). Improved mechanical properties of acrylic bone cement with short titanium fiber reinforcement. J Mater Sci Mater Med. 2006 Aug; , 17(8), 743-8.

[35] Kotha SP, et al. (2006). Improved mechanical properties of acrylic bone cement with short titanium fiber reinforcement. J Mater Sci Mater Med. 2006 Aug; , 17(8), 743-8.

[36] May-Pat, A., et al. (2011). Flores-Gallardo SG. Comparative study on the mechanical and fracture properties of acrylic bone cements prepared with monomers containing amine groups. J Mech Behav Biomed Mater. 2012 Feb; Epub 2011 Nov 17., 6, 95-105.

Chapter 6

All Ceramic Tripolar THA to Prevent Dislocations in Risky Patients

Jean-Yves Lazennec, Adrien Brusson and
Marc Antoine Rousseau

Additional information is available at the end of the chapter

http://dx.doi.org/10.5772/53251

1. Introduction

Dislocation remains one of the most common complications after total hip arthroplasty (THA), especially for ceramic-on-ceramic prostheses. Suboptimal implant positioning, muscular insufficiency, significant lower limb discrepancies, and neurological problems are standard causes for THA dislocations or subluxations [1-3]. Instability may also be linked to 2 specific mechanisms, lever-out (with impingement) and shear-out (without impingement).

Microseparation and edge loading of the femoral ball head on the insert are relevant issues for hard-on-hard bearing surfaces, either ceramic on ceramic or metal on metal [4-5]. Tripolar polyethylene (PE) THAs have been extensively used for more than 20 years in Europe [2, 6-7], and clinical data demonstrate that they provide significant improvement in hip stability. Significant concerns nonetheless remain about PE wear and osteolysis. Recent developments in ceramic matrix composites and the introduction of Biolox Delta® with improved fracture toughness have further reduced the risk of fracture and also extended the design flexibility of the material. A novel tripolar all-ceramic bearing for hip prostheses (CeramConcept, Newark, DE, USA) has been designed and developed to deal with the problems described above. The tripolar delta ceramic (TDC) THA combines the functional advantages of the tripolar PE THA with the tribological advantages of ceramic bearings.

2. The concept

The orientation of the cup in terms of anteversion and inclination has significant consequences on the joint's range of motion and resistance to dislocation [8]. The position of the rotation center in the cup-ball head system affects joint stability: it has been shown that an inset of the rotation center of a few millimeters increases the peak resisting moment against dislocation [9][10]. This benefit in terms of stability has a disadvantage, however: it decreases the range of motion of classical ball-insert systems. The TDC joint allows the center of rotation to be located much deeper inside the insert without significant negative impact on the range of motion [10] [11].

The first all-ceramic tripolar joint was a 22/32 combination including a 22-mm head, a 22/32-mm mobile ceramic head secured with a PE ring, and a 32-mm internal diameter ceramic acetabular insert. Another possibility is a 26/36 combination, including a 26-mm head, a 26/36-mm mobile ceramic head (or "intermediate component" or "bipolar head"), and a 36-mm ceramic acetabular insert. All components were manufactured from Biolox Delta ceramic matrix composite, Ceramtec, Germany.

Tripolar hip prostheses have two bearing surfaces: the outer bearing surface, between the acetabular cup and the intermediate component (bipolar head), and the inner bearing surface, between the intermediate component and the femoral head component (Figures 1-2). The outer surface of the intermediate component is a portion of a solid sphere, the center of which is identical to the center of the acetabular insert during joint loading. The center of the inner bearing surface of the intermediate component (bipolar cup) corresponds to the center of the femoral head and is designed to be inset from the center of the outer bearing surface of the intermediate component (i.e., the center of the acetabular component).

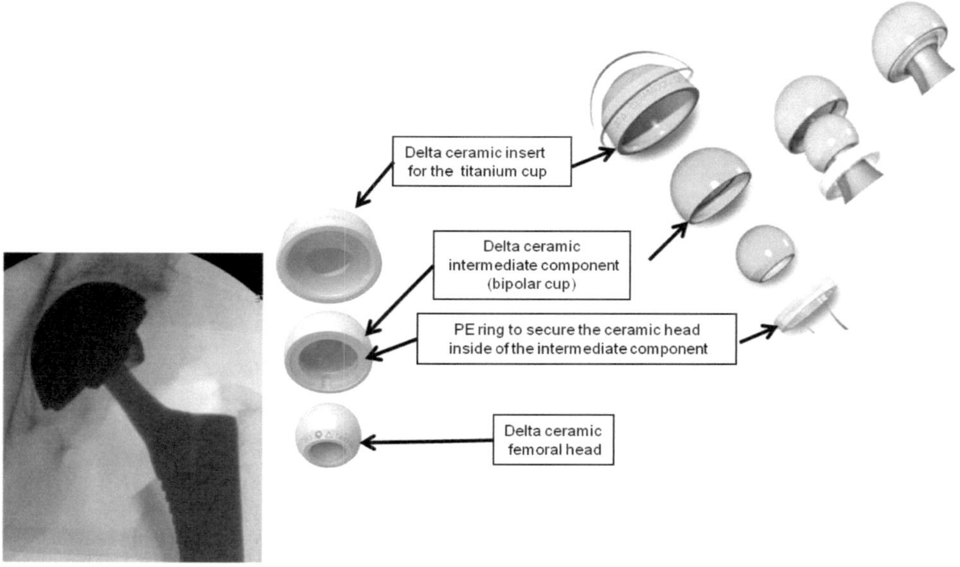

Figure 1. Tripolar hip prostheses have two bearing surfaces: the outer bearing surface, between the acetabular cup and the intermediate component (bipolar head), and the inner bearing surface, between the intermediate component and the femoral head component

http://dx.doi.org/10.5772/53251

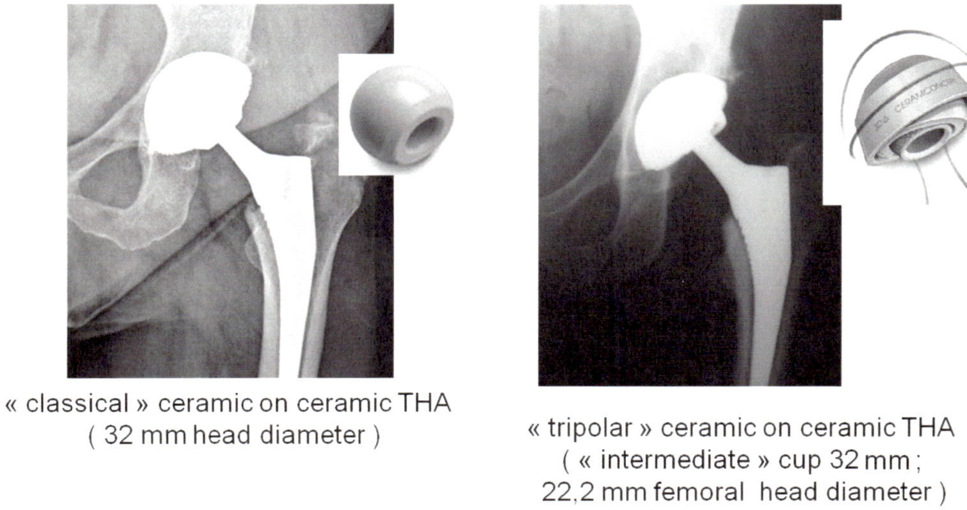

Figure 2. Comparison between a conventional ceramic –ceramic prosthesis and a tripolar delta ceramic prosthesis : Implantation procedures for metal-back or acetabular insert placements or for femoral adjustment are the same. The only originality of the tripolar system is the interposition of a "double femoral ball head" or " bipolar head" on the femoral taper.

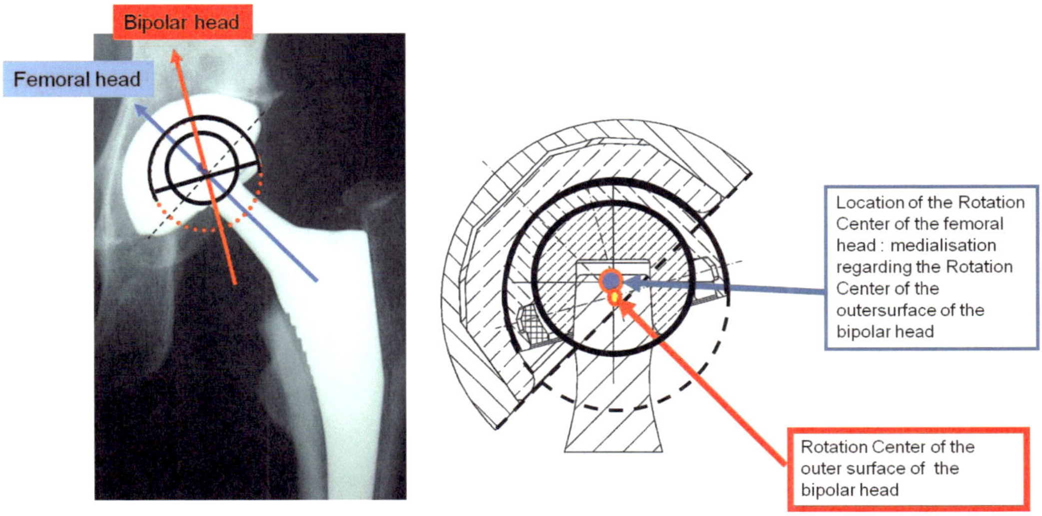

Figure 3. The outer surface of the intermediate component (bipolar head) is a portion of a solid sphere, the center of which is identical to the center of the acetabular insert during joint loading. The center of the inner bearing surface of the intermediate component corresponds to the center of the femoral head and is designed to be inset from the center of the outer bearing surface of the intermediate component (i.e., the center of the acetabular component).

This geometric arrangement thus creates a certain amount of eccentricity between the acetabular component and the femoral head component (Figure 3). If the centers of rotation of the femoral head and of the outer surface of the bipolar head are not aligned when TDC joint loading begins, the intermediate component starts to align itself: the bipolar head (i.e., the intermediate component) can, through the two bearing ceramic delta surfaces, act as a self-adjusting cup and deal with the variations of femoral head and acetabular orientation (Figure 4).

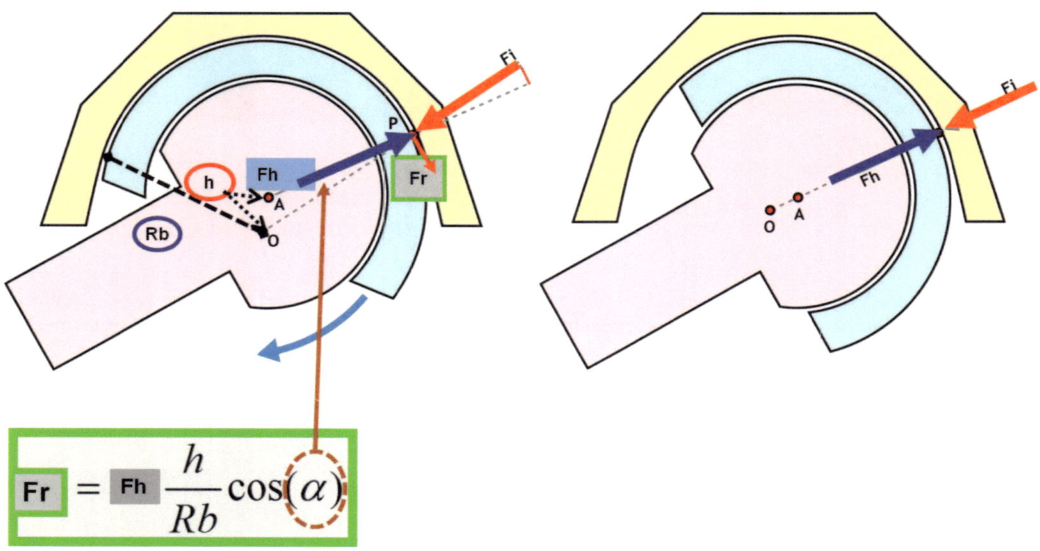

Figure 4. Mechanism of adaptation of the bipolar head in the TCD joint : the non alignment of the rotation centers for the femoral head (A) and the bipolar head (O) induces a self adaptation of the bipolar head. Fh is the contact force which acts on the head at point P. This force is applied on the femoral head through the femoral neck. If friction is neglected, it is necessarily aligned with its centre A. Fi is the reaction force of the acetabular insert upon the bipolar head. If friction is neglected, it is necessarily aligned with its centre O.If Fr and Fi are not mutually in equilibrium, they create a resulting force Fr. The resultant force Fr inducing the adjustment of the bipolar head can be calculated (h is the value of the medialisation of the femoral head center (O A distance) ; Rb is the radius of the bipolar head ; alpha is the angle between Fh et Fi).

3. Preclinical studies

3.1. Evaluation of the mechanical performance of the femoral head and the bipolar head

The mechanical reliability of this device was evaluated by a qualification program according to the criteria defined by CERAMTEC and the standards for marketing authorization. Standard qualification programs were performed on the 22.2-mm ball head and the standard XLW 32/41-mm cup insert. A new program, based on a ball head qualification program, was set up for the bipolar head (intermediate component). Specifications of the bipolar compo-

http://dx.doi.org/10.5772/53251

nent (diameter, roundness, clearance, etc.) are identical to those for the 32-mm ceramic ball head (Figure 5).

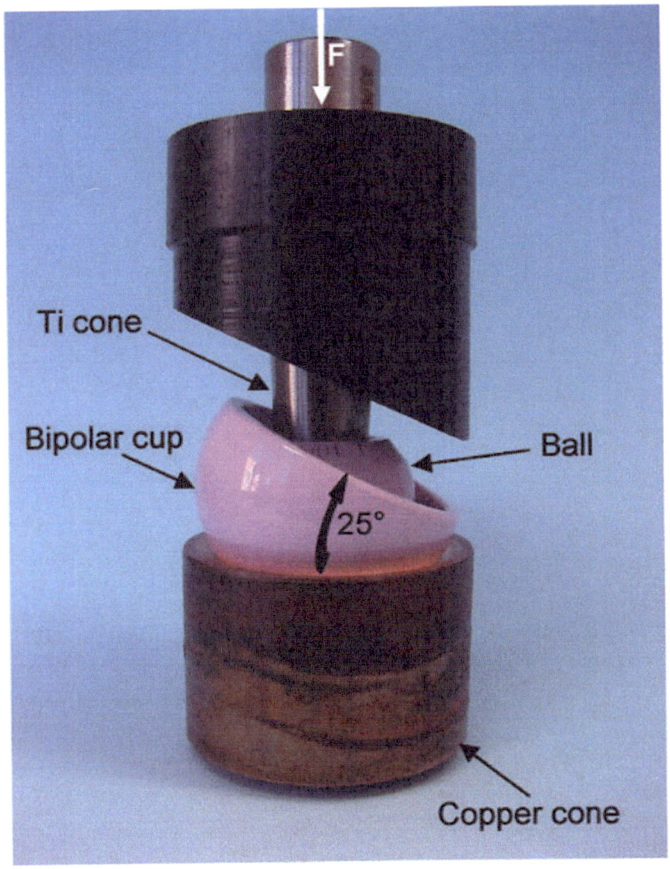

Figure 5. Experimental protocol for burst tests on tripolar delta ceramic (TDC) implants.

The bipolar component has particularly high resistance to fracture, as shown in Table 1 [9].

Static Test (kN)	Avarage value	Minimal value
Avarage value required 46 kN Minimal value required 25 kN	129	58
Post fatigue Test	**Average value**	**Minimal value**
Avarage value required 46 kN Minimal value required 20 kN	91	82

Table 1. Evaluation of the intermediate component: static and post-fatigue tests

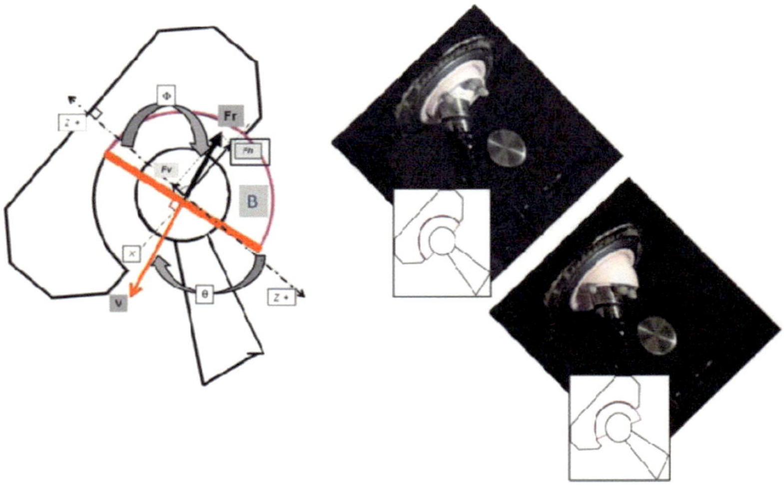

(a)

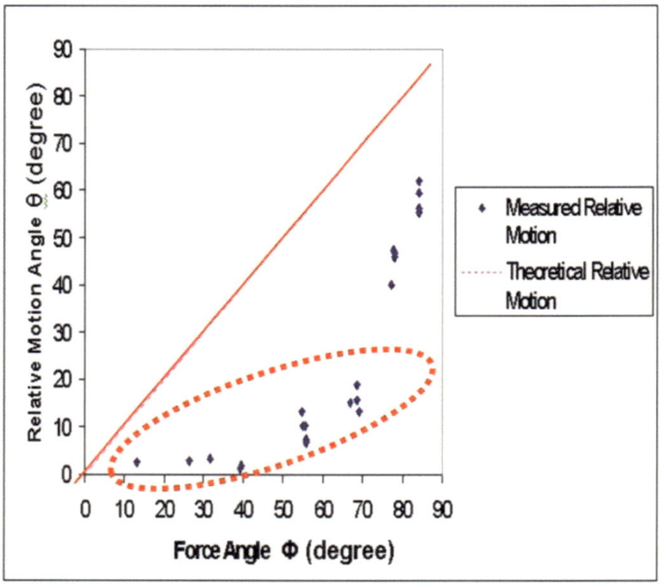

(b)

Figure 6. a) *In-vitro* investigation of the relative motion of the intermediate component for shear-out situations. In shear-out situation, dislocation is supposed to occur without impingement between the acetabular cup and the femoral component. When the direction of the total joint contact force (Fr) goes beyond the edge of the acetabular cup, dislocation occurs. The implementation of an experiment with the tripolar system is more complex than with a classical THA. A series of tests was conducted to record the position of the intermediate component with a motion analysis system. The resultant force on the intermediate component is defined as F_r. The vertical force applied to the intermediate component is defined as F_v; the horizontal force is defined as F_h. The center of the inner bearing surface of the intermediate component (i.e., the center of the femoral head component) is designed to be inset from the outer bearing surface of the intermediate component (i.e., the center of the acetabular component), thus creating a certain amount of eccentricity between the acetabular component and the femoral head component. Theoretically, when the loading on the joint arc surface is not in line with the centers of the arc, self-alignment of the intermediate component will be initiated. Shear-out situation was simulated by applying different magnitudes of F_h while keeping F_v at a fixed value. For a given F_v, as the magnitude of F_h increased, the direction of the resultant force F_r moved toward the edge of the acetabular cup and eventually beyond the edge chamfer. The angle between the direction of Fr and the negative z-axis is defined as Φ; the angle between the direction of the normal vector (V) of the bipolar component (B) and the positive Z-axis is defined as θ. The angle Φ between the resultant force Fr and the negative z-axis was calculated experimentally from the force data recorded by load cells. Reflective markers were rigidly glued to the rim of the intermediate component representing the plane of the bipolar head whose orientation was to be measured. Positional data of the markers implanted on the bipolar component were recorded by motion analysis cameras. Since F_h and F_v were applied in x-z plane, the motion angle between the normal vector of the measured plane and the positive z-axis (θ) was plotted against the resultant force angle (Φ). (b) The dash line 1 represents the θ vs. Φ curve in an idealized theoretical situation (suction force ignored, frictionless). In the ideal situation the normal vector of the intermediate component at any time should seek alignment with the direction of the joint contact force. Dots represent the measured θ vs. Φ curve. Qualitatively, θ increases with the increase of Φ. The rotation of the intermediate component in x-z plane is correlated with the direction of the resultant contact force. At Φ below 40 ° (when the direction of the load was not much deviated from the aligned center-shaft), there was a "toe" area which meant the intermediate component remained in its original horizontal position and did not react to the change of direction of the resultant force F_r.This was due to the effects of surface adhesion and friction : the rotation moment formed by the offset contact forces must first overcome the resistance of suction and friction before it can effectively rotate the intermediate component. As Φ went beyond the toe region, the slope of the experimental curve gradually increased ; the slope of the curve is not exactly superimposable to that of curve 1 because of the suction force and friction.

3.2. Biomechanical tests

- Two typical scenarios (lever-out and shear-out) that can lead to dislocations were investigated. The studies provided evidence that the relative motion of the intermediate component is closely related to the eccentricity between this component and the femoral head [11-12].

We compared the adaptation in impingement situations with lever-out loading between a standard ceramic joint (32-mm ball head/ceramic insert) and the TDC, with a 32-mm self-adjusting cup.

- The variable for assessing dislocation stability was torque during subluxation (resisting moment) against levering the head out of the cup [13]. With the standard system (ceramic ball and socket), dislocation appears as soon as there is contact between the femoral neck and the acetabular insert because of the moment applied. This dislocation by impingement is directly related to range of motion.

The mechanism with the TDC system is different, as are the steps involved. First, the ball head alone rotates. In a second stage, contract forces cause rotation of the bipolar head. Finally, the ball head and the bipolar head rotate together [14]. The moment that must be applied to the joint to obtain luxation is higher than for the conventional system: the increase of this peak resisting moment has been measured at 18.71%

Shear-out loading has also been investigated: the direction of the normal vector (V) of the intermediate component (bipolar head) expresses its relative motion. Adaptation was explored by evaluating the orientation of V in various directions and at various magnitudes of the force to the TDC joint. The orientation of the resultant force (Fr) on the bipolar head is expressed by the angle Φ (Figure 6). Until that angle reaches 40°, the intermediate component remains in its original position, not reacting to the change of direction of this Fr force.

At that point, the intermediate piece adapts and the curve expressing the orientation of vector V changes abruptly.

3.3. Tribological tests

- Simulator studies were carried out under ISO standard conditions, but also under microseparation conditions that replicated head/cup rim contact at heel strike.
- Microseparation is most appropriate for the evaluation of ceramic bearings, as the experimental conditions are optimal for reproducing clinical wear rates and wear mechanisms, including stripe wear, as found on standard ceramic-on-ceramic retrievals. The aim of the tribological tests was to assess the wear characteristics under standard and swing phase microseparation between 200 and 500 μm for a total of 5 million cycles with the Leeds II Physiological Anatomical hip joint simulator [15].
- Under standard conditions, wear was very low on both the tripolar and the conventional ceramic-on-ceramic bearings. The wear of the tripolar all-ceramic hip was less than 0.01 mm^3/million cycles, which is the detection limit for wear measurement, and the conventional ceramic-on-ceramic bearing produced a wear rate of 0.04 mm^3/million cycles. The difference between these very low wear rates is not clinically significant.
- Under microseparation conditions, wear performance differed significantly. In a previous study, conventional Biolox Delta components were tested under microseparation conditions in the same simulator with reported wear rates of 0.32 mm^3/million cycles during bedding-in (0-1 million cycles) that then fell to a steady state wear rate of 0.12 mm^3/million cycles (1-5 million cycles) [8, 12]. Furthermore, stripe wear appeared on the standard Biolox Delta heads and increased the surface roughness Ra from <0.005 μm to between 0.02 μm and 0.13 μm.
- Testing of the TDC joint showed no macroscopic visual evidence of wear. Wear was less than 0.01 mm^3/million cycles (i.e., below the detection limit for wear measurement). No stripe wear was observed; the surface roughness of the ball heads and the outer and inner surfaces of the bipolar head were smoother at the end of the test, indicating that they had undergone a polishing effect.
- The design of the TDC joint with its mobile ceramic head prevented edge loading of the head on the edge of the cup, so significantly reduced wear under these severe, but clinically relevant microseparation conditions [15].

Dislocation tests have been performed to evaluate the resistance of the PE ring in securing the ball head inside the intermediate component. Results were similar to those for similar PE rings that have been used for more than 18 years in standard double-mobility hip joints. The average maximum load for clipping the PE ring was 151.1 N before the tests; it rose to 175.5 N after 5 million cycles of microseparation. The increase in clipping resistance is due to the water load of the ring that occurs in the course of 5 million cycles. The wear volume of the PE rings could not be accurately quantified as it was within the systematic error of the soak control ring. The back side of the PE rings showed no damage, with only a light polishing effect observed in places [9].

http://dx.doi.org/10.5772/53251

4. Clinical data

Clinical results come from the first 2000 consecutive cases in a multicenter study. No specific learning curve was necessary: the surgeons did not change their implantation procedures for metal-back or acetabular insert placements or for femoral adjustment. The only originality of the system is the interposition of a "double femoral ball head" on the femoral taper. Positioning the femoral head on the taper is simple, as the intermediate cup is easily secured in a second step with the PE ring (Figure 7,8,9) [10].

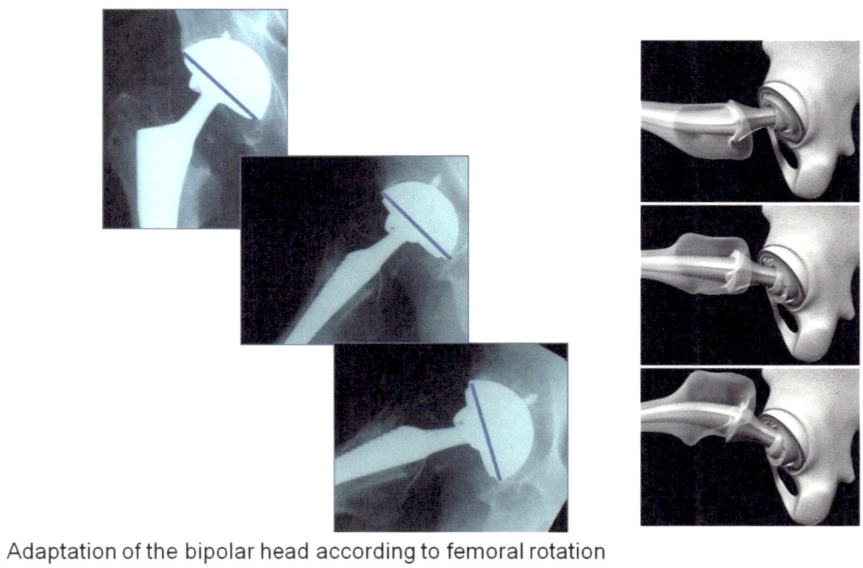

Figure 7. Adapted of the bipolar head according to femoral rotation

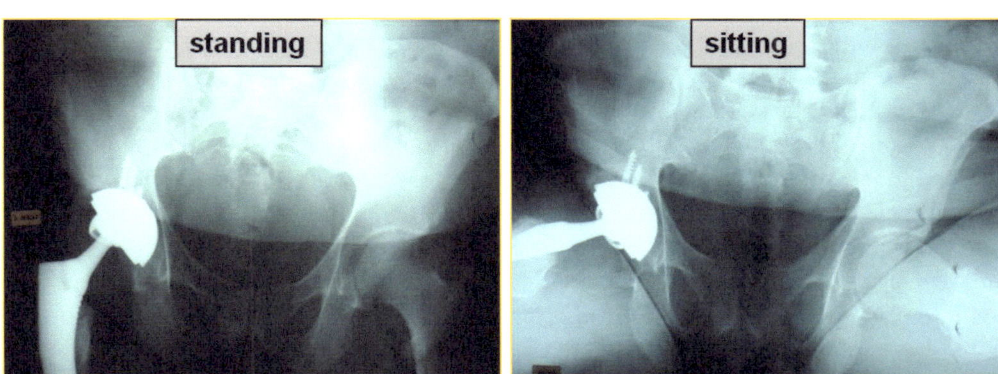

Figure 8. Adaptation of the bipolar head according to standing and sitting position

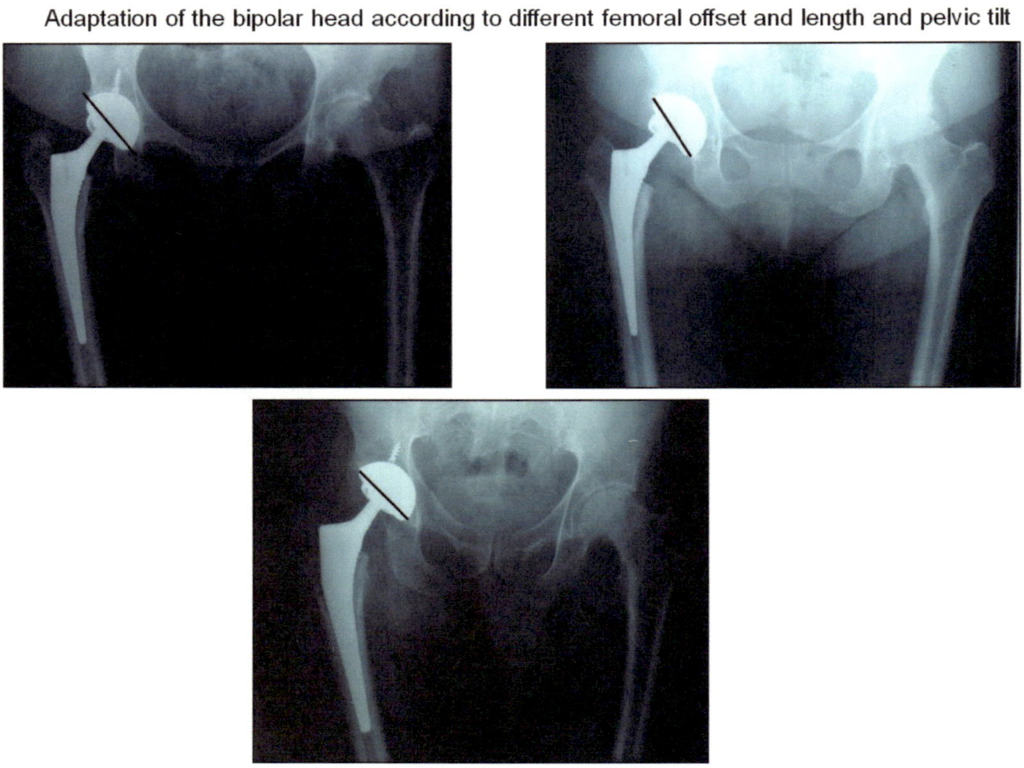

Figure 9. Adaptation of the bipolar head according to different femoral offset and length and pelvic tilt

In our experience, indications for this device are risk of instability, stiff coxarthrosis, osteonecrosis, revisions, oblique pelvis or significant rotational problems, neurological disorders, and some patient problems (alcoholism and psychiatric disorders). The Harris hip score indicates that clinical changes are similar to those with standard THA. The dislocation rate was 0.6%, despite a posterior approach in 87% of the cases. The main explanations were inadequate reconstitution of femoral neck length and/or offset. In a few cases (1.2%), patients described some occasional and irreproducible loud noise from the hip area, similar to that described for standard PE double-mobility systems. Experience with the double mobility PE joints has related this noise to sudden relocation of the intermediate component. The phenomenon is completely different from squeaking in terms of sound characteristics and mechanical aspects. A specific radiologic protocol allowed us to use the EOS® low dose imaging system to observe the adaptation of the intermediate component in standing and sitting positions. The mobility of the intermediate component is consistent with earlier studies and with experimental data. In some patients with significant lower-limb anatomic abnormalities, the tripolar system has been a successfully used as a salvage procedure to resolve cases with complex instability (Figure 10).

http://dx.doi.org/10.5772/53251

		Bipolar cup	Acetabular cup
standing	Frontal inclination	18°	32°
	anteversion	- 46°	45°
sitting	Frontal inclination	41°	36°
	anteversion	43°	42°

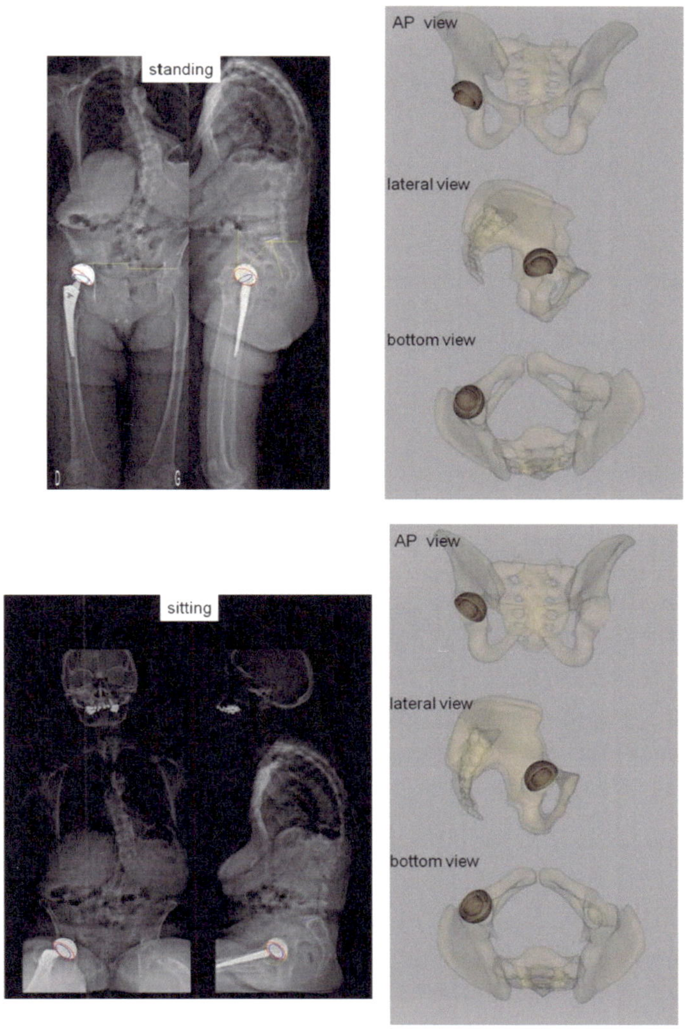

Figure 10. EOS imaging in standing and sitting position. In this case, the scoliosis including a significant pelvic rotation induces a specific adaptation of the intermediate component (bipolar head). One can observe the adaptation of the bipolar head with retroversion in standing position to compensate the hyperanteversion of the femoral neck. The orientation of the bipolar head is significantly different from the acetabular cup anteversion. In sitting position, the adjustment is different and the 2 cups anteversions are equivalent.

5. Conclusions

The use of the tripolar all-delta-ceramic joint appears to be an interesting alternative for optimizing THA function where, as in some cases, no ideal solution can be found for acetabular implantation. The self-adaptation of the intermediate cup can be demonstrated: the additional outer-bearing surface motion creates a second adjustable acetabulum. Its effectiveness against dislocation and microseparation can be explained and documented experimentally. The tripolar ceramic joint provides significant resistance to wear and stripe wear. Nevertheless, it cannot compensate for suboptimal THA implantation resulting in excessive shear-out laxity due to shortening of the head-neck length or lack of femoral offset [3, 16].

Author details

Jean-Yves Lazennec[1], Adrien Brusson[2] and Marc Antoine Rousseau[1]

1 Department of orthopedic and trauma surgery, La Pitié-Salpétrière hospital. Paris, France

2 Department of Anatomy, université Pierre et Marie Curie, Paris, France

References

[1] Jolles, B.M., P. Zangger, and P.F. Leyvraz, Factors predisposing to dislocation after primary total hip arthroplasty: a multivariate analysis. J Arthroplasty, 2002. 17(3): p. 282-8.

[2] Lautridou, C., et al., [Survival of the cementless Bousquet dual mobility cup: Minimum 15-year follow-up of 437 total hip arthroplasties]. Rev Chir Orthop Reparatrice Appar Mot, 2008. 94(8): p. 731-9.

[3] von Knoch, M., et al., Late dislocation after total hip arthroplasty. J Bone Joint Surg Am, 2002. 84-A(11): p. 1949-53.

[4] Ishida, T., et al., Detailed wear mapping of retrieved second-generation metal on metal THR. Annual Meeting of the Orthopaedic Research Society, 2006. Poster No: 1656.

[5] Stewart, T.D., et al., Long-term wear of ceramic matrix composite materials for hip prostheses under severe swing phase microseparation. J Biomed Mater Res B Appl Biomater, 2003. 66(2): p. 567-73.

[6] Grigoris, P., M.J. Grecula, and H.C. Amstutz, Tripolar hip replacement for recurrent prosthetic dislocation. Clin Orthop Relat Res, 1994(304): p. 148-55.

[7] Leclercq, S., S. el Blidi, and J.H. Aubriot, [Bousquet's device in the treatment of recurrent dislocation of a total hip prosthesis. Apropos of 13 cases]. Rev Chir Orthop Reparatrice Appar Mot, 1995. 81(5): p. 389-94.

[8] Lazennec, J.Y., A. Brusson, and M.A. Rousseau, Hip-spine relations and sagittal balance clinical consequences. Eur Spine J, 2011. 20 Suppl 5: p. 686-98.

[9] Lazennec, J.Y., et al., Two ceramic bearing surfaces with a self adjusting cup: a new application of delta ceramics to reduce the risk of dislocation and subluxation bioceramics and alternative bearings. Bioceramics and alternative bearings in joint arthroplasty, 2005. 10th Biolox Symposium

[10] Lazennec, J.Y., et al., All ceramic tripolar Total Hip Arthroplasty: experimental data and clinical results, in Bioceramics and alternative bearings in joint arthroplasty, F. Benazzo, F. Falez, and M. Dietrich, Editors. 2006, Steinkopff. p. 5-9.

[11] Chen Q, et al., Motion of the intermediate component of an eccentric tripolar T.H.P. Annual Meeting of the Orthopaedic Research Society poster 498, 2005. Poster 1181

[12] Krein, S.W. and E.Y. Chao, Biomechanics of bipolar hip endoprostheses. J Orthop Res, 1984. 2(4): p. 356-68.

[13] Bader R, et al., iomechanical study of resistance to dislocation of the ceramic-ceramic delta tripolar joint. Biomaterialen, 2004.

[14] Chen, Q., et al., Technical note: validation of a motion analysis system for measuring the relative motion of the intermediate component of a tripolar total hip arthroplasty prosthesis. Med Eng Phys, 2005. 27(6): p. 505-12.

[15] Jennings, L.M., et al., Wear and friction characteristics of the tripolat all ceramic hip prosthesis. Annual Meeting of the Orthopaedic Research Society poster 498, 2006.

[16] Toni A., S.A., Ceramic on ceramic: long term clinical experience ed. B.i.j. arthroplasty. 2001: Thieme.

Chapter 7

Short-Stem Hip Arthroplasty

Kálmán Tóth and Gellért Sohár

Additional information is available at the end of the chapter

http://dx.doi.org/10.5772/53134

1. Introduction

Total hip arthroplasty has become a remarkably successful operation for treating osteoarthritis in the last half century. The increased need for better quality of life has led the operation to be extended to younger patients. However, long term results showed a rise in the number of revision surgeries. The longer life expectancy of the patient population led to the demand for multiple revision surgeries for the same patient. In revision surgery numerous technical difficulties are encountered because of bone loss due to the loosening. In addition, these solutions are exceptionally expensive. The search for alternatives led to the modification of the primary components. Improvements have introduced changes to achieve more proximal load transfer to the femur in order to reduce proximal stress shielding and thus preserve bone stock for potential revision surgery. As hip resurfacing declines in popularity, it is likely that there will be a corresponding increase in the number of short stem femoral components in use. Metaphyseal stems combine the advantages of straight stem implant design and hip resurfacing.

The aim of this chapter is to outline the recent developments in short (metaphyseal) stem arthroplasty.

2. Concise review of the pertinent literature

2.1. Rationale

Short metaphyseal femoral stems have been developed in order to improve the results of the standard non-cemented stems. Different designs of short stems are available, with differences in operative technique and published outcomes [Mai et al., 2010; McElroy et al., 2011]. The new generation short-stem hip implants are designed to encourage physiological-like loading to minimize stress-strain shielding and therefore implant loosening in the long term.

Traditionally, femoral stems are tapered, anatomical, or cylindrical. The classic tapered stem has rectangular cross-section, 4 corners and 4 flat surfaces that are compressed into the proximal femur. The second, equally popular design consists of anatomically shaped stems designed to match the shape of the proximal femur. The third design, with its different philosophy of fixation, consists of cylindrical, straight, nontapered, and extensively coated stems achieving distal fixation at the isthmus by means of a "scratch fit" between the fully roughened porous surface of the implant and the slightly smaller, underreamed femoral canal [Mai et al., 2010].

Proximal loading short stems have been designed to improve the results of the traditional non-cemented stems. [d'Imporzano & Pierannunzii, 2006; Renkawitz et al., 2008]. In a study by Westphal et al. the migration and cyclic motion were compared between a new short-stemmed hip prosthesis (Proxima™) and two clinically successful shaft prostheses in order to estimate the primary stability of the new stem [Westphal et al., 2006b]. Initially the short stem migrated more than the shaft prostheses. When cortical contact was achieved or the cancellous bone was compacted sufficient stability was acquired. Therefore, correct positioning and good bone quality are important factors for the short stem. Bony ingrowth is more favorable with the short stem because of the lowered cyclic motion after implantation. The effects of stress shielding are reduced by more physiological loading of the femur because of the new stem's lower bending stiffness [Westphal et al., 2006b].

The following advantages have been reported:

1. bone stock and soft tissue (m. gluteus medius et minimus insertation) preservation, in the greater trochanteric and sub-trochanteric regions, at the time of implantation for future revisions [Khanuja et al., 2011; Morrey, 1989] Fig. 1,
2. decreased stress shielding, caused by metaphyseal bone resorption and diaphyseal cortical hypertrophy [Pipino, 2000],
3. stress concentration at the tip of a distal fixation traditional component causes thigh pain, with the short stem this is eliminated [Khanuja et al., 2011; Mai et al., 2010],
4. the iliotibial band's tension band effect provides compression forces both medially and laterally in the proximal femur. [Leali et al., 2002] Fig. 2, lateral cortex provides a strong support as a second compression column [d'Imporzano & Pierannunzii, 2006]
5. transfers load to the metaphysis from a superior to an inferior direction in a physiological manner [Leali et al., 2002; Walker et al., 1999],
6. the method of implantation eases minimally invasive approaches [McElroy et al., 2011] Fig. 1,
7. wide range of indication (over surface arthroplasty risk index grade 3), all types of bone stock with normal femoral morphology are acceptable [Kim et al., 2011],
8. revision surgery becomes easier because of minimally invasive approach, less soft tissue damage, and the intact bone stock below the lesser trochanter [d'Imporzano & Pierannunzii, 2006].

http://dx.doi.org/10.5772/53134

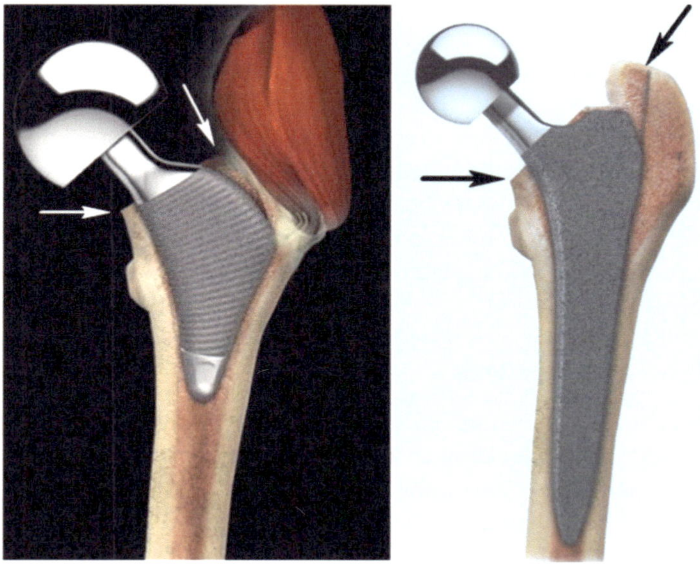

Figure 1. More bone stock and soft tissue preservation (arrows) in the greater trochanteric and sub-trochanteric regions at the time of implantation. Revision surgery becomes easier because of minimally invasive approach and less tissue damage.

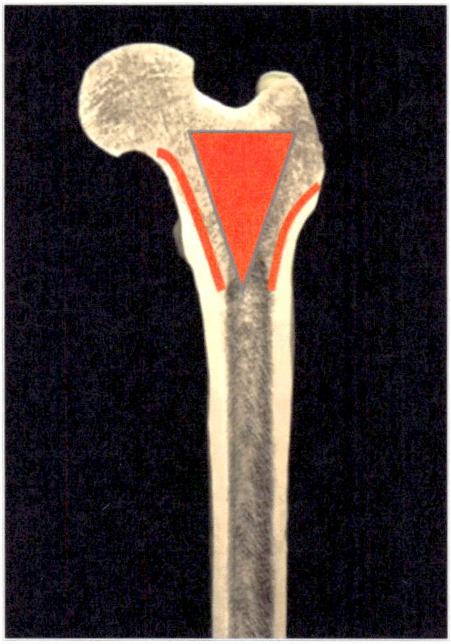

Figure 2. The lateral flare geometry of short stem femoral components loads the proximal wider metaphyseal lateral and medial cortices of the femur. This additional contact area creates a wider base for support and provides a more physiologic load distribution in the proximal femur.

The design and geometry of the implant impacts its ability to transfer loads to the femur [Westphal et al., 2006a]. The lateral flare geometry of short stem femoral components loads the proximal femur more evenly [Walker et al., 1999]. The lateral flare component is stabilized by resting upon the lateral column of cortical bone. This additional contact area creates a wider base for support and provides a more physiologic load distribution in the proximal femur [Leali et al., 2002; Dabirrahmani et al., 2010]. Therefore, femoral components that engage the metaphysis and load the femur both medially and laterally are more stable [Leali et al., 2002]. The stem does not need to be 'press-fitted' into the femur or driven distally. The stem rests upon the proximal wider metaphyseal lateral and medial cortices of the femur [Leali et al., 2002; Walker et al., 1999].

2.2. Outcomes of different short stems

There are no long-term clinical studies available to prove the benefits of these short-stem implants so far. Owing to this lack of clinical data, numerical simulation may be used as a predictor of longer term behaviour. This finite element study predicted both the primary and long-term stability of a short-stem implant. The primary implant stability was evaluated in terms of interface micromotion. This study found primary stability to fall within the critical threshold for osseointegration to occur. Longer term stability was evaluated using a strain-adaptive bone remodelling algorithm to predict the long-term behaviour of the bone in terms of bone mineral density (BMD) changes. No BMD loss was observed in the classical Gruen zones 1 and 7 and bone remodelling patterns were comparable with hip resurfacing results in the literature [Dabirrahmani et al., 2010]

In previous reports on short stems, the HHS values showed an increase of 56 points for the Mayo® stem [Hube et al., 2004] and 33 points for the CUT® stem [Thomas et al., 2004] after a minimum follow-up period of three-months after operation. Our results showed an increase of 39 points with the Proxima™ stem [Tóth et al., 2010]. At a minimum follow-up time of 12 months, an increase in the HHS of 51 [Ender et al., 2007] and 34 points [Thomas et al., 2004] with the CUT® stem, 51 with both the Proxima™ [Ghera & Pavan, 2009] and the Mayo® stem [Morrey, 1989] have been reported. In a similar study [Tóth et al., 2010], we noted a 50 points increase in the HHS with the Proxima™ stem one year post operatively, which is comparable with previous reports.

Some studies reported a vertical or horizontal (varus) migration of short stems requiring a subsequent revision [Ender et al., 2007; Morrey, 1989; Thomas et al., 2004], others described significant radiolucent lines or progressive proximal femoral osteolysis around the short stems without a need for revision [Gilbert et al., 2009; Goebel & Schulz, 2009]. In our reported study [Tóth et al., 2010], no horizontal or vertical migration was found at follow-up at that time, not even with the under-sized and varus positioned stem (Fig. 3). The patient cohort is continuously followed both by radiological and clinical examination. After average follow-up of 4.5 years still no horizontal nor vertical migration was seen.

Thigh pain is a common complaint following traditional non-cemented hip arthroplasty. Among the Proxima™ hip cases evaluated by Tóth et al [Tóth et al., 2010], none of the patients reported any thigh pain even after 4.5 years. Ghera and Pavan reported similar find-

http://dx.doi.org/10.5772/53134

ings with Proxima™ stems [Ghera & Pavan, 2009]. Hube et al also did not find any thigh pain following THA with the Mayo® stem [Hube et al., 2004]. Other studies reported severe thigh pain following short stem implantation (Mayo®, CUT®), requiring revision [Ender et al., 2007; Gilbert et al., 2009; Thomas et al., 2004].

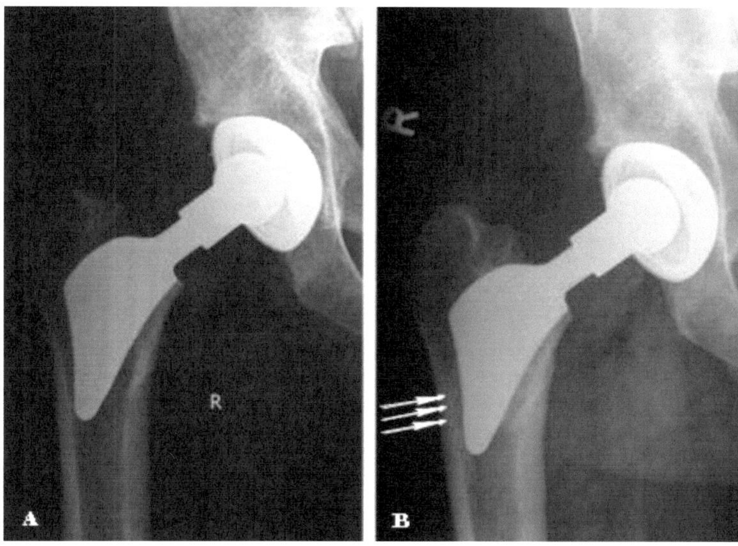

Figure 3. Undersized Proxima™ short-stem in severe varus position (a) immediate postoperative radiograph (b) radiograph 4 year post-op. Even though the long neck is biomechanically disadvantageous, after 4 years the position of the stem is the same. Strengthening of the trabecular structure against the lateral aspect of the stem (arrows) is stimulated by proximal loading (Wolf's law).

Survival of the implanted short stems are summarized in Table 1.

Type	Author	Follow-up	Survival
May® Conservative Stem (Zimmer)	Morrey et al, 2000	5 and 10 years	98.2%
CFP™	Gill et al, 2010	3 years	97%
CFP™	Pons, 2010	3,1 years	100%
Cut® (ESKA)	Steens et al, 2010	6.6 years	98%
Metha™	Synder et al, 2009	1 year	100%
Metha™	Floerkemeier et al, 2012	2.75 years	96%
Proxima™ (DePuy)	Santori et al, 2010	8 years	100%
Proxima™ (DePuy)	Tóth et al, 2010	2.1 years	100%
Proxima™ (DePuy)	Kim et al, 2012	4.1 years	100%
Proxima™ (DePuy)	Ghera et al, 2009	1.7 years	100%
SPS™	Sariali et al 2012	10 years	100%
TaperLoc® Microplasty™	Molli et al 2012	1.8 years	99.7%

Table 1. Reported survival of different short stems

3. Authors' own experience

3.1. Materials and methods

At the Orthopedic Department of the University of Szeged, implantation of the short-stemmed Proxima™ (DePuy; Leeds, UK) began in September 2006. Proxima™ was chosen of all the short stemmed designs on the market because the 36 stem options provide broader variety for the anatomical shape of the femur than the rest. All the 50 procedures were examined clinically and radiologically. Mean age of the patients was 48 (rang from 35 to 61, SD 7) years at time of the surgery. Mean follow-up time was 54 (range from 45 to 61, SD 5) months. Thirty male and 14 female patients were operated on; one female and five male patients had bilateral surgery in two stages. Patients' distribution according to diagnosis was: primary osteoarthritis (OA) in 22, avascular femoral head necrosis in 18, OA with mild dysplasia in 6, post-traumatic OA in 3 and OA secondary to Perthes disease in 1. All procedures were performed by the same surgeon, in the routinely used supine position, from anterolateral approach, with minimally invasive technique. Any intra- or postoperative complications were recorded.

The Proxima™ stem is made of forged titanium alloy, with a Duofix™ HA (porous coating and hydroxyapatite) surface coating. Nine sizes of standard as well as high-offset stems for each side are available. Cementless Duraloc™ porous coated cups (Depuy) with 10° lipped polyethylene liners and 28 mm metal heads were used in all cases.

The indication was hip osteoarthritis or avascular necrosis in young and active patients who were not appropriate candidates for a resurfacing procedure. The following elements were considered contraindications to implantation of a Proixima stem: stem size 1 or 2 for patients with body weight over 100 kg, severe hip dysplasia, previous hip osteotomy or other acquired femoral distortion, cortical index less than 3, severe osteoporosis.

The clinical status of the patients was documented with the Harris Hip Score (HHS) [Harris, 1969]. Low molecular weight heparin was administered for 42 days postoperatively for thromboembolism prophylaxis. Partial weight bearing using crutches was recommended for four weeks post operatively, thereafter full weight bearing with canes was allowed for two additional weeks.

Pre- and post-operative radiographs were taken with identical settings for each patient. Implant migration was assessed according to Martell et al [Martell et al., 1993]. Implant stability was evaluated according to Engh et al [Engh et al., 1987], based on the radiological features of the bone-implant interface. Criteria for radiological loosening of the implant were defined as a radiolucent zone greater than 3 mm, or a horizontal and/or vertical migration greater than 2 mm with an adjacent radiolucent zone [Kim et al., 2003]. Stem alignment was rated as normal if its deviation from the axis of the femoral shaft was 5° or less. A deviation of 6 to 10° was rated as "varus" or "valgus"; a deviation exceeding 10° was rated as "severe varus" or "severe valgus".

3.2. Results

Mean preoperative HHS value was 39 (range: 11 to 71; SD 13). Mean postoperative HHS was 78 at six months (range: 44 to 94; SD 14), 90 at twelve months (range: 52 to 99; SD 13) and 87 at fifty four months (range: 51 to 95; SD 13). We had two complications: an intraoperative fracture was treated by open reduction and fixation with a plate. One patient had dislocation as a result of socket malposition, therefore only the socket's position was adjusted in a revision surgery as the stem had been properly implanted. We did not observe any infection, deep vein thrombosis or pulmonary embolism.

The alignment of the Proxima™ stem on the immediate post-operative radiograph was found to be in severe varus position on two occasions (Fig. 3); nine stems were implanted in varus, and 39 in neutral position. During the follow-up period, no signs of either clinical or radiological loosening were detected.

At the latest follow-up examinations, all respondents stated that they would undergo the operative procedure again. Ninety five percent of the patients were completely satisfied with the outcome of the surgery; the patient who had an intraoperative periprosthetic fracture and the other patient who had a dislocation were satisfied as well.

3.3. Discussion

The number of cases and the length of follow-up are not extensive enough to draw a final conclusion in comparison to traditional arthroplasty procedures. However, it is sufficient to conclude that this procedure greatly differs from standard femoral implantation; therefore a number of factors may be usefully discussed.

3.3.1. Head-neck resection

Attention should be paid to the level of the head-neck resection. A crucial bony surface for fixation of the stem is lost if the cutting plane is more oblique than optimal, i.e. if it is close to the traditional cutting plane. On the medial side the resection should always start at the head-neck junction and run more distally while proceeding laterally, thus creating a wider entrance for the stem (see paragraph 3. below). Ender et al have reported in conclusion of a five-year follow-up of 120 CUT® short-stem implantations, that out of the 11 revision cases, seven femoral necks had ben resected either too diagonally (traditionally) or too widely [Ender et al., 2007].

3.3.2. Positioning

Inadequate hit force during the "round the corner" broaching can result in a varus position of the stem. As no intramedullary guidance is available for the Proxima™ stem due to its metaphyseal location, a varus position is more likely to occur, especially when a minimally invasive approach is used, as visualization of the femoral axis is difficult. It is imperative to perform intraoperative axis measurements during sequential broaching. Until proper experience is acquired the use of fluoroscopy is advisable. Ghera and Pavan reported a study on

65 Proxima™ stem implantations, in which 44 stems were found to be in neutral position, 15 in varus and 6 in valgus [Ghera & Pavan, 2009]. Gilbert et al found that from 34 Mayo® short stems implanted, 14, 19, and 11 cases were neutrally aligned, in varus and in valgus position, respectively [Gilbert et al., 2009]. In our series 2 of 50 Proxima™ stems at the beginning of the learning curve were found to be in severe varus (Fig. 3), 9 in varus and 39 in a neutral position, which seems to be comparable with the previous reports.

3.3.3. Stem sizing

The "round the corner" broaching technique was developed to save bone stock in the lateral segment of the metaphysis. However, it can happen that the broach of the planned size would not fit into the resected part of the femoral neck (Fig. 4).

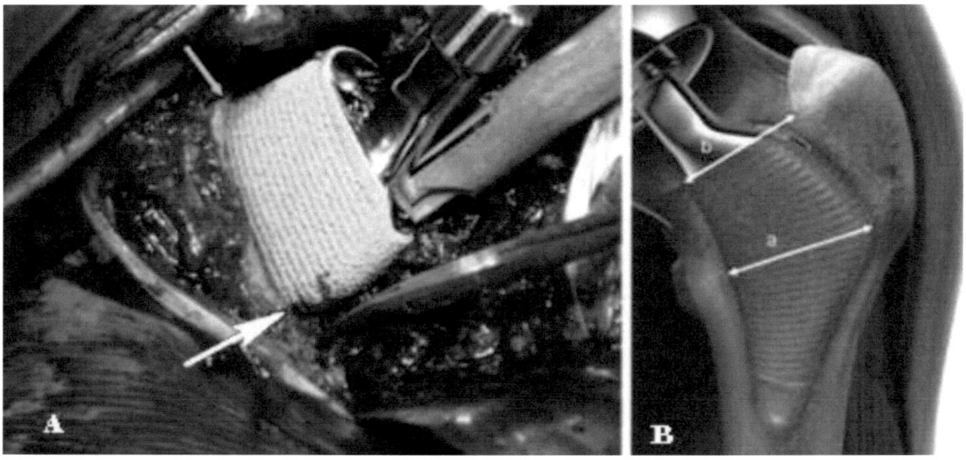

Figure 4. Fitting of the Proxima™ stem into the proximal femoral metaphysis. "Round the corner" technique is used to protect the soft tissues and bone stock, and take advantage of the lateral flare. (a) Intraoperative picture; the cortical bone of the neck is in contact all around with the largest diameter of the stem (arrows) (b) the measured width of the stem (a)is wider than the entrance (b).

In this situation, the following solutions are possible depending on the bone stock quality:

a. When the cancellous bone is weak, the neck in the lateral aspect of the resection plane should be gently enlarged until the stem of the desired size can be implanted. An undersized stem in a weak cancellous bone tends to tilt into varus, and may sink deeper than expected. The deep position of the stem then needs to be corrected by a longer neck, which raises the biomechanically disadvantageous torque force on the short stem (Fig 3).

b. When the cancellous bone is hard, implantation of a Proxima™ stem smaller than the calculated size of the metaphysis is acceptable. Even if the stem does not reach the lateral cortex, the strong and compact cancellous bone can hold the femoral component firmly (Fig. 5).

http://dx.doi.org/10.5772/53134

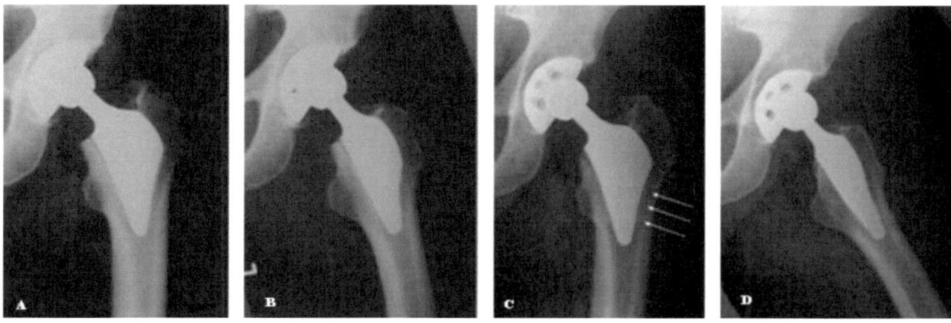

Figure 5. AP and lateral radiographs of a Proxima™ stem in a hard cancellous bone (a-b) immediately after operation (c-d) 24 months post op. The stem is fixed by strong and compact cancellous bone, without loosening.

3.3.4. Cortical index

Calculation of the cortical index: Cortical index = (10 × (a-b))/a, where a is the outer diameter of the femur and b is the inner diameter of the medullary cavity 10 cm below the level of the lesser trochanter (Fig. 6).

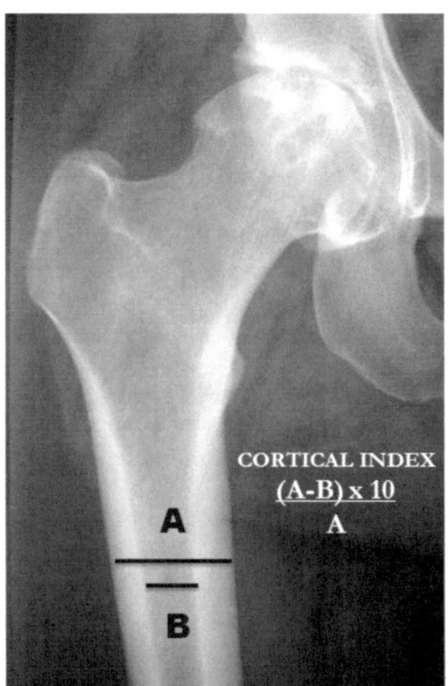

Figure 6. Calculation of the cortical index. Cortical index = (10 × (a-b))/a, where a is the outer diameter of the femur and b is the inner diameter of the medullary cavity 10 cm below the level of the lesser trochanter.

Short-stem hip implantation is contraindicated when cortical index scores are less than 3; in this situation a cemented stem is advisable. If the cortical index is between 3 and 4, an oversized Proxima™ stem would be suggested; if the cortical index exceeds 4, a normal sized Proxima™ stem could be used.

Among the 50 Proxima™ stem implantations, the only intraoperative complication was a spiral femoral shaft fracture. The stem sank deeper into the femoral shaft than the identical sized broach, causing an infraction, which resulted in a complete spiral shaft fracture during the repositioning maneuver. The cortical index of the affected hip was 3.75; the mean cortical index of the other cases was 6.07.

4. Conclusion

Bone-saving hip arthroplasty using metaphyseal stems is gaining importance because the increasing number of young patients, and hip resurfacing is not always indicated. In the last decade, the practice of hip arthroplasty has changed; younger age-group is more frequently undergo surgery because of the need for a better quality of life. The success of non-cemented total hip arthroplasty relies on osteo-integration of the implants. Prerequisite is primary stability, which can be achieved by the fixation principle of "press-fitting" [Morscher et al., 2002]. Clinical studies investigating the migrational behavior of femoral components have shown that the failure rate of uncemented stems correlates with migration [Krismer et al., 1999]. Sychterz found that in vivo bone loss was most extensive in the proximal-medial region [Sychterz et al., 2002]. Following traditional arthroplasty procedures, bone density measurement has shown a bone loss of 16 to 30% [Kim et al., 2003; Schmidt et al., 2002; Sychterz et al., 2002]. Engh's post mortem investigation has found 7 to 52% bone loss around non-cemented femoral components with osteo-integration [Engh et al., 1992]. DXA measurements by Kishida et al. proved that two years after resurfacing procedures 12% raise in bone density developed in the Gruen 7 zone [Kishida et al., 2004].

The previously mentioned facts, along with the experiences obtained from revision surgeries (technical difficulties caused by bone loss due to loosening) and the high cost of the solutions, have led to a change at the level of primary arthroplasty principles to a more preventive approach. As for the material of the prosthesis components, highly cross-linked polyethylene, metal-on-metal and ceramic sliding surfaces have advanced. According to component design, short-shaft stems came into prominence for those young and active patients for whom resurfacing of the hip is contraindicated (large avascular necrosis of the head, osteoporosis, obese patient etc.) The very proximal location of these stems retains the chance for an implantation of a non-revision stem during revision surgery. Short-stem prosthesis with a close anatomical fit to the proximal cortex aim to maximize primary stability, particularly in rotation. It is also proposed that the shorter shaft leads to more physiological loading of the femur, thereby limiting potential bone resorption due to stress shielding. Further advantages are the reduction of the risk of thigh pain and facilitating minimally invasive surgery, particularly when using an anterior approach [Renkawitz et al., 2008].

At our department both resurfacing and short-shaft stem are available for young and active patients. Short stem is implanted when indication criteria are sufficient. The advantages and disadvantages of short-stem arthroplasty are reported through the author's experiences with the metaphyseal stems [Tóth et al., 2010]. It provides vertical stability by the wedge shape of the stem together with the addition of a lateral flare and preservation of the femoral neck. The preservation of the femoral neck provides greater torsional stability and reduces distal migration of the femoral stem. The absence of any diaphyseal fixation attempts to achieve proximal load transfer so as to reduce stress shielding and thigh pain. It also attempts to preserve the femoral canal and femoral elasticity, and ease revision.

The number of cases and the length of follow-up time in the short stem literature are not extensive enough to draw a final conclusion in comparison to traditional arthroplasty procedures. However, it is sufficient enough to conclude that this procedure differs, therefore a number of factors may make sense to be discussed.

Author details

Kálmán Tóth and Gellért Sohár

Department of Orthopaedics, University of Szeged, Faculty of Medicine, Szeged, Hungary

References

[1] Dabirrahmani, D.; Hogg, M., Kohan, L., & Gillies, M. (2010). Primary and long-term stability of a short-stem hip implant. Proceedings of the Institution of Mechanical Engeneers, Part H, Vol.224, No.9, (n.d.), pp. 1109-1119

[2] Ender, S.A; Machner, A., Pap, G., Hubbe, J., Grashoff, H., & Neumann, H.W. (2007). Cementless CUT femoral neck prosthesis: increased rate of aseptic loosening after 5 years. Acta Orthopaedica, Vol.78, (October 2007), pp. 616-621 (doi: 10.1080/17453670710014301)

[3] Engh, C.A.; Bobyn, J.D., & Glassman, A.H. (1987). Porous-coated hip replacement. The factors governing bone ingrowth, stress shielding, and clinical results. The Journal of Bone and Joint Surgery, British Vol.69, (January 1987), pp. 45-55

[4] Engh, C.A.; McGovern, T.F., Bobyn, J.D., & Harris, W.H. (1992). A quantitative evaluation of periprosthetic bone-remodeling after cementless total hip arthroplasty. The Journal of Bone and Joint Surgery, American Vol.74, (August 1992), pp. 1009-1020

[5] Floerkemeier, T.; Tscheuschner, N., Calliess, T., Ezechieli, M., Floerkemeier, S., Budde, S., Windhagen, H., & von Lewinski, G. (2012). Cementless short stem hip arthroplasty METHA® as an encouraging option in adults with osteonecrosis of the

femoral head. Archives of Orthopedic Trauma Surgery, Vol.132, (August 2012), pp. 1125–1131 Epub 2012 May 1

[6] Ghera, S. & Pavan, L. (2009). The DePuy Proxima hip: a short stem for total hip arthroplasty. Early experience and technical considerations. Hip International: The Journal of the Clinical and Experimental Research on Hip Pathology and Therapy, Vol.19, No.3, (July-September 2009), pp. 215-220

[7] Gilbert, R.E.; Salehi-Bird, S., Gallacher, P.D., & Shaylor, P. (2009). The Mayo conservative hip: experience from a district general hospital. Hip International: The Journal of the Clinical and Experimental Research on Hip Pathology and Therapy, Vol.19, No.3, (July-September 2009), pp. 211-214

[8] Gill, I.R.; Gill, K., Jayasekera, N., & Miller, J. (2008). Medium term results of the collum femoris preserving hydroxyapatite coated total hip replacement. Hip International: The Journal of the Clinical and Experimental Research on Hip Pathology and Therapy, Vol.18, No.2, (April-June 2008), pp. 75-80

[9] Goebel, D. & Schulz, W. (2009). The Mayo cementless femoral component in active patients with osteoarthritis. Hip International: The Journal of the Clinical and Experimental Research on Hip Pathology and Therapy, Vol.19, No.3, (July-September 2009), pp. 206-210

[10] Harris, W.H. (1969). Traumatic arthritis of the hip after dislocation and acetabular fractures: treatment by mold arthroplasty. An end-result study using a new method of result evaluation. The Journal of Bone and Joint Surgery, American Vol.51, No.4, (June 1969), pp. 737-755

[11] Hube, R.; Zaage, M., Hein, W., & Reichel, H. (2004). Early functional results with the Mayo-hip, a short stem system with metaphyseal-intertrochanteric fixation. Orthopäde Vol.33, No.11, (November 2004), pp. 1249–1258

[12] Khanuja, H.S.; Vakil, J.J., Goddard, M.S., & Mont, M.A. (2011). Cementless Femoral Fixation in Total Hip Arthroplasty. The Journal of Bone and Joint Surgery, American Vol.93, No.5, (March 2011), pp. 500-509

[13] d'Imporzano, M. & Pierannunzii, L. (2006). Minimally invasive total hip replacement. Journal of Orthopaedic Traumatology, Vol.7, (2006), pp. 42–50

[14] Kim, Y.H.; Oh, S.H., & Kim, J.S. (2003). Primary total hip arthroplasty with a second-generation cementless total hip prosthesis in patients younger than fifty years of age. The Journal of Bone and Joint Surgery, American Vol.85, No.1, (January 2003), pp. 109-114

[15] Kim, Y.H.; Kim, J.S., Park, J.W., & Joo, J.H. (2011). Total hip replacement with a short metaphyseal-fitting anatomical cementless femoral component in patients aged 70 years or older The Journal of Bone and Joint Surgery, British Vol.93, No.5, (May 2011), pp. 587-592

[16] Kim, Y.H. & Oh J.H. (2012). A comparison of a conventional versus a short, anatomical metaphyseal-fitting cementless femoral stem in the treatment of patients with a fracture of the femoral neck The Journal of Bone and Joint Surgery, British Vol.93, No.6, (June 2012), pp. 774–81

[17] Kishida, Y.; Sugano, N., Nishii, T., Miki, H., Yamaguchi, K., & Yoshikawa, H. (2004). Preservation of the bone mineral density of the femur after surface replacement of the hip. The Journal of Bone and Joint Surgery, British Vol.86, No.2, (March 2004), pp. 185-189

[18] Krismer, M.; Biedermann, R., Stöckl, B., Fischer, M., Bauer, R., & Haid, C. (1999). The prediction of failure of the stem in THR by measurement of early migration using EBRA-FCA. Einzel-Bild-Roentgen-Analyse-femoral component analysis. The Journal of Bone and Joint Surgery, British Vol.81, No.2, (March 1999), pp. 273-280

[19] Leali, A.; Fetto, J., Insler, H., & Elfenbein, D. (2002). The effect of a lateral flare feature on implant stability. International Orthopaedics, Vol.26, No.3, (April 2002), pp. 166–169

[20] Mai, K.T.; Verioti, C.A., Casey, K., Slesarenko, Y., Romeo, L., & Colwell C.W. Jr. (2010). Cementless Femoral Fixation in Total Hip Arthroplasty. American Journal of Orthopedics, Vol.39, No.3, (March 2010), pp. 126-130

[21] Martell, J.M.; Pierson, R.H., Jacobs, J.J., Rosenberg, A.G., Maley, M., & Galante J.O. (1993). Primary total hip reconstruction with a titanium fiber-coated prosthesis inserted without cement The Journal of Bone and Joint Surgery, American Vol.75, No. 4, (April 1993), pp. 554-571

[22] McElroy, M.J.; Johnson, A.J., Mont, M.A., & Bonutti P.M. (2011). Short and Standard Stem Prostheses Are Both Viable Options for Minimally Invasive Total Hip Arthroplasty. Bulletin of the NYU Hospital for Joint Diseases, Vol.69(Suppl 1), (n.d.), pp. S68-76

[23] Molli, R.G.; Lombardi, A.V., Jr, Berend, K.R., Adams, J.B., & Sneller, M.A. (2012). A Short Tapered Stem Reduces Intraoperative Complications in Primary Total Hip Arthroplasty. Clinical Orthopedics and Related Research, Vol.470, No.2, (February 2012), pp. 450–461

[24] Morrey, B.F. (1989). Short-stemmed uncemented femoral component for primary hip arthroplasty. Clinical Orthopedics and Related Research, Vol.249, (December 1989), pp. 169-175

[25] Morrey, B.F.; Adams, R.A., & Kessler, M. (2000). A conservative femoral replacement for total hip arthroplasty. A prospective study . The Journal of Bone and Joint Surgery, British Vol.82, No.7, (December 2000), pp. 52-58

[26] Morscher, E.W.; Widmer, K.H., Bereiter, H., Elke, R., & Schenk, R. (2002). Cementless socket fixation based on the ''press-fit'' concept in total hip joint arthroplasty. Acta

Chirurgiae Orthopeadicae et Traumatologiae Cechoslovaca, Vol.69, No.1, (n.d.), pp. 8-15

[27] Pipino F. (2000). The bone-prosthesis interaction. Journal of Orthopaedics and Traumatology, Vol 1 No. 1, (December 2000), pp. 3–9

[28] Pons, M. (2010). Learning curve and short-term results with a short-stem CFP system. Hip International: The Journal of the Clinical and Experimental Research on Hip Pathology and Therapy, Vol.20, No. 2, Suppl.7, (May 2010), pp. 52-57

[29] Renkawitz, T., Santori, F.S., Grifka, J., Valverde, C., Morlock, M.M., & Learmonth, I.D. (2008). A new short uncemented, proximally fixed anatomic femoral implant with a prominent lateral flare: design rationals and study design of an international clinical trial. BMC Musculoskeletal Disorders, Vol.9, (November 2008), pp. 147-152

[30] Santori, F.S. & Santori, N. (2010). Mid-term results of a custom-made short proximal loading femoral component The Journal of Bone and Joint Surgery, British Vol.92, No.9, (September 2010), pp. 1231-1237

[31] Sariali, E.; Mouttet,A., Mordasini, P., & Catonné Y. (2012). High 10-Year Survival Rate with an Anatomic Cementless Stem (SPS) Clinical Orthopedics and Related Research, Vol.470, No.7, (July 2012), pp. 1941-1949 (Epub 2012 Mar 9.)

[32] Schmidt, R.; Muller, L., Kress, A. Hirschfelder, H., Aplas, A., & Pitto, R.P. (2002). A computed tomography assessment of femoral and acetabular bone changes after total hip arthroplasty. International Orthopedics, Vol.26, No. 5, (n.d.), pp. 299-302 (Epub 2002 Jun 28.)

[33] Steens, W.; Skripitz, R., Schneeberger, A.G., Petzing, I., Simon, U., & Goetze, C. (2010). [Cementless femoral neck prosthesis CUT--clinical and radiological results after 5 years]. Zeitschrift für Orthopädie und Unfallchirurgie, Vol.148, No.4, (August 2010), pp. 413-419 (Epub 2010 Aug 16.)

[34] Sychterz, C.J.; Claus, A.M., & Engh, C.A. (2002). What we have learned about long-term cementless fixation from autopsy retrievals. Clinical Orthopedics and Related Research, Vol.405, (December 2002), pp. 79–91

[35] Synder, M.; Drobniewski, M., Pruszczyński, B. & Sibiński, M.(2009). Initial experience with short Metha stem implantation. Ortopedia Traumatologia Rehabilitacja, Vol.11, No.4, (July-August 2009), pp. 317-323

[36] Tóth, K.; Mécs, L., & Kellermann, P. (2010). Early experience with the Depuy Proxima short stem in total hip arthroplasty. Acta Orthopedica Belgica, Vol.76, No.5, (October 2010), pp. 613-618

[37] Thomas, W.; Lucente, L., Mantegna, N., & Grundei, H. (2004). [ESKA (CUT) endoprosthesis.] (in German) Orthopäde, Vol.33, No.11, (November 2004), pp. 1243-1248

[38] Walker, P.S.; Culligan, S.G., Hua, G., Muirhead Allwood S.K., & Bentley G. (1999). The effect of lateral flare feature on uncemented hip stems. Hip International, Vol.9, (1999), pp. 71-80

[39] Westphal, F.M.; Bishop, N., Puschel, K., & Morlock, M.M. (2006a). Biomechanics of a new short stemmed uncemented hip prosthesis, an in-vitro study in human bone. Hip International: The Journal of the Clinical and Experimental Research on Hip Pathology and Therapy, Vol.16, Suppl.3, (n.d.), pp. 22-30

[40] Westphal, F.M.; Bishop, N., Honl, M., Hille, E., Püschel, K., & Morlock, M.M. (2006b). Migration and cyclic motion of a new short-stemmed hip prosthesis – a biomechanical in vitro study. Clinical Biomechanics (Bristil Avon), Vol.21, No.8, (2006), pp. 834–840 (Epub 2006 Jun 27.)

Chapter 8

"Neck-Sparing" Total Hip Arthroplasty

Lee E. Rubin, Scott A. Ritterman and
Timothy McTighe

Additional information is available at the end of the chapter

http://dx.doi.org/10.5772/54830

1. Introduction

Advanced arthritis of the hip joint can lead to profound changes in quality of life. Debilitating pain, stiffness, and altered gait biomechanics all affect the ability to stay mobile and maintain gainful employment; these concerns are magnified in younger patients with hip disease. While symptomatic hip arthritis typically affects older patients, there is a growing subset of active patients in their 30s, 40s, and 50s who are affected and were previously thought of as, "too young for a hip replacement." Over the last several decades, advances in hip replacement surgery are allowing us to rethink that position.

A total hip replacement is one of the most reliably successful procedures in orthopaedics. Long term data has shown that with a well positioned modern prosthesis we can give our patients reliable pain relief that has a very high chance (>80% in most cases) of lasting over twenty years[1, 2]. While this may be very comforting to a 75 year old retired patient with relatively low functional demands, twenty year survival will not suffice for patient in their 30s with advanced arthritis. For this reason in the past, many surgeons were reluctant to perform joint replacement surgeries in young patients for fear of condemning them to multiple revisions over a lifetime of use.

Recent literature on the revision-free survival rates for modern hip implants have shown remarkable success, with 10-year survival rates of 100% for a variety of press-fit, uncemented femoral stem designs at a mean time of 8.2 years from surgery.[3] A 2012 award-winning study from the American Association of Hip and Knee Surgeons showed 100% survival for cross-linked polyethylene bearing surfaces at 10 year follow-up[4]. Another recent paper, looking at the 10-year analysis of various bearing couples, showed respective survival rates of 98.4%, 95.6%, and 87.9% for metal-on-polyethylene, ceramic-on-ceramic, and metal-on-metal groups.

[5] The outstanding results of modern implants and bearing surfaces have given surgeons new confidence when facing the challenging of hip arthroplasty in a young, active patient.

The ideal hip replacement prosthesis for a young patient has several important elements. It would be easily integrated, forming a long lasting bond with the host bone, yet be easily removed if needed. Another aspect of the modern hip prosthesis that has evolved is the actual design of the femoral implant itself. Several implant designs on the market are 'bone sparing,' meaning that less bone is taken off of the head/neck of the femur. Over the past decade, hip resurfacing was a popular procedure in this regard. In a resurfacing procedure, the femoral neck and much of the head are left in place. A metal cap is placed on the end of the femoral head and a metal cup is placed in the acetabulum. Resurfacing procedures have fallen out of favor recently for several reasons, including the difficulty of placing the prosthesis as well as concerns with metal-on-metal articulations.

2. Neck sparing arthroplasty

A "neck-sparing" or "bone-sparing" prosthesis is not a new concept but is one that has been gaining in popularity. This prosthesis is similar in design to other modern prosthesis but preserves more native bone in the femoral neck of the patient during femoral preparation. With a similar idea to the resurfacing, the hope is to allow placement of an implant while leaving a viable option for revision at a later date. These prostheses are proximally porous coated; after the femoral bone cut is made, more femoral neck bone is left in situ, and the proximally coated implant loads and helps maintain this "extra" bone over time. Any modern bearing surface can be utilized by the surgeon. This novel design saves a significant portion of native host bone and will lead to theoretically easier revision surgery when the time comes. A small saw can be slipped around the neck of the prosthesis and the "extra" bone is removed, allowing revision to a primary hip implant rather than the traditional, extensive revision implants currently in use today.

The level of the femoral bone resection varies based on the arthroplasty technique. (Figure 1) A native right proximal hip is visible in Figure 1.1. In hip resurfacing (1.2 A) and "mid-head" resurfacing (1.2 B) (available in Europe), most of the femoral bone is retained. With neck sparing arthroplasty (1.2 C) and conventional total hip arthroplasty (1.2 D), progressively more bone is resected during the operation. With hip revision surgery, native bone is often eroded, leading to an even lower bony resection level (1.2 E). "Neck-sparing" implants allow the surgeon to retain the native bone between cut levels C and D (Figure 1.3), with the concept of native neck bone stock preservation for future revision surgery in the young patient.

The idea of neck retention is not a new concept. Freeman, Townley, Whiteside and Pipino have all advocated saving the femoral neck since the 1980s. Freeman is credited with his classic article "Why Resect The Neck?" as the Godfather of neck retention[6]. His stem retained the femoral neck but was a conventional length straight stem that engaged both the metaphysis and diaphysis. The original stem was designed for cement fixation, with subsequent modifi-

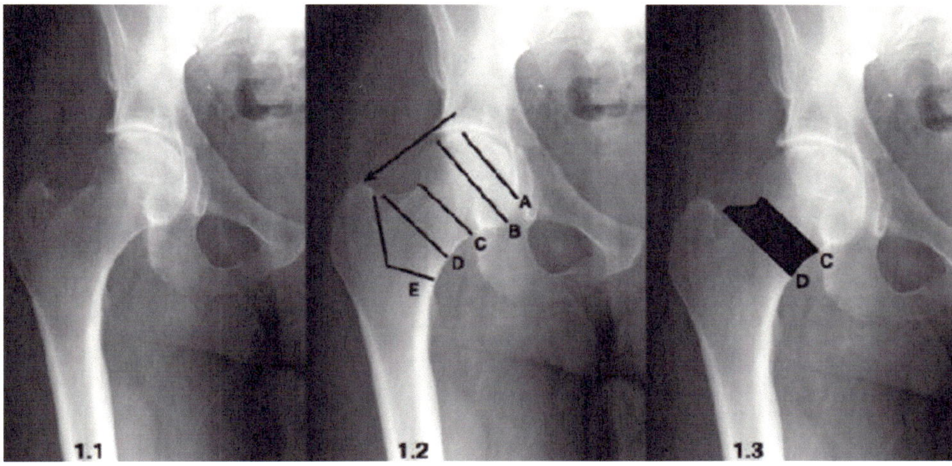

Figure 1. 1.1) Native right proximal hip. 1.2) Bone resection levels for hip resurfacing (A), mid-head resurfacing (B), neck-sparing arthroplasty (C), conventional total hip arthroplasty (D), and revision hip arthroplasty (E). 1.3) Illustration of native bone preserved during neck sparing arthroplasty compared to conventional total hip arthroplasty.

cation to introduce a cementless style stem that was of the same stem length and geometric shape with HA coating, as seen in Figure 2.

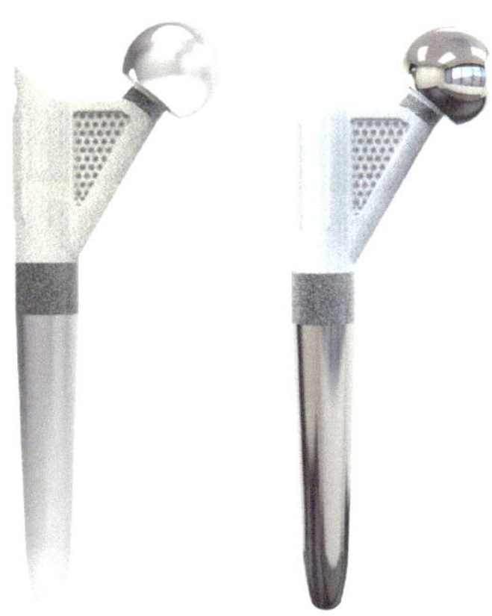

Figure 2. Freeman Femoral Stems. Left: Cemented Right: Cementless

Townley and Whiteside also designed conventional length straight stems that retained the femoral neck, but it was Professor Pipino who first advocated the short curved neck sparing stem to be stabilized by fit and fill of the femoral neck as a cementless press fit stem in 1979. He is also credited with term "tissue-sparing," referring to both saving hard and soft tissue as a surgical strategy. His Biodynamic hip prosthesis was implanted from 1983 to 1996 (Figure 3 Left), until it was replaced by the modified CFP hip stem (Figure 3 Right) Pipino reported outstanding results of his stem design, with 97% satisfactory radiographic results and an implant survival rate of almost 100% at 25 years.[7]

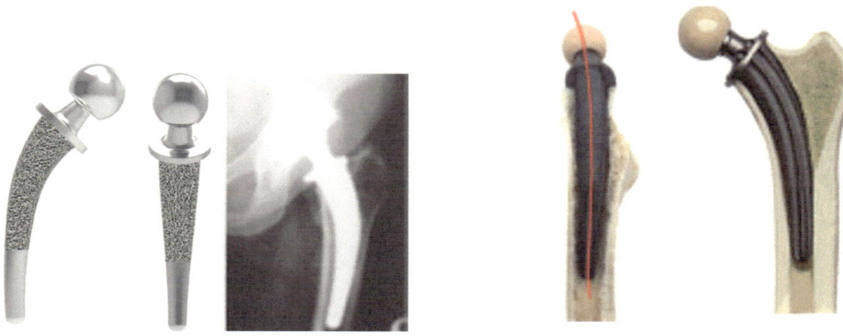

Figure 3. Left: Biodynamic c.c. stem by Howmedica, Right: CFP Stem by Link.

The CFP prosthesis stem is made of titanium alloy, a material better suited for cementless fixation than cobalt-chromium alloy. The left and right stem versions with built-in anatomical anteversion were adapted to the normal anatomy of the proximal femur. The left and right stems were available in six stem sizes along with two stem curvatures; the stem featured bilateral longitudinal ribs to increase surface contact and oppose torsional forces.

To promote osseointegration, the CFP stem has a 70 μm microporous surface with the exception of the short distal portion. In addition, the microporous surface is provided with a special 20 μm hydroxyapatite (calcium phosphate) coating which does not seal the surface but keeps the porous structure intact.

3. Biomechanics of neck sparing stem designs

The natural trabecular pattern of the bone and the trabecular orientation provide support against the natural functional loading, thus creating the necessary functional stability of the individual bone areas within the proximal femur. (Figure 4) The femoral neck and the adjoining medial aspect of the femur in the calcar region show the strongest bone structure with a high load capacity to support the stem. (Figure 5)

Femoral neck retention reduces both torsional and bending moments (forces) at the stem / bone interface. In accordance with Wolff's Law, the reduction of stresses relative to the natural situation would cause bone to adapt itself by reducing its mass, either by becoming more porous (internal remodeling) or by getting thinner (external remodeling).

In Figure 6, The neck on the left has been resected at the conventional level; in the one on the right the neck has been retained. Because the difference in the height of resection the length of the moment arms, the varus- turning moment increases by a factor of four when the neck is

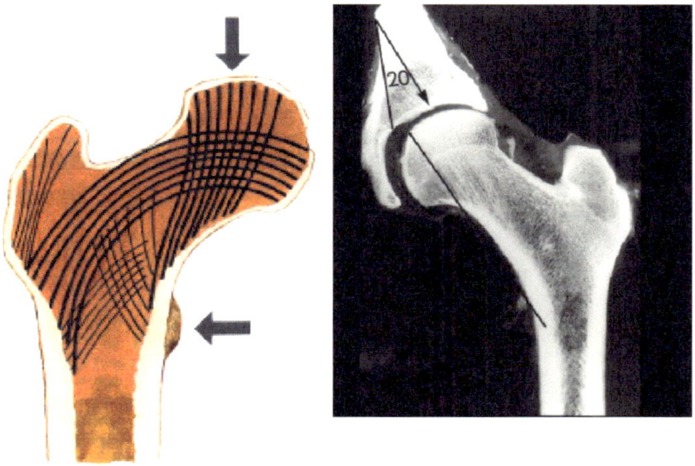

Figure 4. Trabecular bone patterns

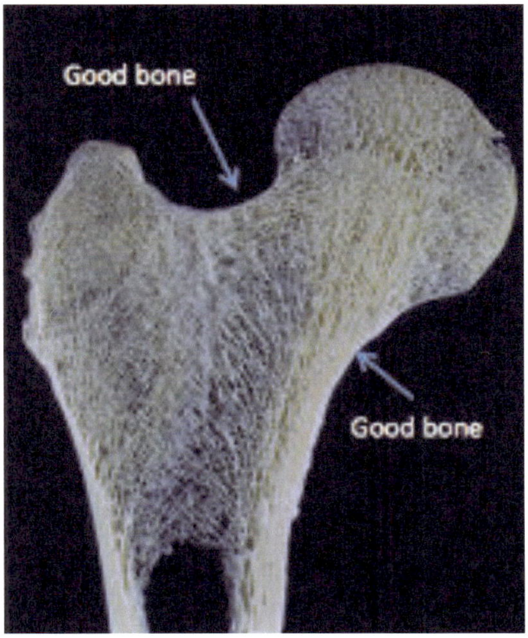

Figure 5. Cross section of the proximal femur

resected (Figure 7). At the same time the area of bone available for supporting the vertical component of the resultant of the forces acting on the implant is almost tripled

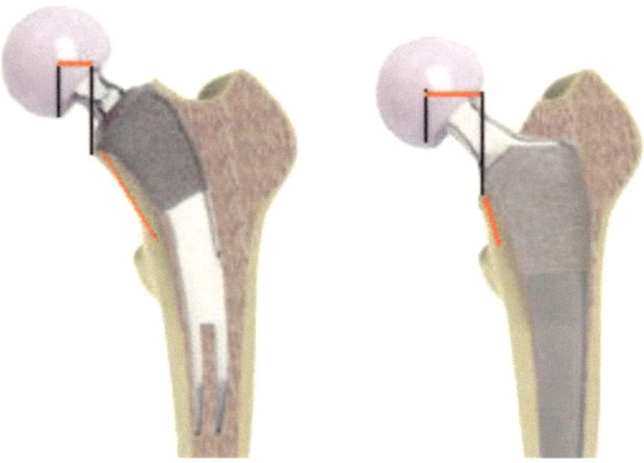

Figure 6. Illustrations comparing neck retention to conventional neck resection bending moment.

The anterior-posterior directed component of the resultant force is represented by an arrow. Neck resection generates a significant torsional moment.

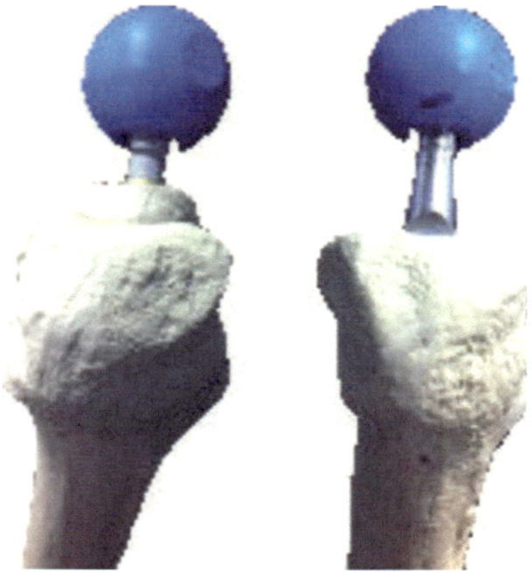

Figure 7. Varus /Valgus turning moment in neck retention vs. conventional neck resection

It is important to remember that not all neck-sparing stems are not all short neck stabilized stems. Historically, neck sparing stems were not short curved neck stabilized by design (Figure 8).

To-date, most neck-sparing stems have been somewhat disappointing in their long-term ability to stimulate and maintain the medial calcar. For that reason, a new short stem neck stabilized design approach was undertaken to improve proximal load transfer and to create a bone or tissue sparing stem that would be simple in design, amenable to reproducible technique and provide for fine tuning joint mechanics while stimulating and maintaining ongoing, in-vivo compressive loads to preserve the medial calcar.

http://dx.doi.org/10.5772/54830

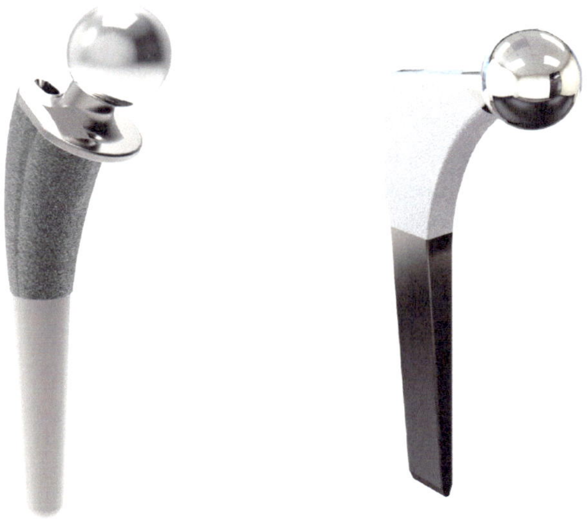

Figure 8. Left: Townley Platform Stem. Right: Whiteside Neck Sparing Stem.

4. "Short" hip arthoplasty stems

The use of short stems is growing. Initial short and mid-term follow up studies of a number of these stems suggest that stable, durable fixation and excellent clinical outcomes can be achieved. As a result, a very large number of short stem designs are available. Until recently, there was no classification system for uncemented short stem implants that would allow for comparisons of clinical and radiographic results.

A number of advantages have been argued to justify the design and clinical usage of short stems; Elimination of femoral proximal-distal mismatch, tissue preservation (hard & soft), facilitation of less invasive surgical exposures, less invasive surgical violation into the femoral canal, less violation into the trochanteric bed, improved proximal bone remodeling, less intraoperative blood loss, less postoperative rehabilitation, less instrumentation and less inventory cost.

All of these advantages are worthwhile if they can be proven to be significant benefits to the clinical outcome and increased survivorship of the device. The real question is can these shorter length devices obtain strong and long-lasting stability of the implant without diaphyseal anchoring?

The European experience with certain styles of conservative designs are years ahead of the U.S. experience. So it is reasonable to look towards Europe for both trends and early to mid-term clinical results. Some of these devices are not available in the U. S. and some are new to their clinical experience. As a result, the Joint Implant Surgery and Research Foundation

(JISRF) developed a short stem classification system based off stabilization contact for implant stability.[8]

JISRF developed this classification system to help identify, differentiate and catalog short stemmed total hip implants by primary stabilization contact points. Not all short stems generate the same radiographic findings and or clinical results. It is also important to appreciate the specific design and appropriate surgical technique for a given design. We believe this classification system helps to clarify some of the design principles and clinical findings. While there will be subcategories within the main categories, (Examples: Neck plugs versus short curved neck stems) but the primary stabilization point determines the same overall category.

5. JISRF classification system for short stems: Implant examples

1. Head Stabilized

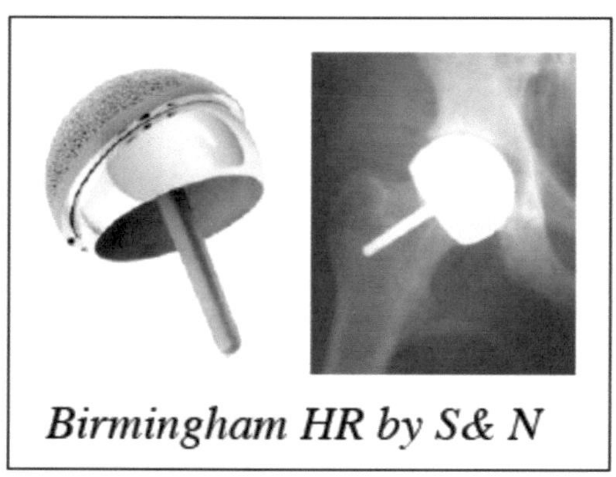

Figure 9. Hip Resurfacing Arthroplasty and "Mid-Head" Resurfacing Arthroplasty (Birmingham System, Smith and Nephew)

2. Neck Stabilized, Figure 11:

http://dx.doi.org/10.5772/54830

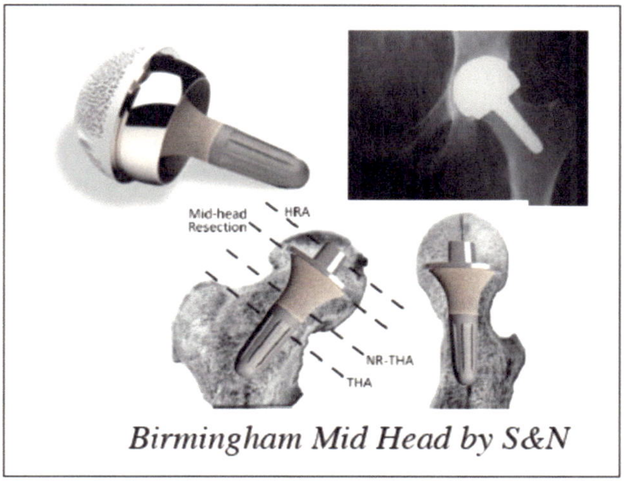

Figure 10. Hip Resurfacing Arthroplasty and "Mid-Head" Resurfacing Arthroplasty (Birmingham System, Smith and Nephew)

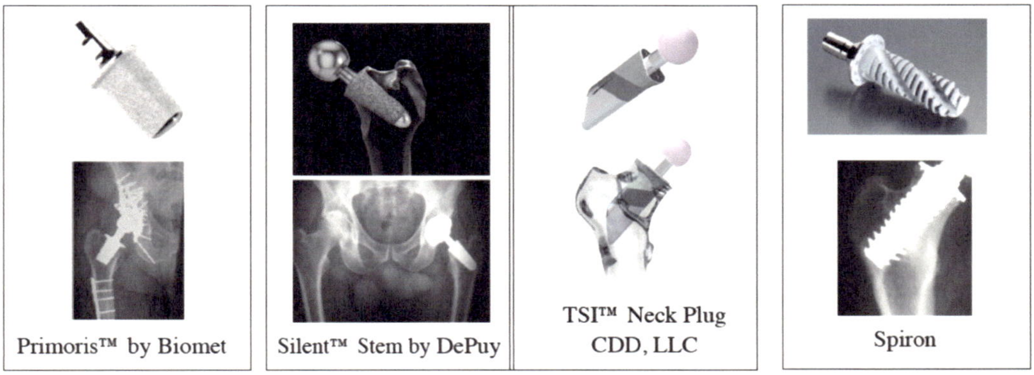

Figure 11. Metaphyseal Stabilized

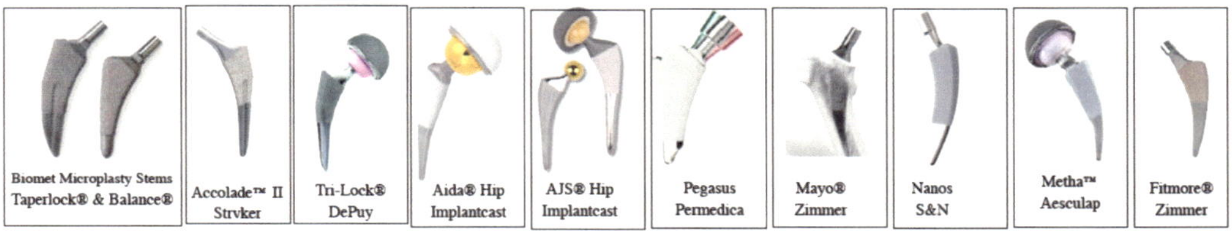

Figure 12. Conventional (Metaphyseal/Diaphyseal) Stabilized: Traditional Arthroplasty Stems

6. Current design rationale for a modular, short, curved neck stabilized stem

Stem Design:

The TSI™ Stem is a simple short curved trapezoidal neck sparing design that is tissue conservative (hard & soft) and features a number of unique and novel elements to improve upon short and long-term survivorship. This novel design has been licensed by Concept, Design and Development, LLC., in Chagrin Falls, Ohio to two commercial partners and has been introduced into the Australian market as the MSA™ Stem and the United States as the Apex ARC™ Stem. (Figure 13)

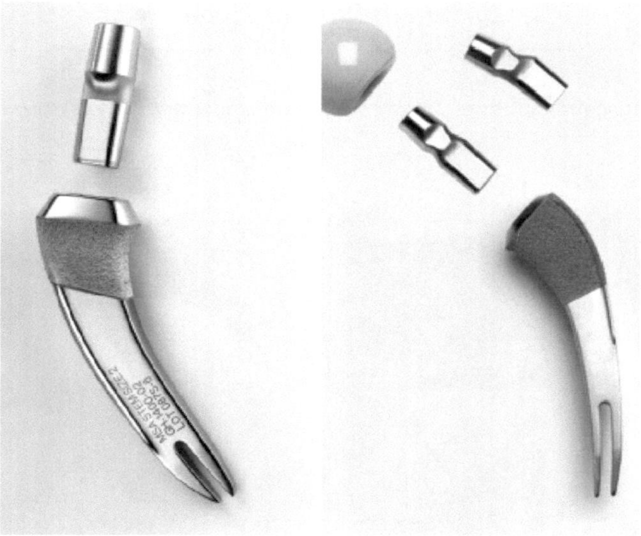

Figure 13. Left: The MSA™ Stem; Right: The Apex ARC™ Stem

The basic curvature of the stem comes from the historical work of Thompson and Müeller. A side-by-side comparison of the Mueller rasp and the ARC™ stem are seen in Figure 14. The medial curve and overall stem length are almost identical.

This simple, yet novel, stem design allows for considerable tissue conservation of both hard and soft tissue. Native bone is preserved in Gruen zones 7, 3,4,5 and zone 1, as seen in Figure 15.

The medial curve reduces the need to remove lateral bone, where one can risk damage to the musculature and increased bleeding by removal of cancellous bone in the greater trochanter (Figure 31). The stem shape is based on a curved trapezoidal design that is intrinsically stable within the cylindrical femur. The torsional stability is enhanced by a lateral "T-Flange" feature, however, this has proven to be too aggressive in the small female profile and has been removed on the size 0 stem.

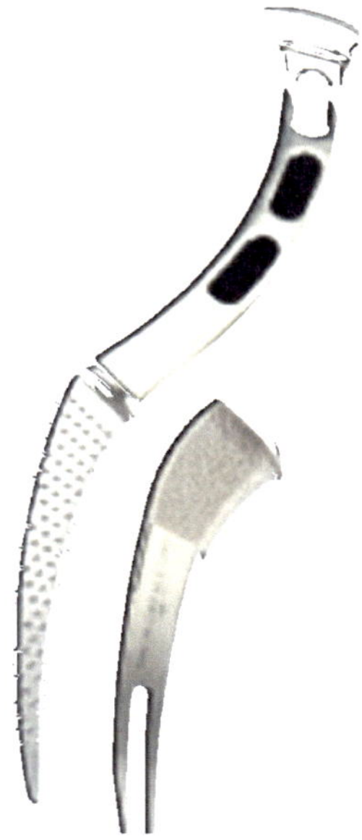

Figure 14. Image of historic Mueller proximal femoral rasp (left) placed adjacent to modern TSI neck-sparing arthroplasty implant (right).

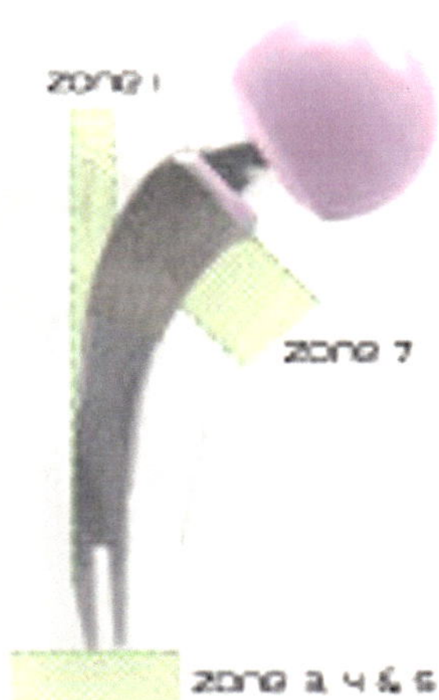

Figure 15. Image demonstrating areas of bone preservation maintained with neck-sparing arthroplasty, including Gruen Zones 1, 3, 4, 5, and 7.

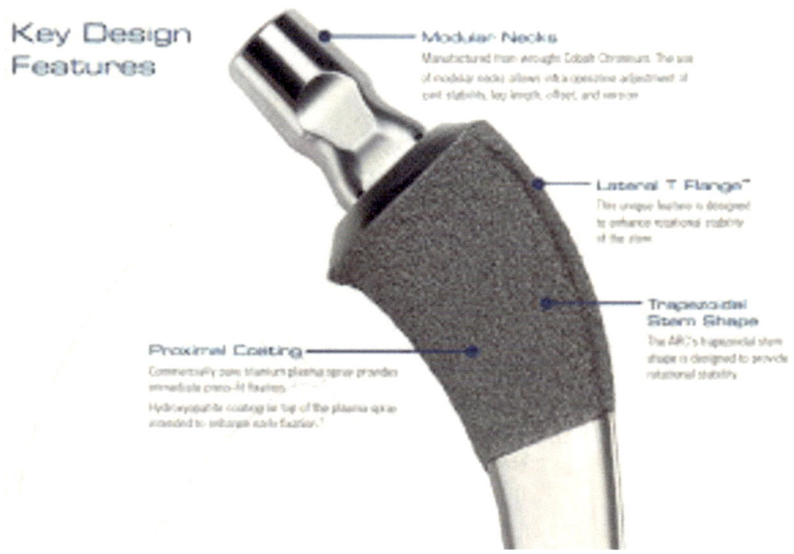

Figure 16. Key Design Features of the ARC™ stem.

A porous titanium coating is applied circumferentially to the upper third of the stem and is a combination of commercially pure titanium applied first using a plasma spray process after which a thin layer of hydroxyapatite (HA) is also applied using a plasma spray process. The proximal portion of the stem also has a patent pending novel conical flair element that is design to off load compressive loads to the medial calcar. (Figure 17) This very unique feature has demonstrated positive stress transfer in both FEA modeling and now clinical observations.

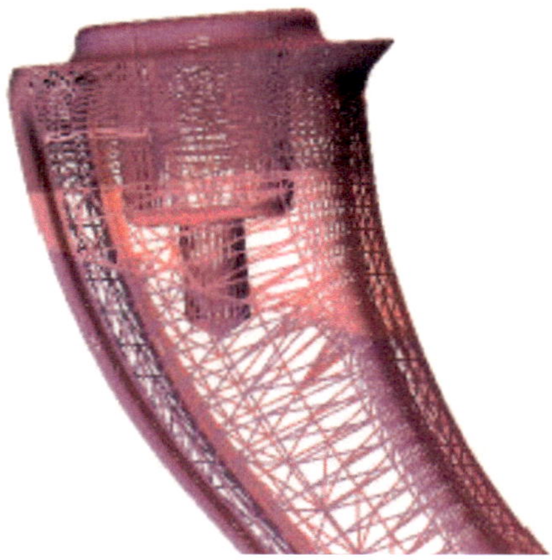

Figure 17. Medial Flare seen on the lateral profile in 3-Dimensional stem rendering

A lateral distal relief of 11º reduces any distal tip contact with the lateral cortex if the stem is in a slight varus position. The sagittal slot reduces distal stiffness reducing the potential of distal load transfer and reduces hoop tension in type A bone by allowing stem to pinch in.

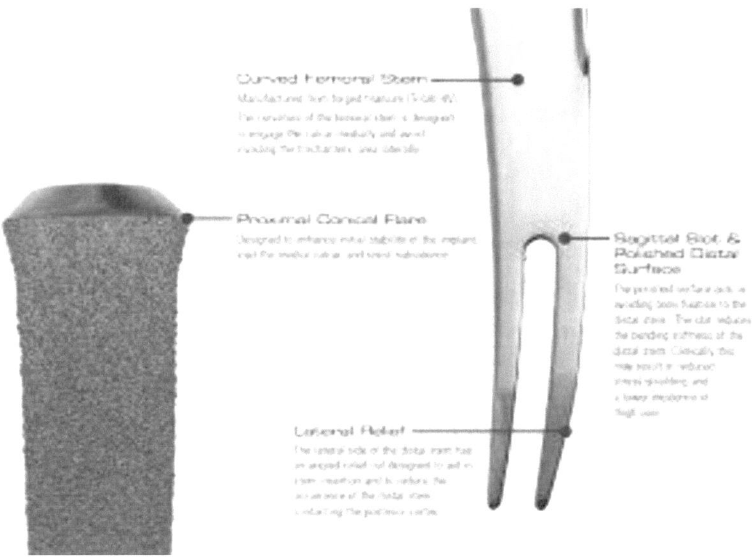

Figure 18. Additional Design Features of the ARC™ stem.

The TSI™ neck stabilized stem with a modular cobalt-chrome neck has demonstrated a reduction of maximum principal tensile stress in the neck stabilization stem was 35% less than that of a monoblock taper style design. (Figure 19) With regards to potential failure mode, the neck sparing feature with a short cobalt-chrome modular neck has basically eliminated potential fatigue failure of the neck, as opposed to other recent titanium modular neck designs that have demonstrated catastrophic fatigue fractures.[9]

7. Stress in the femoral component

The ring of cortical bone saved in the neck sparing stem has significant bio-mechanical advantage. Pipino refers to this as a "tension band." (Figure 20) The principal stress measured in the femoral component was lowest for model with cortical neck ring intact compared to the monoblock conventional cementless stem. (Figure 21)

The stress in the distal femur slightly reduces with the TSI neck sparing stem and reduces even more if the cortical rim remains intact. This data supports the concept that the medial conical flair does offload compression to the proximal femur especially if the cortical ring is intact.

The short TSI™ stem demonstrates better loading patterns as compared to Pipino's first stem (Biodynamic), (Figure 22) which was made of cobalt-chrome material. The x-ray on the right

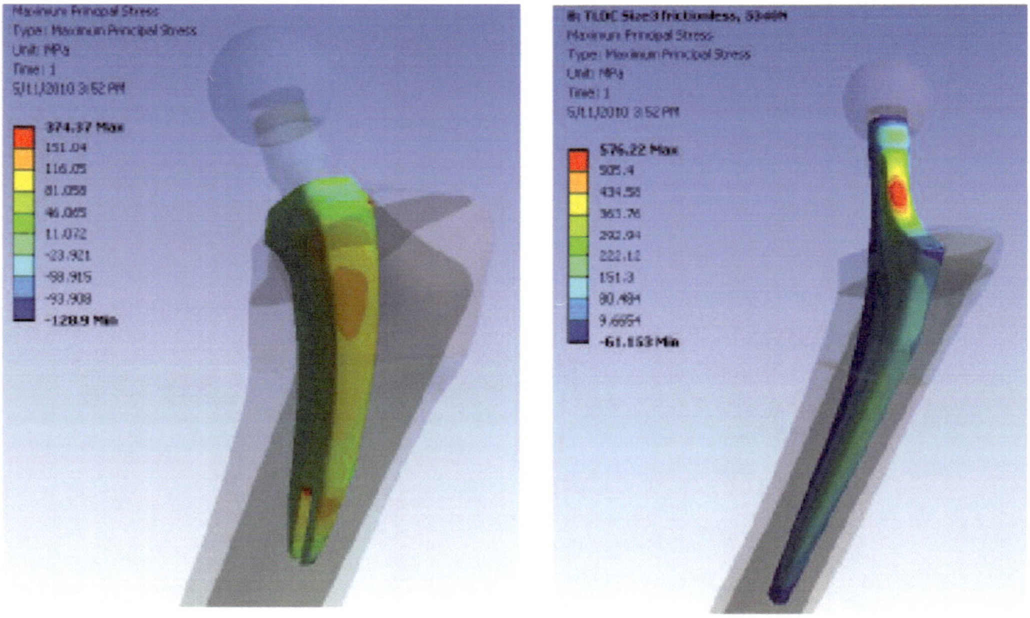

Figure 19. Finite Element Analysis of a short neck-sparing arthroplasty stem (left) compared to a monoblock stem (right). Increased areas of stress foci are highlighted in red.

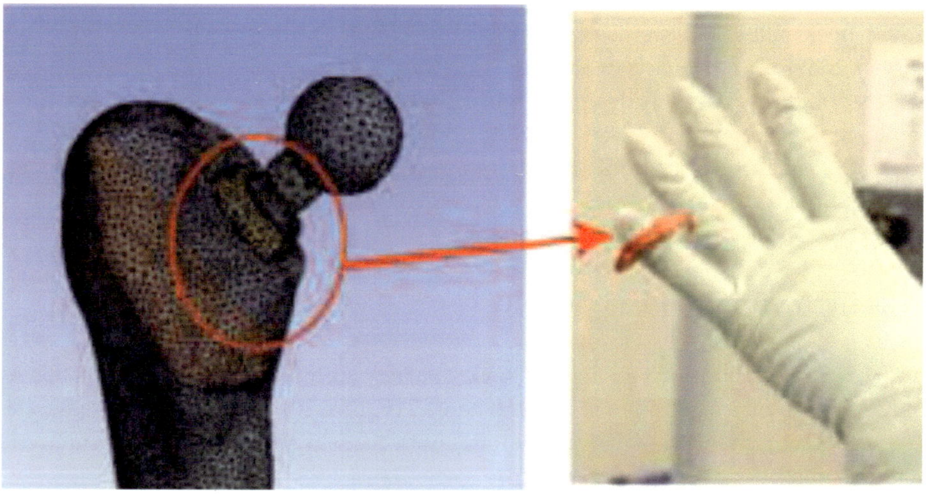

Figure 20. Ring of Proximal Femoral Bone

side of Figure 22 is his current stem CFP which still has had some medial calcar bone resporption issues.

http://dx.doi.org/10.5772/54830

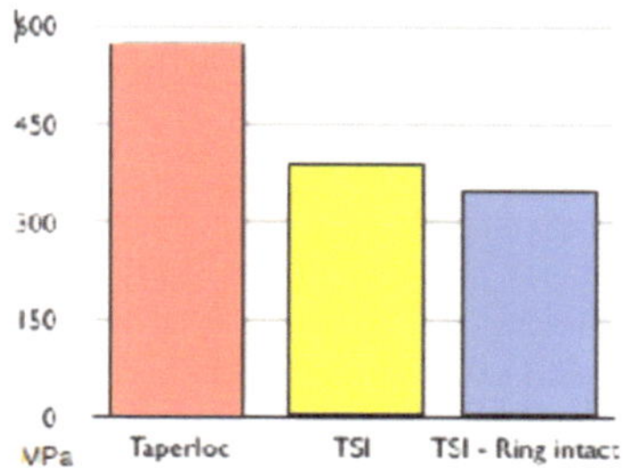

Figure 21. Assessment of proximal femoral stress with axial loading

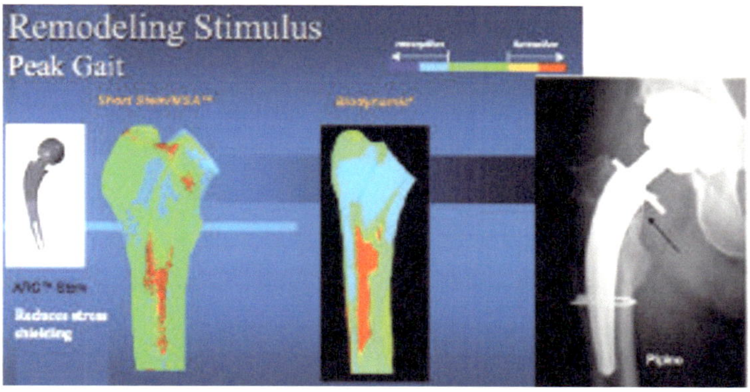

Figure 22. FEA Modeling of ARC™ (Left) compared with the Biodynamic stem (Right), showing normalized loading of the medial calcar on the left, and decreased loading on the right.

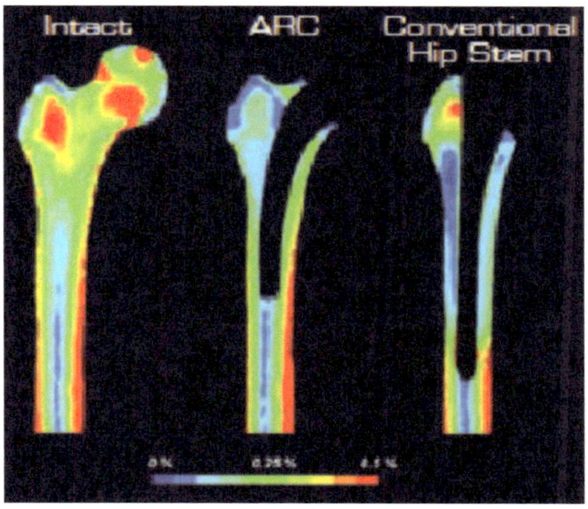

Figure 23. FEA Modeling of an intact femur (left), the ARC™ stem (Center) and a long, extensively coated press-fit stem (right), demonstrating improved proximal strain patterns compared to the AML style conventional cementless stem.

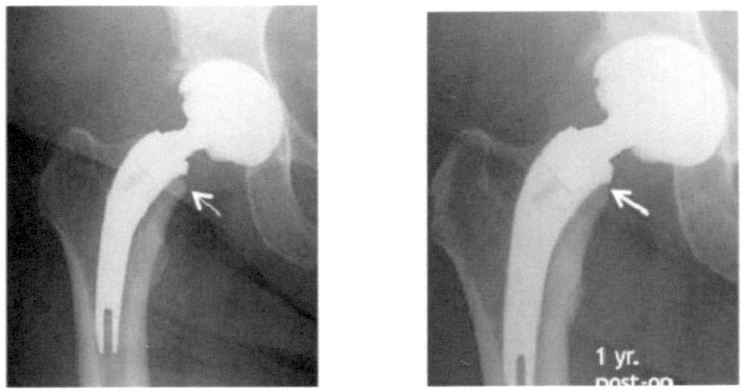

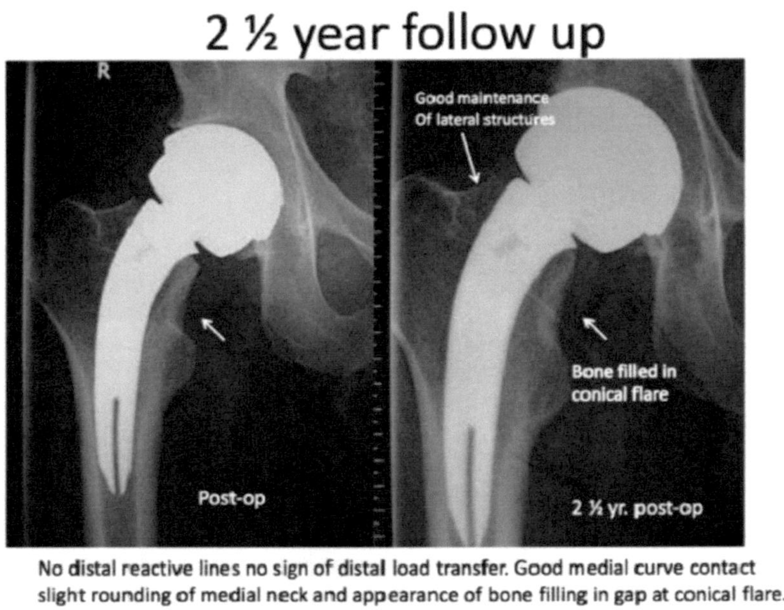

Prof. Ian Woodgate, Sydney, Australia

Figure 24. A and B: Clinical case examples of favorable bone remodeling from the ARC™ stem

8. Proximal neck modularity

Target Restoration of hip mechanics is aided by proximal neck modularity, especially focued on femoral offset, neck length, and combined version. Using monoblock femoral stem designs,

http://dx.doi.org/10.5772/54830

restoration of hip mechanics is difficult to address. Often, accomplishing intra-operative joint stability comes with an increased risk for over-lengthening..

Neck Modularity allows intraoperative fine tuning of joint mechanics, reducing risk of impingement and mitigating risk of accelerated wear and dislocation. This priniciple also aids in access in the event of acetabular revision. Monoblock hip stems are based on proportionality of design. As the stem gets bigger, the neck gets longer. Unfortunately, this scenario is not consistent with the variability seen with proximal femoral geometry, and is illustrated with the radiographs seen in Figure 25.

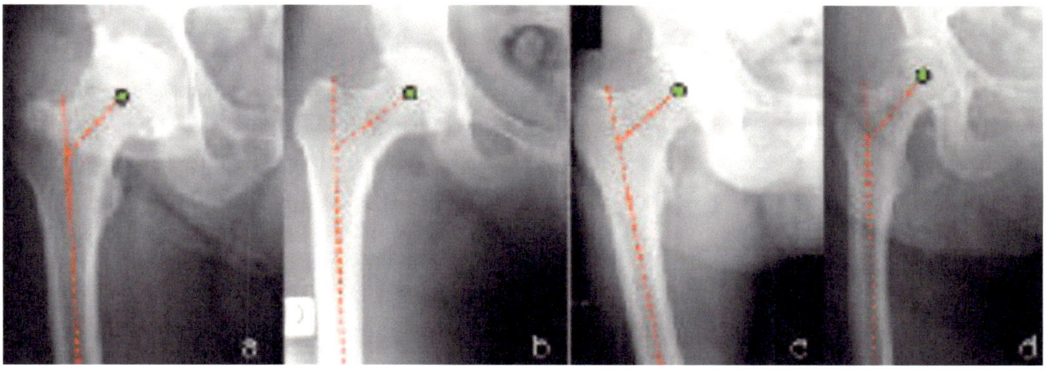

Figure 25. Anatomic variations commonly associated with primary osteo-arthritis patients using a monoblock stem: a: large canal, short neck, low offset, b: thin canal, long neck, high offset, c: large canal, short neck, high offset, d: thin canal, long neck, low offset

Femoral head center location data (Figure 26) shows that a wide variety of offsets and lengths are required to properly balance the soft tissues, but there is often little correlation between head center and stem size. A significant number of small stem diameters (10 or 11.5 mm) required large >45 mm femoral offsets.

One only has to review actual usage data on modular necks to validate the need of proximal modularity. A review of ARC™ Modular Neck Experience (Figure 27) on 1,640 stems implanted from April 2010 to August 2012 demonstrated that a significant variety of stems were selected by surgeons while using the device to fine-tune the biomechanics of the hip joint in vivo.

9. Clinical utilization and outcomes

Case One: A 29 year-old man presented with the acute-onset of debilitating pain in his left hip from osteonecrosis with collapse secondary to chronic steroid use for immunosuppression of severe lupus. (Figure 28). His symptoms developed over 4 weeks and were incapacitating, requiring the use of two crutches and high doses of long-acting narcotic for comfort.

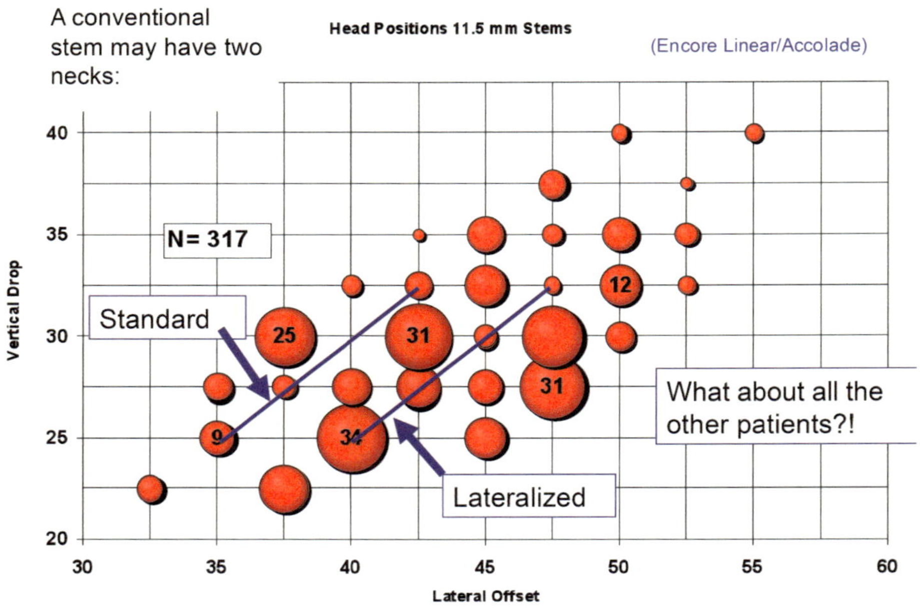

Figure 26. Femoral head location data, mapping a relationship of femoral implant sizing related to vertical drop (vertical axis) and lateral offset (horizontal axis). Most conventional femoral stems are available only in "standard" and "lateral" offsets, which do not match the variety of combined values seen in native anatomy.

Neutral Neck Standard = 33%
Neutral Neck Long = 3% new size
Total Neutral Necks = 36%

8°Varus/Valgus =19%
8°Varus/Valgus Long = 3%
Total 8°Varus/Valgus = 22%

12°Varus Valgus =17%
12°Anteverted/Retroverted = 30% new size
Angled Necks Total = 47%

Figure 27. ARC™ modular neck utilization data, from April 2010 to August 2012.

He was treated with total hip arthroplasty using a neck sparing implant and a ceramic on cross-linked polyethylene bearing surface couple. The implants were inserted via the direct anterior approach with a "bone-sparing technique" allowing retention of 1.5 cm of his proximal femoral bone, with anatomic restoration of his hip center of rotation (Figures 29 and 30). His postoperative course showed complete resolution of his pain with elimination of narcotic use, dramatic improvement in his hip function, and he was able to begin returning to work as a professional chef after less than 8 weeks of recovery.

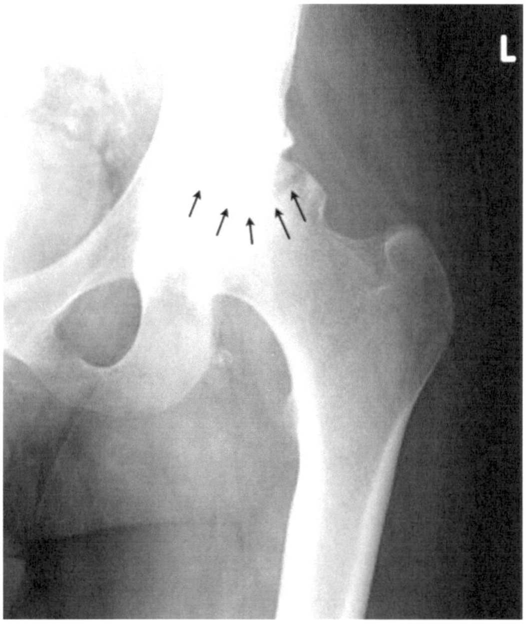

Figure 28. Left Hip Joint with AVN and acute collapse of the dome of the femoral head, indicated by arrows.

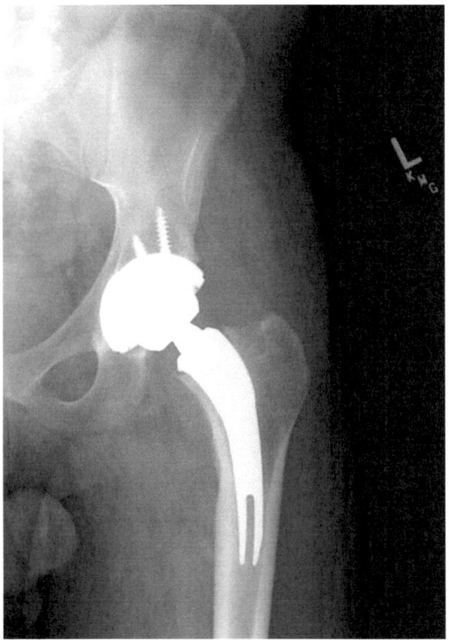

Figure 29. Postoperative AP Left Hip, Showing ARC™ "neck-sparing" arthroplasty in an anatomic position with restoration of hip alignment, offset, and position.

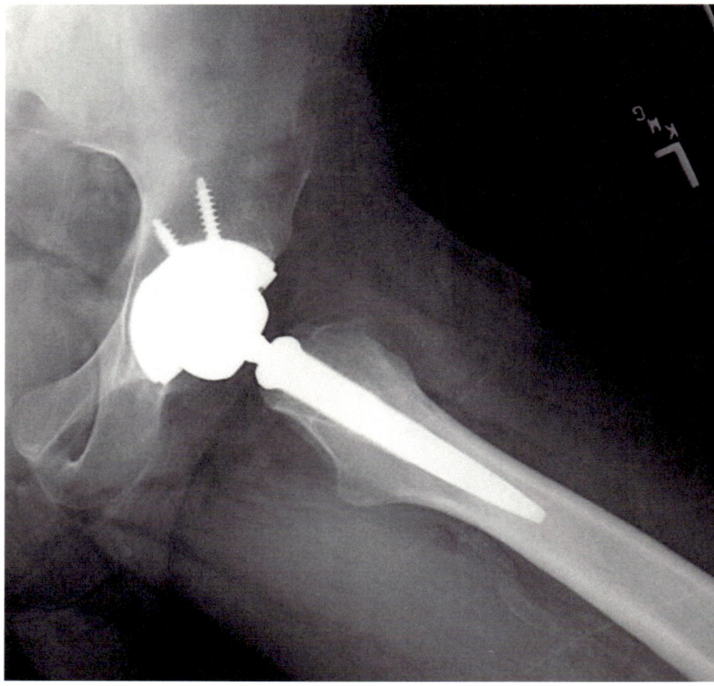

Figure 30. Postoperative Lateral Left Hip demonstrating anatomic prosthesis positioning.

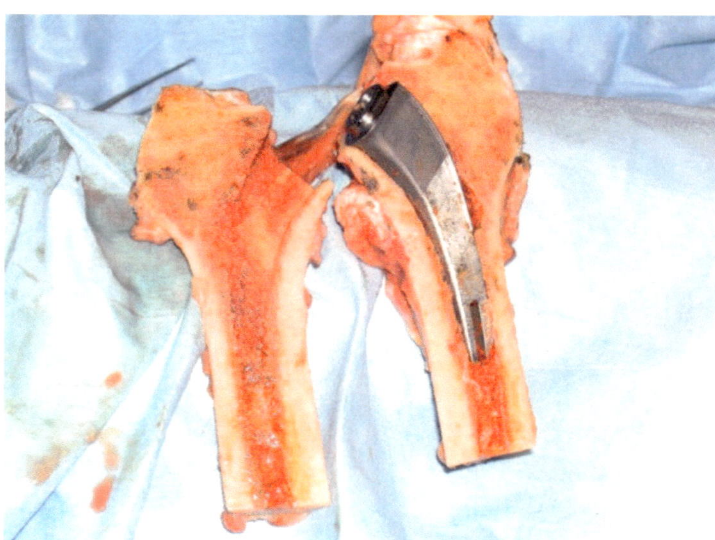

Figure 31. Coronal cross-section of cadaveric left proximal femur, demonstrating neck-sparing prosthesis position along medial calcar, with retained femoral neck and conservation of native trochanteric bone visible.

Case Two: A 32 year-old man presented for evaluation after having been previously diagnosed with advanced bilateral osteonecrosis of his proximal femoral heads. His management had already included a comprehensive medical and metabolic workup to assess for causes for the avascular necrosis, but none had been elucidated. He denied any known exposure to high dose corticosteroids and had no history of alcohol intake. He had previously undergone core decompression procedures at an outside institution on both the right hip (18 months prior) and the left hip (14 months prior) in the recent past, without any significant improvements in his clinical function or symptoms. He underwent simulateneous, bilateral neck-sparing THA, and is walking normally once again after a brief course of rehabilitation. The specific details of his case were described in detail elsewhere.[10]

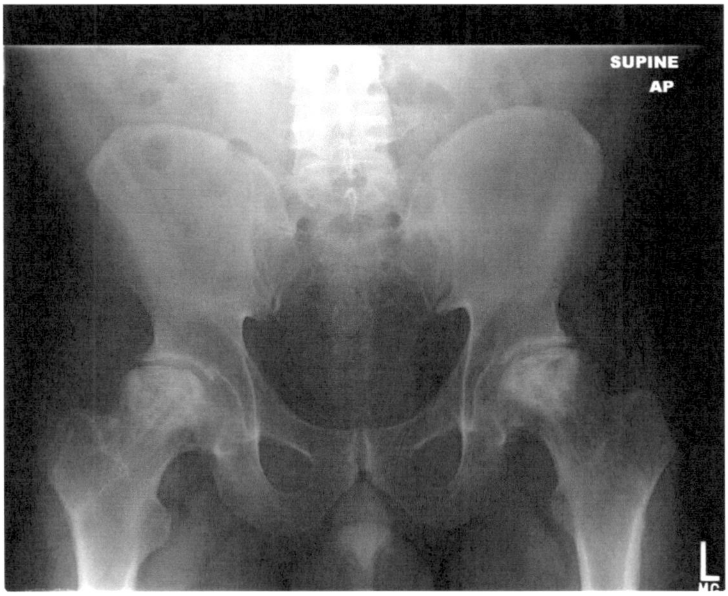

Figure 32. Preoperative AP Pelvis of a 32 year-old male with severe, bilateral, osteonecrosis with associated femoral head collapse and secondary arthrosis.

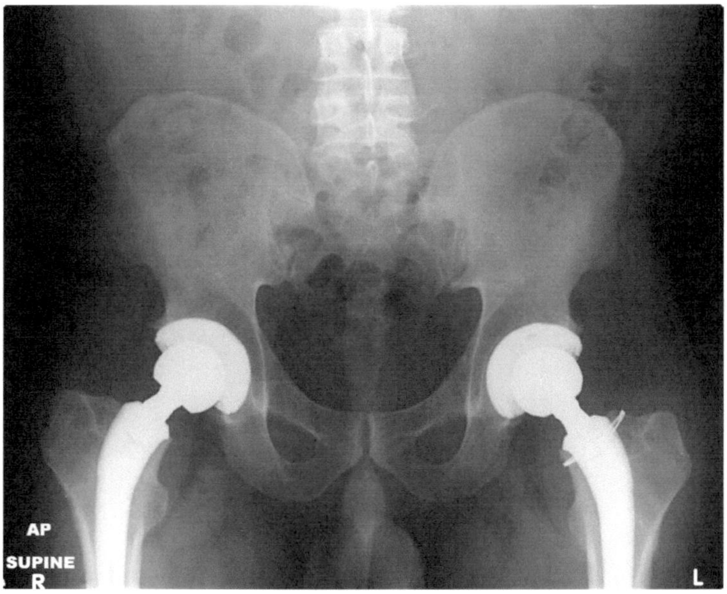

Figure 33. Postoperative AP Pelvis

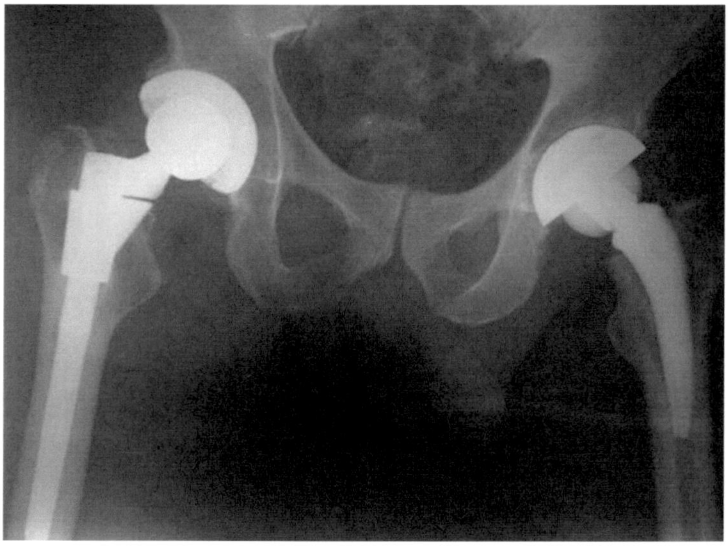

Figure 34. Comparison of historic versus modern femoral stem modularity. Right hip: S-ROM Prosthesis, 1984; Left Hip ARC™ Stem, 2012. (Image Courtesy Louis Keppler, MD and JISRF.)

10. Short-term results of TSI and ARC™femoral stem

Since the introduction of these modular, short, neck-sparing femoral stem designs, the early results of implant utilization have been tracked by their manufacturers and JISRF.[11]

With 1,970 stems implanted worldwide, There have been only 8 stem explants, and an overall femoral stem survival of 99.5% at 29 months. There were 2 traumatic and 1 chronic dislocations, 2 cases of aseptic loosening, 2 infections, and 1 neck/stem disassociation. 10 cases had a leg length discrepancy greater than 7mm. 6 cases had an iatrogenic calcar fracture, and 3 required wiring. 6 patients had subsidence more than 5mm. There were 3 neck exchanges, with 2 performed for cup revisions. There were 3 intra-operative femoral perforations, and 5 cases that of intra-operative calcar fractures resulting in stem bail-out. There have been no known cases of pseudotumors, no elevated peripheral metal ion levels, and no known occurrence of modular neck fracture.

11. Conclusion

Over the next several decades we will continue to see improvements in implant fixation, bioengineering of bearing surface designs, and prosthesis design that will allow us to reliably replace hip joints in younger and more active adult patients. The design of the "neck-sparing" products and bearing surfaces mentioned herein have certainly played a large part in achieving this goal, but continued improvements and careful outcomes monitoring will be needed over the next few decades.

Acknowledgements

Rubin and Ritterman: Unrestricted educational grant from Joint Implant Surgery and Research Foundation. McTighe: Ownership interests, patents, and licensing fees related to Concept, Design, and Development (CDD) and TSI Stem designs.

Author details

Lee E. Rubin[1], Scott A. Ritterman[2] and Timothy McTighe[3]

*Address all correspondence to: lrubin@universityorthopedics.com

1 Division of Adult Reconstruction, Warren Alpert Medical School of Brown University, University Orthopedics, Inc. Providence, Rhode Island, USA

2 Brown University and Rhode Island Hospital, Providence, Rhode Island, USA

3 Joint Implant Surgery and Research Foundation (JISRF), Chagrin Falls, Ohio, USA

References

[1] Moussa, H, Pierre, B, Jacques, D, et al. Alumina-on-Alumina Total Hip Arthroplasty A Minimum 18.5-Year Follow-up Study." J Bone Joint Surg Am (2002). , 84(1), 69-77.

[2] Neumann, L, Freund, K. G, & Sorenson, K. H. Long-Term Results of Charnley Total Hip Replacement." J Bone Joint Surg Br (1994). B (2): 245-251., 76.

[3] Polkowski et alTotal Hip Arthroplasty in the very Young Patient." Journal of the American Academy of Orthopaedic Surgeons. (2012). , 20, 487-497.

[4] Engh, C. A, & Hopper, R. H. Huynh C et. al. A prospective randomized study of cross-linked and non cross-linked polyethylene for total hip arthroplasty at year follow-up. Journal of Arthroplasty (2012). S): 2-7., 10.

[5] Milosev, I, Kovac, S, & Trebse, R. et. al. Comparison of ten-year survivorship of hip prosthesis with use of conventional polyethylene, metal-on-metal, or ceramic-on-ceramic bearings. J Bone Joint Surg Am (2012). , 94(19), 1756-1763.

[6] Freeman, M. A. Why resect the neck? J Bone Joint Surg Br (1986). , 68(3), 346-9.

[7] Pipino, F, & Keller, A. Tissue-sparing surgery: 25 years' experience with femoral neck preserving hip arthroplasty. Journal of Orthopaedics and Traumatology. (2006). , 7(1), 36-41.

[8] Stulberg, S. D, Keggi, J, & Keppler, L. et. al. A classification system for short stemuncemented total hip arthroplasty. Poster Presentation at the International Society for Technology in Arthroplasty. Sydney, Australia, October (2012). , 4-6.

[9] Mctighe, T, & Brazil, D. Memorandum: Modular Necks. Reconstructive Review (2012). , 2(2), 98-101.

[10] Rubin, L. E, Tuttle, J. R, & Ritteman, S. A. Simultaneous bilateral direct anterior total hip arthroplasty utilizing a modular neck-sparing arthroplasty femoral stem. Reconstructive Review (2012). , 2(2), 68-71.

[11] Mctighe, T, Keggi, J, & Keppler, L. et. al. The First 1,200 (1,790) U.S. Short Curved Neck Stabilized Stems. Poster Presentation at the International Society for Technology in Arthroplasty. Sydney, Australia, October (2012). , 4-6.

Chapter 9

The Evolution of Modern Total Knee Prostheses

Eun-Kyoo Song, Jong-Keun Seon,
Jae-Young Moon and Yim Ji-Hyoun

Additional information is available at the end of the chapter

http://dx.doi.org/10.5772/54343

1. Introduction

Many types of prosthesis are used for total knee arthroplasty, and the evolution of knee arthroplasty, which has a history of almost 40 years, involves repetitious cycles of failure and development. During its early stage (1970-1974), instruments of the unicondylar, duocondylar, or hinged types were used, but these were eventually abandoned due to low success rates. A replacement for the total condylar type was successfully developed and became the model for total knee arthroplasty. Recently, unicondylar arthroplasty has produced good results in selected patients, and arthroplasty of the constrained or hinged type have been proven useful for revision surgery or combined surgery, respectively. To solve the problem of the fixed bearing joint, a mobile bearing joint has been developed, and non-cemented fixed knee arthroplasty is receiving renewed attention. Much effort is being expended on the developments of new materials, such as, ceramics and cross-linked polyethylene, on new designs that maximize function and endurance, and on minimally invasive surgery.

2. History of the evolution of total knee arthroplasty

2.1. Interposition and resurfacing knee arthroplasty

During the late 19th and early 20th century, interposition arthroplasty was attempted using soft tissues. In 1860, Verneuil proposed interposition arthroplasty, involving the insertion of soft tissue to reconstruct the joint surface. Since then, pig bladder, nylon, femoral sheath, anterior bursa of the knee, cellophane, and many other materials have been used, but results have been disappointing. The use of metallic interposition arthroplasty began in the late 1930s. Having obtained successful results for mold arthroplasty in the hip joint, Campbell and Smith-Peterson proposed metal femoral mold arthroplasty[2], and McKeever and MacIntosh proposed hemiarthroplasty of the tibia, but all produced unsatisfactory results in terms of minimizing pain, and high rate of failures of the interposition [3], and thus, these procedures were not widely recognized.

Ferguson [1] attempted resection arthroplasty for ankylosis or severe deformity caused by tuberculosis or infection. This procedure involved resecting cartilage from the knee joint and allowing knee joint movement along the subchondral surface. When too little bone was removed, knees spontaneously fused, and when more bone was removed, knee had good motion but poor stability. Accordingly, these operations were attempted in only the most severe cases because their results were poor.

2.2. The hinged prosthesis

In the 1950s, Walldius [4] developed a hinged prosthesis that replaced the joint surfaces of the femur and tibia, as subsequently, modifications of the basic hinged prosthesis design were made by many surgeons. The hinged prosthesis allows the intramedullary stem to align with the artificial knee joint by itself, and is technically easy to perform since all ligaments and soft tissues can be removed due to the mechanical and structural stability of the prosthesis. During the 1950s and 1960s, hinged total knee arthroplasty provided satisfactory results for a longer period of time in more patients than any other knee arthroplasty design used. However, this method could not be widely used since this type of simple hinged prosthesis cannot replace the complex movements of the knee joint and because of a high failure rate due to early loosening caused by overloading the prosthesis and bone contact surface or by infection.

2.3. The bicompartmental prosthesis

In 1971, Gunston [5] developed polycentric knee arthroplasty. This was done by adopting the concepts of low friction hip arthroplasty espoused by Charnley. Gunston's knee arthroplasty retained the collateral and cruciate ligaments to help absorb stress, and consisted of relatively flat tibial interposition of high-density polyethylene and a round femoral prosthesis, which replaced the posterior portion of femoral condyles. These components were fixed to bones with bone cement, and replaced the complex movements of 'femoral roll-back'. Polycentric knee arthroplasty was initially successful due to improved mobility and movement range, but the fixation it provided was not sufficient.

Geomedic knee arthroplasty was introduced by Coventry et al. at the Mayo Clinic in 1972[6], and consisted of a polyethylene tibial instrument which was of one structure and was in joint with the femoral condyles. This design was initially devised to sustain the cruciate ligament, but joint mobility was limited because of pathologic posterior cruciate ligament in some cases. The main limitation of this design was rapid and excessive loosening.

Freeman et al.[7] at Imperial College Hospital (London) designed a femoral and tibial prosthesis to work in a 'roller-in-trough' manner by the strength of collateral ligament. The anterior and posterior cruciate ligaments were usually removed, and the tibial prosthesis did not have an intramedullary stem to minimize the risk of infection and to maximize knee joint function for salvage procedures. However, the loosening of the tibial prosthesis became a major drawback.

In the mid 1970s, duocondylar interposition was designed to resemble the anatomic structure of the knee joint [8]. The femoral prosthesis connected with two unicondylar prostheses via an anterior bridge, and formed a joint, which was considerable wider than previous polycentric knee arthroplasties, with two flat tibial instruments. However, the design had the drawbacks of frequent destruction or deformity of the tibial prosthesis.

2.4. The tricompartmental prosthesis

In the early 1970s, three types of condylar prostheses were developed, which opened the era of modern knee arthroplasty. First, in 1976, Ranawart et al. [8] at the Hospital for Special Surgery, developed the duocondylar prosthesis; second, Coventry et al.[6] developed the geometric prosthesis; and third, Townley [9] developed the anatomic prosthesis. The condylar prosthesis developed by Ranawart et al. preserved the anterior and posterior cruciate ligaments, provided stability of the knee joint, and used bone cement for fixation to bone. However, the geometric and anatomic types were not produced continuously due to early loosening of fixation. The duocondylar type was further developed to produce the first total condylar prosthesis with a tibial stem by Walker et al. in 1976 [10] at the Hospital for Special Surgery and became the early model for today's posterior cruciate ligament substitution knee arthroplasty. The total condylar prosthesis is a design that removes anterior and posterior cruciate ligaments. The femoral prosthesis, which is made of chrome cobalt, has a symmetric femur with a double curve, which has a flat patellar trochlear groove. The tibial prosthesis is completely made of polyethylene, has good conformity in the flexion and extension states, has anterior and posterior lips in the tibial joint surface, and has eminence in the mid joint surface which provides anteroposterior and mediolateral stability. There is also a stem in the tibial prosthesis, which can endure asymmetric loading. The patellar prosthesis is of the half-ball type and is completely made of polyethylene, with a fixation lug in the middle, which is fixed with bone cement. The features of this early total condylar knee are used in most of today's prostheses. Along with these total condylar prostheses, the duopatellar prosthesis was developed, which preserves the posterior cruciate ligament. This prosthesis is anatomically similar to the normal knee joint with respect to the femoral prosthesis trochlear groove, and forms a joint with a polyethylene patellar prosthesis. The early tibial prosthesis model could be separated into medial and lateral parts, but later a form communicating the bilateral parts was developed. The duopatellar prosthesis was developed into the kinematic condylar prosthesis, which was widely used in the 1980s[11]. Early total condylar prostheses did not allow roll-back in the flexed position and the tibial portion was located posteriorly, which reduced the mobility range when the flexion gap was not balanced. According to early clinical reports, the average mobile angle was 90-100 degrees. To solve this problem, Insall et al. [12] added a cam to the femoral prosthesis and a post to the tibial prosthesis for posterior cruciate ligament substitution knee arthroplasty to accelerate the posterior location of the femoral prosthesis when flexed at about 70 degrees, thus enhancing flexion. These Insall-Burnstein and kinematic interpositions became the foundation of modern knee arthroplasty. Despite the developments of modern joint replacement designs, complications of the femoro-patellar joint were frequent after knee arthroplasty in the 1980s and 1990s, which led to the development of today's knee arthroplasty which increases contact surface in the femoro-patellar joint and prevents lateral displacement of patellar bone.

2.5. Unicompartmental knee arthroplasty

Although it has been used since its introduction in 1950s, the results of unicompartmental knee arthroplasty (Figure 1) remain controversial. In the early 1970s, several authors reported unsatisfactory results for unicompartmental knee arthroplasties but over the next decade, better surgical techniques and proper patient selection improved results [13]. Unicompartmental knee arthroplasty can be used in cases with up to moderate arthritis and when diseased is confined to one compartment. Along with Repicci and Eberle's [14] minimally invasive techniques, unicompartmental knee arthroplasty has aroused much interest. As compared with total knee arthroplasty, the unicompartmental knee arthroplasty has the advantage of preserving anterior and posterior cruciate ligaments and of recovering almost the full range of motion of the normal knee joint. It also boasts a small amount of bone loss and theoretically enables easier revision surgery [15]. The recently reported long-term endurance of unicompartmental knee arthroplasty is about 85-95%, which is similar to that of total arthroplasty. Therefore, if patients are properly selected and an adequate technique is used, it may be a good surgical option.

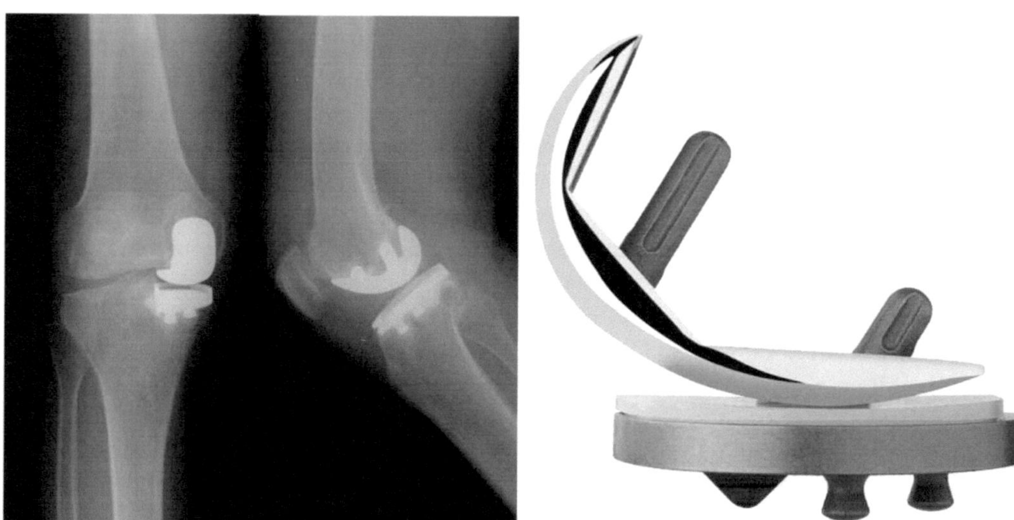

Figure 1. Unicompartmental Knee System (Courtesy of Zimmer)

http://dx.doi.org/10.5772/54343

2.6. Patellar resurfacing

Patellar resurfacing was described as early as 1955. The first patellar resurfacing materials were metallic components, but this design was limited because of problems concerning metal to cartilage articulation. Subsequently, the polyethylene patellar prosthesis was developed and satisfactory results were obtained. Present day knee arthroplasty became total knee replacement when patellar component was added.

3. Spectrum of prosthesis designs

Nowadays, many types of prostheses are used for total knee arthroplasty. However, controversy exists regarding which prostheses are the most appropriate for individual surgeons and specific patients. Therefore, we compare the advantages and disadvantages of each type of interposition knee arthroplasty.

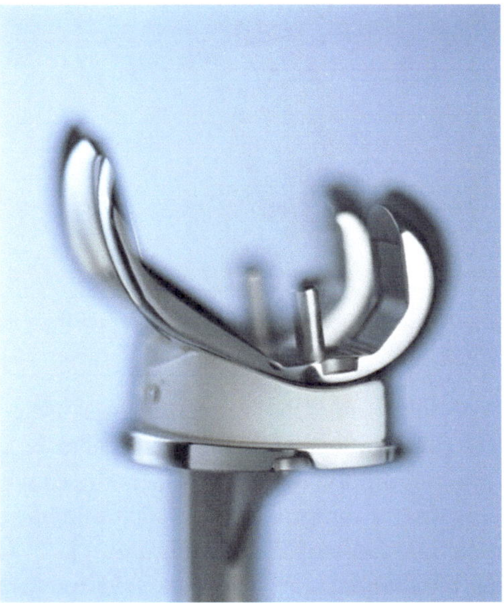

Figure 2. Posterior cruciate ligament retention type prosthesis (Courtesy of DePuy)

3.1. Posterior cruciate ligament retention versus substitution

All knee arthroplasties require anterior cruciate ligament removal, but retention of the posterior cruciate ligament depends on the type of arthroplasty. The preservation type, in which posterior cruciate ligament is preserved, is considered better than the replacement type for performing functions, such as, climbing stairs, and has the advantage of simplifying revision surgery due to less loss of bone (Figure 2). However, knee joints with degenerative arthritis usually show soft tissue contracture, and when preserving the posterior cruciate ligament, the soft tissue balance is not easy to achieve, which possibly increases the risk of early failure due to polyethylene insert overloading caused by posterior cruciate ligament unbalanced tension [16].

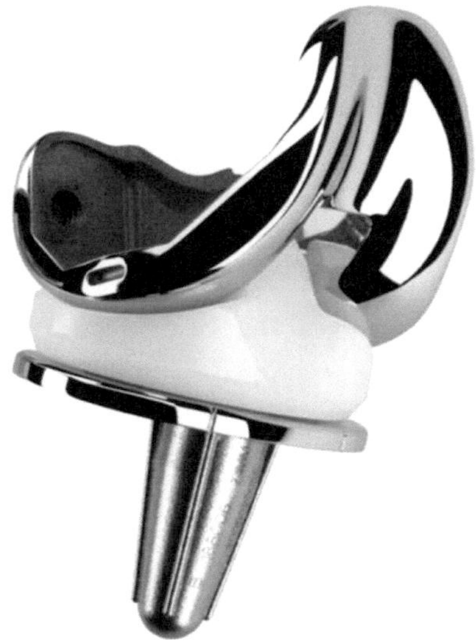

Figure 3. Posterior-substitution prosthesis showing that the post-and-cam mechanism offers no restraint to varus or valgus stability (Courtesy of Biomet)

When the posterior cruciate ligament substitution type is used, even degenerative knee joints with relatively severe deformities can achieve ligament balance, and when flexed at 60-70 degrees, the post of the tibial polyethylene contacts the cam of the femoral component and induces posterior placement of femoral bone, which allows relatively satisfactory rollback and can achieve sufficient knee joint flexion (Figure 3) [17]. However, bone loss at the intercondylar notch makes revision surgery difficult, and fracture may occur intra-operatively or post-operatively in patients with small femurs. From the biomechanical perspective, neither posterior cruciate ligament preservation nor substitution types can totally replace the biomechanics of the normal knee joint. Furthermore, many clinical studies have concluded that there is no significant difference between these two types of prosthesis.

3.2. Mobile versus fixed bearing total knee arthroplasty

Traditional fixed bearing knee arthroplasties have produced good clinical results at 10-15 years postoperatively. Unfortunately, problems associated with polyethylene wear can occur in the long-term, especially in young patients. This wear can be reduced by reducing

http://dx.doi.org/10.5772/54343

contact stress at the joint surface and by improving the wear characteristics of the material used. Contact stress may be reduced by increasing conformity between the femoral component and the polyethylene insert. The development of mobile-bearing articulating polyethylene surfaces in implants for patients undergoing total knee arthroplasty reflects the efforts made by designers to optimize wear while addressing the complexities of function. However, the trade-off for conformity and free mobile range in fixed bearing knee arthroplasty makes marked improvements in contact stress near impossible. To solve this problem, mobile bearing interposition knee arthroplasty was invented to reduce contact stress but to preserve freedom of movement. In 1986, Goodfellow and O'Connor [18] invented Oxford knee arthroplasty, which is a mobile bearing knee arthroplasty of the bicondylar type (Figure 4), and subsequently, Beuchel and Pappas [19] invented the meniscus sustaining bearing, which boasts low contact stress. However, in the case of the mobile bearing insert, the bearing can be dislocated when flexion extension gaps are inadequate. In Europe, this mobile bearing prosthesis has been used for decades with good clinical results, but recent reports have found no significant differences between this mobile bearing prosthesis and fixed bearing polyethylene.

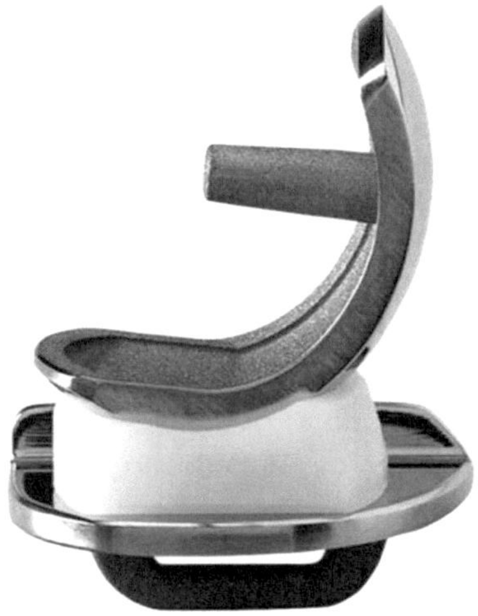

Figure 4. Mobile bearing knee prosthesis, which reduces contact stress but preserves freedom of movement (Courtesy of Biomet)

3.3. Non-cemented versus cemented knee prostheses

Concern over the long-term tolerance of bone cement fixation led to the development of a non-cemented fixation design in 1980. Hungerford et al. [20] invented the initial porous-coated anatomic design, others include, the Miller-Galante, Miller-GalanteII, Tricon-M, Genesis, and Ortholoc prostheses. These implant designs have a surface topography that is conducive to bone ingrowth. Most are coated or textured so that the new bone actually grows into the surface of the implant. They may also use screws or pegs to stabilize the implant until bone ingrowth occurs. However, because they depend on new bone growth for stability, non-cemented implants require a longer healing time than cemented replacements.

Non-cemented implants, unfortunately, showed higher failure rates than cemented knee arthroplasties due to aseptic loosening and bone loss. In all knee replacement implants, metal rubs against the polyethylene insert, and although the metal is polished and the polyethylene is treated to resist wear, the loads and stresses of daily movements generate microscopic particle debris, which in turn, can trigger inflammatory responses that result in osteolysis or loosening.

Because non-cemented implants have not been used as long as cemented implants, comparisons after long-term use are not possible. However, some studies have shown that non-cemented fixation has success rates comparable to those of cemented fixation [21]. Nevertheless, non-cemented knee arthroplasty has not widely adopted, but recent material developments have resulted in materials that enhance bone ingrowth which has led to the use of non-cemented knee arthroplasty in young patients.

3.4. Constrained condylar knee prostheses

Revision total knee arthroplasty is often associated with poorer outcomes due to bone loss and ligament damage, which can result in ligamentous laxity and imbalance. A constrained condylar knee design was developed to resist coronal moments in the plane caused by soft-tissue deficiency. Constrained condylar knee designs have the advantage of allowing changes in the center of rotation during flexion, and thereby, theoretically impart less tangential anterior-posterior stress across the prosthetic interface [22]. An early model of constrained condylar knee design was proposed by Insall et al, although similar to posterior cruciate ligament substitution knee arthroplasty, the polyethylene post is thicker and longer, which provides stability for valgus and varus movements as well as not posterior movements [23]. These early models were developed into Legacy Constrained Condylar Knee (Figure 5)[24]. Excessive constraint is a problem when the LCCK is used and this causes failure by loosening the prosthesis. Thus, in difficult knee arthroplasty cases, usage may be determined during surgery by taking into consideration the need for constraint. For example, in severe valgus knee joints, the LCCK polyethylene insert may be a good candidate, but posterior cruciate substitution tibial bearing is recommended over the constrained type.

3.5. Cross-linked polyethylene bearing

The development of arthroplasty design and materials has led to long-term endurance, but the not infrequent need for revision due to polyethylene wear has been a cause of patient dissatisfaction. To reduce polyethylene wear, a cross-linked polyethylene bearing was developed and used in hip replacements in 1990s, and thus, its effectiveness has been proven. Its resistance to wear provides a promising solution for arthroplasty patients, especially today's more active, physically demanding patients. However, in knee arthroplasty, it has neither been widely used nor widely studied. Recently improved resistance in posterior cruciate substitution knees have been reported to lead to cam and post delamination, pitting, cracking or fractures [25].

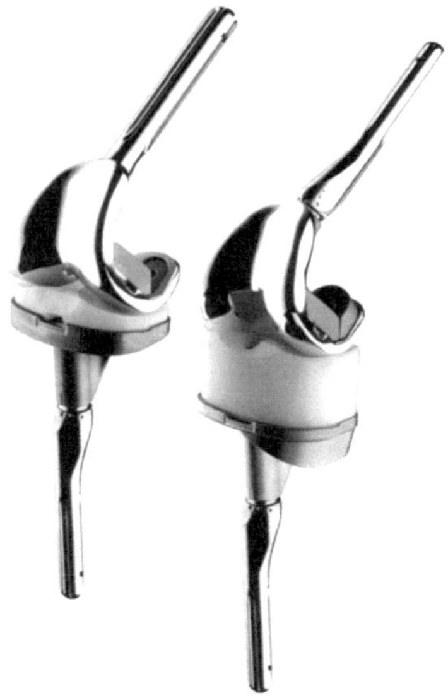

Figure 5. The Legacy Constrained Condylar Knee Prosthesis (Courtesy of Zimmer)

3.6. High flexion type knee prostheses

Generally, postoperative knee motion range for total knee arthroplasty is less than 120 degrees. Recently, to obtain motion ranges similar to those of the normal knee joint, high flexion femoral prostheses with a thickened posterior portion of femoral prostheis and a wider contact surface with the bearing are being used to reduce contact pressure and wear (Figure 6). To prevent collision between the patellar ligament and bearing at high degrees of flexion, a high flexion bearing with an oblique cutting of the anterior bearing has been developed. Furthermore, many authors have reported that high flexion knee arthroplasty can result in smaller contact loadings and wider ranges of motion than previous knee arthroplasties. For example, Huang et al. [26] found that mean flexion in patients with a high-flexion prosthesis was approximately 10° greater than in patients with a standard posterior stabilized implant. Laskin [27] has also published similar findings. In addition to pain reduction and restoration of function, survivorship is also a decisive contributor to the success of TKA. Thanks to its extended posterior condyle radius, which has been broadened all round, the NexGen CR-Flex system offer a larger contact surface during deep bending, and therefore, spreads contact stress over a large area. However, some authors [28, 29] have reported no increase of flexion when using high-flexion prostheses.

In particular, in a clinical study that used both knee implants, high flexion knee arthroplasty did not show a significant increase in knee joint flexion range. This issue needs to be proven by long-term follow up over 10 to 15 years [30].

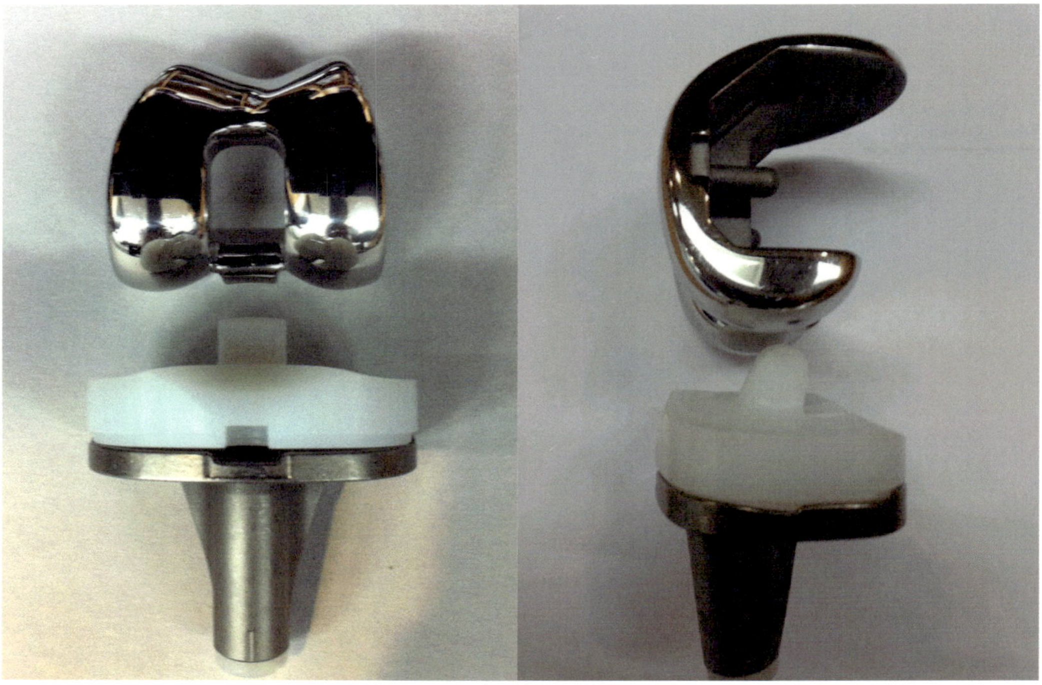

Figure 6. High flexion type prosthesis (Courtesy of Zimmer)

3.7. Ultracongruent polyethylene bearings

The most important thing to remember when performing posterior cruciate ligament preserving knee arthroplasty is to balance the posterior cruciate ligament and prevent instability by ligament disruption when flexed. For these reasons, deep-dished polyethylene insert (also called ultracongruent insert) was developed. This bearing insert has moderate conformity in coronal and sagittal planes, which can prevent edge loading caused from paradoxical anterior translation due to elevation of the anterior lip of the prosthesis, prevent elevation in flexion, and prevent posterior subluxation (Figure 7). Ultracongruent bearings can reduce cam-and-post wear or fracture that may occur after posterior cruciate ligament substitution knee arthroplasties, and can prevent bone loss at the intercondylar cutting site. This bearing represents a new concept in that it can also maintain the posterior cruciate ligament and provide moderate conformity in total knee arthroplasty. Further long-term clinical follow-up is required along with comparative clinical trials of posterior cruciate ligament preservation, substitution, and sacrificing techniques.

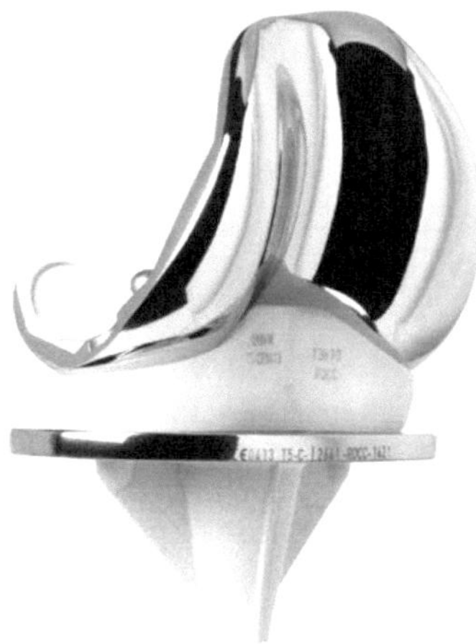

Figure 7. Ultracongruent polyethylene bearing (Courtesy of Biomet)

4. Conclusion

The history of prostheses evolution follows a repetitive course of development and failure. The continuous and rapid developments of biomechanics and of materials in the 20th century hugely expanded the information available. Furthermore, spectrums of designs are currently being used for total knee arthroplasty.

Most knee replacements are now being performed with PCL-retaining or PCL-substituting prosthesis that have their merits and limitations, as discussed above. New mobile-bearing devices, which address the issue of functional complexity, have been developed and have the potential to prolong implant durability. Nonetheless, prosthesis materials and the historical and current results of different types of prosthesis remain topics of discussion with respect to their indications and contraindications. In the future, the new implant will be developed by applying the pros and removing the cons based on the implant history.

Author details

Eun-Kyoo Song, Jong-Keun Seon, Jae-Young Moon and Yim Ji-Hyoun

Department of Orthopedic Surgery, Chonnam National University Hwasun Hospital, Hwasun, Korea

References

[1] Ferguson, W. Excision of the knee joint: recovery with a false joint and a useful limb. Med Times Gaz (1861).

[2] Campbell, W. C. Interposition of vitallium plates in arthroplasties of the knee. Preliminary report. By Willis C. Campbell, (1940). Clin Orthop Relat Res 1988;, 226, 3-5.

[3] MacIntosh DLHemiarthroplasty of the knee using a space occupying prosthesis for painful varus and valgus deformities. J Bone Joint Surg Am (1958).

[4] Walldius, B. Arthroplasty of the knee joint using an endoprosthesis. Acta Orthop Scand (1957). Suppl:19.

[5] Gunston, F. H. Polycentric knee arthroplasty: prosthetic simulation of normal knee movement. J Bone Joint Surg Br (1971). , 53, 272-277.

[6] Coventry, M. B, Finerman, G. A, Riley, L. H, Turner, R. H, & Upshaw, J. E. A new geometric knee for total knee arthroplasty. Clin Orthop Relat Res (1972). , 83, 157-162.

[7] Freeman, M. A, Swanson, S. A, & Todd, R. C. Total replacement of the knee using the Freeman-Swanson knee prosthesis. Clin Orthop Relat Res (1973). , 94, 153-170.

[8] Ranawat, C. S, Insall, J, & Shine, J. Duo-condylar knee arthroplasty: hospital for special surgery design. Clin Orthop Relat Res (1976). , 120, 76-82.

[9] Townley, C. O. The anatomic total knee resurfacing arthroplasty. Clin Orthop Relat Res (1985).

[10] [10] Walker, P. S, Ranawat, C, & Insall, J. Fixation of the tibial components of condylar replacement knee prostheses. J Biomech (1976). , 9, 269-275.

[11] Rand, J. A, Chao, E. Y, & Stauffer, R. N. Kinematic rotating-hinge total knee arthroplasty. J Bone Joint Surg Am (1987). , 69, 489-497.

[12] Insall, J. N, Lachiewicz, P. F, & Burstein, A. H. The posterior stabilized condylar prosthesis: a modification of the total condylar design. Two to four-year clinical experience. J Bone Joint Surg Am (1982). , 64, 1317-1323.

[13] Laskin, R. S. Unicompartmental tibiofemoral resurfacing arthroplasty. J Bone Joint Surg Am (1978). , 60, 182-185.

[14] Repicci, J. A, & Eberle, R. W. Minimally invasive surgical technique for unicondylar knee arthroplasty. J South Orthop Assoc (1999). , 8, 20-27.

[15] Jung, Y. B, & Lee, Y. S. Principles of unicompartmental knee arthroplasty. J Korean Orthop Assoc (2004). , 39, 108-114.

[16] Martin, S. D, Mcmanus, J. L, Scott, R. D, & Thornhill, T. S. Press-fit condylar total knee arthroplasty: 5- to 9-year follow-up evaluation. J Arthroplasty (1997). , 12, 603-614.

[17] Freeman, M. A, & Railton, G. T. Should the posterior cruciate ligament be retained or resected in condylar nonmeniscal knee arthro-plasty? The case for resection. J Arthroplasty (1988). Suppl: SS12., 3.

[18] Goodfellow, J. W, & Connor, O. J. Clinical results of the Oxford knee: surface arthroplasty of the tibiofemoral joint with a meniscal bearing prosthesis. Clin Orthop Relat Res (1986). , 205, 21-42.

[19] Buechel, F. F, & Pappas, M. J. Long-term survivorship analysis of cruciate-sparing versus cruciate-sacrificing knee prostheses using meniscal bearings. Clin Orthop Relat Res (1990). , 260, 162-169.

[20] Hungerford, D. S, Kenna, R. V, & Krackow, K. A. The porous-coated anatomic total knee. Orthop Clin North Am (1982). , 13, 103-122.

[21] Baker, P. N, Khaw, F. M, Kirk, L. M, Esler, C. N, & Gregg, P. J. A randomised controlled trial of cemented versus cementless press-fit condylar total knee replacement: 15-year survival analysis. J Bone Joint Surg Br (2007). , 89, 1608-14.

[22] Kim, Y. H, & Kim, J. S. Revision total knee arthroplasty with use of a constrained condylar knee prosthesis. J Bone Joint Surg Am. (2009). , 91, 1440-7.

[23] Ranawat, C. S, & Sculco, J. P. History of the development of total knee prosthesis at the hospital for special surgery. In: Ranawat CS, editor. Total condylar knee arthroplasty: technique, results, and complications. Berlin: Springer Verlag; (1985). , 3-6.

[24] Easley, M. E, Insall, J. N, Scuderi, G. R, & Bullek, D. D. Primary constrained condylar knee arthroplasty for the arthritic valgus knee. Clin Orthop Relat Res (2000). , 380, 58-64.

[25] Oral, E, Malhi, A. S, Wannomae, K. K, & Muratoglu, O. K. Highly cross-linked ultra-high molecular weight polyethylene with improved fatigue resistance for total joint arthroplasty: recipient of the 2006 Hap Paul Award. J Arthroplasty (2008). , 23, 1037-44.

[26] Huang, H. T, Su, J. Y, & Wang, G. J. The early results of high-flex total knee arthroplasty: a minimum of 2 years of follow-up. J Arthroplasty (2005). , 20, 674-9.

[27] Endres, S, & Wilke, A. Early experience with the NexGen® CR-Flex Mobile knee arthroplasty system: results of year follow-up. Orth Rev (2010). , 2.

[28] Laskin, R. S. The effect of a high-flex implant on postoperative flexion after primary total knee arthroplasty. Orthopedics (2007). Suppl): , 86-8.

[29] Kim, Y. H, Sohn, K. S, & Kim, J. S. Range of motion of standard and highflexion posterior stabilized total knee prostheses: a prospective, randomized study. J Bone Joint Surg Am (2005). A:1470-5., 87.

[30] Endres, S, & Wilke, A. High flexion total knee arthroplasty- mid-term follow up of 5 years. Open Orthop J. (2011). , 14, 138-42.

Chapter 10

Optimization of Tuberosity Healing in Prosthetic Reconstruction of Proximal Humerus Fractures

Moby Parsons

Additional information is available at the end of the chapter

http://dx.doi.org/10.5772/53727

1. Introduction

Achieving successful clinical outcomes after hemiarthroplasty for 4-part proximal humerus fractures remains a sobering challenge for even the experienced shoulder reconstruction surgeon or traumatologist. Despite what appears to be secure tuberosity fixation at the time of wound closure, serial postoperative radiographs often reveal progressive displacement and/or resorption of the greater tuberosity.[1-3] This results in a situation akin to a posterior-superior rotator cuff tear, where most patients cannot generate sufficient cuff strength to stabilize the humeral head against the superior pull of the deltoid. Secondary mechanical consequences, including shoulder weakness, superior instability and trapezial substitution can compromise outcomes both in terms of shoulder function and pain in such circumstances.[4, 5] Stiffness and cuff dysfunction frequently render the functional results only fair and many patients must accept a limited goals end result.[6-8]

It is well established that restoration of shoulder function after hemiarthroplasty for fracture depends on successful tuberosity healing in combination with proper reconstruction of the head-tuberosity and head-shaft relationships.[1, 7-9] In the native proximal humerus, the edge of the articular cartilage of the superior head is directly adjacent to the cuff insertion and the two are nearly confluent. The dome of the head is about 5-8 mm above the supraspinatus footprint. Restoring this confluence between the cuff insertion and the prosthetic head while maintaining appropriate tuberosity offset relative to the center of rotation is essential for proper cuff mechanics. Restoring proper head height, medial offset, posterior offset and retrotorsion is also critical to achieving soft tissue balance that will provide both strength and stability.

Despite the introduction of fracture-specific prostheses, translating successful anatomical reconstruction into shoulder function is not guaranteed by the theoretical solutions these newer designs propose for complex fracture treatment. Realistically, outcomes after hemiarthroplasty for fracture are a blend of appropriate prosthesis selection and use, optimal management of tuberosity fixation, respect for the biology of fracture healing and application of an appropriate rehabilitation protocol that does not jeopardize these other aims. As follows is a discussion about principles for optimizing tuberosity reduction, fixation and healing using horizontal cable cerclage in combination with a press-fit, porous coated fracture-specific prosthesis. This technique can be applied in the setting of hemiarthroplasty or reverse shoulder arthroplasty for fracture.

2. Why does failure of tuberosity healing occur?

As with fractures in other bones, successful union of the tuberosities after humeral hemiarthroplasty requires an optimal biological and mechanical environment for bone healing. Failure occurs for several potential reasons alone or in combination. Firstly, aggressive mobilization techniques during exposure may devascularize and further destabilize the tuberosities by stripping periosteal attachments. These periosteal attachments are critical to the blood supply of the greater tuberosity when the posterior circumflex humeral artery has been severed by the fracture pattern. This is generally the case when fracture severity warrants prosthetic reconstruction. Secondly, violation of the rotator interval capsule during exposure and head retrieval disrupts the remaining bridge of tissue that links the tuberosities. This further destabilizes the tuberosities by dissociating the transverse force couple that counteracts their individual deforming forces.

Thirdly, thermal damage from cement may further damage the endosteal blood supply of the humerus, and cement blocks the marrow cavity and areas where the fracture fragments may interdigitate. Fourthly, conventional suture fixation constructs often fail to achieve sufficiently rigid fixation to permit healing. Poor bone quality and fracture comminution increase the likelihood of suture loosening, which occurs early in the postoperative period. Finally, prosthesis designs that do not provide an adequate template for recreation of the cortical shell of the proximal humerus and those that do not allow direct fixation of the tuberosities to the body of the prosthesis will invite a degree of micromotion that is not compatible with fracture union.

3. Features of the EPOCA prosthesis

For fracture hemiarthroplasty, the author prefers the EPOCA Shoulder System (Synthes, Westchester, PA). The EPOCA shoulder prosthesis has several features that make it an ideal choice for use in reconstructing proximal humerus fractures. The design of the humeral prosthesis is based on extensive anatomical studies with the goal of restoring the normal structural relationships between the head, tuberosities and shaft.[10] The rationale behind the design of the EPOCA system is that aspects of the proximal humeral anatomy that are

http://dx.doi.org/10.5772/53727

highly variable across the population should be adjustable while those aspects with minimal variation should be standardized. Features with a high variation include head radius, size of the humeral medullary canal, medial offset and tuberosity offset. Features with a low variation include neck-shaft angle and the ratio of head height to radius. To this end, the system offers 5 stem sizes (6 - 14mm in 2 mm increments) and 10 head diameters (40 – 58 mm in 2 mm increments). There are also standard (115 mm) and long (215 mm) stem lengths. Independent adjustment of medial and posterior offset can be achieved by a dual eccentricity (Eccenter) that allows the head to be placed in an infinite number of X-Y positions within a 6 mm orbit relative to the humeral component. This ensures precise reconstruction of the proximal humeral anatomy and center of rotation.

The EPOCA stem comes in both a press fit and cemented option (Figure 1). The former has porous coating on the proximal half, the roughness of which may help promote tuberosity adherence and security. The tapered wedge geometry has a prominent calcar design that helps the stem self-center, self-rotate and self-lock as it is inserted. Thus, even in a fracture situation, a press-fit stem can be used and achieve excellent stem stability without the need for cement fixation.

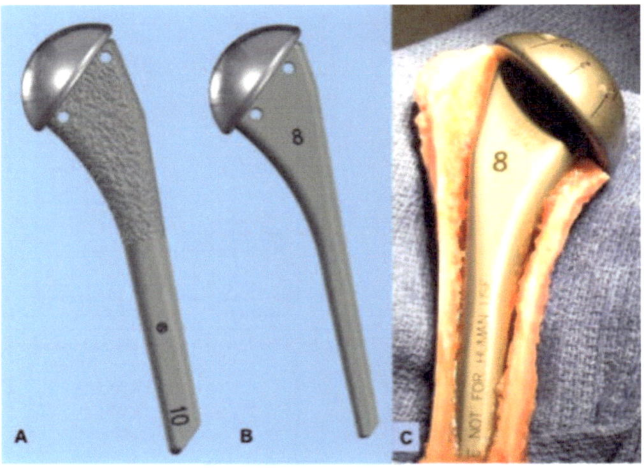

Figure 1. The EPOCA stem comes in press-fit, porous coated (A) and smooth, cemented (B) options. Both have a tapered wedge geometry with a prominent calcar design that promotes metaphyseal fill (C). Medial and lateral holes in the proximal stem allow cerclage directly through the prosthesis rather than around its medial calcar portion. These features permit use of the press-fit stem in the setting of fracture due to the rotational stability afforded by the stem geometry.

The proximal body of the stem has both a medial and lateral hole through which cables can be passed for tuberosity cerclage (Figure 1). This construct improves rotational stability of the cerclage fixation compared to cables or sutures passed around the calcar section of the prosthesis. In the latter case, the fixation is not directly linked to the stem so that the tuberosities can still move independently of the prosthesis when the arm is rotated about the axis of the humerus. By passing fixation through the stem of the prosthesis, the tuberosities are compressed directly to the stem so that the construct rotates as a single unit during arm rotation. The improved stability of this fixation obviates the need for multiple other sutures, specifically vertical sutures between the shaft and bone-tendon junction that tend to result in the common mistake of tuberosity over-reduction.

4. Preoperative planning

When the decision to operate has been made, the surgeon needs to consider a variety of factors in deciding the best method of treatment for the given fracture pattern. Aspects of the patient's medical and social history are important to consider. The following patients factors may bear on the decision to attempt fixation versus prosthetic replacement: age, hand-dominance, physical demands, expectations, compliance, smoking history, and medical comorbidity.

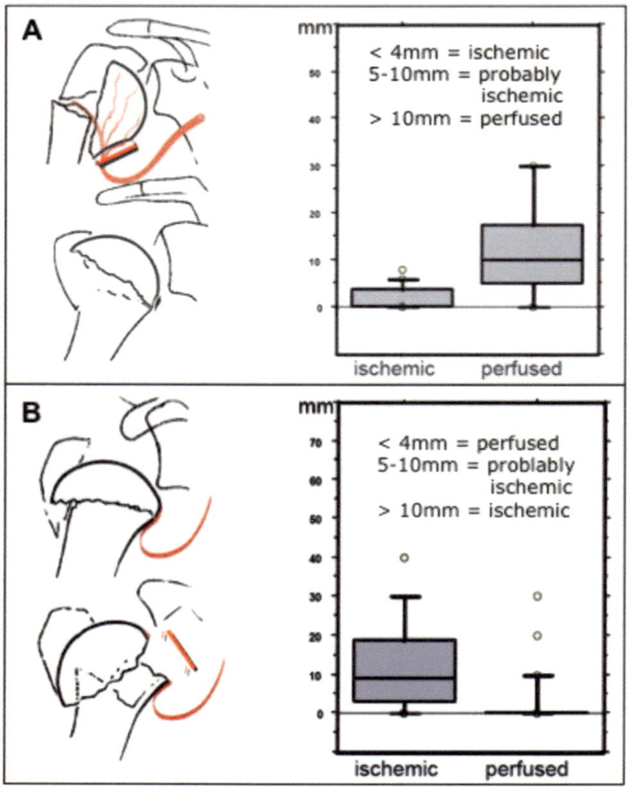

Figure 2. Head perfusion is best assessed by the length of the medial metaphyseal extension (A) and the displacement of the medial periosteal hinge (B). If the metaphyseal extension is less than 5mm and/or the displacement of the medial hinge is more than 5-10mm, the head is likely ischemic.

It is essential when assessing these fractures to have a thorough understanding of the fracture "personality" and this usually demands a CT scan with coronal and sagittal reconstructions that allow for 3-D rendering. Such imaging can be invaluable in determining the location and degree of comminution, the integrity of the articular surface, the exact relationship between the head, tuberosity and shaft, as well as prognostic indicators of head vascularity. In the latter case, the length of the medial metaphyseal extension and the displacement of the medial periosteal hinge are most predictive of head perfusion (Figure 2).

This collective information can help the surgeon determine if fixation is both warranted and feasible. Feasibility depends on factors such as bone quality and comminution, fracture complexity, availability of the necessary implants and surgeon skill. If stable, anatomical fixation is not possible, then prosthetic replacement is warranted. While reverse shoulder arthroplasty has become increasingly popular in this setting, there remains a role for hemiarthroplasty in younger and more physically demanding patients. Of note, the technique described herein can be used for secure tuberosity fixation during reverse arthroplasty for fracture where outcome can also be improved by successful tuberosity healing allowing restoration of active external rotation.

5. Surgical technique

The patient is positioned as for a shoulder arthroplasty such that the scapula is supported but the arm can be brought over the side of the bed to expose the humeral shaft. The fracture is exposed through a standard delto-pectoral approach taking the cephalic vein laterally with the deltoid. The anterior deltoid is elevated off the coracoacromial (CA) ligament and a sharp angled lever is placed behind the ligament. This helps "roll" the deltoid laterally to expose the proximal humerus.

The clavipectoral fascia is excised en bloc from the CA ligament proximally to the pectoralis major tendon distally and the conjoint tendon medially to the deltoid laterally. Once this layer has been removed, the humeroscapular motion interface is accessible and adhesions in this interval can be freed using blunt dissection. One must avoid overzealous dissection to prevent stripping of any residual periosteal attachment of the tuberosities to the shaft. A curved ring retractor can then be placed beneath the deltoid and a right-angle retractor beneath the conjoint tendon.

The biceps tendon is then identified and followed proximally. It should be sutured to the pectoralis major tendon to preserve native tension and then tenotomized at the superior aspect of the bicipital groove. Because the bicipital groove and a portion of the anterior greater tuberosity usually remain attached to the lesser tuberosity fragment, it is critical to preserve the rotator interval capsule (Figure 3A). Thus, it should not be routinely divided above the transverse humeral ligament as many conventional techniques recommend (Figure 3B). Preservation of the rotator interval will help stabilize the tuberosity repair by leaving a soft tissue bridge between the anterior and posterior fragments. This helps neutralize the individual deforming forces that lead to loosening and failure of fixation. In a majority of cases there is a longitudinal split in the supraspinatus tendon where the anterior bundle remains attached to the lesser tuberosity fragment. Maintenance of this attachment is critical to maximize the potential for cuff function postoperatively. Exposure of the humeral head and glenoid can be achieved by extending the longitudinal cuff split medially. This can be repaired side-to-side at the conclusion of the case and does not jeopardize the cuff insertion to the bone.

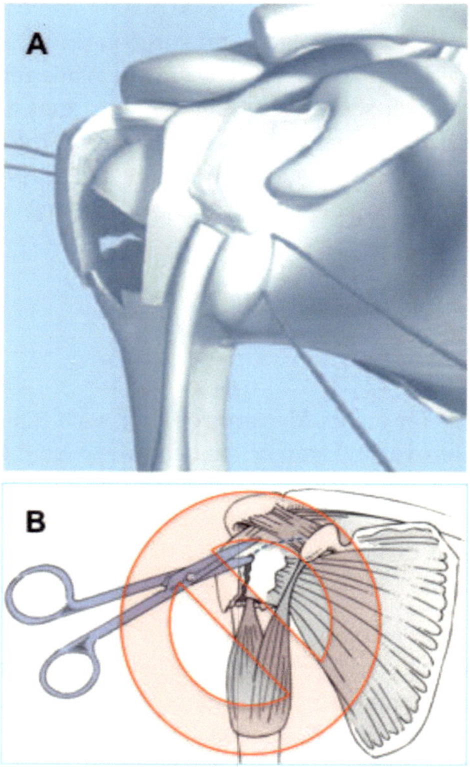

Figure 3. In a typical 4-part fracture, the bicipital groove and anterior most portion of the greater tuberosity remains attached to the anterior, lesser tuberosity fragment (A). The anterior bundle of the supraspinatus tendon remains attached to this anterior fragment, separated by a longitudinal split in the tendon at the level of the fracture plane. The rotator interval capsule remains intact and should not be violated as is current convention (B).

Heavy braided suture is placed through the bone tendon interface of each of the subscapularis (SC), supraspinatus (SS) and infraspinatus (IS) tendons. It is essential when placing the posterior sutures that excessive traction is not applied so that soft tissue attachments between the tuberosity and shaft are maintained. Overly aggressive tuberosity mobilization injures the periosteal blood supply and reduces the likelihood of eventual healing. As much as possible, the greater tuberosity should be left in-situ posteriorly.

The humeral head can then be retrieved from the joint through the split in the SS tendon. The head can then be "keyed in" to the shaft to determine the location of the medial metaphyseal extension. The length of this extension is then measured and this length represents the distance above the calcar that the prosthetic head should sit to restore proper head height (Figure 4). This is a simple, reliable and accurate method of determining head height that can be cross-referenced with other accepted methods per the surgeon's discretion. The humeral head is then sized against the prosthetic head trials. One should typically downsize if the native head is in between trial head sizes so as not to overstuff the joint. Cancellousautograft is then harvested from the humeral head for supplemental bone grafting of the tuberosities to aid in restoration of tuberosity offset.

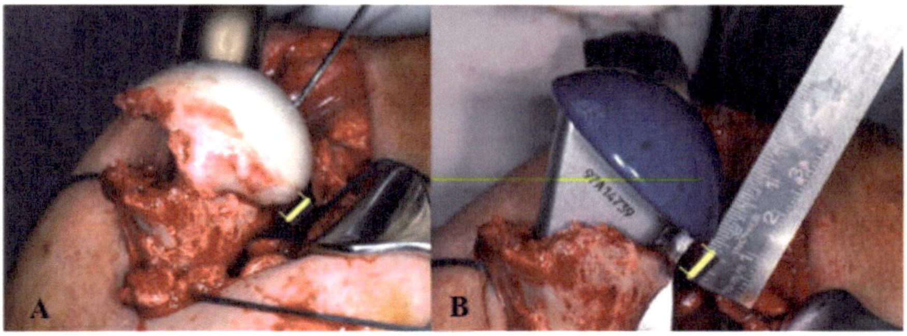

Figure 4. The length of the medial metaphyseal extension can be used as an accurate and reproducible method of determining the height at which the prosthesis should be seated to recreate proximal humeral anatomy. The native head can be keyed onto the shaft to determine this height (A). The prosthesis height and medial offset should be set to reproduce the native shoulder anatomy (B).

Prior to stem implantation, it is important to place the cerclage cables through the greater tuberosity in an inside-out fashion (Figure 5) At a level approximately 5 mm below the bone-tendon junction, a 2 mm drill bit is used to make the medial and lateral holes through the tuberosity bone. Again, care should be taken to leave the tuberosity in-situ when these holes are drilled to protect soft-tissue attachments. A Synthes 1 mm needled, beadless cable is then passed through each of the holes. The cable crimp must be taken off before the cable is placed and the crimp saved on the back table so that it is not inadvertently lost. The needle can be bounced off of the curved deltoid retractor and the cable retrieved on the dorsal tuberosity surface. The needle is removed and the cables are then tagged with a hemostat and parked posteriorly for later tuberosity repair.

A distally-angled Fukuda retractor is next placed behind the glenoid to inspect the joint. The root of the biceps should be excised and the glenoid articular surface checked for concomitant fracture. The labrum should be preserved to aid in stability and load distribution. Aggressive capsular releases are not necessary in fracture reconstruction as would be performed during shoulder arthroplasty for degenerative disease, and the temptation to perform a circumferential subscapularis release should be avoided. This will only jeopardize the anterior circumflex humeral artery, which provides vascularity to the anterior tuberosity fragment, and disrupt the important rotator interval "bridge."

The humeral shaft is then exposed by placing the arm in extension, adduction and external rotation. Two blunt Hohman retractors, posteriorly and medially, are used to leaver the shaft anteriorly. If necessary, the medullary canal is opened with the cylindrical starter rasp. Further reaming is not necessary as the EPOCA system uses impaction broaches to prepare the canal. Starting with the smallest broach, proper stem rotation is determined by orienting the laser-etched center line of the broach with a point 8 mm posterior to the deepest point of the bicipital. This point has been shown to correspond to the equatorial plane of the humeral head (Figure 6A & B).[10] The broach is seated to the level that restores the head height according to the pre-determined metaphyseal extension length. Proper retrotorsion of the humeral stem can be confirmed by inserting the 6 mm rod into the broach and measuring roughly 25 degrees relative to the forearm axis with the goniometer.

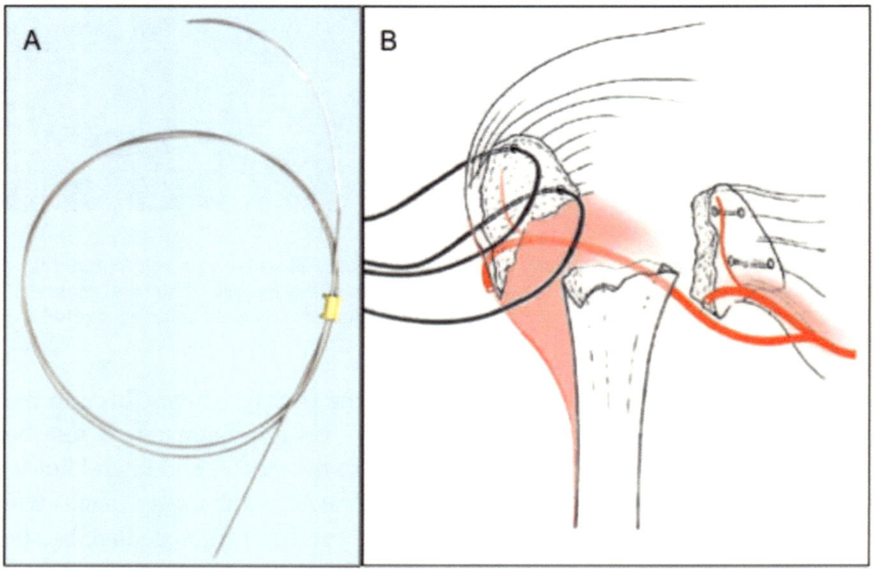

Figure 5. The Synthes beadles, needled cable should be used (A); cables should be placed prior to instrumentation of the humeral shaft with care taken not to disrupt periosteal attachments between the tuberosities and the humeral shaft (B).

Progressively larger broaches are introduced until distal (diaphyseal) canal fill is achieved. A curved curette can be used to remove cancellous bone along the medial humeral metaphyseal region to help fully seat the desired broach if necessary. The pronounced calcar design allows the broach to self-center, self-align and self-lock in the proper height and orientation, obviating the need for cumbersome jigs to position the trial stem. Once the stem size has been determined, the trial stem is impacted to the proper height using light progressive taps with the mallet to prevent fracture of the shaft by the wedge-shaped stem.

In a majority of cases, an optimal fit can be achieved allowing the use of a press-fit stem. In the occasional case, one stem size is over-recessed relative to the calcar and the next size too big for the diaphysis. In these cases, the surgeon has two choices. The first is to attempt impaction grafting the smaller stem to the proper height using autograft from the humeral head and the smaller impaction broach. With the diaphyseal portion of the broach inserted only slightly into the canal, small croutons of bone graft can be placed circumferentially around the canal opening and progressively impacted into the metaphysis. This process can be repeated until a snug fit is achieved with the broach. In patients with severely osteoporotic bone, a stable press-fit may not be possible without undue risk of humeral shaft fracture. The second option is to cement the final prosethsis in a conventional manner. In such a case, the final chosen stem will be one size smaller than the broach and trial stem to allow for a circumferential cement mantle.

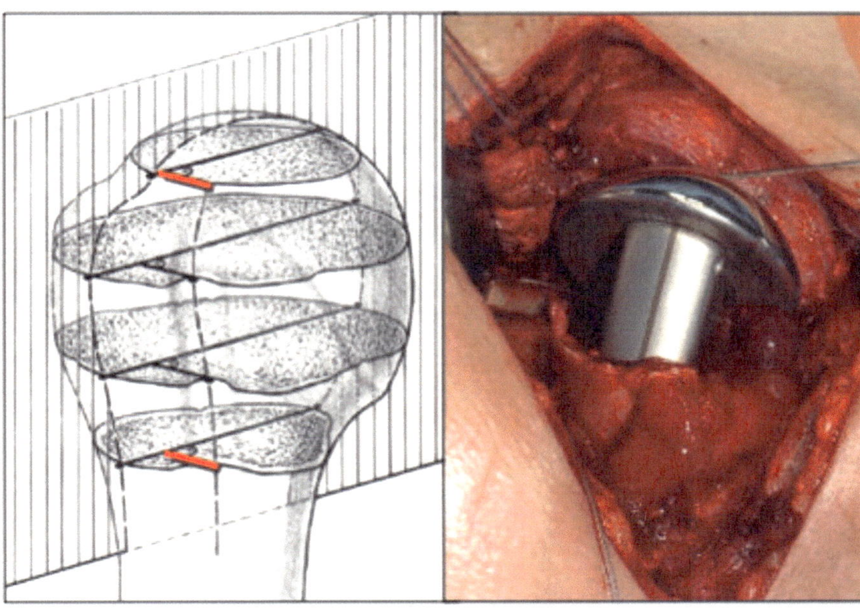

Figure 6. The equatorial plane of the humeral head bisects the edge of the articular cartilage adjacent the rotator cuff at a point approximately 8mm posterior to the deepest point of the bicipical groove (A); This is also true in the metaphyseal region and can be used to orient the trial stem into the proper retrotorsion. When the laser etch on the back of the stem is 8mm posterior to the bicipital groove on the proximal aspect of the humeral shaft, the retrotorsion should measure roughly 25-30 degrees relative to the forearm axis (B).

The Eccenter is then placed on the trial stem followed by the trial humeral head. The 2.5 mm hex driver is used to dial the Eccenter with respect to the stem while the head can be manually rotated on the Eccenter. The combined dual eccentricity of this design allows the head to be placed in an infinite number of antero-posterior (AP) and medio-lateral (ML) offset positions within a 6mm orbit (Figure 7A). More importantly it allows independent adjustment of the medial and posterior offset to more accurately restore the patient's native anatomy and center of rotation. Optimal medial offset is achieved by recreating the medial calcar line without step off (Figure 7B). In the AP plane, slight posterior offset is desirable to accommodate the larger greater tuberosity and restore native posterior offset of the humeral head relative to the humeral medullary canal. Once the head position has been chosen, the head and Eccenter can be locked using the 2.0 mm hex driver. The trial prosthesis is then reduced into the joint to confirm a congruent stable fit with the glenoid. After the offset number of the head is recorded, the head is removed and the offset letter of the Eccenter is then recorded so that the construct can be replicated with the final components.

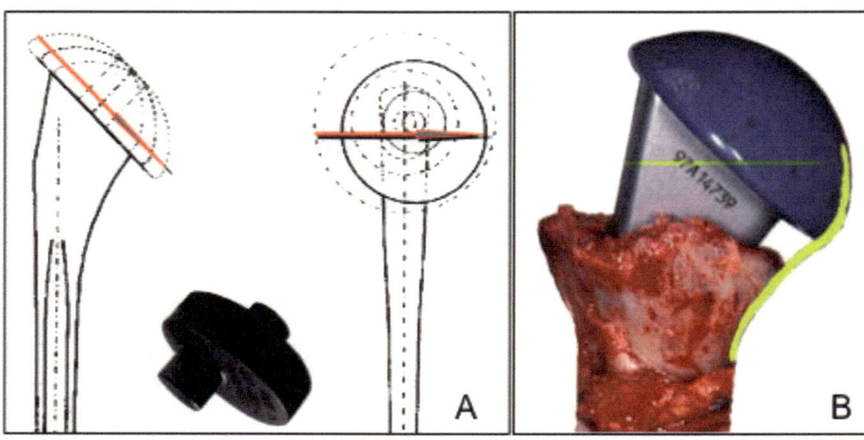

Figure 7. The Eccenter in combination with the humeral head provides a dual offset that allows independent adjustment of the medial and posterior offset for optimal head positioning (A); The medial offset should be adjusted to recreate the normal calcar line relative to the humeral shaft (B).

The final component is then assembled using the press and inserted as a monoblock. The diaphyseal portion of the stem is placed into the medullary canal. Prior to fully seating the component, the cables are passed through the medial and lateral holes from posterior to anterior (Figure 8A). The 3 mm retrotorsion bar is then used to cross-check proper rotation and the component is then fully press fit to the pre-determined height.

The prosthesis is then reduced into the glenoid. Two holes are then drilled into the lesser tuberosity fragment using the 2.0 mm drill. These holes should be placed slightly below the bone tendon junction and correspond to positions of the cables exiting the stem. A 14 gauge angiocath can then be inserted from outside to inside through these holes as a transit to shuttle the cables through the bone fragment. Prior to final tuberosity reduction, bone graft from the humeral head is packed around the stem to fill any voids and augment the often fragile cortical sleeve of the tuberosity fragments. A #2 non-absorbable suture is next used to reapproximate the longitudinal SS split. This aids in fine tuning the tuberosity reduction.

Care must be taken not to over-reduce the tuberosities especially distally. Rather than being pulled down and fixed to the humeral shaft with vertical sutures, the tuberosities should be pushed up to restore the native position of the superior rotator cuff insertion relative to the edge of the prosthetic head. Once this position has been optimized, the tuberosities can be securely fixed with horizontal cable cerclage (Figure 8B).

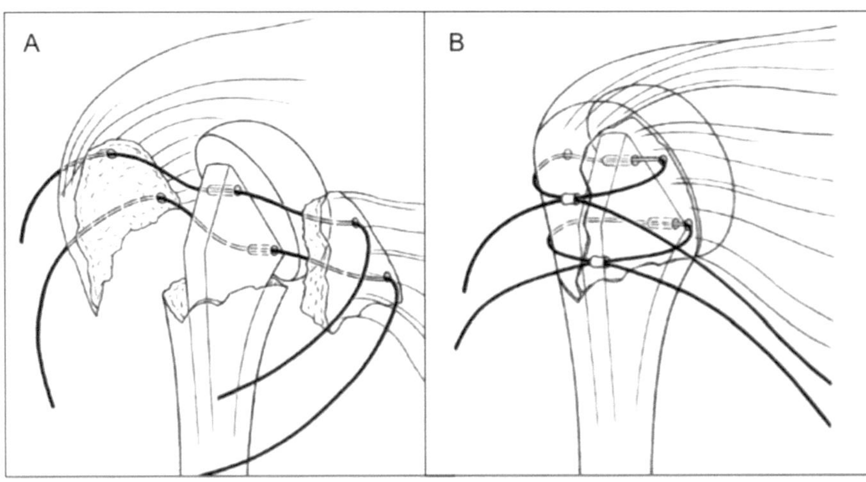

Figure 8. The cables should be passed through the prosthesis from back to front before final prosthesis seating. After holes are drilled into the lesser tuberosity fragment, these cables are then passed from inside to outside through the lesser fragment (A). Once the joint is reduced and the tuberosities situated to recreate the proper head-tuberosity relationship, the cables can be tightened and crimped to effect a horizonal cerclage directly to the prosthesis (B).

Both ends of each cable are threaded through their respective crimps, which are positioned over the bicipital groove. The cables are then spaced superiorly and inferiorly on the tuberosities. The superior cable must be placed below the bone tendon junction so that it does not subluxate over the humeral head. To tension the beadless cable, the crimp must be stabilized on one side by either a hemostat or by the accessory locking portion of the Synthes tensioner. The tensioner is then placed on the opposite side and tensioned until a firm embrace is achieved (roughly 20-30 kg). Overtensioning should be avoided so to prevent deforming or crushing the fragile bone and to avoid devascularization. After crimping and cutting the cables to length, the biceps tendon can be used to cover the crimps by a soft tissue tenodesis to the cuff.

Further tuberosity fixation is not necessary and usually only promotes overreduction and devascularization. A single vertical suture, however, can be passed from the shaft around the superior cable to prevent it from slipping over the head. After copious irrigation, the wound is closed in layers over a drain, followed by a sterile compressive dressing and sling. Postoperative radiographs are obtained in the recovery room to confirm an optimal reconstruction (Figure 9).

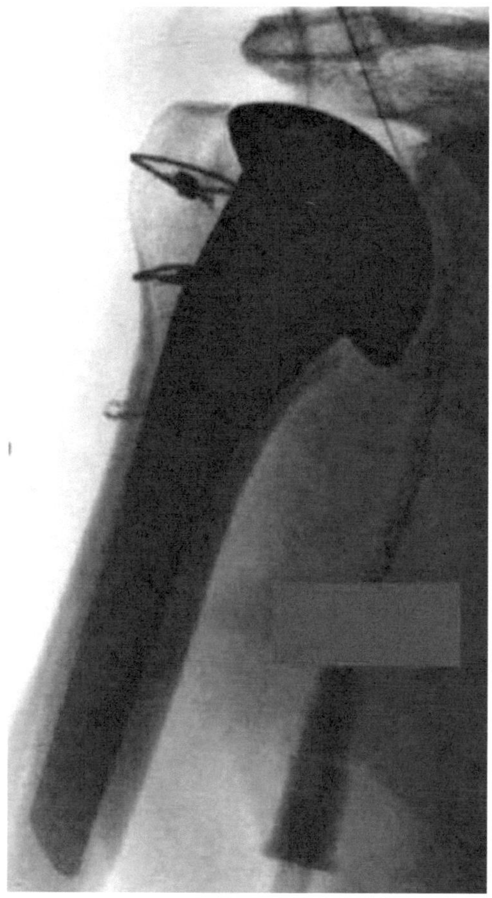

Figure 9. Postoperative AP film showing stable tuberosity reduction with anatomical reconstruction of the calcar line, head height and tuberosity height and offset.

6. Postoperative protocol

Active use of the arm is avoided for 6 weeks to allow tuberosity healing but passive motion exercises must be started early to maximize postoperative function. Although some advocate no passive motion for several weeks, stiffness remains a significant problem that limits the final outcome of these procedures. Because dense adhesions form in the subacromial space and humeroscapular motion interface, nonoperative and operative treatment of post-surgical adhesive capsulitis in the presence of prosthesis is a substantial challenge that is often marginal in its success. Codman's exercises and positional exercises such as gentle table slides or resting the arm in an abducted position can be started as soon as patients are comfortable. Patients are instructed to steadily increase their passive range on a self-directed basis. Formal physical therapy is often avoided in the early stages to prevent overly aggressive applied stress that might jeopardize tuberosity fixation.

Serial x-rays and clinical status are checked at approximately 2, 4 and 8 weeks postoperatively. Active-assisted range of motion can be added around 6 weeks assuming stable tuberosity fixation. Progressive active range of motion and active use can be started at 8 weeks based on radiographic evidence of tuberosity healing and patient compliance.

7. Discussion

Prosthetic replacement for the fractured proximal humerus follows the same biological and mechanical principles that have evolved from experience in fracture fixation in other areas. Surgeons should approach this case with the same tenets and goals as any fracture case and not abandon these principles given the insertion of a prosthesis. Preservation of soft tissue and periosteal attachments is critical to maintaining blood supply to the fracture fragments. Preservation of the endosteal blood supply and avoidance of suture strangulation are also important. Finally, fixation must be sufficiently rigid to reduce micromotion to a level that permits fracture healing. The use of horizontal cable cerclage for tuberosity fixation using the above-described technique in combination with a press-fit, porous humeral stem addresses each of these critical elements to optimize the chance for successful healing in these difficult cases.

Nils et al performed a meta-analysis of fracture hemiarthroplasty outcomes. Although the quality of existing reports was deemed to be insufficient to make formal recommendations about the role of hemiarthroplasty in the fracture setting, the authors did note that "tuberosity healing has influenced functional outcome in all series mentioning this parameter."[7] Boileau et al followed 66 patients after hemiarthroplasty for fracture and found tuberosity malposition and migration in 50% of cases leading to unsatisfactory results including superior migration, stiffness, weakness and pain.[1] Greiner and associated found that tuberosity malposition correlates with the development of fatty infiltration of the cuff muscles and this occurrence was significantly associated with poorer clinical outcomes in patients after hemiarthroplasty for fracture.[11] Huffman and colleagues studied the biomechanics of tuberosity malposition in 4-part fractures and determined that inferior placement (tuberosity overreduction) has a significant negative impact on the mechanical advantage of the deltoid during shoulder abduction.[5]

Taken together, these reports demonstrate that complications related to failure of tuberosity reduction and fixation are frequent, have a negative impact on normal shoulder kinematics, and result in inferior outcomes for pain and function. This fact has remained true despite advances in the development of fracture-specific prostheses, improved suture material and purportedly improved suture constructs. Borowsky and colleagues recently reported on failure modes of suture repair and found that tuberosity migration occurs early and in many cases was over 1 centimeter.[2] Given the frequency of clinical reports of tuberosity migration, it seems clear that currently accepted methods of suture repair fail to achieve a biological and mechanical environment that is suitable for bone healing, particularly in osteoporotic bone. Cable cerclage on the other hand has 4.8 times the circular embracing strength of conventional suture material and does not succumb to creep as suture material is proven to do.[12] Cables also have a prone track record in fracture fixation in long bones, such as periprosthetic fractures, and in fixation of trochanteric osteotomy in revision hip arthroplasty. Thus, their application to tuberosity fixation has a solid mechanical and clinical foundation.[13] Krause et al retrospectively compared cable fixation to nonabsorbable suture fixation and found that consistently better radiographic and functional results were achieved when cables were used with the Epoca stem. [12]

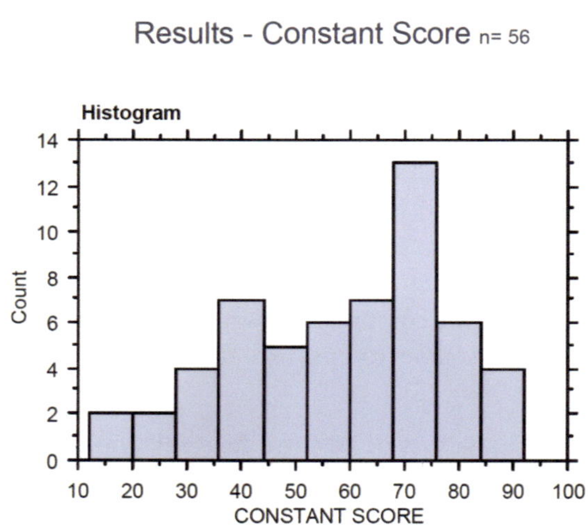

Figure 10. Histogram of Constant Scores in a consecutive series of 56 patients s/p fracture hemiarthroplasty with cable cerclage

The technique described above has been refined through Prof. Ralph Hertel's extensive use of this prosthesis in the fracture setting. Between 1997 and 2002, 60 patients were followed prospectively following humeral hemiarthroplasty for fracture.(R Hertel, unpublished data) The mean age was 68 years (range 39 – 88 years) and there were 26 males and 34 females. Four patients were lost to follow-up leaving 56 patients available for review with an average follow-up interval of 40 months (range 12 – 92 months). Successful tuberosity healing was achieved in 49 patients with displacement or resorption in 7 patients. Five patients underwent an additional operation to refix the tuberosities. A total of 31 patients achieved active forward elevation above 120 degrees. The histogram in Figure 10 demonstrates the range of Constant Scores in this series of patients. These results, while not as favorable as those achieved in arthroplasty for degenerative joint disease, do demonstrate that relatively robust shoulder function can be restored by hemiarthroplasty given tuberosity healing and successful patient rehabilitation. Stiffness remains a problem with neither an optimal preventative strategy nor a reliably effective treatment.

8. Technique for the reverse prosthesis

There is growing interest in fracture reconstruction using a reverse prosthesis which may afford better active elevation in cases where tuberosity healing is unpredictable and will potentially be unsuccessful. Even in these cases, however, the surgeon should attempt to achieve stable tuberosity fixation to improve the possibility for rotational movement which aids in positioning the hand in space. Specifically, if active external rotation can be achieved through reattachment of the greater tuberosity, patients may achieve greatly improved the functional outcomes with a reverse arthroplasty.

Similar to primary shoulder arthroplasty, fracture specific systems are now available to address this reverse arthroplasty for fracture. As with primary systems, however, their design does not guarantee successful tuberosity fixation and the principles outlined above still apply to reconstruction with a reverse prosthesis. In addition to the importance of sound technique which preserves the optimal biological conditions for fracture healing, tuberosity fixation with horizontal cable cerclage can also be used to achieve a stable reconstruction with a reverse prosthesis. In such cases, the technical steps are essentially identical to those outlined for primary fracture hemiarthroplasty. Figure 11 demonstrates cable cerclage of the tuberosities in a fracture reconstruction using a reverse prosthesis.

As the indication of reverse shoulder arthroplasty for fracture and fracture sequel has gained more traction and as experience with this technique has grown, clinical studies are now available to report on the outcomes of this procedure including comparative studies with conventional hemiarthroplasty. Boyle and colleagues compared 313 fracture hemiarthroplasty patients to 55 fracture reverse patients and found that Oxford Shoulder Scores at 5 years postoperatively were superior in the reverse group.[14] Young et al, however, we unable to realize any gains in range of motion, American Shoulder and Elbow Surgeons Score or Oxford Shoulder Score in patient who underwent a reverse reconstruction compared to those who underwent hemiarthroplasty for fracture cases.[15] Cazeneuve et al reported on 35 patients who underwent reverse reconstruction for fracture or fracture dislocation.[16] Complications including neurological injury, infection, instability and progressive scapular notching led to a complication rate of 24% and stiffness was noted to be a functionally limiting problem. Bufquin et al also reported stiffness with mean active elevation of only 97 degrees and mean active external rotation of only 30 degrees.[17] Tuberosity migration also occurred in 53% of cases. Lenarz and colleagues reported on 30 patients status post reverse arthroplasty for fracture and mean achieved active elevation of 139 degrees and mean active external rotation of 27 degrees with a 10% complications rate.[18]

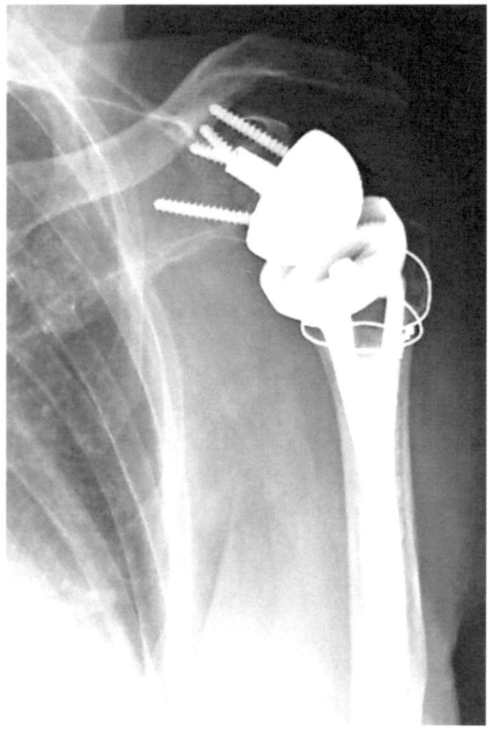

Figure 11. AP view showing horizontal cable cerclage tuberosity fixation in reverse arthroplasty for fracture.

Collectively these early outcomes are somewhat sobering relative to the anticipated advantages that reverse shoulder replacement might achieve in fracture cases. They prove the complexity of these cases and the challenges they present to the shoulder reconstruction surgeon. As design modifications continue to improve reverse systems and as experience with reverse arthroplasty in the fracture setting increases, surgeons can hopefully look forward to future advancements in our ability to provide improved function restoration in these difficult cases. Nevertheless, strict adherence to surgical techniques that preserve the biology of fracture healing, that maximize stability of fragment fixation and that permit early rehabilitation to encourage recovery of function are all critical regardless of the theoretical merits of any specific system in terms of biomechanics and design.

Acknowledgements

The concepts and techniques put forth in this manuscript represent the work of Professor Ralph Hertel, Department of Orthopaedics, Lindenhofspital, Berne Switzerland. He is the principle clinical design surgeon of the EPOCA prosthesis.

Author details

Moby Parsons

Address all correspondence to: impiv@comcast.net

Seacoast Orthopedics & Sports Medicine, Somersworth, NH, USA

References

[1] Antuna, S. A., J. W. Sperling, and R. H. Cofield. 2008. Shoulder hemiarthroplasty for acute fractures of the proximal humerus: a minimum five-year follow-up. J Shoulder Elbow Surg 17:202-209.

[2] Berend, K. R., A. V. J. Lombardi, T. H. Mallory, D. J. Chonko, K. L. Dodds, and J. B. Adams. 2004. Cerclage wires or cables for the management of intraoperative fracture associated with a cementless, tapered femoral prosthesis: results at 2 to 16 years. J Arthroplasty 19:17-21.

[3] Boileau, P., S. G. Krishnan, L. Tinsi, G. Walch, J. S. Coste, and D. Mole. 2002. Tuberosity malposition and migration: reasons for poor outcomes after hemiarthroplasty for displaced fractures of the proximal humerus. J Shoulder Elbow Surg 11:401-412.

[4] Borowsky, K., V. Raghuprasad, L. Wear, T. Stevenson, N. Marsden, N. Trent, and A. Bennett. 2010. Failure modes of suture repair of the tuberosities in hemiarthroplasty for four part fracture of the shoulder. 11th International Congress of Shoulder and Elbow Surgery 59.

[5] Boyle, M. J., S. M. Youn, C. M. Frampton, and C. M. Ball. 2012. Functional outcomes of reverse shoulder arthroplasty compared with hemiarthroplasty for acute proximal humeral fractures. J Shoulder Elbow Surg

[6] Bufquin, T., A. Hersan, L. Hubert, and P. Massin. 2007. Reverse shoulder arthroplasty for the treatment of three- and four-part fractures of the proximal humerus in the elderly: a prospective review of 43 cases with a short-term follow-up. J Bone Joint Surg Br 89:516-520.

[7] Cazeneuve, J. F., and D. J. Cristofari. 2010. The reverse shoulder prosthesis in the treatment of fractures of the proximal humerus in the elderly. J Bone Joint Surg Br 92:535-539.

[8] Cazeneuve, J. F., and D. J. Cristofari. 2011. Long term functional outcome following reverse shoulder arthroplasty in the elderly. OrthopTraumatolSurg Res 97:583-589.

[9] Compito, C. A., E. B. Self, and L. U. Bigliani. 1994. Arthroplasty and acute shoulder trauma. Reasons for success and failure. ClinOrthopRelat Res 27-36.

[10] Demirhan, M., O. Kilicoglu, L. Altinel, L. Eralp, and Y. Akalin. 2003. Prognostic factors in prosthetic replacement for acute proximal humerus fractures. J Orthop Trauma 17:181-8; discussion 188-9.

[11] Dimakopoulos, P., N. Potamitis, and E. Lambiris. 1997. Hemiarthroplasty in the treatment of comminuted intraarticular fractures of the proximal humerus. ClinOrthopRelat Res 7-11.

[12] Goldman, R. T., K. J. Koval, F. Cuomo, M. A. Gallagher, and J. D. Zuckerman. 1995. Functional outcome after humeral head replacement for acute three- and four-part proximal humeral fractures. J Shoulder Elbow Surg 4:81-86.

[13] Greiner, S. H., G. Diederichs, I. Kroning, M. Scheibel, and C. Perka. 2009. Tuberosity position correlates with fatty infiltration of the rotator cuff after hemiarthroplasty for proximal humeral fractures. J Shoulder Elbow Surg 18:431-436.

[14] Hawkins, R. J., and P. Switlyk. 1993. Acute prosthetic replacement for severe fractures of the proximal humerus. ClinOrthopRelat Res 156-160.

[15] Hertel, R., U. Knothe, and F. T. Ballmer. 2002. Geometry of the proximal humerus and implications for prosthetic design. J Shoulder Elbow Surg 11:331-338.

[16] Huffman, G. R., J. M. Itamura, M. H. McGarry, L. Duong, J. Gililland, J. E. Tibone, and T. Q. Lee. 2008. Neer Award 2006: Biomechanical assessment of inferior tuberosity placement during hemiarthroplasty for four-part proximal humeral fractures. J Shoulder Elbow Surg 17:189-196.

[17] Krause, F. G., L. Huebschle, and R. Hertel. 2007. Reattachment of the tuberosities with cable wires and bone graft in hemiarthroplasties done for proximal humeral fractures with cable wire and bone graft: 58 patients with a 22-month minimum follow-up. J Orthop Trauma 21:682-686.

[18] Lenarz, C., Y. Shishani, C. McCrum, R. J. Nowinski, T. B. Edwards, and R. Gobezie. 2011. Is reverse shoulder arthroplasty appropriate for the treatment of fractures in the older patient? Early observations. ClinOrthopRelat Res 469:3324-3331.

[19] Lervick, G. N., R. M. Carroll, and W. N. Levine. 2003. Complications after hemiarthroplasty for fractures of the proximal humerus. Instr Course Lect 52:3-12.

[20] Loebenberg, M. I., D. A. Jones, and J. D. Zuckerman. 2005. The effect of greater tuberosity placement on active range of motion after hemiarthroplasty for acute fractures of the proximal humerus. Bull HospJt Dis 62:90-93.

[21] Mighell, M. A., G. P. Kolm, C. A. Collinge, and M. A. Frankle. 2003. Outcomes of hemiarthroplasty for fractures of the proximal humerus. J Shoulder Elbow Surg 12:569-577.

[22] Nijs, S., and P. Broos. 2009. Outcome of shoulder hemiarthroplasty in acute proximal humeral fractures: a frustrating meta-analysis experience. ActaOrthopBelg 75:445-451.

[23] Park, M. S., Y. K. Lee, K. H. Yang, and S. J. Shin. 2003. Management of periprosthetic femoral fractures. J Arthroplasty 18:903-906.

[24] Plausinis, D., Y. W. Kwon, and J. D. Zuckerman. 2005. Complications of humeral head replacement for proximal humeral fractures. Instr Course Lect 54:371-380.

[25] Reuther, F., B. Muhlhausler, D. Wahl, and S. Nijs. 2010. Functional outcome of shoulder hemiarthroplasty for fractures: A multicentre analysis. Injury 41:606-612.

[26] Robinson, C. M., R. S. Page, R. M. Hill, D. L. Sanders, C. M. Court-Brown, and A. E. Wakefield. 2003. Primary hemiarthroplasty for treatment of proximal humeral fractures. J Bone Joint Surg Am 85-A:1215-1223.

[27] Shah, N., H. J. Iqbal, S. Brookes-Fazakerley, and C. Sinopidis. 2010. Shoulder hemiarthroplasty for the treatment of three and four part fractures of the proximal humerus using Comprehensive(R) Fracture stem. IntOrthop

[28] Smith, A. M., R. M. Mardones, J. W. Sperling, and R. H. Cofield. 2007. Early complications of operatively treated proximal humeral fractures. J Shoulder Elbow Surg 16:14-24.

[29] Stiehl, J. B. 2006. Extended osteotomy for periprosthetic femoral fractures in total hip arthroplasty. Am J Orthop (Belle Mead NJ) 35:20-23.

[30] Voos, J. E., J. S. Dines, and D. M. Dines. 2010. Arthroplasty for fractures of the proximal part of the humerus. J Bone Joint Surg Am 92:1560-1567.

[31] Wretenberg, P., and A. Ekelund. 1997. Acute hemiarthroplasty after proximal humerus fracture in old patients. A retrospective evaluation of 18 patients followed for 2-7 years. ActaOrthopScand 68:121-123.

[32] Young, S. W., B. S. Segal, P. C. Turner, and P. C. Poon. 2010. Comparison of functional outcomes of reverse shoulder arthroplasty versus hemiarthroplasty in the primary treatment of acute proximal humerus fracture. ANZ J Surg 80:789-793.

[33] Zyto, K., M. Kronberg, and L. A. Brostrom. 1995. Shoulder function after displaced fractures of the proximal humerus. J Shoulder Elbow Surg 4:331-336.

Chapter 11

The LP-ESP Lumbar Disc Prosthesis: Concept, Development and Clinical Experience

Jean-Yves Lazennec, Alain Aaron, Adrien Brusson,
Jean Patrick Rakover and Marc Antoine Rousseau

Additional information is available at the end of the chapter

http://dx.doi.org/10.5772/53726

1. Introduction

Because of its impairment of patients' personal, social, and professional lives, degenerative disk disease has become an important public health problem with multiple dimensions. The current therapeutic strategy remains controversial and is also a medical and surgical challenge. Conservative treatment, based mostly based on physical therapy, constitutes the first-line approach, but persistent symptomatic disease may be treated surgically in selected patients [1-4]. Lack of pain relief, stiffening of the lumbar spine, non-union, sagittal balance misalignment, bone graft donor site morbidity, and, last but not least, adjacent segment disease are the pitfalls of intervertebral fusion that led to the idea of total disk replacement (TDR) [5-12]. Since 1966 and Fernström's first TDR implantation [13], many designs and concepts have been proposed [14-23]. The devices are usually articulated implants, and their mobility depends on the designs of the bearing surfaces. Ball-and-socket two-piece prostheses have 3 degrees of freedom in every rotation around a single fixed center of rotation. Three-piece devices allow additional translation components, providing 5 degrees of freedom. Articulated TDRs have demonstrated their clinical utility in several patient series. Specifically, the non-inferiority of TDR versus fusion is now generally accepted [18-20, 24]. However, in vitro testing of the two types of implants reveals that both designs have biomechanical advantages and limitations.

Because the healthy human intervertebral disk has a deformable elastic structure with 6 degrees of freedom, elastomeric one-piece intervertebral prostheses might be the most physiological implant for mimicking physiologic levels of shock absorption and flexural stiffness. Designing such a device is challenging, especially when we remember the Acroflex® prostheses: the elastic rubber failed so rapidly in vivo that only 28 were implanted in all [25-26].

The LP-ESP® (lumbar disk prosthesis-elastic spine pad) was developed over a 20-year period. Improvements in technology have made it possible to solve the problem of the bond between the elastic component and the titanium endplates. After successful in vitro and in vivo evaluation, the LP-ESP has been authorized for clinical use in Europe since 2005. The goal of this paper is to present its innovative concept and the clinical results and radiological outcomes over its 7 years of use. In addition to measuring range of motion, we were specifically interested in the quality of the kinematics and thus investigated the mean center of rotation at both the instrumented and adjacent levels. Changes in spinal posture were also a major point of the study.

2. Implant design

The design of the LP ESP® prosthesis is based on the principle of the silent block bush (Figure 1). The LP-ESP ® is a one-piece deformable implant including a central core made of silicone gel with microvoids and surrounded by polycarbonate urethane (PCU) securely fixed to titanium endplates. The endplates have five anchoring pegs to provide primary fixation and are covered by a textured T 40 titanium layer (60 μm thick) and hydroxyapatite to improve bone ingrowth (Figure 2).

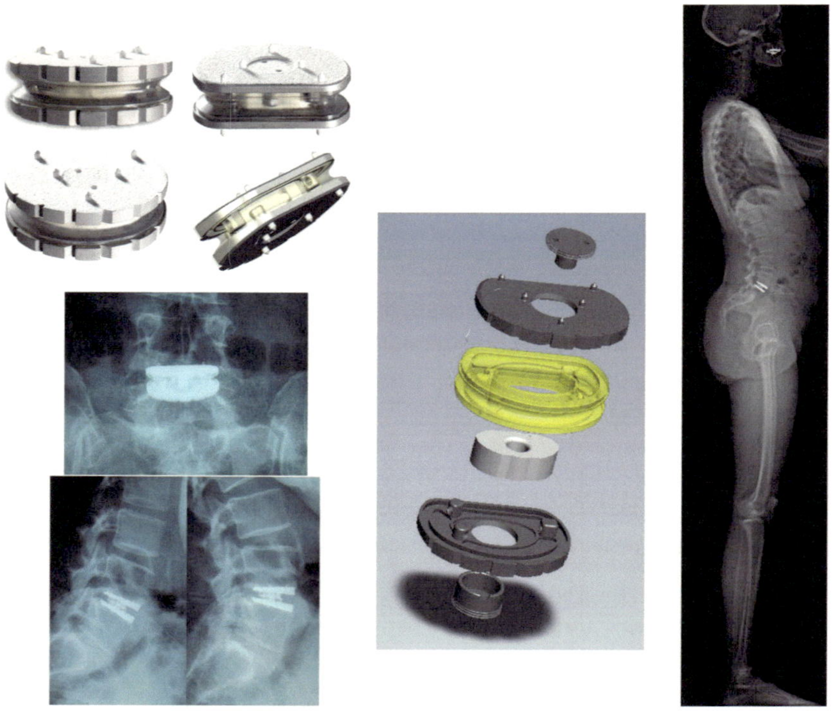

Figure 1. The design of the LP ESP® prosthesis is based on the principle of the silent block bush

http://dx.doi.org/10.5772/53726

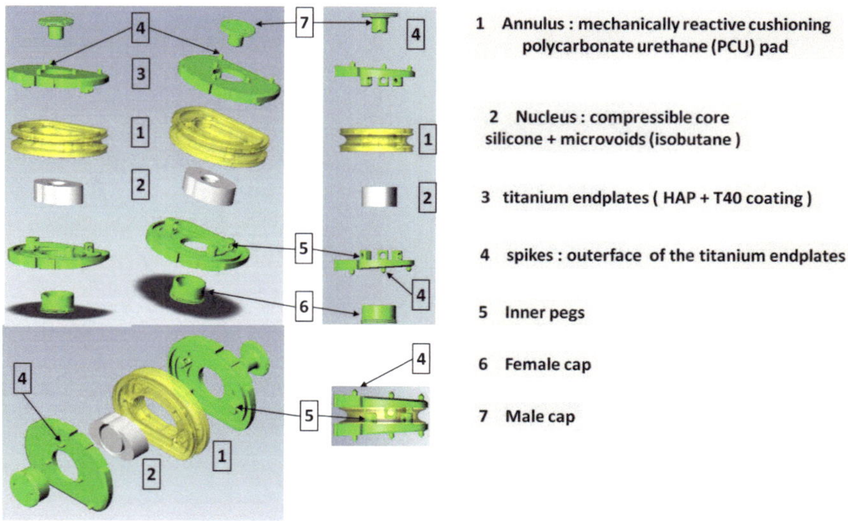

Figure 2. The LP-ESP ® is a one-piece deformable implant including a central core made of silicone gel with microvoids and surrounded by polycarbonate urethane (PCU) securely fixed to titanium endplates.

Depending on the size, the titanium endplates differ in thickness and angulation. The prostheses are available in two thicknesses (10 and 12 mm), each with 3 angles of lordosis (7°, 9°, and 11°). Regardless of the model, however, the mechanically active cushion and the mechanical properties of the prosthesis are the same: The differences in thickness of the lordotic angle do not affect the prosthesis's mobility or its cushioning, even shock-absorbing, effect.

Accordingly, the peripheral cushion (that is, the annulus) is securely fixed to the titanium alloy endplates by adhesion-molding technology. This attachment is reinforced by a peripheral groove without the addition of glue. This process of fixation avoids fluid infiltration and the risk of fatigue fractures of the interface, despite the very different mechanical properties of the polymer and the metal endplates. The PCU annulus is stabilized by supplementary pegs located on the internal surface of both metal endplates. The geometry and position of the pegs, between the peripheral groove and the central area of the endplates, were planned to control rotational mobility (Figures 3 and 4). The polymer molding was designed to prevent all direct contact between the upper and lower pegs.

The core or nucleus is composed of a compressible silicone structure containing isobutane microbubbles. This core is injected after the annulus surrounding it has been molded. Two titanium caps allow the core to be contained at the moment of the injection. These two pieces are firmly secured to the titanium plates: they also play a mechanical role by their contactless fit, because they contribute to limiting shearing during antero-posterior and medio-lateral translation. The cushioning and compressing effects are obtained on the one hand by the contactless interlocking of the male and female caps and, on the other hand, by crushing the annulus between the two metal plates. The same components limit the shearing effect when the endplates are inclined to the horizontal (Figure 5).

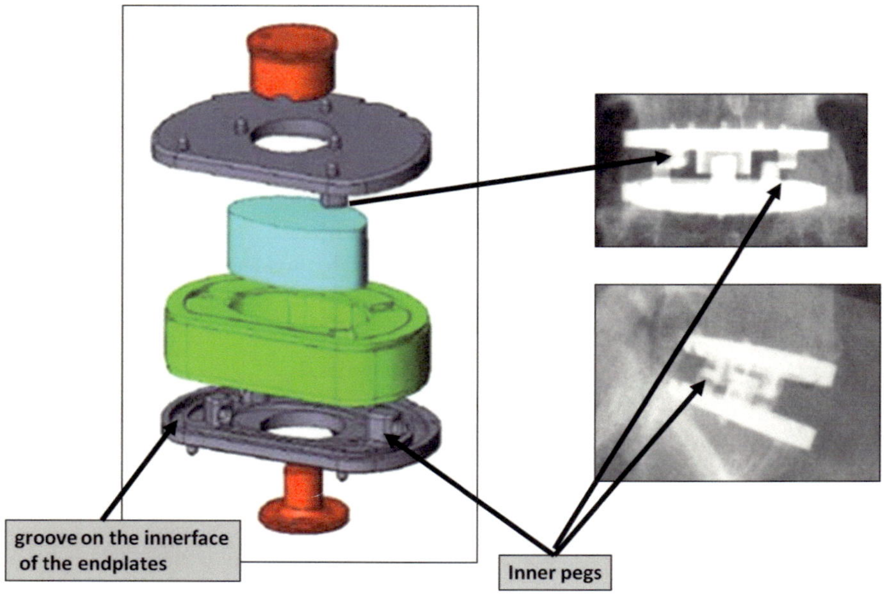

Figure 3. The LP-ESP ® is a one-piece deformable implant including a central core made of silicone gel with microvoids and surrounded by polycarbonate urethane (PCU) securely fixed to titanium endplates.

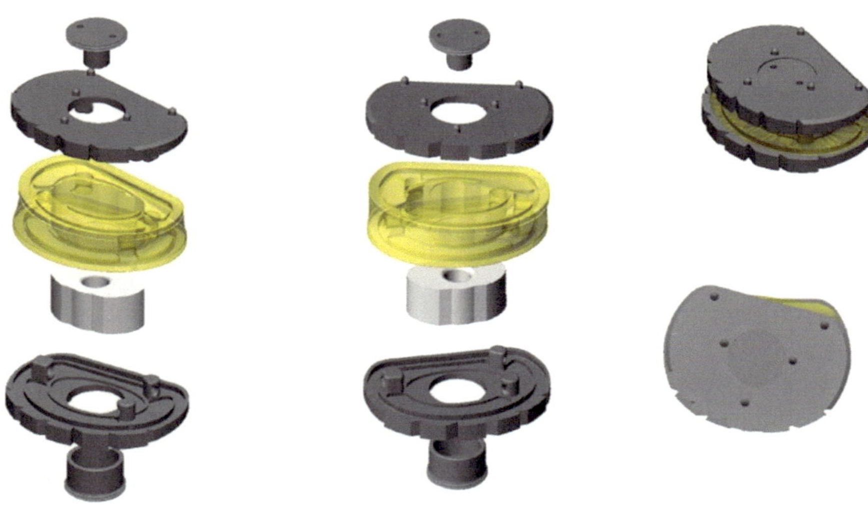

Figure 4. The geometry and position of the pegs, between the peripheral groove and the central area of the end-plates, are planned to control rotational mobility

This design and the adhesion-molding technology differentiate the LP ESP prosthesis from other monoelastomeric prostheses, for which the constraints of shearing during rotations or movement are absorbed at the plastic/titanium interface because of the molding technology

http://dx.doi.org/10.5772/53726

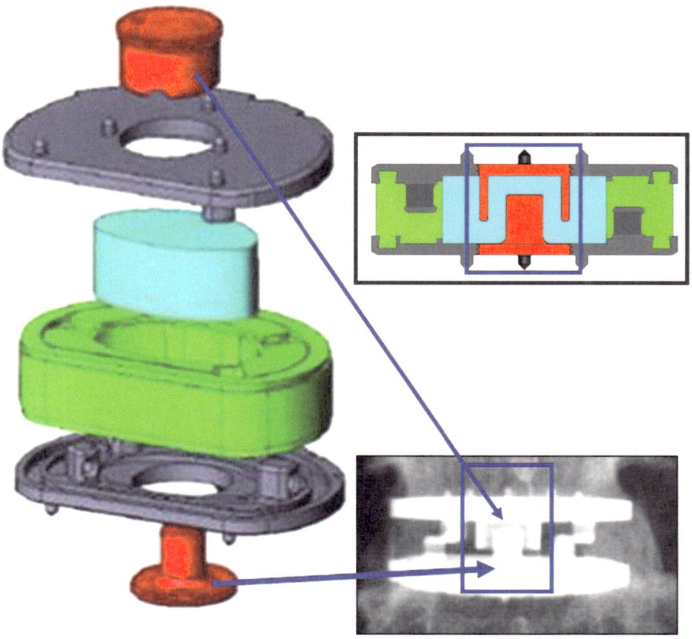

Figure 5. The cushioning and compressing effects are obtained on the one hand by the contactless interlocking of the male and female caps and, on the other hand, by crushing the annulus between the two metal plates.

used in their design. The attachment is obtained by the penetration of the polymer through small holes in the endplates. This process creates multiple interfaces and potential fatigue lesions of the anchoring mechanism due to inhomogeneous loading during flexion-extension, lateral inclination, and rotation. Thus, in these designs, the plastic monobloc cushion secured to the titanium plates flows into the space between them during compression, creating an area of friction and wear.

On the whole, in the LP ESP, the constraints of the interface between the PCU cushion and its titanium seating are reduced. These are principally constraints of compression:

- between the exterior of the male cap and the interior of the female cap for translations;
- between the pegs for the rotation ;
- between the titanium endplates for flexion.

The principle of the LP ESP® makes it possible to reproduce the anisotropy of the healthy disk, and the design allows modification of the return torque (without modifying the other parameters of the prosthesis. For example:

- bringing the pegs closer together increases stiffness in rotation without modifying either translation or compression;

- diminishing the clearance between the male and female caps increases the stiffness of translation without modifying either rotation or compression;
- modifying the ratio between the small and large diameters of the elliptic form of the cushion changes the ratios of the return torques between flexion/extension and lateral flexion without modifying stiffness in compression or rotation.

3. Manufacturing process

The manufacture of this complex implant includes 6 stages, each with its own quality control for each piece:

- Stage 1: Machining titanium (TA6V) plates and male and female caps and 3-dimensional check of each unit.
- Stage 2: Preparation of the annulus made of PCU.
  - Electrochemical treatment of the interior surfaces of the TA6V plates
  - Preparation and quality control of materials including drying PCU granules at 85°C for 4 h to reduce their humidity to less than 0.1%
  - Molding the PCU annulus between the two titanium endplates with a 22-ton vertical injection press (the endplates are pre-positioned in a mold that makes it possible to define the external geometry and to preserve the ovoid-shaped housing of the core).
  - Visual check of each unit, followed by testing compression of the implant without its core.
- Stage 3: Preparation of the core.
  - Placement of the female cap by screwing it in
  - Injection of a silicone-based component through the opening of the male cap
  - Screwing in the male cap as the injection starts
  - Cold polymerization
- Stage 4: Implant checks.
  - dimensional check of each unit,
  - testing rigidity while compressed by an axial load)
  - destructive testing of the first and last pieces of each lot by axial traction of the 2 metal endplates and then visual examination of the polymer parts (annulus and core).
- Stage 5:Two-stage spraying for final preparation of the anchoring endplates:
  - the T40 coating by plasma in a vacuum
  - and the layer of hydroxyapatite by plasma in a controlled atmosphere (inert gas)

http://dx.doi.org/10.5772/53726

Testing is performed as required by the standards:

ASTM F 1185-03 (2009) Standard Specification for Hydroxylapatite Composition for Surgical Implants

ISO 5832-2:1999 Surgical implants-- Metal-based products -- Part 2: Non-alloy titanium

ASTM F 1044: Standard test method for Shear Testing of Calcium Phosphate Coatings and Metallic Coatings

ASTM F 1147: Standard test method for Tension Testing of Calcium Phosphate and Metallic Coatings

ASTM F 1609: Standard Specification for Calcium Phosphate Coating for Implantable Materials.

ISO 13779-1: Hydroxyapatite - Part 1: Hydroxyapatite-based ceramic.

ISO 13779-2: Hydroxyapatite - Part 2: Hydroxyapatite-based coatings.

ISO/CD 13779: Hydroxyapatite - Chemical analysis and characterization of crystallinity and phase purity

- Stage 6: processing in a class 100 clean room workstation
- Stage 7: sterilization by gamma radiation (min: 25 kgray; max: 40 kgray) according to a special validated process

4. Design stages

After an initial patent application in 1994 by R. ROY CAMILLE, different avenues of research were explored, with the scientific expertise of the CEA (Commissariat à l'Energie Atomique, Fontenay aux Roses,France) and the industrial expertise of FH Industry for further R & D (Heimsbrunn, France).

The preliminary stages involved optimizing the choice of PCU, the development of the attachment of the annulus to the metal endplates without chemical adhesives, the definition of the pegs and caps, and the implementation of reliable techniques for polymer molding and injection.

Biocompatibility tests were performed by BIOMATECH, a subsidiary of NAMSA (Northwood, Ohio, USA).

Human implantation began in 2004 with the first generation of LP ESP® implants, which used endplates without lordosis (40 implantations, all complying with the Huriet Act, which defines French ethical requirements) (Figure 6).

A second generation of implants with lordotic endplates (7°, 9°, and 11°) was introduced in 2005 — LP ESP 1 (Figure 7).

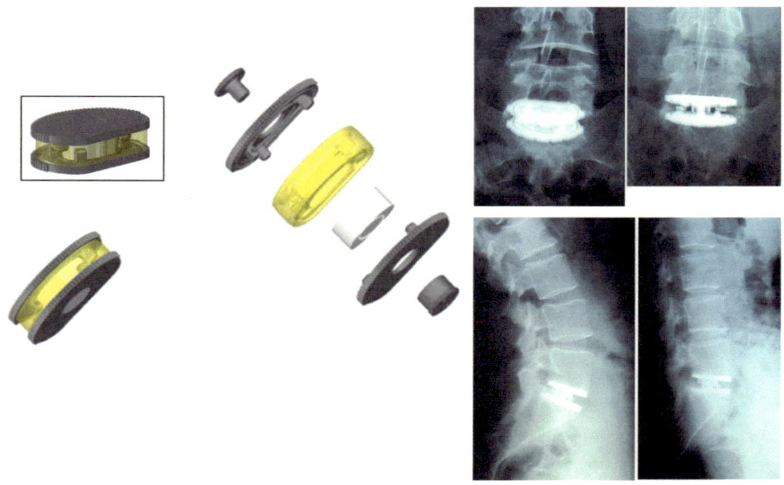

Figure 6. First generation of lumbar ESP® (2004) : endplates without lordosis

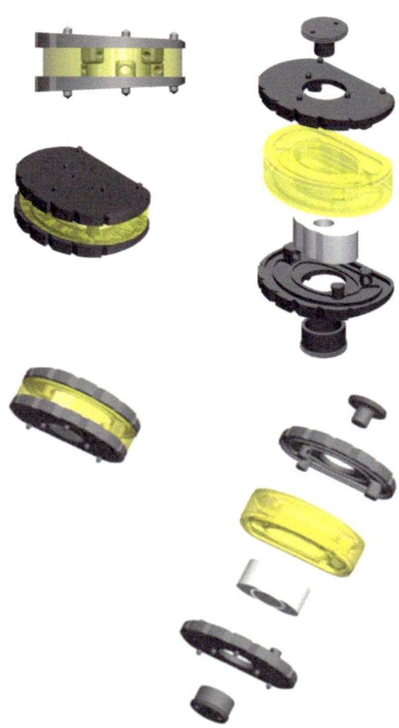

Figure 7. Second generation of lumbar ESP® (2005) : the shape of the endplates provides lordosis

http://dx.doi.org/10.5772/53726

A final change was made to the PCU annulus in 2006: its periphery is no longer rectilinear but was recessed somewhat during the molding process. This change did not modify the attachment of the cushion of the LP ESP 2® prosthesis but made it possible to reduce its stiffness during compression by 30% without changing its characteristics for flexion/extension, lateral incline, or rotation (Figure 8).

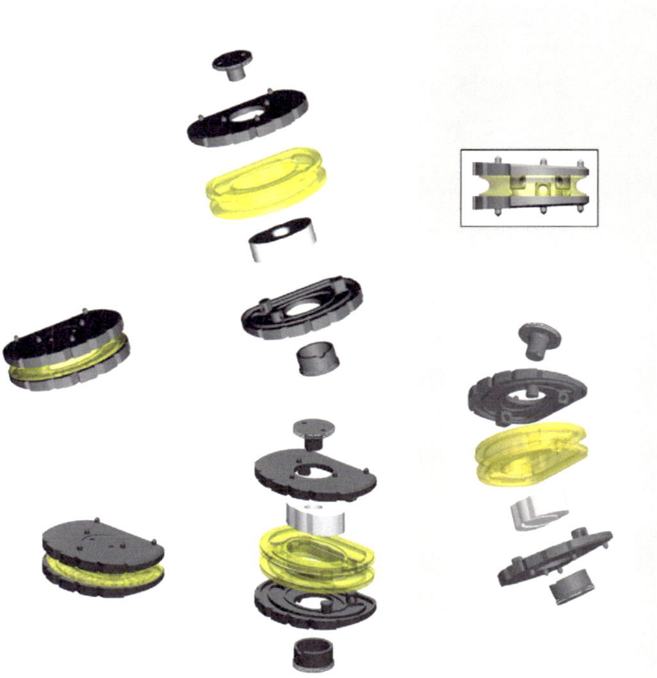

Figure 8. Last generation of lumbar ESP® (2006) : anterior recess in the PCU annulus to reduce stiffness during compression

This ESP prosthesis received CE marking in 2005, making it the first elastomeric lumbar prosthesis to be validated and authorized for marketing.

5. Mechanical properties

The "silent block bush" design of the LP ESP® prosthesis avoids the disadvantage of centers of rotation that are fixed or controlled by the implant design, as observed in disk prostheses based on an articulated design. In addition, in each direction solicited, the prosthesis offers resistance that increases with the amplitude of the movement. In this sense, the LP ESP® cannot be compared to first-generation implants. It meets the mechanical criterion of 6 degrees of freedom and provides a cushioning effect while restoring elastic recovery properties. Its mechanical properties are close to those reported in the literature for the normal disk (see Table 1).

Pure moments applied in increments up to a maximum value of 10 N-m	References	Level	Natural disk
flexion extension	Panjabi [27]	L4/L5	6°
		L5/S1	4°
	Campana	L1/L2	4°
		L4/L5	7°
	Yamamoto [28]	L1/L2	5°
		L4/L5	7.5°
lateral flexion	Panjabi	L4/L5	4°
		L5/S1	2°
	Campana [29]	L1/L2	4.1°
		L4/L5	6.1°
	Yamamoto	L1/L2	5°
		L4/L5	5.7°
Torsion	Panjabi	L4/L5	2°
		L5/S1	1°
	Campana	L1/L2	2.4°
		L4/L5	3.4°
	Yamamoto	L1/L2	2.3°
		L4/L5	2.2°
axial compression	Gardner- Morse [30]		2420 N/mm
Variable according to the loading speed, values retained for 0.1 m/s	Virgin [31]		3000 N/mm
	Kemper [32]		1835 N/mm
	Bouzakis [33]		1700 N/mm
Elastic recovery»			yes

Table 1. Comparison of the mechanical properties of the LP ESP 2° prosthesis with those of the natural disk

6. Biomechanical assessment

The originality of the concept of the ESP® prosthesis led to innovative and intense testing of various sorts.

6.1. Structural tests

a. Creep tests

After continuous compression to 1250 kN for 2928 hours (122 days), the height loss was 0.2 mm. In the 8 hours following load removal, the residual height loss was 0.1 mm.

b. Influence of the pegs included in the PCU annulus to control rotations

Tests were performed for combined compression and rotation: the pegs included in the PCU annulus absorb approximately 50% of the torque.

c. Assessment of the cohesion of the prosthetic cushion and the metal endplates:

The tests were performed for mediolateral and anteroposterior exertion applied to one of the metal endplates, with the other plate attached to the test machine (figure 9). For implants 12- and 10-mm thick, respectively, a force of 450 and 800 N was required to obtain a gap of 1 mm between the 2 endplates in the anteroposterior direction and 550 and 600 N in the mediolateral direction.

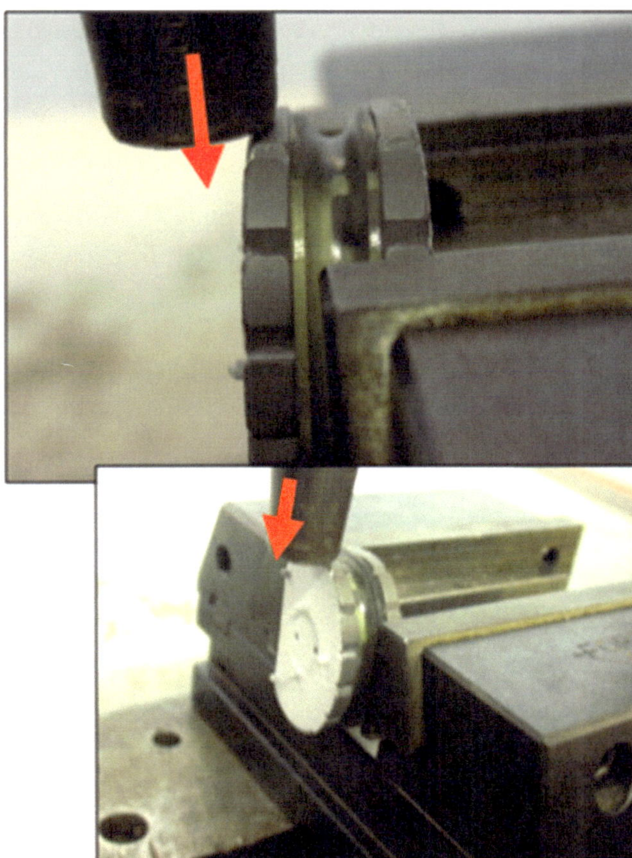

Figure 9. Assessment of the cohesion of the prosthetic cushion and the metal endplates: the tests were performed for mediolateral and anteroposterior exertion applied to one of the metal endplates, with the other plate attached to the test machine

d. Maximum compression tests

These tests were inspired by the experimental protocol of Virgin [31], who stated that a natural healthy disk is irreversibly injured by a load of 3 to 11 kN. After application of a force of 4,800 N (100 h) and then 9,200 N (64 h), we did not observe irreversible destruction of the implants. Compression tests and then compression-shearing at an angle of 45° were performed on the same samples to obtain successive compressions of 2 mm, 3 mm, and 6 mm. These tests show the implant's excellent tolerance of these compression–shearing mechanisms.

e. Tests to validate the final stage of coating on the exterior side of the metal plates

Adding a further final coating of porous titanium and spraying hydroxyapatite on the implant in its permanent form causes its temperature to rise. During the coating process, the disc is cooled by compressed air so that the ambient temperature remains stable at 21°C. Tests were performed to verify the absence of any effect from this rise on the mechanically active cushion in view of the known risk of PCU deterioration at 120°C. These tests demonstrated that the temperature did not reach a level of risk to the PCU.

6.2. Fatigue and wear tests

Wear tests were conducted in a 3-axis motion simulator according to the following protocol:

- 10 million cycles of flexion, extension, and lateral tilting
- Frequency = 4 Hz
- Loads of 135 to 1350 N
- Inclination of the prosthesis at 45° to reproduce the sagittal orientation of the disk in functional situations (Figure 10)
- In a demineralized water bath at 37° C

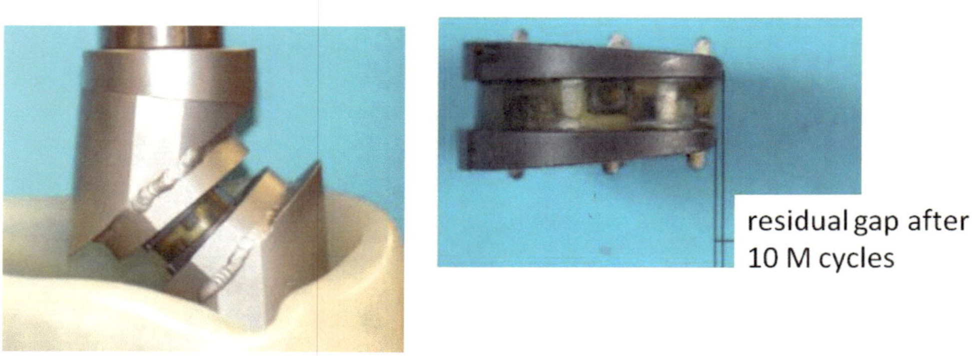

Figure 10. Wear tests were conducted in a 3-axis motion simulator (frequency = 4 Hz, loads of 135 to 1350 N), The inclination of the prosthesis was 45° to reproduce the sagittal orientation of the disk in functional situations. The gap between the metal plates was measured after each series of 10 million cycles.

Tests have even been extended to 40 million cycles without any observation of signs of mechanical failure. No loss of cohesion was seen. The residual gap between the metal endplates was 0.55 mm after 20 million cycles and 0.78 mm after 40 million cycles. Loss of mass after 20 million cycles was less than 0.5 % (very low absorption of saline solution and slight degradation of the endplates coating).

6.3. Biostability tests

This test was conducted according to the requirements of IS0 standard 10993-13/ biological evaluation of medical devices, Part 13: Identification and quantification of the decay products of polymer-based medical devices.

The biostability of the implant was assessed by analysis of the particles collected during the filtration of the demineralized water bath, after a wear test of 10 million cycles under a load of 1350 N. This study used a scanning electron microscope (SEM LEO1455VP), equipped with an energy-selective spectrometer (EDS OXFORD). No particles from the component materials of the prosthesis were found.

The tests looking for salted out or released matter showed the emission of <1 mg/kg methylene diphenyl 4-4 diisocyanate and of 64.9 mg/kg of 4-4 methylene diamine. These results are consistent with the data in the literature [34].

6.4. PCU aging test

The specific PCU used for the LP ESP prosthesis is not oxidized during storage (bionate 80A (DSNM Biomedical,The Netherlands) according to master file MAF844). Kurz demonstrated that five years of shelf aging has little effect on the mechanical properties of the PCU and concludes that the bionate 80A material has greater oxidative stability than ultra-high molecular weight polyethylene following gamma irradiation in air and exposure to a severe oxidative challenge [35]. Tests were performed after artificial aging in water at 80°C followed by 10 million compression cycles at loads ranging from 150 to 1250 N. In the absence of published standards in the literature, the temperature was determined in comparison with that recommended for aging plastics, including UHMWPE (ASTM standard F 2003: Accelerated aging of ultra-high molecular weight polyethylene after gamma irradiation in air) and the axial load is that recommended by ISO standard 18192 (Intervertebral spinal disk prostheses — Part 1: Loading and displacement parameters for wear testing and corresponding environmental conditions for test) for wear tests. It was not observed significant changes in the stiffness of the implants tested.

No modification of the Fournier transform infrared spectrum or any modification of the mean molecular weight (ASTM standard D 5296) was observed. The chemical composition and organization of the atomic bonds therefore remained identical because oxidation or natural cross-linkage would have modified the atomic organization and thus the spectrum. These results are consistent with the literature [34].

7. Biocompatibility tests

They were performed by Biomatech (*Chasse-sur-Rhône, France).*

All the materials were studied separately and in their final assembly, meeting the specifications for biocompatibility tests described in ISO standard 10993 (Biological Evaluation of Medical Devices).

Cytotoxicity test according to ISO standard 10993-5

Sensitization test according to ISO standard 10993-10

Test of irritation or intradermal reaction according to ISO standard 10993-10; acute systemic toxicity according to ISO standard 10993-11 Chromosomal genotoxicity (Hearts test, and chromosomal anomalies according to ISO standard 10993-3)

The implants also meet the criteria of the FDA's subacute sensitization test (following FDA - Guidelines for Toxicity Tests Chapter IV).

8. Clinical results

8.1. Evaluation process:

As of today, more than 2000 LP ESP II prostheses have been implanted. No complication related to the materials has been reported. Our clinical experience is based on prospective studies of clinical and radiologic assessment. The time points were 3, 6, 12, and 36 months. The intensity of back pain was evaluated with a Visual Analog Scale (VAS). Disability was assessed with the Oswestry Disability Index (ODI) [36-37, 39]. FDA criteria consider an improvement in the ODI at 2 years equal to or greater than 15% as success. The SF 36 was used to assess global health status [40]; the quality of life dimension of this test (SF-36) is composed of two subscores, the physical component summary (PCS) and the mental component summary (MCS), expressed as percentages [40-44]. The results of this score were compared to data known for a normal population [45]. In addition, the GHQ28 was used to investigate psychological distress [46].

Radiographs of the lumbar spine were prospectively collected for the studies. The time points for the radiological evaluation were 3, 6, and 12 months. The X-ray films were digitalized with the VXR12® scanner (Vidar System Corporation) and analyzed with Spineview® software (Surgiview Corporation, Paris, France), the precision and reliability of which has previously been reported [47]. The analysis was performed by a single observer who was not involved in patient selection, surgical procedures, or follow-up examinations. Kinematics parameters were studied at the level of implantation and the adjacent upper level on the flexion/extension X-rays. Range of motion (ROM) was measured to describe angular mobility quantitatively. As Champain et al. [47] has reported 2° accuracy for the measurement of ROM with Spineview®, we considered that the prosthesis had no motion if the measured range of motion was less than 3°. For mobile levels, the mean center of rotation (MCR) was recorded to assess motion qualitatively, as previously described. An orthogonal coordinate system centered at the posterior superior corner of the lower vertebra, with the X axis along the posterior wall and the Y axis along the endplate, was used to describe the location of the MCR. The percentage of MCRs in a correct or normal location was determined according to the method of Tournier et al [48].

Lateral views in standing position (lumbar spine including femoral heads) were used to assess the sagittal balance indicators, as defined by Duval and Beaupere [49].

- Sacral slope (SS): angle between the endplate of S1 and the horizontal line,
- Pelvic tilt (PT): the angle between the vertical line and the line connecting the center of the S1 endplate to the center of the femoral head. The middle of the line connecting the two femoral heads was used when those were not exactly superimposed;
- Segmental lordosis (SL): the angle between the upper endplate of the superior vertebra and the lower endplate of the inferior vertebra (for L5S1, the upper L5 endplate and the upper S1 endplate).

8.2. Clinical results

Clinical outcomes can be assessed from one of our prospective series of 120 patients. The mean operative time was 92 min (standard deviation, SD: 49 min). The mean blood loss was 73 cc (SD: 162 cc).

Analysis of the VAS showed a preoperative baseline of 6.6, a strong decrease to 3.7 points at 3 months, and a stable score of 3.6 through 36 months. The VAS thus decreased by 45%.

The baseline preoperative ODI score was 47.3%; it decreased regularly to 19.5% at 36 months, that is, a reduction of 40%. Overall, 77% of the patients had an ODI score at 36 months that improved by more than 15 points compared with the preoperative score. At 36 months after surgery, 90% of the patients showed an improvement of more than 15% compared with the preoperative value and 83% more than 25% (Tables 2 and 3).

The baseline preoperative GHQ28 score was 64.2; it began to fall at 3 months and remained at 52.2 at 36 months. This indicates an improvement of this psychological score of 18.7%.

The preoperative baseline SF 36 PCS score was 32.3%; it increased to 48.8% at 3 months and reached 56.8% at 36 months, for an increase of 24,5%.

The preoperative baseline SF 36 MCS score was 42.9%; it increased regularly and reached 57.9% at 36 months, for an increase of 15%.

Mean±SD	PRE OP	3 MO	6 M	12 M	24 M
VAS	6.6±1.7	3.7±1.9	3.4±2.1	3.5±2.3	3.4±2.4
ODI (%)	47.6±14.6	30.3±17.6	24.5±17.6	21.8±16.3	20.6±17.3
GHQ 28	64.2±15.6	52.5±14.7	52.7±15.8	52.2±15.4	50.6±15.4
SF 36 PCS (%)	32.4±34.8	48.4±39	51.9±39.3	55.6±39.8	59±39.2
SF 36 MCS (%)	42.3±34.0	50.8±34.6	52.8±35.6	53±36.3	58.7±34.6

Table 2. Description of the different evaluations performed

improvement/preoperative status	3 M	6 M	12 M	24 M
ODI improvement of 15 points	53	69	72	76
ODI improvement of 15%	72	82	85	85
ODI improvement of 25%	59	75	82	83

Table 3. Improvement in ODI score compared with preoperative score (in % of the population)

8.3. Radiological outcome

The radiological results can be analyzed from another prospective series of 41 patients (20 L5S1 and 21 L4L5 implantations) for whom postural and kinematic indicators can be evaluated.

Table 4 summarizes the changes in the radiological indicators of sagittal balance over time. Patients did not have major balance disorders before or after implantation. SS, PT, SL, and DH all changed significantly between the preoperative period and all other time points.

	Pre-op	3 months	6 months
Pelvic incidence (PI)		54.1° ± 14.6	
Sacral slope (SS)	36.5° ± 10.6	39.2° ± 5.7	40.8° ± 8.5
Pelvic tilt (PT)	16.7° ± 7.8	15.1° ± 6.7	13.2° ± 8.2
Segmental lordosis (SL)	19.4° ± 6.7	26.6° ± 5.3	27.9° ± 6.9
Discal height (DH)	28.5% ±10.3	50.7% ± 7.4	50.3% ± 5.0

Table 4. Radiological parameters in standing position over time (mean + SD). Changes in SS, PT, SL, and DH were significant between the preoperative measurements and all other time points.

The average range of motion in flexion-extension at the one-year follow-up was 5.0° (SD: 4.8°) (Table 5). The ROM increased significantly from 3 to 12 months, from 3.4 ° to 5.0°. With the 3° cut-off point, 66% of patients demonstrated mobility at one-year. The average ROM for the mobile prostheses was 6.9° (SD: 4.5). The average ROM of the prosthesis was 6.4° (SD: 4.9) at L5S1 and 7.9° (SD: 3.3) at L4L5.

	3 months	6 months
ROM at the prosthetic level	3.4° (2.5)	3.1° (2.8)
% of mobile prostheses	66%	60%
ROM of the mobile prostheses	4.4° (2.1)	4.6° (2.8)
ROM at the adjacent upper level	7.5° (5.1)	7.5° (4.2)

Table 5. Range of motion of the prosthesis and the upper adjacent disk over time. Mean (SD). The instrumented level reached a physiological range of motion similar to the adjacent level above it at between 6 and 12 months.

The MCR was in a normal location for 43% at 3 months, 42% at 6 months, and 87.5% at 12 months. Another prospective series of 74 implants seen at least 2 years after surgery allows analysis of the prostheses with more than 5° of mobility in flexion-extension: the mean mobility at L4L5 was 8.2° and at L5S1, 7.6°, for a global mean mobility of 7.9°. Table 6 compares these values with data from the literature for the same criterion of minimum mobility at 5°.

Author	Year	Follow-up	Type of Prothesis	L3-L4 ROM	L4-L5 ROM	L5-S1 ROM	Global ROM
Gioia [50]	2007	2	Charité III	8	10.3	8	8.7
Bertagonil [51]	2005	2	Prodisc	-	-	-	6.5
Guyer [52]	2009	2	Charité	-	6.5	6	6.3
		5		-	6	6.3	6.2
David [53]	1993	1	Charité	2	9.4	6.4	5.9
Siepe [54]	2007	1	Charité III	-	7.2	5.9	6.5
Zigler [55]	2012	5	Prodisc	-	-	-	7.7
Delamarter [56]	2011	2	Prodisc L	7.8	6.2		7.0
the series	2012	2	LP ESP	-	8.2*	7.6*	7.9*

Table 6. Mobility described in the literature of implants restoring more than 5° of segmental mobility

9. Discussion

The geometry of the LP ESP® prosthesis allows limited rotation and translation with resistance to motion aimed at avoiding overload of the posterior facet joints. The center of rotation can vary freely during motion. This viscoelastic prosthesis achieves 6 degrees of freedom including vertical translation; it provides a cushion and may allow shock absorption. It thus differs substantially from other current prostheses, which are 2- or 3-piece devices involving 1 or 2 bearing surfaces and providing 3 or 5 degrees of freedom, with no or very little resistance, and no elastic return. A 20-year research program has demonstrated that this concept provides mechanical properties very close to those of a natural disk.

In addition, the biostability of the implant was demonstrated: no particles from the component materials of the prosthesis were found after a wear test of 10 million cycles under a load of 1350 N.

These experimental data should be considered in relation to previously reported results from Nechtow et al. [57] of wear rates of 16.59 ± 0.96 mg/million cycles for ProDisc_ L and 19.35 ± 1.16 mg/million cycles for Charite, and from Grupp et al. [58] of wear rates ranging from 0.14 ± 0.06 mg/million cycles to 2.7 ± 0.3 mg/million cycles for Active L.

Moreover, the size and morphology of the UHMWPE particulates observed in these studies are similar to those described in total hip and knee replacements [59], the osteolytic potential of which is well known.

Seven years after the first implantation, we can document in a solid and detailed fashion the course of clinical outcomes and the radiological postural and kinematical behavior of this prosthesis. The clinical data show early and stable improvement of clinical status, while the radiological data show immediate improvement of local lordosis and discal height at the instrumented level and associated adaptation of the sacral slope. At 3 and 12 months, 66% of cases had physiological mobility at the instrumented level, with secondary self-adjustment of the center of rotation in flexion/extension.

We acknowledge that more studies with more patients and more follow-up would be useful in the future to assess long term reliability. Nonetheless, the series reported here describe the outcomes that might be expected by surgeons and patients over the first 7 years. These encouraging results are basically similar to the clinical results reported by Tropiano [60] et al. with the Prodisc II® and the clinical data of the SB Charite®, as reported by McAffee et al [61]. Although the preoperative radiological parameters showed no major imbalance in spinal posture compared to the global population, SS, PT, and SL improved significantly immediately after implantation. These results are consistent with those reported in literature with articulated prostheses [48, 62, 63].

We note that publications do not appear to report significant sagittal misalignments after prosthetic implantation, whereas lumbar fusion may deleteriously alter the sagittal balance of the spine, including a decrease in the SS and lumbar lordosis [6,7]. The increased segmental lordosis might be related to the lordotic shape of the prosthesis but also probably to the fact that arthroplasty, in contrast to fusion, allows the lumbar spine to find a new balance spontaneously. It has not yet been demonstrated, however, that this self-adaptation of the sagittal balance protects against adjacent level degeneration. Unlike arthrodesis, the preservation or restoration of some mobility with a total disk replacement aims at limiting overload of the adjacent levels.

The optimal ROM after TDR for limiting adjacent segmental disease has not yet been established. Huang et al [64] reported a series of 42 Prodisc I® implantations with 8.7 years of follow-up, and 24% of the junctional levels showed radiological signs of degeneration. In their study, the mean ROM of the disk prostheses adjacent to junctional disease was significantly lower than the mean ROM of the prostheses adjacent to a radiologically normal disk, i.e., 1.6° versus 4.7°. Prevalence of junctional degeneration was 0% among patients with ROM of 5° or more and 35% among those with less than 5°. The authors did not conclude that 5° was the trigger value for avoiding adjacent degeneration, as 65% of patients with less than 5° did not develop adjacent segmental degeneration. In our series, the LP-ESP® device provides mobility levels similar to those with articulated prostheses such as Prodisc, which vary according to the series from 3.8° to 13.2° [62, 64].

We recognize that assessing spinal kinematics with static X-rays in flexion and extension is subject to bias, given the same-day variations due to inconsistent effort during flexion/extension [65]. Nonetheless, flexion/extension X-rays are easily available and cause less irradiation than continuous motion analysis with in vivo fluoroscopy. Quality of movement is also an issue. The LP-ESP is a novel one-piece deformable but cohesive interbody spacer that provides 6 full degrees of freedom about the 3 axes. This allows instantaneous axis rotation change freely, as in the normal disk, while preventing facet overloading.

MCR, initially defined by Pearcy [66], is a pivot point about which a vertebra appears to move and is thought to reflect the quality of movement of a segment. As disk arthroplasty develops, this indicator appears to be an informative parameter for studying the quality of spinal movement imposed by the prosthesis. The coordinates of the MCR for LP-ESP® prosthesis appears similar to those of the natural disk described in literature. After one year of follow-up, we found the MCR in a physiological area in 87.5% of the patients. With the same methods, Tournier et al. [48] reported a normal MCR for 51% of patients receiving the Maverick®, 66% of those with the Prodisc® (both of which have 3 degrees of freedom), and 80% with the SB Charite® (5 degrees of freedom). These results suggest that less constrained prostheses, i.e., those with more than 3 degrees of freedom, are associated with more normal MCR locations. In addition, we observed that the MCR location tends to improve during the first year. However, this must be interpreted while bearing in mind the uncertainty of the MCR measurement reported by Tournier et al., specifically at the L5-S1 level.

10. Conclusion

The concept of the LP-ESP® prosthesis is different from that of the articulated devices currently used in the lumbar spine; it allows 6 degree of freedom with elastic return and is intended to respect the spontaneous instantaneous axis of rotation and to reduce facet forces. Our series provide encouraging clinical results about pain, function, kinematic behavior and radiological sagittal balance after implantation of the LP-ESP ®.

Author details

Jean-Yves Lazennec[1,2,4], Alain Aaron[3], Adrien Brusson[4], Jean Patrick Rakover[5] and Marc Antoine Rousseau[1,2]

1 Department of Orthopedic and Trauma Surgery, La Pitié-Salpétrière Hospital, Paris, France

2 Biomechanics Lab, Arts et Métiers Paritech, Paris, France

3 FH Orthopedics, Heimsbrunn, France

4 Department of Anatomy, Universite′ Pierre et Marie Curie, Paris, France

5 Clinique du Pré, Le Mans, France

References

[1] Fritzell, P, et al. (2001). Volvo Award Winner in Clinical Studies: Lumbar fusion versus nonsurgical treatment for chronic low back pain: a multicenter randomized controlled trial from the Swedish Lumbar Spine Study Group. Spine (Phila Pa 1976), 2001. 26(23): discussion 2532-4., 2521-2532.

[2] Resnick, D. K, Malone, D. G, & Ryken, T. C. Guidelines for the use of discography for the diagnosis of painful degenerative lumbar disc disease. Neurosurg Focus, (2002). , E12.

[3] Wetzel, F. T, et al. The treatment of lumbar spinal pain syndromes diagnosed by discography. Lumbar arthrodesis. Spine (Phila Pa 1976), (1994). , 792-800.

[4] Thalgott, J. S, et al. Anterior lumbar interbody fusion with titanium mesh cages, coralline hydroxyapatite, and demineralized bone matrix as part of a circumferential fusion. Spine J, (2002). , 63-69.

[5] Moore, K. R, Pinto, M. R, & Butler, L. M. Degenerative disc disease treated with combined anterior and posterior arthrodesis and posterior instrumentation. Spine (Phila Pa 1976), (2002). , 1680-1686.

[6] Kumar, M. N, Baklanov, A, & Chopin, D. Correlation between sagittal plane changes and adjacent segment degeneration following lumbar spine fusion. Eur Spine J, (2001). , 314-319.

[7] Rao, R. D, David, K. S, & Wang, M. Biomechanical changes at adjacent segments following anterior lumbar interbody fusion using tapered cages. Spine (Phila Pa 1976), (2005). , 2772-2776.

[8] Kim, Y. E, et al. Effect of disc degeneration at one level on the adjacent level in axial mode. Spine (Phila Pa 1976), (1991). , 331-335.

[9] Weinhoffer, S. L, et al. Intradiscal pressure measurements above an instrumented fusion. A cadaveric study. Spine (Phila Pa 1976), (1995). , 526-531.

[10] Dekutoski, M. B, et al. Comparison of in vivo and in vitro adjacent segment motion after lumbar fusion. Spine (Phila Pa 1976), (1994). , 1745-1751.

[11] Eck, J. C, Humphreys, S. C, & Hodges, S. D. Adjacent-segment degeneration after lumbar fusion: a review of clinical, biomechanical, and radiologic studies. Am J Orthop (Belle Mead NJ), (1999). , 336-340.

[12] Rahm, M. D, & Hall, B. B. Adjacent-segment degeneration after lumbar fusion with instrumentation: a retrospective study. Journal of Spinal Disorders, (1996). , 392-400.

[13] Fernstrom, U. Arthroplasty with intercorporal endoprothesis in herniated disc and in painful disc. Acta Chir Scand Suppl, (1966). , 154-159.

[14] Cunningham, B. W, et al. General principles of total disc replacement arthroplasty: seventeen cases in a nonhuman primate model. Spine (Phila Pa 1976), (2003). , S118-S124.

[15] Cunningham, B. W, et al. Total disc replacement arthroplasty using the AcroFlex lumbar disc: a non-human primate model. Eur Spine J, (2002). Suppl 2: , S115-S123.

[16] Frelinghuysen, P, et al. Lumbar total disc replacement part I: rationale, biomechanics, and implant types. Orthop Clin North Am, (2005). , 293-299.

[17] Auerbach, J. D, et al. Evaluation of spinal kinematics following lumbar total disc replacement and circumferential fusion using in vivo fluoroscopy. Spine (Phila Pa 1976), (2007). , 527-536.

[18] Awe, O. O, et al. Impact of total disc arthroplasty on the surgical management of lumbar degenerative disc disease: Analysis of the Nationwide Inpatient Sample from 2000 to 2008. Surg Neurol Int, (2011). , 139.

[19] Blumenthal, S, et al. A prospective, randomized, multicenter Food and Drug Administration investigational device exemptions study of lumbar total disc replacement with the CHARITE artificial disc versus lumbar fusion: part I: evaluation of clinical outcomes. Spine (Phila Pa 1976), (2005). discussion E387-91., 1565-1575.

[20] Szpalski, M, Gunzburg, R, & Mayer, M. Spine arthroplasty: a historical review. Eur Spine J, (2002). Suppl 2: , S65-S84.

[21] Goel, V. K, et al. Effects of charite artificial disc on the implanted and adjacent spinal segments mechanics using a hybrid testing protocol. Spine (Phila Pa 1976), (2005). , 2755-2764.

[22] Hochschuler, S. H, et al. Artificial disc: preliminary results of a prospective study in the United States. Eur Spine J, (2002). Suppl 2: , S106-S110.

[23] Galbusera, F, et al. Design concepts in lumbar total disc arthroplasty. Eur Spine J, (2008). , 1635-1650.

[24] Errico, T, Sasso, R, & Mize, e. a. G, Total disc replacement for treating lumbar discogenic back pain: A prospective randomized multicenter study of FlexiCore vs. 360 spinal fusion. Spine J 2008;. (2008). Suppl 1)): , 15S-16S.

[25] Fraser, R. D, et al. AcroFlex design and results. Spine J, (2004). Suppl): , 245S-251S.

[26] Enker, P, et al. Artificial disc replacement. Preliminary report with a 3-year minimum follow-up. Spine (Phila Pa 1976), (1993). , 1061-1070.

[27] Panjabi, M. M, et al. Mechanical behavior of the human lumbar and lumbosacral spine as shown by three-dimensional load-displacement curves. J Bone Joint Surg Am, (1994). , 413-424.

[28] Yamamoto, I, et al. Three-dimensional movements of the whole lumbar spine and lumbosacral joint. Spine (Phila Pa 1976), (1989). , 1256-1260.

[29] Campana, S, et al. Relationships between viscoelastic properties of lumbar intervertebral disc and degeneration grade assessed by MRI. J Mech Behav Biomed Mater, (2011). , 593-599.

[30] Gardner-morse, M. G, & Stokes, I. A. Structural behavior of human lumbar spinal motion segments. J Biomech, (2004). , 205-212.

[31] Virgin, W. J. Experimental investigations into the physical properties of the intervertebral disc. J Bone Joint Surg Br, (1951). B(4): , 607-611.

[32] Kemper, A. R, Mcnally, C, & Duma, S. M. The influence of strain rate on the compressive stiffness properties of human lumbar intervertebral discs. Biomed Sci Instrum, (2007). , 176-181.

[33] Bouzakis, K. D, et al. Loading simulation of lumbar spine vertebrae during a compression test using the finite elements method and trabecular bone strength properties, determined by means of nanoindentations. J Musculoskelet Neuronal Interact, (2004). , 152-158.

[34] Christenson, E. M, et al. Poly(carbonate urethane) and poly(ether urethane) biodegradation: in vivo studies. J Biomed Mater Res A, (2004). , 407-416.

[35] Kurtz, S. M, Siskey, R, & Reitman, M. Accelerated aging, natural aging, and small punch testing of gamma-air sterilized polycarbonate urethane acetabular components. J Biomed Mater Res B Appl Biomater, (2010). , 442-447.

[36] Page, S. J, et al. Scaling of the revised Oswestry low back pain questionnaire. Arch Phys Med Rehabil, (2002). , 1579-1584.

[37] Fairbank, J. C, et al. The Oswestry low back pain disability questionnaire. Physiotherapy, (1980). , 271-273.

[38] Niskanen, R. O. The Oswestry Low Back Pain Disability Questionnaire. a two-year follow-up of spine surgery patients. Scand J Surg, (2002). , 208-211.

[39] Sanjaroensuttikul, N. The Oswestry low back pain disability questionnaire (version 1.0) Thai version. J Med Assoc Thai, (2007). , 1417-1422.

[40] Ware, J. E, & Jr, C. D. Sherbourne, The MOS 36-item short-form health survey (SF-36). I. Conceptual framework and item selection. Med Care, (1992). , 473-483.

[41] Brazier, J. E, et al. Validating the SF-36 health survey questionnaire: new outcome measure for primary care. BMJ, (1992). , 160-164.

[42] Leplege, A, et al. The French SF-36 Health Survey: translation, cultural adaptation and preliminary psychometric evaluation. J Clin Epidemiol, (1998). , 1013-1023.

[43] Mchorney, C. A, Haley, S. M, & Ware, J. E. Jr., Evaluation of the MOS SF-36 Physical Functioning Scale (PF-10): II. Comparison of relative precision using Likert and Rasch scoring methods. J Clin Epidemiol, (1997). , 451-461.

[44] Veresciagina, K, Ambrozaitis, K. V, & Spakauskas, B. Health-related quality-of-life assessment in patients with low back pain using SF-36 questionnaire. Medicina (Kaunas), (2007). , 607-613.

[45] Leplege, A, et al. Manuel de l'utilisateur et guide d'interprétation des scores de la SF-36, ed. P. ESTEM. (2001).

[46] De Mont-marin, F, et al. Validation of a French version of the General Health Questionnaire (GHQ-28) in a diabetic population]. Encephale, (1993). , 293-301.

[47] Champain, S, et al. Validation of new clinical quantitative analysis software applicable in spine orthopaedic studies. Eur Spine J, (2006). , 982-991.

[48] Tournier, C, et al. Total disc arthroplasty: consequences for sagittal balance and lumbar spine movement. Eur Spine J, (2007). , 411-421.

[49] Duval-beaupere, G, Schmidt, C, & Cosson, P. A Barycentremetric study of the sagittal shape of spine and pelvis: the conditions required for an economic standing position. Ann Biomed Eng, (1992). , 451-462.

[50] Gioia, G, Mandelli, D, & Randelli, F. The Charité III Artificial Disc lumbar disc prosthesis: assessment of medium-term results. Journal of Orthopaedics and Traumatology, (2007). , 134-139.

[51] Bertagnoli, R, et al. The treatment of disabling single-level lumbar discogenic low back pain with total disc arthroplasty utilizing the Prodisc prosthesis: a prospective study with 2-year minimum follow-up. Spine (Phila Pa 1976), (2005). , 2230-2236.

[52] Guyer, R. D, et al. Prospective, randomized, multicenter Food and Drug Administration investigational device exemption study of lumbar total disc replacement with

the CHARITE artificial disc versus lumbar fusion: five-year follow-up. Spine J, (2009). , 374-386.

[53] David, T. Lumbar disc prosthesis. Surgical technique, indications and clinical results in 22 patients with a minimum of 12 months follow-up. Eur Spine J, (1993). , 254-259.

[54] Siepe, C. J, et al. Total lumbar disc replacement in athletes: clinical results, return to sport and athletic performance. Eur Spine J, (2007). , 1001-1013.

[55] Zigler, J. E. Five-Year Results of the ProDisc-L Multicenter, Prospective, Randomized, Controlled Trial Comparing ProDisc-L With Circumferential Spinal Fusion for Single-Level Disabling Degenerative Disk Disease. Seminars in Spine Surgery, (2012). , 25-31.

[56] Delamarter, R, et al. Prospective, randomized, multicenter Food and Drug Administration investigational device exemption study of the ProDisc-L total disc replacement compared with circumferential arthrodesis for the treatment of two-level lumbar degenerative disc disease: results at twenty-four months. J Bone Joint Surg Am, (2011). , 705-715.

[57] Nechtow et al. Nechtow W, Hintner M, Bushelow M, Kaddick C (2006) Intervertebral disc replacement mechanical performance depends strongly on input parameters. 52nd Orthopaedic Research Society. Abstract 0118

[58] Grupp TM, Yue JJ, Garcia R Jr, Basson J, Schwiesau J, Fritz B, Blömer W (2009) Biotribological evaluation of artificial disc arthroplasty devices: influence of loading and kinematic patterns during in vitro wear simulation. Eur Spine J 18(1):98–108

[59] Ingham E, Fisher J (2000) Biological reactions to wear debris in total joint replacement. Proc Instn Mech Engrs 214:21–37

[60] Tropiano, P, et al. Lumbar disc replacement: preliminary results with ProDisc II after a minimum follow-up period of 1 year. J Spinal Disord Tech, (2003)., 362-368.

[61] McAfee PC, Cunningham B, Holsapple G, Adams K, Blumenthal S, Guyer RD, Dmietriev A, Maxwell JH, Regan JJ, Isaza J (2005) A prospective, randomized, multicenter Food and Drug Administration investigational device exemption study of lumbar total disc replacement with the CHARITE artificial disc versus lumbar fusion: part II: evaluation of radiographic outcomes and correlation of surgical technique accuracy with clinical outcomes. Spine (Phila Pa 1976) 30:1576–1583 (discussion E388–90)

[62] Chung, S. S, et al. The effect of lumbar total disc replacement on the spinopelvic alignment and range of motion of the lumbar spine. J Spinal Disord Tech, (2006)., 307-311.

[63] Le Huec J., et al.The effect of single-level, total disc arthroplasty on sagittal balance parameters: a prospective study. Eur Spine J, (2005)., 480-486.

[64] Huang, R. C, et al. Range of motion and adjacent level degeneration after lumbar total disc replacement. Spine J, (2006)., 242-247.

[65] Ensink, F. B, et al. Lumbar range of motion: influence of time of day and individual factors on measurements. Spine (Phila Pa 1976), (1996)., 1339-1343.

[66] Pearcy, M. J, & Bogduk, N. Instantaneous axes of rotation of the lumbar intervertebral joints. Spine (Phila Pa 1976), (1988)., 1033-1041.

Section 3

Diagnostic Techniques

Chapter 12

X-Ray Digital Tomosynthesis Imaging: An Appropriate Reconstruction Algorithm for Arthroplasty

Tsutomu Gomi, Hiroshi Hirano and
Masahiro Nakajima

Additional information is available at the end of the chapter

http://dx.doi.org/10.5772/53248

1. Introduction

Digital tomosynthesis is a limited-angle method for image reconstruction. In this technique, a projection dataset of an object acquired at regular intervals during a single acquisition pass is used to reconstruct planar sections post priori. Tomosynthetic slices exhibit high resolution in planes that are parallel to the detector plane. Digital tomosynthesis enhances the existing advantages of conventional tomography, including low radiation dose, short examination time, and easy, low-cost availability of longitudinal tomographs, which do not include the partial volume effect. Furthermore, digital tomosynthesis provides the additional benefits of digital imaging (Ziedses et al 1971, Miller et al 1971, Grant et al 1972, Baily et al 1973, Kruger et al 1983, Sone et al 1991, Sone et al 1995) as well as the tomographic benefits of computed tomography (CT) at a decreased radiation dose and cost in an approach that is easily implemented in conjunction with chest radiography. This technique was developed by improving the old technique of geometric tomography, which is unpopular for chest imaging because of positioning difficulties, high radiation dose, and residual blur due to out-of-plane structures. Digital tomosynthesis overcomes these difficulties by enabling the reconstruction of numerous image slices from the data acquired from a single low-dose image. Digital tomosynthesis images are invariably affected by blurring because of objects lying outside the plane of interest and those superimposed on the focused image of the fulcrum plane by the limited acquisition angle. This results in poor object detectability in the in-focus plane. This technique has been investigated in angiography and the imaging of chest, hand joints, lungs, teeth and breasts (Stiel et al 1993, Duryea et al 2003, Sone et al 1995, Niklason et al 1997, Dobbins et al 2003).

Imaging by X-ray CT has improved over the past three decades and is now a powerful tool in medical diagnostics. It has become an essential, non-invasive imaging technique since the advent of spiral CT imaging in the 1990s, which led to shorter scan times and improved three-dimensional (3D) spatial resolution. CT provides a high resolution in the tomographic plane but limited resolution in the axial direction. However, the quality of images generated by a CT scanner can still be reduced by the presence of metal objects in the field-of-view. Imaging patients with metal implants such as marker pins, dental fillings or hip prostheses is susceptible to artifacts, generally in the form of bright and dark streaks, cupping, capping and so on. This artifact susceptibility is mostly due to quantum noise, scattered radiation and beam hardening (Hsieh 1995). Metal artifacts influence the image quality by reducing the contrast and obscuring details, thus hindering the ability to detect structures of interest and possibly leading to misdiagnosis. In addition, CT values are reduced, which can lead to errors while using these data e.g. for attenuation correction in positrin emission tomography (PET)/CT imaging (Kamel et al 2003). The metallic components of arthroplasty devices are high-contrast objects that generate artifacts when imaged using CT scans. These artifacts can make it extremely difficult or impossible to interpret images obtained by these devices. The presence of artifacts, along with the partial volume effect, severely limits the potential for the objective quantification of total joint replacement with CT.

Methods for reducing metal artifacts aim to improve the quality of images, affected by them. Recently, modified- iterative (Wang et al 1996, 1999, 2000, Man et al 2000) or wavelet-reconstruction techniques have produced promising results. However, these methods cannot be combined with the fast, robust filtered backprojection (FBP) algorithm, which is the standard reconstruction technique (Robertson et al 1997) implemented in modern CT scanners.

Digital tomosynthesis using the FBP algorithm shows satisfactory overall performance, but its effectiveness depends strongly on the region of the image. This type of digital tomosynthesis gives good results independent of the type of the metal present in the patient and effectively removes noise artifacts, especially at greater distances from the metal objects (Gomi et al 2008). In addition, flexibility in choosing digital tomosynthesis imaging parameters on the basis of the desired final images and generation of high-quality images may be beneficial.

In this study, we focus on the potential application of digital tomosynthesis using a different algorithm for an enhanced performance, which is used for imaging hip prosthesis phantoms (titanium) and human hip prostheses. The present study was performed to evaluate the clinical application of digital tomosynthesis in imaging these objects using the relatively commercial tomosynthesis method. Digital tomosynthesis was compared to the use of conventional reconstruction for tomosynthesis (FBP), metal-artifact-reduction processing reconstruction for tomosynthesis, iterative reconstruction for tomosynthesis [simultaneous iterative reconstruction technique; SIRT (Gordon et al 1970)], adaptive statistical iterative reconstruction CT and non-metal-artifact-reduction processing CT (conventional FBP reconstruction) scans of a hip prosthesis phantom and human hip prosthetic case.

2. Image reconstruction

2.1. Tomosynthesis

Existing tomosynthesis algorithms can be divided into three categories: (1) backprojection algorithms, (2) FBP algorithms, and (3) iterative algorithms. The backprojection algorithm is referred to as a shift-and-add (SAA) process, in which the projection images obtained at different angles are electronically shifted and added to generate an image plane, focused at a certain depth below the surface. The projection shift is adjusted such that the visibility of features in the selected plane is enhanced, whereas that in other planes is blurred. By using a digital detector, the image planes at all depths can be retrospectively reconstructed from one set of projections. The SAA algorithm is valid only if the motion of the X-ray focal spot is parallel to the detector (Gomi et al 2012).

In FBP algorithms, which are widely used in CT, many projections acquired at greater than 360º are used to reconstruct cross-sectional images. The number of projections typically ranges between a few hundred and approximately one thousand. The Fourier central slice theorem is fundamental to the FBP theory. In two-dimensional (2D) CT imaging, projecting an object corresponds to sampling it perpendicular to the X-ray beam in Fourier space (Kak et al 1988). For many projections, information of the object is well sampled, and the object can be restored by combining the information from all the projections. In 3D cone-beam imaging, the information of the object in Fourier space is related to the Radon transform of the object. The relationship between the Radon transform and cone-beam projections has been studied properly, and solutions to the cone-beam reconstruction have been provided (Smith 1985). The FBP algorithm generally provides highly precise 3D reconstruction images when an exact-type algorithm is employed (Feldkamp et al 1984). Therefore, this method has been adopted for the image reconstruction of 3D tomography and multi-detector cone-beam CT.

An iterative algorithm performs reconstruction recursively (Ruttimann et al 1984, Bleuet et al 2002), unlike the one-step operation in backprojection and FBP algorithms. During the iterative reconstruction, a 3-D object model is repeatedly updated until it converges to the solution, which optimizes an objective function. The objective function defines the criteria of the reconstruction solution. The objective function in SIRT are applied iteratively so that the projections of the reconstructed volume, computed from an image-formation model, resemble the experimental projections. A linear-projection model is a first-order approximation of the nonlinear image-formation process, occurring in tomosynthesis. Furthermore, although the noise is not white, the SIRT formula for white noise produces good estimates of the underlying structures.

Metal artifacts influence the image quality by reducing the contrast and obscuring the detail, thereby impairing the ability to detect structures of interest and making diagnosis impossible. Artifacts due to high-attenuation features in hip prostheses are observed in digital-tomosynthesis reconstruction because of the small number of projections and narrow angular range, typically employed in tomosynthesis imaging developed artifact-reduction methods on the basis of a modified Shepp–Logan reconstruction filter kernel by considering the additional weight of the direct current components in the frequency domain (Gomi et al 2009). Processing increases the ratio of low-frequency components in an image (Fig. 1). Artifact was reduced using basic and FBP algorithms. It provides a filtering method that can be used in combination with the backprojection algorithm to yield sliced images with the desired properties via tomosynthesis.

The tomosynthesis system (SonialVision Safire II, Shimadzu Co., Kyoto, Japan) comprised an X-ray tube with a 0.4-mm focal spot and a 362.88 × 362.88-mm digital flat-panel detector composed of amorphous selenium. Each detector element was 150 × 150 μm in size. Tomography was performed linearly with a total acquisition time of 6.4 s {80 kVp, 250 mA, 20 ms/view, effective dose: 1.33 mSv [International Commission on Radiological Protection (ICRP) 60], 0.69 mSv (ICRP 103)} and an acquisition angle of 40 degree. Projection images were sampled during a single tomographic pass (74 projections) using a matrix size of 1440 × 1440 with 12 bits per image and were used to reconstruct tomograms of a desired height. The reconstructed images (0.272 mm/pixel) were obtained with a 4-mm slice thickness at 1-mm reconstruction intervals. An antiscatter grid was used (focused type, grid ratio 12:1). The distance from the source to the isocentre was 980 mm and that from the isocentre to the detector was 1100 mm (3.0-mm aluminium equivalent filtration). The tomosynthesis images were reconstructed using FBP with the conventional Shepp–Logan filter kernel.

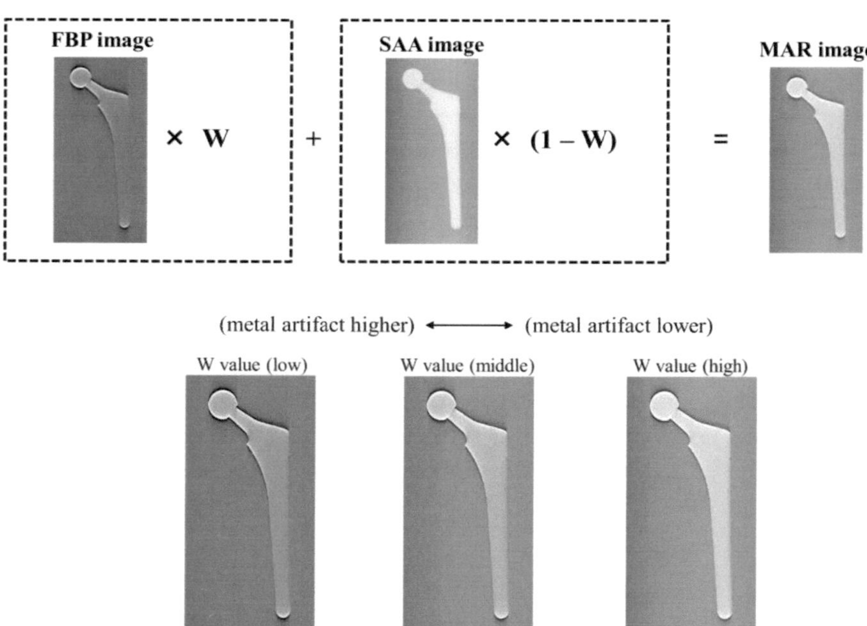

Figure 1. Concept of the metal-artifact-reduction processing method for tomosynthesis. The image is weighted by multiplying the different weight coefficients and adding them to the shift-added image and the conventional FBP image.

2.2. CT

The presence of metal artifacts has been a major problem in X-ray CT. Metal parts in the field-of-view attenuate most of the X-ray photons and generate dark and bright streaks after FBP, which is currently the selected reconstruction method for CT. These artifacts severely degrade the image quality, particularly near metal surfaces. Metal-artifact reduction has important applications in orthopaedic, oncologic, and dental imaging.

Iterative reconstruction algorithms, with and without the incorporation of a priori information, have been used to reconstruct incomplete projections. Although previous results using iterative reconstruction were unsatisfactory, a recently developed iterative-deblurring method has produced an image reconstruction of the incomplete data with few artifacts. Iterative reconstruction, which has recently become available on commercial CT scanners, enables metal-artifact-noise reduction without trade-off in spatial resolution (Main et al 2010). However, iterative reconstruction has unfavourable effects. Its use alters the texture of the image noise and can yield an unusually homogenous image. This may not be immediately appealing to most radiologists, who are usually accustomed to FBP images (Hara et al 2009). Moreover, an excessive degree of iterative reconstruction may obscure fine and subtle findings (Yanagawa et al 2010).

In computation with iterative reconstruction, the image has an initial condition of values, which are iteratively optimized according to the rules of the model. The FBP image is used for the initial condition in adaptive statistical iterative reconstruction (GE Healthcare Corp.; the initial value of each pixel) for the following reasons: it is presumably close to the final optimized solution (lessening the need for iterations), it is a valid indicator of specific-slice image noise and it can be obtained rapidly. For modelling and using iterative reconstruction, minimum convergence is achievable with adaptive statistical iterative reconstruction. However, a fully converged, 100% adaptive statistical iterative reconstruction image, has a noise-free appearance with an unusually homogeneous attenuation. Because some noise is inherent in CT, the use of 100% adaptive statistical iterative reconstruction may not be immediately appealing to most of the radiologists. However, blended images containing a linear mixture of the original FBP and this reconstruction can exhibit markedly decreased noise while retaining a more typical CT appearance. This blended image can be adjusted from 1% to 100% in adaptive statistical iterative reconstruction. The 40% level was chosen because 40% adaptive statistical iterative reconstruction should produce a diagnostically acceptable image with less noise than a full-dose FBP image. We selected the blending ratios of 20%, 40%, and 60% according to the results of a previous study (Hara et al 2009). In the conventional FBP reconstruction, standard reconstruction kernels were used.

CT scan was performed on a multi-slice CT scanner (64-slice Discovery CT 750HD scanner; GE Healthcare Corp., Milwaukee, WI) with 120 kVp, 150 mA, 0.625 mm × 64 collimation, and a 1-s gantry rotation time at a beam pitch of 0.984 [effective dose, 5.4 mSv (ICRP 60), 4.1 mSv (ICRP 103)]. The clinical task was to assess the hip prostheses. A 4-mm thick slice is generally used in clinical practice. In this study, we applied the slice thickness used during the screenings; therefore, the axial reconstructed images were obtained with a 4-mm slice thickness at 1-mm reconstruction intervals (512 × 512 pixels and 140-mm field-of-view).

3. Evaluation

In the study, the artifact-reduction performance was evaluated using the intensity profile, artifact spread function (ASF) and root-mean-square error (RMSE). The intensity profiles were compared using different reconstruction methods in the in-focus plane. Wu et al. proposed an ASF metric to quantify the artifacts observed in planes outside the focus image plane (Wu et al 2003). These artifacts are generated from real features located in the focus image plane and resemble the real feature. The artifacts exhibited in the image plane are defined by the ASF as $\frac{N_{artifact}(z)-N_{BG}(z)}{N_{artifact}(z_0)-N_{BG}(z_0)}$, where z to the base of 0 is the location of the in-focus plane of the real feature and z is the location of the off-focus plane. N to the base of artifact (z0) (z) and *NBG*(z0) are the average pixel intensities of the feature and the image background in the in-focus plane, respectively. *Nartifact*(z) and *NBG*(z) are the average pixel intensities of the artifact and the image background in the off-focus plane, respectively. Another important metric to be considered is RMSE, which can be computed by obtaining the root of the summation of the square of the standard deviation and the square of the bias. The errors in the image plane are defined in terms of RMSE as $RMSE = \sqrt{\sum_{i=1}^{n}(X-x_i)^2/n}$, where X is the observed image, x_i is the referenced image, and n is the number of compounds in the analysed set.

4. Results

4.1. Hip prosthesis phantoms (titanium)

A comparison of the intensity profiles and RMSEs of the tomosynthesis and CT images revealed that tomosynthesis (metal-artifact-reduction processing and the iterative algorithm) decreased the number of metal and beam hardening artifacts in the reconstructed images. Furthermore, this technique yielded a higher contrast detectability than the existing FBP algorithm. In the reconstructed images obtained from metal-artifact-reduction processing, the quantum noise structure decreased, and the noise structure was slightly smoother (Figs. 2–6).

The chart in Fig. 7 shows the ASF results for the prosthetic case. This chart shows ASF versus the distance from the in-focus slice in millimetres. There were nine reconstructed slices. The chart demonstrates that tomosynthesis with metal-artifact-reduction processing (W = high) removes the highest number of metal artifacts. Examining Fig. 7 through the entire thickness of the specimen shows that the order of ASF performance of the algorithm is as follows: (1) tomosynthesis (metal-artifact-reduction processing with FBP, W = high); (2) CT (20%, 40%, and 60% adaptive statistical iterative reconstruction and conventional FBP); (3) tomosynthesis (iterative algorithm, 100 iterations); and (4) tomosynthesis (conventional FBP).

http://dx.doi.org/10.5772/53248

4.2. Human hip prostheses

To demonstrate the potential benefits of digital tomosynthesis compared with CT in imaging hip prostheses, we used one clinical case, a 52-year-old female with total hip arthroplasty. The use of digital tomosynthesis improved the visualisation of the underlying tissue detail by blurring the overlying structures. CT provided information [multiplanar reformation (MPR) of images] on the hip prostheses, as shown in Fig. 8. MPR of CT images suffered from string artifacts in all regions. In addition, due to strong beam hardening and scattering, the femur region was poorly displayed. The artifacts in CT images, produced by FBP, were realistic and resembled actual patient images. The more metal was present in the field-of-view (metal-backed and bilateral prostheses), the more metal artifacts were produced. Reconstruction of the incomplete projection data by using iterative deblurring produced an essentially metal-artifact-free image for soft tissues and outperformed the FBP methods. The hip prostheses present on the digital tomosynthesis images could be removed effectively by blurring in the 74-projection digital tomosynthesis image. This allowed better visualisation of the tissue detail directly below the hip prostheses structures.

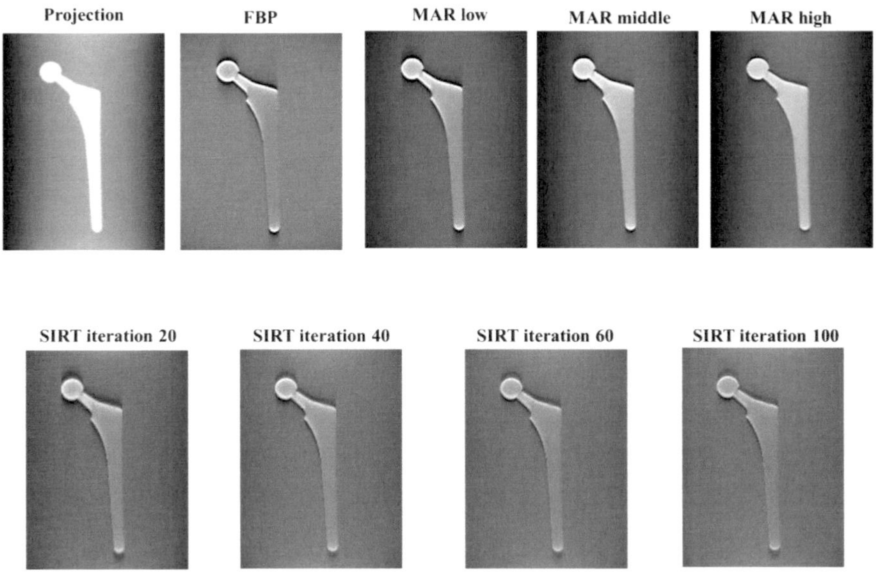

Figure 2. Comparison between tomosynthesis images and those obtained by metal-artifact-reduction processing, conventional FBP and SIRT imaging algorithms in the in-focus plane. (Reference is projection image.)

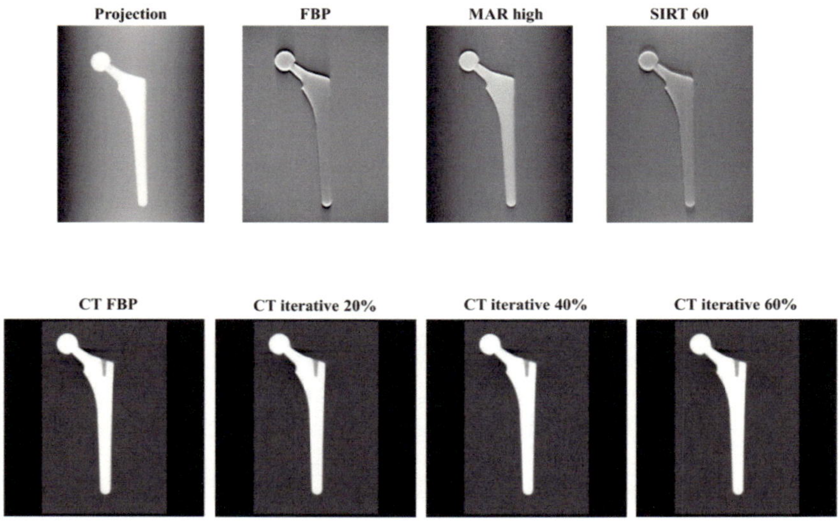

Figure 3. Comparison between excellent tomosynthesis images and those obtained by metal-artifact-reduction processing (W = high), conventional FBP, SIRT imaging algorithms (60 iterations) in the in-focus plane and CT images (conventional FBP and iterative reconstruction). Metal-artifact-reduction processing provided a better visualisation of the hip prosthesis phantom by eliminating, blurring and reducing the artifacts, above, and the visualized planes, below.

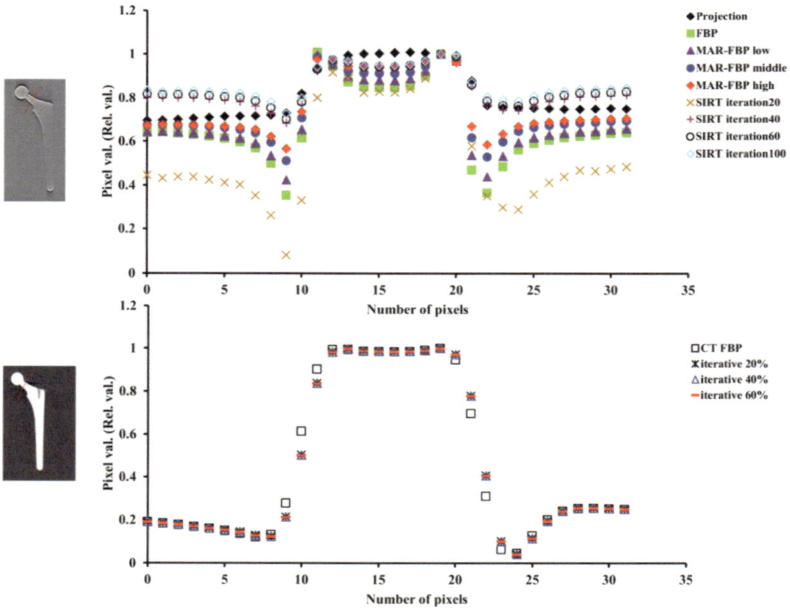

Figure 4. Comparison between intensity profiles using tomosynthesis and CT in the in-focus plane. Artifacts (part of undershooting) are reduced by metal-artifact-reduction processing and SIRT technique for tomosynthesis.

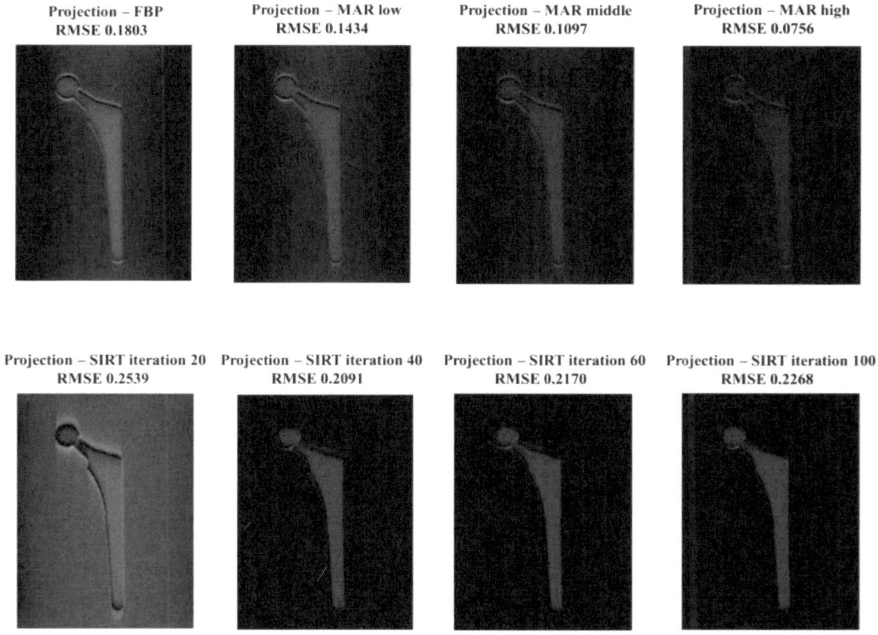

Figure 5. Comparison between tomosynthesis error images and RMSE of the images obtained by metal-artifact-reduction processing (W = low, medium and high), conventional FBP and SIRT imaging algorithms in the in-focus plane. (Reference is the projected image.)

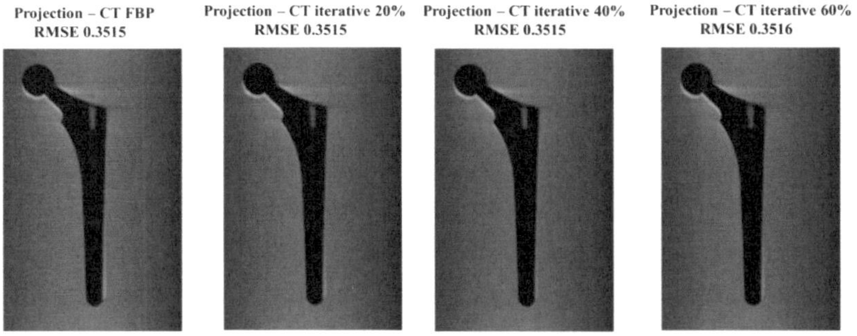

Figure 6. Comparison between CT error images and RMSE of images obtained from conventional FBP and iterative reconstruction algorithms in the in-focus plane. (Reference is the projected image.)

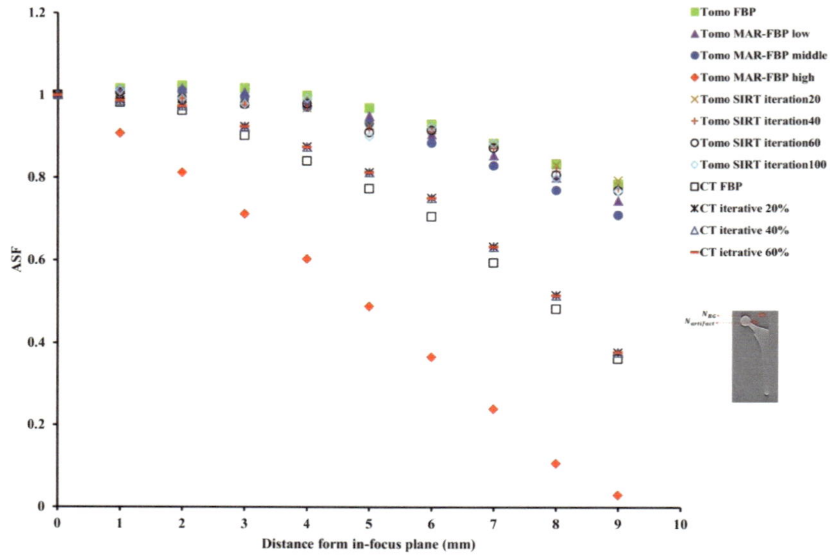

Figure 7. Comparison between ASF versus distance from the in-focus plane for tomosynthesis and CT. ASF chart demonstrates that tomosynthesis with metal-artifact-reduction processing results in the maximum removal of metal artifacts.

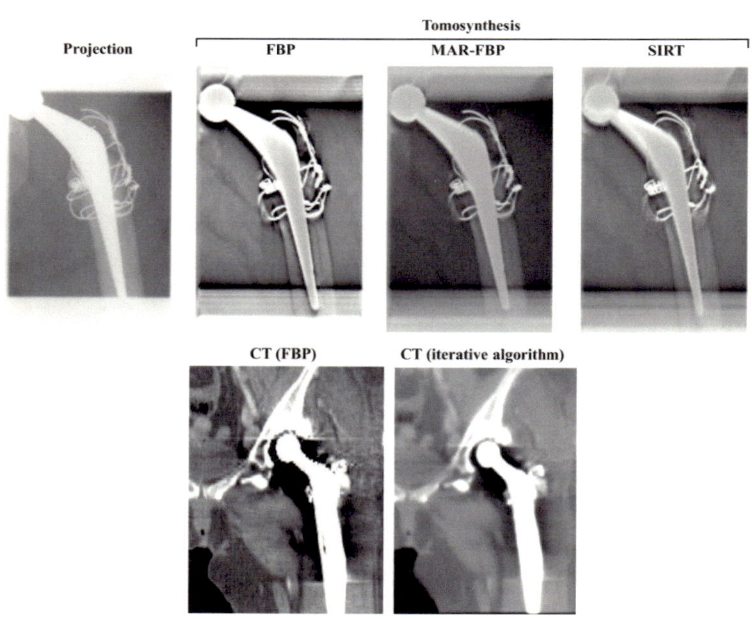

Figure 8. Case patient (52-year-old woman; coxarthrosis, after total hip arthroplasty). The use of metal-artifact-reduction processing tomosynthesis allowed a better visualisation of the left hip joint prosthesis by blurring the anatomic structures above and below the visualized planes. (MAR; metal-artifact-reduction)

5. Conclusion

Applicaton of metal-artifact-reduction processing digital tomosynthesis in imaging prostheses appears promising. The results of a prosthesis study suggest that digital tomosynthesis (metal-artifact-reduction processing and an iterative reconstruction algorithm) can produce improved image quality compared with that by conventional FBP tomosynthesis by removing the overlying structures and providing limited 3D information. In addition, the digital tomosynthesis method apparently facilitates the significant improvement of images corrupted by metal artifacts. Metal-artifact-reduction processing digital tomosynthesis provided higher quality images compared to those by CT. Metal-artifact-reduction processing digital tomosynthesis is the best solution when the high-attenuation feature causing the artifacts can be segmented accurately from the projection.

On the whole, metal-artifact-reduction processing performed satisfactorily, but its effectiveness depended strongly on the image region. Metal-artifact-reduction processing digital tomosynthesis images yielded good results, which were independent of the type of metal present in the phantom study or patient, and showed good removal of metal artifacts, particularly at greater distances from the metal objects. Flexibility in selecting the imaging parameters in metal-artifact-reduction processing digital tomosynthesis on the basis of the desired final images and realistic imaging conditions may be beneficial.

Author details

Tsutomu Gomi[1], Hiroshi Hirano[2] and Masahiro Nakajima[3]

1 School of Allied Health Sciences, Kitasato University, Japan

2 Department of Radiology, Shinshu University Hospital, Japan

3 Department of Radiology, Dokkyo Medical University Hospital, Japan

References

[1] Gordon R, Bender R, Hermen GT. (1970) Algebraic reconstruction techniques (ART) for three-dimensional electron microscopy and x-ray photography. Journal of theoretical biology, 29, pp.471-481 ISSN 0022-5193

[2] Ziedses des, Plante BG. (1932) Eine neue methode zur differenzierung in der roentgenographie (planigraphie). Acta radiologica, 13, pp.182-92, ISSN 0284-1851

[3] Miller ER, McCurry EM, Hruska B. (1971) An infinite number of laminagrams from a finite number of radiographs. Radiology, 98, pp.249-255, ISSN 0033-8419

[4] Grant DG. Tomosynthesis. (1972) A three-dimensional radiographic imaging technique. IEEE transactions on bio-medical engineering, 19, pp.20-8, ISSN 0018-9294

[5] Baily NA, Lasser EC, Crepeau RL. (1973) Electrofluoro-plangigraphy. Radiology, 107, pp.669-671 ISSN 0033-8419

[6] Kruger RA, Nelson JA, Ghosh-Roy et al. (1983) Dynamic tomographic digital subtraction angiography using temporal filteration. Radiology, pp.863-867, ISSN 0033-8419

[7] Sone S, Kasuga T, Sakai S et al. (1991) Development of a high-resolution digital tomosynthesis system and its clinical application. Radiographics, 11, pp.807-822, ISSN 0271-5333

[8] Stiel G, Stiel LG, Klotz E et al. (1993) Digital flashing tomosynthesis: A promising technique for angiographic screening. IEEE transactions on medical imaging, 12, pp. 314-21, ISSN 0278-0062

[9] Duryea J, Dobbins JT, Lynch JA. (2003) Digital tomosynthesis of hand joints for arthritis assessment. Medical Physics, 30, pp.325-33, ISSN 0094-2405

[10] Sone S, Kasuga T, Sakai F, et al. (1995) Image processing in the digital tomosynthesis for pulmonary imaging. European Radiology, 5, pp.96-101, ISSN 0938-7994

[11] Niklason LT, Christian BT, Niklason LE, et al. (1997) Digital tomosynthesis in breast imaging. Radiology, 205, pp.399-406, ISSN 0033-8419

[12] Dobbins JT III, Godfrey DJ. (2003) Digital x-ray tomosynthesis: curent state of the art and clinical potential. Physics in medicine and biology, 48, R65-106, ISSN 0031-9155

[13] Kak A, Slaney M. (1988) Principles of computerized tomographic imaging. IEEE, ISBN 0-89874-494-X, New York

[14] Smith DB. (1985) Image reconstruction from cone-beam projections: necessary and sufficient conditions and reconstruction methods. IEEE transactions on medical imaging, M1-4, pp.14-25, ISSN 0278-0062

[15] Feldkamp LA, Davis LC, Kress JW. (1984) Practical cone-beam algorithm. Journal of the Optical Society of America, A1, pp.612-619, ISSN 0030-3941

[16] Ruttimann U, Groenhuis R, Webber R. (1984) Restoration of digital multilane tomosynthesis by a constrained iteration method. IEEE transactions on medical imaging, MI-3, pp.141-8, ISSN 0278-0062

[17] Bleuet P, Guillemaud R, Magin I. Et al. (2002) An adapted fan volume sampling scheme for 3D algebraic reconstruction in linear tomosynthesis. IEEE transactions on nuclear science, 49, pp.2366-72, ISSN 0018-9499

[18] Hsieh J. (1995) computed tomography technology and applications; Image artifacts causes and correction, In: Medical CT and ultrasound, LW Goleman, JB Fowlkes, pp. 487-518, Advanced Medical Publishing ISBN 1-883526-03-5, Madison

[19] Kamel EM, Burger C, Buck A, et al. (2003) Impact of metallic dental implants on CT-based attenuation correction in a combined PET/CT scanner. European Radiology, 13, pp.724-8, ISSN 0938-7994

[20] Wang G, Snyder DL, O'Sullivan JA, et al. (1996) Iterative debluring for metal artifacts reduction. IEEE transactions on medical imaging, 15, pp.657-664, ISSN 0278-0062

[21] Wang G, Vannier MW, Cheng PC. (1999) X-ray cone-beam tomography for metal artifacts reduction and local region reconstruction. Microscopy and microanalysis, 5, pp.58-65, ISSN 1431-9276

[22] Wang G, Frei T, Vannier MW. (2000) A fast iterative algorithm for metal artifact reduction in x-ray CT. Academic Radiology, 7, pp.607-614, ISSN 1076-6332

[23] Man B De, Nuyts J, Dupont P, et al. (2000) Reduction of metal streak artifacts in x-ray computed tomography using a transmission maximum a posteriori algorithm. IEEE transactions on nuclear science, 47, pp.997-981, ISSN 0018-9499

[24] Robertson DD, Yuan J, Wang G, et al. (1997) Total hip prosthesis metal-artifact suppression using iterative deblurring reconstruction. Journal of computer assisted tomography, 21, pp.293-298, ISSN 0363-8715

[25] Wu T, Stewart A, Stanton M, McCauley T, et al. (2003) Tomographic mammography using a limited number of low-dose cone-beam projection images. Medical Physics, 30, pp.265-380, ISSN 0094-2405

[26] Gomi T, Hirano H. (2008) Clinical potential of digital linear tomosynthesis imaging of total joint arthroplasty. Journal of Digital Imaging, 21, pp.312-22, ISSN 0897-1889

[27] Gomi T, Hirano H, Umeda T. (2009) Evaluation of the X-ray digital linear tomosynthesis reconstruction processing method for metal artifact reduction. Computerized Medical Imaging and Graphics, 33, pp.257-274, ISSN 0895-6111

[28] Hara AK, Paden RG, Silva AC et al. (2009) Iterative reconstruction technique for reducing body radiation dose at CT. American Journal of Roentgenology, 193, pp. 764-771, ISSN 0361-803X

[29] Marin D, Nelson RC, Schindera ST et al. (2010) Low-tube-voltage, high-tube-current multidetector abdominal CT: improved image quality and decreased radiation dose with adaptive statistical iterative reconstruction algorithm-initial clinical experience. Radiology, 254, pp.145-153, ISSN 0033-8419

[30] Yanagawa M, Honda O, Yoshida S et al. (2010) Adaptive statistical iterative reconstruction technique for pulmonary CT: image quality of the cadaveric lung on standard- and reduced-dose CT. Academic Radiology, 17, pp.1259-1266, ISSN 1076-6332

[31] Gomi T, Hirano H, Nakajima M. (2012) Recent advance in arthroplasty. "Chapter 6 x-ray digital linear tomosynthesis imaging of arhtoroplasty", pp.95-108, INTECH, ISSN 978-953-307-990-5, Croatia

Section 4

Results of Arthroplasty by Etiology

Chapter 13

Hip and Knee Arthroplasty in the Patient with Inflammatory Arthritis

Andrew Gordon, Hosam E. Matar and
J. Mark Wilkinson

Additional information is available at the end of the chapter

http://dx.doi.org/10.5772/54743

1. Introduction

The term inflammatory arthritis refers to an inflammatory arthropathy in patients suffering from one of a number of chronic inflammatory conditions including rheumatoid arthritis (RA), and the seronegative spondyloarthropathies of ankylosing spondylitis (AS), psoriatic arthritis (PsA), spondyloarthritis associated with inflammatory bowel disease and undifferentiated spondyloarthritis. This chapter will focus on a review of the surgical management of patients with RA, AS, and PsA, as these represent the most common of the inflammatory arthropathies.

Knowledge of the inflammatory arthritidies is important for lower limb arthroplasty surgeons as awareness of both the local changes within the affected joints and how extra-articular manifestations can adversely affect anaesthesia, surgery and rehabilitation is necessary to ensure good surgical outcomes. In addition to the local and systemic manifestations of the inflammatory diseases, patients may be prescribed multiple medications, including disease modifying anti-rheumatic drugs (DMARDs) or biological therapies that may affect the local surgical site or affect the patient systemically and have an impact on rehabilitation and patient outcome. In addition, quality of life and functional outcome of patients with chronic inflammatory arthropathies may also be reduced compared to simple osteoarthritis because of the chronicity and systemic nature of the inflammatory disease. Finally, the choice of implant and the method of fixation may affect implant survival and revision burden.

The term inflammatory arthropathy covers a wide spectrum of diseases which ultimately manifest themselves with joint destruction, systemic features and disability. In the following section the pathophysiology, presentation, diagnosis and medical treatments for the inflammatory conditions will be considered separately to the treatment of hip and knee 'inflammatory arthritis'.

2. Rheumatoid arthritis

2.1. Epidemiology and pathophysiology

Rheumatoid arthritis (RA) is the most common chronic inflammatory condition and affects 3% of women and 1% of men, and has its peak age of onset between 35 and 45 years. The aetiology of RA remains unclear but involves environmental and heritable factors. Several susceptibility loci reside in the HLA region on chromosome 6 and within this region, normal genetic variation may increase a patient's susceptibility to or severity of rheumatoid disease. Although many genetic variants have been identified [1-4], the impact of individual variants on the risk of developing RA is low. Research into the functional mechanisms by which these genetic variants confer disease susceptibility is on-going, with the ultimate goal of identifying discrete biological pathways which pathologically induce chronic inflammation. From this research, medical therapies to specifically target RA may be further developed. Environmental triggers which may increase the risk of RA include smoking, high alcohol intake, coffee, vitamin D levels and low socio-economic group [5-10].

The underlying pathophysiology of RA is of over-activation of intra and extra-cellular inflammatory cascades including over the expression of tumour necrosis factor and other inflammatory cytokines including interleukin (IL) 6 and IL-1 [11-14]. The cells that drive the inflammatory response include B and T lymphocytes, macrophages and synovial cells [15]. The activation of inflammatory pathways result in persistent synovial inflammation with subsequent joint and periarticular bone destruction.

2.2. Presentation

2.2.1. Joint features

Patients with RA typically present with a persistent symmetrical polyarthritis. The small joints of the hand and foot are most commonly affected, although any synovial joint may be involved. The natural history of the affected joint is one of low grade chronic inflammation with periods of intense pain and stiffness during a 'flare.' Between flares, joint stiffness is usually worst in the morning or after a period of rest.

2.2.2. Systemic features

Extra articular manifestations (EAM) of RA affect many organ systems and can be classified by the Malmö criteria [16] into severe and non-severe (Table 1). EAM may be present in up to 41% of patients with RhA and up to 22% of patients may develop the severe EAMs [17]. These EAMs must be considered in any patient presenting to the orthopaedic surgeon and investigated further in conjunction with rheumatology and anaesthetic specialists prior to any

http://dx.doi.org/10.5772/54743

surgery. In addition, patients with RA may suffer from general malaise, anorexia, anaemia, weight loss and depression.

Affected tissue or organ	EAM		Co-morbidities
	Not severe	Severe	
Skin	Nodules Raynaud's phenomenon	Petechiae, purpura, ulcers, gangrene	Cancer
Pulmonary system	Bronchiolitis obliterans Organizing pneumonia	Pleuritis Interstitial lung disease	Lung carcinoma
Heart	Valvular heart disease Myocarditis Arrhythmias	Pericarditis Coronary vasculitis and aortitis	Hypertension Heart failure Ischaemic heart disease
Nervous system	Non identified	Mono/polyneuritis multiplex Central nervous system vasculitis	Depressive syndrome Cervical myelopathy
Eyes	Secondary Sjögren's syndrome Sicca syndrome	Episcleritis or scleritis Retinal vasculitides	None identified
Haematological system	None identified	Felty's syndrome	Non-Hodgkin lymphoma Lymphadenopathy Splenomegaly
Kidneys	None identified	Glomerulonephritis Interstitial nephritis Amyloid deposition	None identified
Bone	None identified	None identified	Osteoporosis

Table 1. Extra-articular manifestations (EAM) in rheumatoid arthritis (RA). (Reproduced with permission from Prete M *et al* [17]).

2.3. Diagnosis

Diagnostic criteria have been designed to differentiate RA from other joint diseases. In 1987 the American College of Rheumatology (ACR) published seven diagnostic criteria to aid the diagnosis [18]. For a patient to be diagnosed with RA, four of the seven criteria have to be present and morning stiffness, arthritis in three or more joints, symmetrical arthritis and hand arthritis had to be present for at least 6 weeks (Table 2).

	ACR Criteria for Rheumatoid Arthritis
1	Morning stiffness (present for at least 1 hour)
2	Arthritis of 3 or more joints.
3	Arthritis of hand joints (>1 swollen joint)
4	Symmetrical arthritis
5	Rheumatoid Nodules
6	Serum Rheumatoid factor
7	Radiographic changes

Table 2. The American College of Rheumatology diagnostic criteria for Rheumatoid Arthritis [18].

However, the ACR classification has been criticised for its low sensitivity and specificity for early RA [19], a time which is critical since early pharmacological intervention increases remission rate. Further, early treatment can limit the severity of the disease and prevent bony destruction [9]. This has led to the development of another classification system by the ACR and the European League Against Rheumatism (ELAR) (Table 3) [20]. This more recent classification system assesses joint involvement, and duration of symptoms along with serological markers including acute-phase reactants and detection of antibodies against citrullinated peptides (ACPA). The detection of ACPA antibodies increases the sensitivity of the serological tests greater than the detection of rheumatoid factor. The common radiographic features of RA are shown in Table 4.

	ACR/EULAR 2010 criteria
1	Joint involvement (0-5) One medium to large joint (0) Two to ten medium to large joints (1) One to three small joints (large joints not counted((2) Four to ten small joints (large joints not counted) (3) More than ten joints (at least one small joint) (5)
2	Serology (0-3) Negative RF and negative ACPA (0) Low positive RF and low positive ACPA (2) High positive RF or high positive ACPA (3)
3	Acute-phase reactants (0-1) Normal CRP and normal ESR (0) Abnormal CRP or abnormal ESR (1)
4	Duration of symptoms (0-1) Less than 6 weeks (0) Greater than 6 weeks (1)

Table 3. The 2010 American College of Rheumatology &European League Against Rheumatism classification criteria for Rheumatoid Arthritis [20].

http://dx.doi.org/10.5772/54743

Soft tissue overlying the joint
Swelling
Effusion
Rheumatoid nodules
Intra-articular changes
Global joint space narrowing
Marginal erosions
Secondary osteoarthritic change (osteophytes, sclerosis, cysts)
Peri-articular changes
Juxta-articular osteoporosis
Metaphyseal cysts (geodes)
Periostitis (common at the digits, rare at large joints)
Joint mal-alignment (alignment abnormalities due to ligament incompetence, joint subluxation, joint dislocation)

Table 4. Common radiographic features in rheumatoid arthritis [48]

2.4. Medical management

The classes of medication therapies used in rheumatoid and in other inflammatory arthropathies include simple analgesics non-steroidal anti-inflammatories (NSAIDs), disease modifying anti-rheumatic drugs (DMARDs), glucocorticosteroids and biological agents.

In RA, reduction of pain and stiffness may be achieved with the use of simple analgesics and NSAIDs. However, the long-term use of NSAIDs is limited by their cardiac and renal toxic effects and their lack of impact on disease progression [9]. DMARDs are the first line of treatment for rheumatoid disease. Although they are a heterogeneous group of drugs, they all decrease pain and stiffness, improve function, and may limit disease progression and induce disease remission. The most frequent DMARD used in RA remains methotrexate. Others include sulfasalazine, leflunomide, hydroxychloroquine, and gold. Serious adverse effects are associated with these potential agents and require careful monitoring. Hepatotoxicity, pancreatitis, interstitial lung disease, blood dyscrasias, marrow aplasia, induction of autoimmune diseases and acute kidney injury are all adverse effects of DMARDs. In particular, methotrexate can induce bone marrow suppression, induction of liver enzymes and folic acid depletion, necessitating concurrent folic acid supplementation.

Glucocorticosteroids may be used as an effective local treatment when given intra-articularly. They may also be administered systemically for controlling acute flares, as they reduce synovitis, however with longer term use the adverse effects of osteoporosis, increased risk of infection and chronic adrenal suppression limit their use.

To date, five anti-tumour necrosis factor (anti-TNF) antibodies have been licenced as biological therapy for RA. They act in one of two ways, Enterocept blocks the effect of TNF by acting as a soluble TNF receptor whereas Infliximab, Golimumab, Adalimumab and Certolizumab are monoclonal antibodies which bind and block TNF. A recent meta-analysis of the efficacy of the TNF blocking agents concluded that TNF blockers as a monotherapy were efficacious but only as much as the DMARD methotrexate [21]. Combination therapy of methotrexate and an anti-TNF were more efficacious than either of the treatments in isolation. Adverse reactions and complications of anti-TNF treatment has been widely reported and includes local injection site reactions, infusion reactions, reactivation of latent infections, especially tuberculosis and an increased risk of sepsis, both local and systemic. Other biological approaches to disease modification include depletion in B cell numbers that drive inflammation using Rituximab, a monoclonal antibody to a protein found of the surface of B cells.

3. Ankylosing spondylitis

3.1. Epidemiology and pathophysiology

Ankylosing spondylitis (AS) is a chronic seronegative autoimmune arthropathy and is the most common of the spondyloarthritis subtypes. It predominantly affects the axial skeleton especially the sacroiliac joints and the spine, however the lower limb joints, the entheses and peripheral joints may be affected. AS typically starts in the third decade of life, has a prevalence of up to 1.2% and is 2.5 times more common in men than women [22, 23]. All of the spondyloarthropathies have a strong heritable component to susceptibility, most strongly with the HLAB27 variant on chromosome 6. 90-95% of patients with ankylosing spondylitis are positive for HLAB27. However, only 5% of subjects carrying this variant develop a spondyloarthropathy.

3.2. Bony features

Bony changes in AS commonly include new bone formation which arises from the cortical surfaces. Bony spurs from the vertebral bodies (syndesmophytes) extend vertically and may bridge across the intervertebral disc ultimately leading to a rigid 'bamboo' spine appearance. Entheses are also affected by new bone formation and patients may develop bony spurs in the Achilles tendon or plantar fascia. In addition, patients with AS have an increased risk of osteoporosis which can lead to devastating spinal fractures and cord compromise. The hip joint is more commonly affected than the knee joint in AS, 20% of patients who develop AS during adolescence go onto total hip arthroplasty (THA) [24].

3.3. Systemic features

AS is a systemic disease and extra-articular features (EAMs) are present in up to 40% of patients [25]. The most common EAMs include anterior uveitis, inflammatory bowel disease, lung disease, cardiac abnormalities (including conduction defects, valvular disease and cardiomyopathy) and renal disease secondary to deposition of IgA and renal amyloid [25].

3.4. Diagnosis

The main clinical manifestations of AS are pain and stiffness within the axial skeleton. A number of radiographic grading systems have been developed in AS, however magnetic resonance imaging (MRI) is more sensitive and can detect inflammation within the sacroiliac joints before radiographic changes are apparent [26, 27]. The clinical diagnosis of AS can approach a sensitivity of 70% and a specificity of 81% if two of the four criteria developed by Rudwaleit *et al* are present [28] (Table 5). Other investigations that aid the diagnosis include typing for HLAB27 and C-reactive protein however this may be elevated in only 50% of cases [27]. Serum alkaline phosphatase is elevated in severe disease.

In established disease, lumbar spine and pelvis plain radiographs may show squaring of the lumbar vertebrae (a consequence of inflammatory bone remodelling), syndesmoses and structural changes within the sacroiliac joint. MR imaging reveals bony oedema, inflammation and bony erosions within the sacroiliac joints before radiographic changes are apparent.

New criteria for inflammatory back pain in young to middle-aged adults (<50 yrs) with chronic back pain
Morning stiffness >30 minutes
Improvement in back pain with exercise but not with rest
Awakening because of back pain during the second half of the night only
Alternating buttock pain
The criteria are fulfilled at least two of four of the parameters are present (sensitivity 70.3%, specificity 81.2%).

Table 5. Clinical criteria for the diagnosis of Ankylosing Spondylitis [25].

3.5. Medical management

Simple NSAIDs and cyclooxygenase-2 inhibitors are used to control pain and stiffness. In addition NSAIDs may limit the osteoprolific component of the disease as they block the osteoblastic effects of prostaglandin E2. Again the adverse effects of long term NSAIDs however limit protracted use. Intense physiotherapy may assist individual patients but its role has not been proven to be of benefit when evaluated in Cochrane systematic reviews [29].

As with RA, AS is a systemic disease and the DMARDs methotrexate, sulphasalazine and leflunomide have been used to treat symptoms and prevent or slow disease progression. Clinical results and results from RCTs unfortunately have been disappointing. Methotrexate may be effective at treating the peripheral joint disease but its use for axial disease has not been proven. Similar results are seen with other DMARs as well perhaps reflecting a different pathophysiology in AS compared to RhA.

The recent introduction of anti-TNF biological agents has greatly aided the medical management of AS. RCTs have shown that these agents control symptoms, improve function and limit or halt disease progression. The adverse reactions of these drugs have been previously documented but in selected patients therapy is well tolerated both in the short term and up to 6 years [30, 31].

4. Psoriatic arthritis

4.1. Epidemiology and pathophysiology

Psoriatic arthritis (PsA) is usually a seronegative spondyloarthropathy associated with psoriasis. Five subsets were described by Moll and Wright in 1973 [32] and are widely used in clinical practise, these include; distal interphalangeal arthritis, asymmetrical oligoarthritits, symmetrical arthritis, spondylitis and arthritis mutilans. The prevalence of psoriasis in Western Europe is 2-3% and up to 30% of patients with psoriasis develop an arthritis [33]. However this prevalence varies considerably due to geographic variation and variation in diagnostic criteria.

PsA has a strong genetic component to susceptibility, and has been linked to the MHC region and HLA-B28, HLA-B39 and HLA-B27. This latter association is much weaker in PsA than ankylosing spondylitis [34, 35]. As with the other major spondyloarthropathies, upregulation of the T-cells and increased expression of inflammatory cytokines are features of the disease. A bacterial or traumatic environmental trigger has been proposed with PsA, however no conclusive evidence for this has been found to date [36, 37].

4.2. Presentation

PsA differs from RA in that fewer joints are affected, and the pattern of joint involvement is commonly asymmetric, and involves the distal interphalangeal joints and nail lesions [38]. Dactylitis, spondylitis and sacroiliitis are common features of PsA, the involved joints are tighter, contain less fluid and are less tender than those in RA [38]. The systemic features of PsA are less significant than RhA but patients may still suffer from EAMs of anterior uveitis and a disease pattern similar to SAPHO (synovitis, acnes, pustulosis, hyperostosis and oseitis). The incidence of and mortality from cardiovascular complications is increased in patients with PsA which is thought to be secondary to an increase in atherosclerosis [39, 40].

4.3. Diagnosis

Many diagnostic criteria have been used to detect psoriatic arthropathy, the most recent in 2006 by the Classification Criteria for Psoriatic Arthritis (CASPAR) group [41] (Table 6). The sensitivity and specificity for psoriatic arthritis may reach 98.7 and 91.4 respectively [42]. No single laboratory finding in PsA is diagnostic however acute phase reactants are elevated in approximately 50% of cases [43].

4.4. Medical management

Methotrexate, retinoids and psoralen combined with ultraviolet A (PUVA) treatment appear to be most effective at treating skin and joints together [43]. The role of biological agents remains unclear with limited data evaluating their use in PsA [33].

http://dx.doi.org/10.5772/54743

Category	Point
Current psoriasis	2
Personal history of psoriasis	1
Family history of psoriasis	1
Typical psoriatic nail dystrophy (onycholysis, pitting, hyperkeratosis)	1
Negative rheumatoid factor	1
Current dactylitis or history of dactylitis (recorded by a rheumatologist)	1
Hand or foot plain radiography: evidence of juxta-articular new bone formation, appearing as ill-defied ossification near joint margin (excluding osteophytes)	1

Table 6. Caspar Classification of Psoriatic Arthritis [41]

5. Surgical interventions for inflammatory arthritis

Optimal management of the patient with inflammatory arthropathy requires a multidisciplinary approach both in primary and secondary care. The hospital management of the inflammatory arthropathies is predominantly led by the rheumatologist with support from physiotherapy, occupational therapy, the surgeon, dieticians, social workers, orthotists and chiropodists. Community care is also paramount to maintain and optimise pain control and function. The multidisciplinary approach comprises general practitioners, district nursing, occupational therapy and social workers. Patients also often require support through housing agencies for home adaptation, community care workers and employment services [44].

In the lower limb, patients with inflammatory arthritis can present with a combination of progressive pain, restricted movement, instability particularly in the knee joint and progressive loss of function. Arthroplasty should be considered when optimal medical and non-drug supportive therapies have failed.

5.1. Pre-operative assessment

The systemic features of RA and the spondyloarthropathies need to be thoroughly identified through a detailed history, examination and appropriate investigations (Table 7). Abnormalities which may affect fitness for surgery or rehabilitation need to be discussed with the anaesthetist, rheumatologist and where necessary other relevant medical and allied professionals. Cardiovascular pathology maybe silent because of low physical demand. The incidence of silent myocardial infarction is six times that of the general population and is responsible for much of the 10 year reduced life expectancy in the rheumatoid population versus the background population [45]. Any abnormalities within the history in a patient with inflammatory arthritis therefore need to be investigated further.

History	Disease onset Pattern and temporal sequence of joints involved Presence and persistence of joint swelling Pain: site, severity and radiation Morning stiffness and duration Functional difficulties Presence of non-articular features (e.g. nodules) Systemic features (e.g. anorexia, fatigue, weight loss) Psychological effects Full review of systems Previous anaesthetic and surgical history Drugs and allergies
Examination	Complete medical Evidence of joint inflammation Joint damage, range of motion, and previous surgical scars Tendon and ligamentous damage Presence of extra-articular features (e.g. plenomegaly, leg ulcers, vasculitis) Grip strength General health, anaemia, muscle atrophy Dental inspection, assessment of mouth opening ability, dysphonia Neurological assessment for cervical myelopathy and peripheral neuropathy
Investigations	Full blood count, urea, creatinine, electrolytes, and liver function tests Chest radiograph, lateral cervical spine flexion and extension radiographs Electrocardiogram Urine dipstick; culture to exclude occult infection Pulmonary function tests in patients with limiting lung disease Echocardiogram in patients with limiting cardiac involvement

Table 7. Preoperative assessment of the Rheumatoid Patient, Wilkinson *et al* [48]

Airway management in the rheumatoid patient may also present difficulties because of laryngomalacia and atlanto-axial subluxation (AAS). AAS may be anterior, posterior, vertical, lateral/rotatory and sub-axial. The less common posterior and lateral subluxations place the spinal cord in jeopardy during extension of the neck. Cervical pathology is common. In a review of rheumatoid patients awaiting orthopaedic surgery, Neva *et al* found that 44% of patients had cervical spine subluxation or previous fusion [46]. Interestingly, they found no difference in neck pain, headaches or upper limb radiculopathy between patients with or without cervical spine instability. Flexion and extension views of the cervical spine or computed tomography (CT) scanning may aid AAS diagnosis and although this diagnosis may not change anaesthetic practise it will ensure that neck handling is kept to a minimal and ensure that staff with adequate training are present for anaesthesia [45]. Further cervical spine difficulties are encountered in the AS patient who may have fixed spinal deformities. These

http://dx.doi.org/10.5772/54743

fixed deformities in the presence of osteoporosis place patients at high risk of fracture and subsequent neurological deficit. The anaesthetist needs to be made aware of these issues before surgery. Cervical spine involvement is not common in psoriatic arthritis and the most common clinical feature is a decrease in range of movement secondary to apophysial joint ankylosis [47]. Radiographically, the prevalence of anterior atlanto-axial instability is less than 10%. Published data with regards to the incidence of cervical spine involvement with spondyloarthritis secondary to inflammatory bowel disease is extremely limited.

Finally, patients with chronic inflammatory disease often have anaemia both as a result of their disease or secondary to medication. Optimising pre-operative haemoglobin levels, intraoperative cell salvage and reinfusion post-operative drains should be planned before surgery is undertaken.

5.2. The order of surgery

Patients with inflammatory arthritis often present with many symptomatic joints of both the upper and lower limbs. Careful consideration to the order of surgical intervention requires assessment on an individual level. Surgical priority should be given to structures that are at high risk of failure (for example symptomatic cervical spine instability or imminent tendon rupture). In general, lower limb surgical procedures precede those of the upper limb as post-operative rehabilitation using crutches can compromise upper limb reconstructive surgery. Within the lower limb, total knee arthroplasty implant positioning and rotational alignment is simpler once femoral length and rotation have been restored with a total hip arthroplasty [48], however generally the order of surgery should be dictated by managing the most painful and functionally limiting joints first. In patients with severe forefoot disease, consideration should be given to undertaking forefoot arthroplasty prior to hip or knee joint replacement (Figure 1).

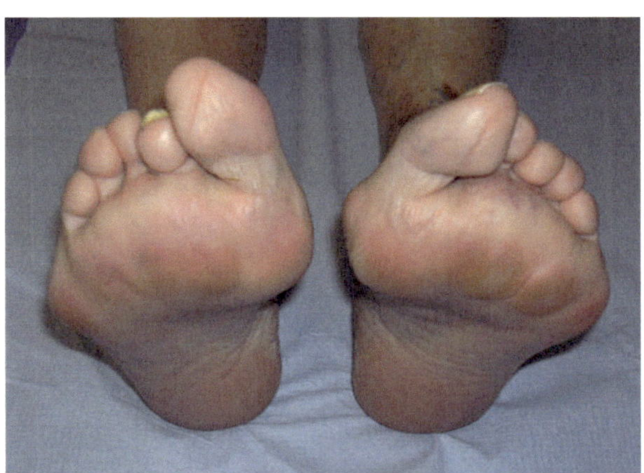

Figure 1. Soles of the feet in a patient with rheumatoid arthritis. There is distal subluxation of the forefoot fad pad with exposure of subluxed metatarsal heads and resultant callosity formation.

5.3. The perioperative management of medical therapies

The adverse effect profile of many of the medications used to control symptoms and influence disease progression in inflammatory arthropathy may affect a wide variety of organ systems and an awareness of these and of their potential drug interactions is required.

NSAIDs increase the risk of gastric ulceration and patients may benefit from perioperative gastric protection with proton pump inhibitors. Long term use may also impair renal function increasing the risk of acute kidney injury secondary to post-operative dehydration.

The risk of an Addisonian crisis, an insufficient adrenal response to stress, is increased in patients with long term glucocorticosteroid use. Exognous steroid use results in adrenal atrophy secondary to suppression of corticotropin-releasing hormone and adrenocorticotropic hormone (ACTH). Patients in Addisonian crisis may present with symptoms ranging from lethargy, abdominal pain and syncope to coma. Biochemically, hypoglycaemia, hyponatraemia, hyperkalaemia and hypercalcaemia may be present. Local practice governs the regimen of hydrocortisone supplementation in the perioperative period, however typical dosing includes 100mg of intravenous hydrocortisone at induction of anaesthesia and 100mg 6 or 8 hourly for 3 days. Lower dosing regimens with a total of 150mg per day are also used [48].

While the effects of NSAIDs and glucocorticoids are well understood, there is no consensus on the perioperative management of the DMARDs. A randomised controlled trial in RA patients revealed that the infection rate was lower in patients continuing methotrexate versus those who stopped methotrexate prior to surgery (2% versus 15% respectively) [49]. A recent systematic review of the use of methotrexate in RA patients undergoing elective orthopaedic surgery found that continuing methotrexate was not associated with increasing risk of surgery complications, and led to fewer disease flares in the perioperative period [50]. Disease activity is also better controlled when methotrexate weekly administration remains un-interrupted [51]. Also, a study examining late infection rates with uninterrupted methotrexate use found no evidence of increased risk of late deep infection in 65 patients undergoing elective orthopaedic surgery over 10 years of follow up [52].

There is, to date, no clear evidence on the perioperative risk of orthopaedic infections in patients receiving biological agents, such as anti-TNF therapy [53]. A review of the limited published data in this area reveals much heterogeneity. RA patients have shown no increase in superficial wound infection rates following arthroplasty surgery with the continued use of biological agents [54, 55]. Conversely other studies have shown an increased rate of post-operative infection [56]. In a retrospective review of 81 total hip arthroplasties (THA) and 339 total knee arthroplasties (TKA), there was an increased odds ratio for superficial skin infection of up to 9.8 with continued use of anti-TNF therapy [57]. In a much larger Japanese study [58], 1626 patients treated with biological agents versus 29,903 patients not on a biological agent, reported an odds ratio for superficial infection of 2.1 with the use of biological agents even when these were stopped prior to surgery. The general recommendations of the American College of Rheumatology (ACR) guidelines in 2008 [59] and its update in 2012 [60] on the perioperative management of DMARDs are as follows:

http://dx.doi.org/10.5772/54743

i. Methotrexate: continue perioperatively for all procedures.

ii. Sulfasalazine: discontinue 1 day before surgery, resume 3 days after surgery.

iii. Leflunomide: discontinue 2 days before surgery, resume 2 weeks after surgery.

iv. Hydroxychloroquine: continue perioperatively for all procedures.

v. Biological agents (eg. Anti-TNF- α): discontinue 1 week before surgery, resume 2 weeks after surgery. The ACR guidelines also recommend that the time period for cessation of biological agents is dependent upon the half-life of the biological agent used. Gilson et al. [110] recommends that the cessation of anti-TNF therapy should allow levels to fall by 5 half-lives prior to surgery in order to ensure that the drug has been eliminated.

6. Surgical challenges and choice of implant in inflammatory arthritis

Patients with inflammatory arthritis may be regular attenders to primary and secondary care. A good rapport and doctor-patient relationship is essential to gain trust and understanding and help to manage patients expectations. Some orthopaedic challenges stem from the general chronicity of the inflammatory disease or from the medications used to treat it. Others are joint-specific.

6.1. General features

Many patients will have had previous hip or knee procedures or had surgery at other sites. The overall function of these sites, as well as the presenting joint, must be assessed as they may affect rehabilitation and outcome. Soft tissue pathology may manifest as joint contracture, tendon attenuation or rupture, ligamentous instability, skin loss, chronic ulceration, vascular or neurological insufficiency, or a combination of these features (Figure 2). Previous surgical scars, especially around the knee, may affect planning, exposure and outcome after surgery. Bony disease can result in extensive bone loss secondary to erosive disease, avascular necrosis, or osteoporosis with increased fracture risk and deformity and challenges in establishing primary implant fixation.

6.2. Surgical challenges for hip arthroplasty

Surgical challenges at the hip include acetabular protrusio, focal bone loss and osteoporosis. Flexion contractures may be present in patients who have been chair-bound for a considerable time prior to seeking treatment for their joint disease.

Protrusio may be primary, or secondary, and can occur with or without medial wall defects and is common in all inflammatory arthritidies (Figure 3). Protrusio was first recognised by Otto in 1816 [61] and it was 1935 when Overgaard [62] presented the first useful classification into primary and secondary, since modified by Gilmour [63]. Other classifications have also emerged e.g. Charnley [64] and Hirst [65].

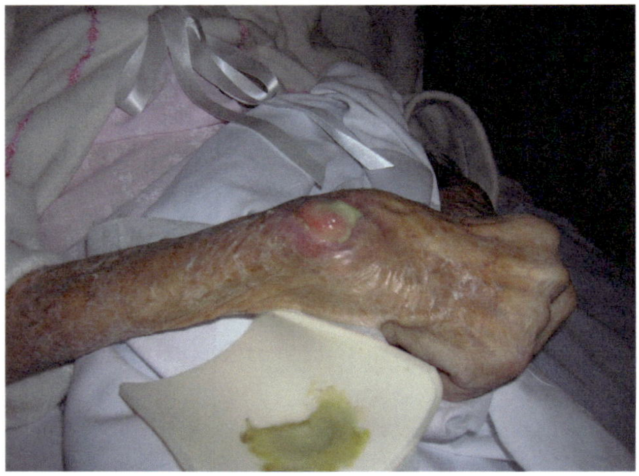

Figure 2. Thin skin, ligamentous damage, infection, and soft tissue loss at the wrist in a patient with rheumatoid arthritis. Similar problems at the foot are common, and may impact on hip and knee reconstructive options.

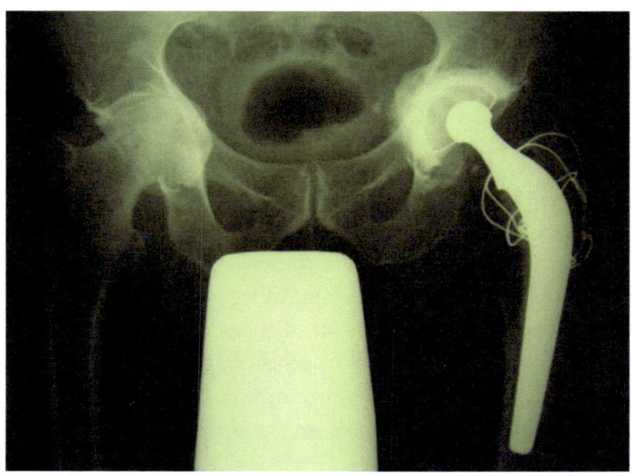

Figure 3. Plain radiograph of the pelvis in a patient with rheumatoid arthritis. On the right side there is protrusio acetabuli, on the left this has been treated with cemented total hip arthroplasty plus impaction of morsellised allograft to the protrusio defect.

Charnley graded protrusio acetabuli by measuring the distance between the medial wall of the acetabulum and the iliopectineal line. In Grade I protrusio the medial acetabular wall is medial to the line by 1-5mm, Grade II 6-15mm and Grade III greater than 15mm. Edstein and Murphy recognised that using the ilioischial line as a reference point that there was sex specific variation of the medial wall of the acetabulum, in males the medial wall was 2mm lateral to the line and females were 1mm medial [66]. Hirst graded the protrusio taking into account this sex related variation [65](Table 8).

http://dx.doi.org/10.5772/54743

Grade	Men	Women
I	3-8 mm	6-11 mm
II	8-13 mm	12-17 mm
III	>13 mm	>17 mm with fragmentation

Table 8. Protrusio acetabuli classification by Hirst [65]

In Grade III cases dislocation of the femoral head may be difficult and the surgeon should be confident with his/her ability to divide the femoral neck in situ and remove the femoral head as a secondary procedure. The normal anatomy of the sciatic nerve may also be altered and it should be actively sought for in posterior approaches to the hip. Anatomical restoration of the centre of hip rotation lateral to Kohler's line is essential. Anatomical restoration optimises hip biomechanics and prevents impingement; therefore further deepening of the acetabulum should be avoided. Medial wall supplementation and anatomical restoration can be achieved with the use of bone grafting or metal augmentation. Hirst [65] initially described the use of 2mm thick femoral head slices impacted into the medial acetabular wall and Rosenburg *et al* have reported a 90% survival rate at 12 years using morsellised impaction bone grafting [67]. Larger defects require medial wall supplementation. The clinical results of support with metal mesh in these large defects is poor [68] and therefore cage supplementation prior to impaction bone grafting is needed. These systems report good outcomes, up to 95% survival at 9 year follow-up [69], in revision surgery for large defects. However there are few long term studies assessing the clinical and radiographic outcomes of primary hip arthroplasty in Grade III protrusio defects in inflammatory arthritis. Studies utilising trabecular metal supplementation are awaited.

6.3. Choice of implant for hip arthroplasty

Cemented or cementless THA components may be used in patients with RA. A study from the Finish Arthroplasty register found comparable long-term results between cemented and cementless components in 4,019 patients who were over 55 years when revision for any reason was used as an end point [70]. Similarly, in a study of 2,557 patients under the age of 55 years there were no significant differences in overall survival between different components [71]. The 15-year survival rate for cementless proximally circumferentially porous-coated stems was 87% and for cemented stems was 81%. However, the 15-year survivorship for cementless cups was poorer than cemented cups, 67% versus 80%, respectively.

In another study from the Danish Hip Arthroplasty registry [72], 1,395 (1,661 primary hips) patients with RA were followed for up to 14 years and results were compared with 64,858 patients with osteoarthritis (RA: cemented cups 47%, cemented stems 73%, OA: cemented cups 43%, cemented stems 68%). There was no difference in survival of cups between primary THAs in rheumatoid versus osteoarthritis patients. In contrast, there was better overall survival of stems in rheumatoid versus osteoarthritis patients, both for revision due to aseptic loosening (adjusted relative risk = 0.58; 95% CI: 0.34-0.99) and for any reason (adjusted relative risk = 0.63; 95% CI: 0.45-0.88).

In a 10-year follow up study of 75 patients with RA (106 hips) who received a cemented THA, stem survival was 98% and cup survival was 92% [73]. In cemented Charnley THA in young patients with rheumatoid arthritis (63 patients, 100 hips) versus osteoarthritis (54 patients, 66 hips), 25-year survivorship of the femoral component was 85% in patients with rheumatoid arthritis versus 74% in patients with osteoarthritis, and of the acetabular component was 79% versus 59%, respectively [74]. Finally, in a recent systematic review of 23 small case series and 5 national implant registers of THA in rheumatoid patients there was no evidence in favour of cemented components over cementless ones [75].

The role of resurfacing arthroplasty in RA remains unclear. In a recent international register study, 47 rheumatoid patients (54 hips) were gender and age matched with 131 osteoarthritis patients (138 hips) and all had uncemented acetabular and cemented femoral hip resurfacing with Birmingham Hip Resurfacing implant. At 8-year average follow up, the survival rate was 96.3% in the RA group and 97.8% in OA group [76]. In another small series of 10 patients (13 hips) who had metal-on-metal resurfacing, no failures were reported at short term 3-year follow up [77]. However, recent data on the survival of resurfacing prostheses in general suggests avoiding this type of prosthesis in women, and in smaller men, phenotypic characteristics that are common in the rheumatoid population.

6.4. Surgical challenges for Total Knee Arthroplasty (TKA)

Soft tissue destruction leading to ligamentous instability, focal bone loss particularly of the femoral condylar bone leading to loss of height within the lateral compartment and fixed valgus deformity (Figure 4a and b), and periarticular osteoporosis are common features in the rheumatoid knee [48]. Valgus deformities with a variable degree of hyperextension rather than fixed flexion are commonly seen. Varus deformities are often secondary to osteoarthritic changes with a degree of fixed flexion [78]. The surgical challenge is to ensure correct soft tissue balance to avoid unequal loading and asymmetric stresses on the implant and eventual loosening. A stepwise approach to the release of contracted tissue is required [79-81]. A medial parapatellar or a lateral approach is used and structural bone grafting or prosthetic augmentation blocks may be required to restore large bone defects [48, 82]. Soft tissue insufficiency and ligamentous imbalance often favours the use of a cruciate sacrificing, rather than a posterior cruciate-retaining prosthesis. The survivorship of cruciate retaining prostheses is reported as poor in some series [83][84]. In cases of ligamentous incompetence a fully constrained prosthesis may be required [85]. The role of patella resurfacing in the rheumatoid patient is unclear. In a randomised controlled trial of 26 patients with RA who had bilateral TKA and patellar replacement performed in one randomly selected knee in each patient demonstrated improved pain and function in the patella resurfacing group [86].

http://dx.doi.org/10.5772/54743

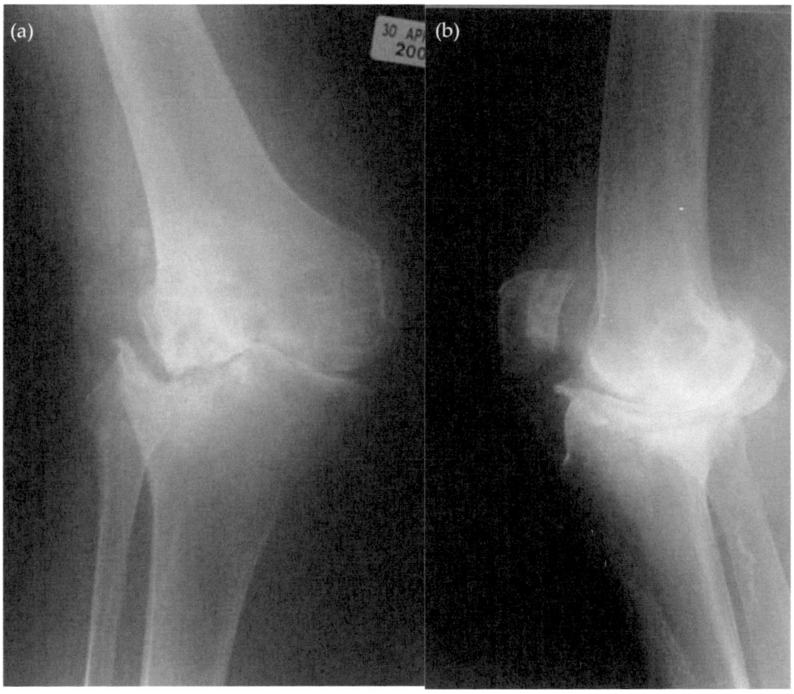

Figure 4. Plain anteroposterior (a) and lateral (b) radiographs of the knee in a patient with rheumatoid arthritis. Degenerative changes are present in all 3 joint compartments. There is collapse of the lateral compartment with resultant valgus deformity. Erosion of the anterior aspect of the distal femoral metaphysis due to pannus is also seen.

6.5. Choice of implant for knee arthroplasty

Cemented TKA has been considered the gold standard prosthesis for the rheumatoid patient. The 10-year revision rate of cemented TKA between 2001 and 2010 in rheumatoid patients reported to the Swedish Knee Arthroplasty register was 4% [87]. Fifteen-year survival rate of cemented Kinematic TKA was 93.7% in 25 rheumatoid patients (36 knees) [88]. However, recent survivorship data on cementless TKA also show good results, with a survival rate of 96.8 % at 10 years in a cohort of 112 patients (179 knees) [89]. The cementless Hi-Tech Knee II cruciate-retaining prosthesis was evaluated in 31 Japanese patients with RA with an average 8-year follow up and a reported survival rate 96.9% [90]. Similarly, 16-year survival rate of cementless low contact stress TKA in 47 patients was 94% [91]. Unicompartmental prostheses are not appropriate for RA patients as the degenerative changes are pan-articular, and their use is associated with high failure rates [92].

7. Complications of hip and knee arthroplasty in inflammatory arthritis

When compared to the general arthroplasty population, patients with inflammatory arthritis have more comorbidities and are taking more prescription medication. This is reflected by the higher risk of systemic and surgery specific complications. Mortality rates in rheumatoid patients are 1.5-1.6 fold higher than in the general population [93]. In a ten-year survivorship analysis from the Scottish register, greater mortality rate was associated with rheumatoid disease. Cardiovascular disease is the most commonly attributed cause of death, although other complications, such as infection, pulmonary and renal disease, are also more prevalent in the rheumatoid population [94].

In a population based study on risk of revision for infection in THA and TKA from the Norwegian Arthroplasty register, data from 6,629 (2,462 TKA, 4,167 THA) patients with RA were compared with 102,157 osteoarthritis patients (21,832 TKA, 80,325 THA). On an average 8-9 year follow up, rheumatoid patients with TKA had a 1.6 times higher risk of revision for infection than osteoarthritis patients, whereas there was no difference in the THAs [95]. In a population based study from Mayo clinic, 462 patients with RA (657 total joint replacements) the prosthetic infection rate at 4 years follow up was 3.7% [96]. Da Cunha *et al* [97] found no significant difference in infectious complications when compared perioperative infections in 49 rheumatoid patients (28 TKA, 47 THA) with 75 gender and age matched osteoarthritis patients (56 TKA, 75 THA).

A retrospective review of nearly 5 million patients demonstrated that RA was an independent risk factor for pulmonary embolism and deep vein thrombosis (DVT) in hospital patients, with a relative risk of 2.25 and 1.9 respectively [98]. In a recent comparative study, the risk of DVT was compared in 199 patients (238 knees) with RA and 156 patients (169 knees) with osteoarthritis and was found to be higher in the osteoarthritis group [99]. Earlier studies have also demonstrated lower risk in rheumatoid patients, which has been attributed to the use of NSAIDs [100]. The use of NSAIDs is also believed to cause lower incidence of heterotopic ossification in the rheumatoid patient as compared with those with osteoarthritis [101].

The risk of dislocation is also reported as higher in RA patients in a recent population based study from the Scottish National arthroplasty register, 62,175 total hip arthroplasties performed from April 1989 to March 2004 [102]. This is supported by the results of a prospective study assessing dislocation 2-years following THA in inflammatory arthritis patients [103]. Finally, periprosthetic fractures are reported more common in RA patients compared to OA, this can be explained by the poor bone quality and comorbidities [104, 105]

7.1. Functional outcomes

Successful functional outcome requires realistic understanding of goals and expectations of surgery with active inclusion of the patient in the decision making process [109]. In measuring the success of lower limb arthroplasty in patients with inflammatory arthritis, condition-specific outcome measures should be used. Scoring systems have been developed to measure disease activity and functional deficit. The American College of Rheumatology has developed the "ACR20 response score" [106], this was modified and adapted by the European League Against Rheumatism "EULAR score"[107]. The ACR score is considered the gold standard and it is based on seven clinical end points: swollen joint count, tender joint count, the physician's assessment of disease activity, the patient's assessment of disease activity, pain, and physical function, and levels of an acute-phase reactant (either the C - reactive protein levels or the erythrocyte sedimentation rate). The "ACR20 response" [106], defined as at least 20% improvement in in both the tender joint count and the swollen joint count and at least 20% improvement in 3 of the 5 other core set measures listed above. ACR20 aims to provide an objective assessment of disease status and is used in longitudinal studies to measure the effectiveness of medical and surgical interventions. The use of these scores helped to provide objective assessment of patients outcomes, better preoperative scores are associated with better surgical outcome [108].

The outcome of surgery is influenced by the local pathology, nature of the procedure and the severity of the disease [53, 88, 110]. In a systematic review of patients characteristics affecting the surgical outcome of total joint arthroplasty, older age was related to worse function particularly among women, whilst age and sex did not influence the outcome of pain [111]. There is good evidence that an increase in joint damage is associated with an increase in functional disability [112] and joint surgery has improved the function and quality of life of patients with RA [113].

However, when compared to patients with osteoarthritis, those with inflammatory arthritis have a slower, more gradual functional improvement in clinical outcomes scores [114]. Functional outcomes following THA are poorer in rheumatoid compared with non-inflammatory arthritis [73], this is perhaps explained by the multiple joints involvement in this group and its effects on functional outcomes [115]. Nevertheless, following THA in 50 rheumatoid patients, Harris hip score improved from 22 to 82 at 9 years mean follow up [116], and from 25 to 89 at 11 years follow up in another cohort of 20 patients [117].

Studies on TKA in rheumatoid patients have also reported good long term functional outcomes. When using the knee society score, 46 patients (71 knees) achieved 77% 'Good' or 'Excellent' at 10 years follow up [118]. In another study, 25 patients (36 knees) achieved 78% 'Good' or 'Excellent' at 15 year follow up [88]. However, when compared with osteoarthritis patients who had TKA, 207 rheumatoid patients younger than 55 years achieved less postoperative improvement [119]. On the other hand, when assessing patient satisfaction following TKA, there was a significantly better subjective outcome in rheumatoid versus osteoarthritis patients [120].

8. Conclusions

Hip and knee reconstruction are important surgical interventions in the management of the patient with inflammatory arthritis. Evidence to date suggests that both cemented and cemented prosthesis give good long term results. The functional benefit achieved in an individual patient will be affected by the systemic nature of the disease, and other joint involvement. Because inflammatory arthropathy involves the whole joint, partial and uni-compartmental joint replacement should be avoided. The perioperative management of the patient with inflammatory arthropathy requires multidisciplinary input, and recognition and appropriate management of comorbidities that are common in this patient group. Finally, an awareness of the pharmaceutical and biological agents taken by the patient, and their appropriate peri-operative management is important to minimise the risk of iatrogenic complications.

Author details

Andrew Gordon[1], Hosam E. Matar[1] and J. Mark Wilkinson[2]

*Address all correspondence to: a.gordon@sheffield.ac.uk

*Address all correspondence to: hematar@doctors.org.uk

*Address all correspondence to: j.m.wilkinson@sheffield.ac.uk

1 Department of Orthopaedics The Northern General Hospital, Sheffield, United Kingdom

2 Academic Unit of Bone Metabolism, University of Sheffield, Sheffield, United Kingdom

References

[1] Ceccarelli F, D'Alfonso S, Perricone C, Carlomagno Y, Alessandri C, Croia C, et al. The role of eight polymorphisms in three candidate genes in determining the susceptibility, phenotype, and response to anti-TNF therapy in patients with rheumatoid arthritis. Clinical and Experimental Rheumatology 2012;Epub ahead of print

[2] de Rooy DP, Yeremenko NG, Wilson AG, Knevel R, Lindqvist E, Saxne T, et al. Genetic studies on components of the Wnt signalling pathway and the severity of joint destruction in rheumatoid arthritis. Annals of Rheumatic Diseases 2012;Epub ahead of print.

[3] Han SW, Sa KH, Kim SI, Lee SI, Park YW, Lee SS, et al. CCR5 gene polymorphism is a genetic risk factor for radiographic severity of rheumatoid arthritis. Tissue Antigens 2012;80:416-23.

[4] Orozco G, Goh CL, Al Olama AA, Benlloch-Garcia S, Govindasami K, Guy M, et al. Common genetic variants associated with disease from genome-wide association studies are mutually exclusive in prostate cancer and rheumatoid arthritis. British Journal of Urology International 2012.

[5] Bergstrom U, Jacobsson LT, Nilsson JA, Berglund G, and Turesson C. Pulmonary dysfunction, smoking, socioeconomic status and the risk of developing rheumatoid arthritis. Rheumatology (Oxford) 2011;50:2005-13.

[6] Lundberg K, Bengtsson C, Kharlamova N, Reed E, Jiang X, Kallberg H, et al. Genetic and environmental determinants for disease risk in subsets of rheumatoid arthritis defined by the anticitrullinated protein/peptide antibody fine specificity profile. Annals of Rheumatic Diseases 2012.

[7] Mikuls TR, Cerhan JR, Criswell LA, Merlino L, Mudano AS, Burma M, et al. Coffee, tea, and caffeine consumption and risk of rheumatoid arthritis: results from the Iowa Women's Health Study. Arthritis & Rheumatism 2002;46:83-91.

[8] Ruiz-Esquide V and Sanmarti R. Tobacco and other environmental risk factors in rheumatoid arthritis. Reumatologia Clinica 2012.

[9] Scott IC, Steer S, Lewis CM, and Cope AP. Precipitating and perpetuating factors of rheumatoid arthritis immunopathology: linking the triad of genetic predisposition, environmental risk factors and autoimmunity to disease pathogenesis. Best Practice & Research Clinical Rheumatology 2011;25:447-68.

[10] Song GG, Bae SC, and Lee YH. Association between vitamin D intake and the risk of rheumatoid arthritis: a meta-analysis. Clinical Rheumatology 2012.

[11] Bhardwaj N, Santhanam U, Lau LL, Tatter SB, Ghrayeb J, Rivelis M, et al. IL-6/IFN-beta 2 in synovial effusions of patients with rheumatoid arthritis and other arthritides. Identification of several isoforms and studies of cellular sources. Journal of Immunology 1989;143:2153-9.

[12] Cope AP, Aderka D, Doherty M, Engelmann H, Gibbons D, Jones AC, et al. Increased levels of soluble tumor necrosis factor receptors in the sera and synovial fluid of patients with rheumatic diseases. Arthritis & Rheumatism 1992;35:1160-9.

[13] Houssiau FA, Devogelaer JP, Van DJ, de Deuxchaisnes CN, and Van SJ. Interleukin-6 in synovial fluid and serum of patients with rheumatoid arthritis and other inflammatory arthritides. Arthritis & Rheumatism 1988;31:784-8.

[14] Waage A, Kaufmann C, Espevik T, and Husby G. Interleukin-6 in synovial fluid from patients with arthritis. Clinical Immunology and Immunopathology 1989;50:394-8.

[15] Brennan FM, Foey AD, and Feldmann M. The importance of T cell interactions with macrophages in rheumatoid cytokine production. Current Topics in Microbiology and Immunology 2006;305:177-94.

[16] Turesson C, Jacobsson L, and Bergstrom U. Extra-articular rheumatoid arthritis: prevalence and mortality. Rheumatology (Oxford) 1999;38:668-74.

[17] Prete M, Racanelli V, Digiglio L, Vacca A, Dammacco F, and Perosa F. Extra-articular manifestations of rheumatoid arthritis: An update. Autoimmunity Reviews 2011;11:123-31.

[18] Arnett FC, Edworthy SM, Bloch DA, McShane DJ, Fries JF, Cooper NS, et al. The American Rheumatism Association 1987 revised criteria for the classification of rheumatoid arthritis. Arthritis & Rheumatism 1988;31:315-24.

[19] Banal F, Dougados M, Combescure C, and Gossec L. Sensitivity and specificity of the American College of Rheumatology 1987 criteria for the diagnosis of rheumatoid arthritis according to disease duration: a systematic literature review and meta-analysis. Annals of Rheumatic Diseases 2009;68:1184-91.

[20] Funovits J, Aletaha D, Bykerk V, Combe B, Dougados M, Emery P, et al. The 2010 American College of Rheumatology/European League Against Rheumatism classification criteria for rheumatoid arthritis: methodological report phase I. Annals of Rheumatic Diseases 2010;69:1589-95.

[21] Aaltonen KJ, Virkki LM, Malmivaara A, Konttinen YT, Nordstrom DC, and Blom M. Systematic review and meta-analysis of the efficacy and safety of existing TNF blocking agents in treatment of rheumatoid arthritis. PLoS One 2012;7:e30275.

[22] Braun J, Bollow M, Remlinger G, Eggens U, Rudwaleit M, Distler A, et al. Prevalence of spondylarthropathies in HLA-B27 positive and negative blood donors. Arthritis & Rheumatism 1998;41:58-67.

[23] Feldtkeller E, Khan MA, van der Heijde D, van der Linden S, and Braun J. Age at disease onset and diagnosis delay in HLA-B27 negative vs. positive patients with ankylosing spondylitis. Rheumatology International 2003;23:61-6.

[24] Braun J and Sieper J. Ankylosing spondylitis. Lancet 2007;369:1379-90.

[25] El Maghraoui A. Extra-articular manifestations of ankylosing spondylitis: prevalence, characteristics and therapeutic implications. European Journal of Internal Medicine 2011;22:554-60.

[26] Hermann KG, Landewe RB, Braun J, and van der Heijde DM. Magnetic resonance imaging of inflammatory lesions in the spine in ankylosing spondylitis clinical trials: is paramagnetic contrast medium necessary? The Journal of Rheumatology 2005;32:2056-60.

[27] Oostveen J, Prevo R, den BJ, and van de Laar M. Early detection of sacroiliitis on magnetic resonance imaging and subsequent development of sacroiliitis on plain radiography. A prospective, longitudinal study. The Journal of Rheumatology 1999;26:1953-8.

[28] Rudwaleit M, Metter A, Listing J, Sieper J, and Braun J. Inflammatory back pain in ankylosing spondylitis: a reassessment of the clinical history for application as classificatoin and diagnositc criteria. Arthritis & Rheumatism 2006;54:569-78.

[29] Dagfinrud H, Kvien TK, and Hagen KB. The Cochrane review of physiotherapy interventions for ankylosing spondylitis. The Journal of Rheumatology 2005;32:1899-906.

[30] Saougou I, Markatseli TE, Voulgari PV, and Drosos AA. Maintained clinical response of infliximab treatment in ankylosing spondylitis: a 6-year long-term study. Joint Bone Spine 2010;77:325-9.

[31] Woodward LJ and Kam PC. Ankylosing spondylitis: recent developments and anaesthetic implications. Anaesthesia 2009;64:540-8.

[32] Moll JM and Wright V. Psoriatic arthritis. Seminars in Arthritis and Rheumatism 1973;3:55-78.

[33] Woolacott N, Bravo Vergel Y, Hawkins N, Kainth A, Khadjesari Z, Misso K, et al. Etanercept and infliximab for the treatment of psoriatic arthritis: a systematic review and economic evaluation. Health Technology Assessment 2006;10:1-239.

[34] Khan MA. Update on spondyloarthropathies. Annals of Internal Medicine 2002;136:896-907.

[35] Winchester R, Minevich G, Steshenko V, Kirby B, Kane D, Greenberg DA, et al. HLA associations reveal genetic heterogeneity in psoriatic arthritis and in the psoriasis phenotype. Arthritis & Rheumatism 2012;64:1134-44.

[36] Scarpa R, Del PA, di GC, della VG, Lubrano E, and Oriente P. Interplay between environmental factors, articular involvement, and HLA-B27 in patients with psoriatic arthritis. Annals of Rheumatic Diseases 1992;51:78-9.

[37] Wang Q, Vasey FB, Mahfood JP, Valeriano J, Kanik KS, Anderson BE, et al. V2 regions of 16S ribosomal RNA used as a molecular marker for the species identification of streptococci in peripheral blood and synovial fluid from patients with psoriatic arthritis. Arthritis & Rheumatism 1999;42:2055-9.

[38] Gladman DD, Stafford-Brady F, Chang CH, Lewandowski K, and Russell ML. Longitudinal study of clinical and radiological progression in psoriatic arthritis. Journal of Rheumatology 1990;17:809-12.

[39] Eder L, Zisman D, Barzilai M, Laor A, Rahat M, Rozenbaum M, et al. Subclinical atherosclerosis in psoriatic arthritis: a case-control study. The Journal of Rheumatology 2008;35:877-82.

[40] Tam LS, Tomlinson B, Chu TT, Li M, Leung YY, Kwok LW, et al. Cardiovascular risk profile of patients with psoriatic arthritis compared to controls--the role of inflammation. Rheumatology (Oxford) 2008;47:718-23.

[41] Taylor W, Gladman D, Helliwell P, Marchesoni A, Mease P, and Mielants H. Classification criteria for psoriatic arthritis: development of new criteria from a large international study. Arthritis & Rheumatism 2006;54:2665-73.

[42] Chandran V, Schentag CT, and Gladman DD. Sensitivity of the classification of psoriatic arthritis criteria in early psoriatic arthritis. Arthritis & Rheumatism 2007;57:1560-3.

[43] Cantini F, Niccoli L, Nannini C, Kaloudi O, Bertoni M, and Cassara E. Psoriatic arthritis: a systematic review. International Journal of Rheumatic Diseases 2010;13:300-17.

[44] Sandles L. An holistic approach to the management of rheumatoid disease. Occupatonal Therapy in Rheumatology. London: Chapman and Hall; 1990, p. 41-50.

[45] Samanta R, Shoukrey K, and Griffiths R. Rheumatoid arthritis and anaesthesia. Anaesthesia 2011;66:1146-59.

[46] Neva MH, Hakkinen A, Makinen H, Hannonen P, Kauppi M, and Sokka T. High prevalence of asymptomatic cervical spine subluxation in patients with rheumatoid arthritis waiting for orthopaedic surgery. Annals of Rheumatic Diseases 2006;65:884-8.

[47] Shen FH, Samartzis D, Jenis LG, and An HS. Rheumatoid arthritis: evaluation and surgical management of the cervical spine. Spine Journal 2004;4:689-700.

[48] Wilkinson JM, Haslam P, and Getty CJM. (ii) Hip and knee reconstruction in the rheumatoid patient. Current Orthopaedics 2007;21:330–9.

[49] Grennan DM, Gray J, Loudon J, and Fear S. Methotrexate and early postoperative complications in patients with rheumatoid arthritis undergoing elective orthopaedic surgery. Annals of Rheumatic Diseases 2001;60:214-7.

[50] Loza E, Martinez-Lopez JA, and Carmona L. A systematic review on the optimum management of the use of methotrexate in rheumatoid arthritis patients in the perioperative period to minimize perioperative morbidity and maintain disease control. Clinical and Experimental Rheumatology 2009;27:856-62.

[51] Heldmann F and Braun J. Perioperative use of methotrexate. Clinical and Experimental Rheumatology 2010;28:S110-3.

[52] Sreekumar R, Gray J, Kay P, and Grennan DM. Methotrexate and post operative complications in patients with rheumatoid arthritis undergoing elective orthopaedic surgery-a ten year follow-up. Acta Orthopaedica Belgica 2011;77:823-6.

[53] da Cunha BM, Maria Henrique da Mota L, and Dos Santos-Neto LL. Risk of orthopedic surgical site infections in patients with rheumatoid arthritis treated with antitumor necrosis factor alfa therapy. International Journal of Rheumatology 2012;2012:369565.

[54] Talwalkar SC, Grennan DM, Gray J, Johnson P, and Hayton MJ. Tumour necrosis factor alpha antagonists and early postoperative complications in patients with inflammatory joint disease undergoing elective orthopaedic surgery. Annals of Rheumatic Diseases 2005;64:650-1.

[55] Wendling D, Balblanc JC, Brousse A, Lohse A, Lehuede G, Garbuio P, et al. Surgery in patients receiving anti-tumour necrosis factor alpha treatment in rheumatoid arthritis: an observational study on 50 surgical procedures. Annals of Rheumatic Diseases 2005;64:1378-9.

[56] Giles JT, Bartlett SJ, Gelber AC, Nanda S, Fontaine K, Ruffing V, et al. Tumor necrosis factor inhibitor therapy and risk of serious postoperative orthopedic infection in rheumatoid arthritis. Arthritis & Rheumatism 2006;55:333-7.

[57] Momohara S, Kawakami K, Iwamoto T, Yano K, Sakuma Y, Hiroshima R, et al. Prosthetic joint infection after total hip or knee arthroplasty in rheumatoid arthritis patients treated with nonbiologic and biologic disease-modifying antirheumatic drugs. Modern Rheumatology 2011;21:469-75.

[58] Suzuki M, Nishida K, Soen S, Oda H, Inoue H, Kaneko A, et al. Risk of postoperative complications in rheumatoid arthritis relevant to treatment with biologic agents: a report from the Committee on Arthritis of the Japanese Orthopaedic Association. Journal of Orthopaedic Science 2011;16:778-84.

[59] Saag KG, Teng GG, Patkar NM, Anuntiyo J, Finney C, Curtis JR, et al. American College of Rheumatology 2008 recommendations for the use of nonbiologic and biologic disease-modifying antirheumatic drugs in rheumatoid arthritis. Arthritis & Rheumatism 2008;59:762-84.

[60] Singh JA, Furst DE, Bharat A, Curtis JR, Kavanaugh AF, Kremer JM, et al. 2012 update of the 2008 American College of Rheumatology recommendations for the use of disease-modifying antirheumatic drugs and biologic agents in the treatment of rheumatoid arthritis. Arthritis Care & Research (Hoboken) 2012;64:625-39.

[61] Otto AW. Ein Becken, mit kugelformig augedehnten Pfannen. In: E Heft editor. Seltene Beobachtungen zur Anatomie, Physiologie und Pathologie gehorig. Breslau: Verlag Willibald August Holaufer; 1816, p. 19–20.

[62] Overgaard K. Otto's disease and other forms of protrusio acetauli. Acta Radiologica 1935;16 390-419.

[63] Gilmour J. Adolescent deformities of the acetabulum: an investigation into the nature of protrusio acetabuli. British Journal of Surgery 1939;26:670-99.

[64] Sotelo-Garza A and Charnley J. The results of Charnley arthroplasty of hip performed for protrusio acetabuli. Clinical Orthopaedics and Related Research 1978:12-8.

[65] Hirst P, Esser M, Murphy JC, and Hardinge K. Bone grafting for protrusio acetabuli during total hip replacement. A review of the Wrightington method in 61 hips. Journal of Bone and Joint Surgery (Br) 1987;69:229-33.

[66] Edelstein G and Murphy WA. Protrusio acetabuli: radiographic appearance in arthritis and other conditions. Arthritis & Rheumatism 1983;26:1511-6.

[67] Rosenberg WW, Schreurs BW, de Waal Malefijt MC, Veth RP, and Slooff TJ. Impacted morsellized bone grafting and cemented primary total hip arthroplasty for acetabular protrusion in patients with rheumatoid arthritis: an 8- to 18-year follow-up study of 36 hips. Acta Orthopaedica Scandinavica 2000;71:143-6.

[68] Buttaro MA, Comba F, Pusso R, and Piccaluga F. Acetabular revision with metal mesh, impaction bone grafting, and a cemented cup. Clinical Orthopaedics and Related Research 2008;466:2482-90.

[69] Jones L, Grammatopoulos G, and Singer G. The Burch-Schneider cage: 9-year survival in Paprosky type 3 acetabular defects. Clinical and radiological follow-up. Hip International 2012;22:28-34.

[70] Mäkelä KT, Eskelinen A, Pulkkinen P, Virolainen P, Paavolainen P, and Remes V. Cemented versus cementless total hip replacements in patients fifty-five years of age or older with rheumatoid arthritis. Journal of Bone and Joint Surgery (Am) 2011;93:178-86.

[71] Eskelinen A, Paavolainen P, Helenius I, Pulkkinen P, and Remes V. Total hip arthroplasty for rheumatoid arthritis in younger patients: 2,557 replacements in the Finnish Arthroplasty Register followed for 0-24 years. Acta Orthopaedica Scandinavica 2006;77:853-65.

[72] Rud-Sørensen C, Pedersen AB, Johnsen SP, Riis AH, and Overgaard S. Survival of primary total hip arthroplasty in rheumatoid arthritis patients. Acta Orthopaedica Scandinavica 2010;81:60-5.

[73] Creighton MG, Callaghan JJ, Olejniczak JP, and Johnston RC. Total hip arthroplasty with cement in patients who have rheumatoid arthritis. A minimum ten-year follow-up study. Journal of Bone and Joint Surgery (Am) 1998;80:1439-46.

[74] Sochart DH and Porter ML. The long-term results of Charnley low-friction arthroplasty in young patients who have congenital dislocation, degenerative osteoarthrosis, or rheumatoid arthritis Journal of Bone and Joint Surgery (Am) 1997;79:1599–617.

[75] Zwartelé RE, Witjes S, Doets HC, Stijnen T, and Pöll RG. Cementless total hip arthroplasty in rheumatoid arthritis: a systematic review of the literature. Archives of Orthopaedic and Trauma Surgery 2012;132:535-46.

[76] Aulakh TS, Kuiper JH, Dixey J, and Richardson JB. Hip resurfacing for rheumatoid arthritis: independent assessment of 11-year results from an international register. International Orthopaedics 2011;35:803-8.

[77] Wisk LE and Amstutz HC. Metal-on-metal hip resurfacing in rheumatoid patients. A report on thirteen hips with minimum 3 year follow-up. Hip International 2011;21:59-65.

[78] Mihalko WM, Saleh KJ, Krackow KA, and Whiteside LA. Soft-tissue balancing during total knee arthroplasty in the varus knee. Journal of the American Academy of Orthopaedic Surgeons 2009;17:766-74.

[79] Kanamiya T, Whiteside LA, Nakamura T, Mihalko WM, Steiger J, and Naito M. Ranawat Award paper. Effect of selective lateral ligament release on stability in knee arthroplasty. Clinical Orthopaedics 2002;404:24-31.

[80] Peters CL, Mohr RA, and Bachus KN. Primary total knee arthroplasty in the valgus knee: creating a balanced soft tissue envelope. Journal of Arthoplasty 2001;16:721-9.

[81] Wang W and Niu D. Balancing of soft tissues in total knee arthroplasty for patients with rheumatoid arthritis with kneeflexion contracture. Zhongguo Xiu Fu Chong Jian Wai Ke Za Zhi 2008;22:1173-6.

[82] Clarke HD, Fuchs R, Scuderi GR, Scott WN, and Insall JN. Clinical results in valgus total knee arthroplasty with the "pie crust" technique of lateral soft tissue releases. Journal of Arthoplasty 2005;20:1010-4.

[83] Archibeck MJ, Berger RA, Barden RM, Jacobs JJ, Sheinkop MB, Rosenberg AG, et al. Posterior cruciate ligament-retaining total knee arthroplasty in patients with rheumatoid arthritis. Journal of Bone and Joint Surgery (Am) 2001;83:1231-6.

[84] Miller MD, Brown NM, Della Valle CJ, Rosenberg AG, and Galante JO. Posterior cruciate ligament-retaining total knee arthroplasty in patients with rheumatoid arthritis: a concise follow-up of a previous report. Journal of Bone and Joint Surgery (Am) 2011;93:e130(1-6).

[85] Morgan H, Battista V, and Leopold SS. Constraint in primary total knee arthroplasty. Journal of the American Academy of Orthopaedic Surgeons 2005;13:515-24.

[86] Kajino A, Yoshino S, Kameyama S, Kohda M, and Nagashima S. Comparison of the results of bilateral total knee arthroplasty with and without patellar replacement for rheumatoid arthritis. A follow-up note. Journal of Bone and Joint Surgery (Am) 1997;79:570-4.

[87] Swedish knee arthroplasty register annual report 2011 (www.ort.lu.se/kneeS). 2011.

[88] Ito J, Koshino T, Okamoto R, and Saito T. 15-year follow-up study of total knee arthroplasty in patients with rheumatoid arthritis. Journal of Arthoplasty 2003;18:984-92.

[89] Woo YK, Kim KW, Chung JW, and Lee HS. Average 10.1-year follow-up of cementless total knee arthroplasty in patients with rheumatoid arthritis. Canadian Journal of Surgery 2011;54:179–84.

[90] Yamanaka H, Goto K, and Suzuki M. Clinical results of Hi-tech Knee II total knee arthroplasty in patients with rheumatoid athritis: 5- to 12-year follow-up. Journal of Orthopaedic Surgery and Research 2012;22:9.

[91] Sharma S, Nicol F, Hullin MG, and McCreath SW. Long-term results of the uncemented low contact stress total knee replacement in patients with rheumatoid arthritis. Journal of Bone and Joint Surgery (Br) 2005;87:1077–80.

[92] Robertsson O, Knutson K, Lewold S, Goodman S, and Lidgren L. Knee arthroplasty in rheumatoid arthritis. A report from the Swedish Knee Arthroplasty Register on 4,381 primary operations 1985–1995. Acta Orthopaedica Scandinavica 1997;68:545-53.

[93] Sokka T, Abelson B, and Pincus T. Mortality in rheumatoid arthritis: 2008 update. Clinical and Experimental Rheumatology 2008;26:S35-61.

[94] Clement ND, Jenkins PJ, Brenkel IJ, and Walmsley P. Predictors of mortality after total knee replacement: a ten-year survivorship analysis. Journal of Bone and Joint Surgery (Br) 2012;94:200-4.

[95] Schrama JC, Espehaug B, Hallan G, Engesaeter LB, Furnes O, Havelin LI, et al. Risk of revision for infection in primary total hip and knee arthroplasty in patients with rheumatoid arthritis compared with osteoarthritis: a prospective, population-based study on 108,786 hip and knee joint arthroplasties from the Norwegian Arthroplasty Register. Arthritis Care & Research (Hoboken) 2010;62:473-9.

[96] Bongartz T, Halligan CS, Osmon DR, Reinalda MS, Bamlet WR, Crowson CS, et al. Incidence and risk factors of prosthetic joint infection after total hip or knee replacement in patients with rheumatoid arthritis. Arthritis & Rheumatism 2008;59:1713-20.

[97] da Cunha BM, de Oliveira SB, and Santos-Neto L. Incidence of infectious complications in hip and knee arthroplasties in rheumatoid arthritis and osteoarthritis patients. Revista Brasileira de Reumatologia 2011;51:609-15.

[98] Matta F, Singala R, Yaekoub AY, Najjar R, and Stein PD. Risk of venous thromboembolism with rheumatoid arthritis. Journal of Thrombosis and Haemostasis 2009;101:134-8.

[99] Niki Y, Matsumoto H, Hakozaki A, Mochizuki T, and Momohara S. Rheumatoid arthritis: a risk factor for deep venous thrombosis after total knee arthroplasty? Comparative study with osteoarthritis. Journal of Orthopaedic Science 2010;15:57-63.

[100] Buchanan RR and Kraag G. Is there a lower incidence of deep venous thrombosis after joint replacement in rheumatoid arthritis? The Journal of Rheumatology 1980;7:551-4.

[101] Eggli S and Woo A. Risk factors for heterotopic ossification in total hip arthroplasty. Archives of Orthopaedic and Trauma Surgery 2001;121:531-5.

[102] Meek RM, Allan DB, McPhillips G, Kerr L, and Howie CR. Late Dislocation after Total Hip Arthroplasty. Clinical Medicine & Research 2008;6:17-23.

[103] Zwartelé RE, Brand R, and Doets HC. Increased risk of dislocation after primary total hip arthroplasty in inflammatory arthritis: a prospective observational study of 410 hips. Acta Orthopaedica Scandinavica 2004;75:684-90.

[104] Lindahl H, Malchau H, Oden A, and Garellick G. Risk factors for failure after treatment of a periprosthetic fracture of the femur. Journal of Bone and Joint Surgery (Am) 2006;88:26-30.

[105] Pap G and Neumann HW. Periprosthetic fractures in patients with rheumatoid arthritis. Zeitschrift fur Rheumatologie 2007;66:22-7.

[106] Felson DT, Anderson JJ, Boers M, Bombardier C, Furst D, Goldsmith C, et al. American College of Rheumatology: preliminary definition of improvement in rheumatoid arthritis. Arthritis & Rheumatism 1995;38:727–35.

[107] van Gestel AM, Prevoo ML, van 't Hof MA, van Rijswijk MH, van de Putte LB, and van Riel PL. Development and validation of the European League Against Rheumatism response criteria for rheumatoid arthritis. Comparison with the preliminary American College of Rheumatology and the World Health Organization/International League Against Rheumatism Criteria. Arthritis & Rheumtism 1996;39:34-40.

[108] Fortin PR, Penrod JR, Clarke AE, St-Pierre Y, Joseph L, Bélisle P, et al. Timing of total joint replacement affects clinical outcomes among patients with osteoarthritis of the hip or knee. Arthritis & Rheumatism 2002;46:3327-30.

[109] Sledge CB. Introduction to surgical management of patients with arthritis. In: S Ruddy, ED Harris, and CB Sledge editors. Kelley's textbook of rheumatology. Philadelphia: W.B.Saunders, p. 1691–8.

[110] Gilson M, Gossec L, Mariette X, Gherissi D, Guyot MH, Berthelot JM, et al. Risk factors for total joint arthroplasty infection in patients receiving tumor necrosis factor alpha-blockers: a case-control study. *Arthritis Research & Therapy* 2010;12:R145.

[111] Santaguida PL, Hawker GA, Hudak PL, Glazier R, Mahomed NN, Kreder HJ, et al. Patient characteristics affecting the prognosis of total hip and knee joint arthroplasty: a systematic review. Canadian Journal of Surgery 2008;51:428-36.

[112] Bombardier C, Barbieri M, Parthan A, Zack DJ, Walker V, Macarios D, et al. The relationship between joint damage and functional disability in rheumatoid arthritis: a systematic review. Annals of Rheumtic Diseases 2012;71:836-44.

[113] Benoni AC, Bremander A, and Nilsdotter A. Patient-reported outcome after rheumatoid arthritis-related surgery in the lower extremities: a report from the Swedish National Register of Rheuma Surgery (RAKIR). Acta Orthopaedica 2012;83:179-84.

[114] Nguyen-Oghalai TU, Ottenbacher KJ, Caban M, Granger CV, Grecula M, and Goodwin JS. The impact of rheumatoid arthritis on rehabilitation outcomes after lower extremity arthroplasty. Journal of Clinical Rheumatology 2007;13:247-50.

[115] Bischoff-Ferrari HA, Lingard EA, Losina E, Baron JA, Roos EM, Phillips CB, et al. Psychosocial and geriatric correlates of functional status after total hip replacement. Arthritis & Rheumatisim 2004;51:829-35.

[116] Katsimihas M, Taylor AH, Lee MB, Sarangi PP, and Learmonth ID. Cementless acetabular replacement in patients with rheumatoid arthritis: a 6- to 14-year prospective study. Journal of Arthroplasty 2003;18:16–22.

[117] Tang WM and Chiu KY. Primary total hip arthroplasty in patients with rheumatoid arthritis. International Journal of Orthopaedics 2001;25:13-6.

[118] Kristensen O, Nafei A, Kjaersgaard-Andersen P, Hvid I, and Jensen J. Long-term results of total condylar knee arthroplasty in rheumatoid arthritis. Journal of Bone and Joint Surgery (Br) 1992;74:803-6.

[119] Ritter MA, Lutgring JD, Davis KE, Faris PM, and Berend ME. Total knee arthroplasty effectiveness in patients 55 years old and younger: osteoarthritis vs. rheumatoid arthritis. Knee 2007;14:9-11.

[120] Bullens PH, van Loon CJ, de Waal Malefijt MC, Laan RF, and Veth RP. Patient satisfaction after total knee arthroplasty: a comparison between subjective and objective outcome assessments. Journal of Arthroplasty 2001;16:740-7.

Chapter 14

Total Joint Arthroplasty for Hemophilia

Hideyuki Takedani

Additional information is available at the end of the chapter

http://dx.doi.org/10.5772/53232

1. Introduction

Hemophilia is hereditary x-chromosomal recessive disorders. Hemophilia A is caused by deficiency or absence of coagulation factor VIII and hemophilia B is caused by that of coagulation factor IX. The prevalence is reported as one in 5000 in the male population and one in 10000 overall. These diseases are classified into three categories according to serum coagulation factor activity; severe (<1%), moderate (1-5%), or mild (>5%). The particular hemophilic manifestation is intra-articular bleeding. Intra-articular bleeding is usually occurred by trauma but also often spontaneously. Approximately 5% of first bleeding episodes in hemophilic boys are into a joint. The average age of first intra-articular bleeding is 1.91±0.91 years old and the median age of that is 1.63 years old [1]. A joint in which four or more recurrent bleedings have occurred in the prior 6 months is defined as target joint. In the United States, 2.3% of children 2-5 years of age enrolled in the Universal Data Collection Project have target joints [2]. Most of target joints have hemophilic synovitis, which is characterized by inflammation, angiogenesis and fibrosis [3] and develop hemophilic arthroplasty which is characterized by cartilage and bone destruction.

The average annual intra-articular bleeding number were higher in the episodic-therapy group than in the prophylaxis group and the relative risk of MRI-detected joint damage with the episodic was 6-fold greater compared with prophylactic group [4]. Therefore, it is a clear the relationship between intra-articular bleeding and hemophilic arthropathy. However, the number and volume of intra-articular bleedings which result in target joint and arthropathy is not understood. Experimental pathgenetic studies were reported and many points of the pathogenesis are still remained as poorly understood points [2,5,6].

As for radiological evaluation methods of hemophilic arthropathy, there are three major systems. De Palma classification is classical progressive system and popular in Japan. This system classified hemophilic arthropathy from grade 0 (normal) to grade IV (end-stage) [7].

Arnold-Hilgartner classification is also classical progressive system and classified from stage 0 (normal) to stage V (end-stage) [8]. Pettersson score is recommend additive scoring system by World Federation of Hemophilia (WFH) [9]. 8 categories in this system have 0 (normal) to 2 (worse) points and totally scored from 0 (normal) to 13 points (worst). There are classical and authorized good systems but it may need to improve them, because their inter-observer reliabilities were poor [10].

As for MRI evaluation methods, there were several reports since 2000 [11-13], and WFH recommended MRI scale and modified version were published from the international prophylaxis study group [14, 15].

The causative mechanism of hemophilia was recognized in the 1950s [16], and concentrates for coagulation factor replacement became generally available since 1960s, however the easy administration of the concentrates resulted in transmission of viral infection including hepatitis C (HCV) and Human immunodeficiency virus infection (HIV) during the 1980s [17]. Also, the appearance of allo-immune antibody (inhibitor) against deficient coagulation factor is severe adversity. Product development such as recombinant concentrates has especially improved therapeutic safety and availability [18], resulting in the possibility of performing elective orthopedic surgery and prevention of bleeding episodes. The routine administration of prophylactic treatment has undoubtedly resulted in a greatly improvement in the quality of life and life expectancy of hemophilic patients. However, many of young hemophilic adults still have severe destructive joints as a result of repeated intra-articular bleeding during their early years.

For hemophilic arthropathy, there are two major surgical options which are synovectomy for early stage (hemophilic synovitis) and total joint arthroplasty (TJA) for end stage. At progressive stage, there are not good surgical options so that several usual orthopedic options are tried: anti-inflammatory drugs, corticosteroids, joint infusion of hyaluronic acid or corticosteroids, braces and rehabilitation. However many of them are progressed to end-stage. Total joint arthroplasty (TJA) is effective procedure in the management of hemophilic arthropathy for them [19].

2. Major surgery for hemophilia

In our hospital, 126 major surgeries for 80 patients have been performed between June 2006 and June 2012 in which were 96 surgeries for 63 hemophilia A, 28 surgeries for 16 hemophilia B, and 2 surgeries for 2 other coagulation disorders. 18 surgeries with inhibitor were included. The average age at operation was 39.03 years (13 ~ 60 years). As for virus infection, HBs antigen positive ratio was 1.5% (2/126 surgeries), HCV antibody positive ratio was 89.7% (113/126), HIV antibody positive ratio was 33.3% (42/126) and both HCV and HIV antibody positive ratio was 31.7% (41/126).

Major surgery such as TJA is never easily undertaking in hemophilic patients. It required bleeding control at peri-operative periods, management for viral infection and inhibitor, and treatment for complication subsequently to bleeding.

As for bleeding control, guidelines were published[20, 21], in which the aim serum factor level at peri-operative period is explained clearly. However it is difficult without the support of hematologists so that major surgeries are usually performed at hemophilia centers.

As for HIV infection, CD4 cell counts had been important factor as major influence factor on bacterial infection in the early literatures [22-25]. HIV medical treatment has drastically improved during the last decade. In the recent literatures [26-29] and our experience, there was no evidence to suggest that bacterial deep infection at surgical site was influenced on the decline of CD4 cell counts. However HIV-positive patients whose CD4 cell counts is less than 50 cell/mm3 have a considerable risk of the occurrence of opportunistic infection at peri-operaive periods.

Most hemophilia adult patients infected hepatitis C virus at 1980s and long period of the virus carrier results in hepatic insufficiency and hepatoma. The treatment for chronic hepatitis has also improved, however it was not good enough to control it. According to our clinical experiences, severe hepatic insufficiency has been influenced on the fatal ratio after major surgery.

Between 10-30% of patients with hemophilia A and 2-5% of patients with hemophilia B develop an inhibitor to FVIII or FIX [30]. Intra-articular bleedings in inhibitor patients have a more negative impact on their joint function and daily life. They desire to reduce the pain and improve function at affected joint. However surgical treatments may be deferred until patients suffer from increasingly severe pain and progressive physical incapacity find no other options, due to the higher bleeding risks associated with surgery [31]. In fact, there are some surgical reports for inhibitors, but many of them are a few cases reports [32]. Guidelines for inhibitor [33] were also published, but bleeding control plan at peri-operative periods is not established. We believe surgical treatments for inhibitor should be performed at hemophilic center.

Delayed wound healing is the major complication subsequently to bleeding. In hemophilia B mice, dermal wound healing is delayed and can be treated with factor IX replacement therapy to restore thrombin generation. This delay is associated with bleeding into granulation tissue [34]. In our hospital, there were 3.3% delayed wound healings.

3. Total joint arthroplasty

TJA has been available as a final option in the end-stage hemophilic arthropathy with significantly reduced quality of life. The major objectives of TJA are to reduce the pain in the affected joint and improve the joint function. These effects are influenced on the adjacent joints beneficially. In addition, the frequency and number of the intra-articular bleeding is significantly reduced. Thereby, their life-style and quality of life significantly improved. The indications are adult hemophilia patients with severe destructive arthropathy and subjective dysfunction. Adult means the patient's epiphyses are closed. We have performed total hip arthroplasty for 18 years boy. Their dysfunction have been started from childhood and made worse gradually. They are satisfied to live on their ability even if they have severe destructive arthropathies. These cases are not indication subjectively. Total knee or hip arthroplasty (TKA, THA) are generally performed and total elbow and ankle arthroplasty (TEA, TAA) are rarely performed. However the most common affected joints are elbow, knee and ankle. The average of operation is around forty [35, 36]. In our hospital, 81 total joint arthroplasty were performed included 59 TKAs, 20 THAs, 1TEA and 1TAA and average age were 44.5. (figure 1, 2)

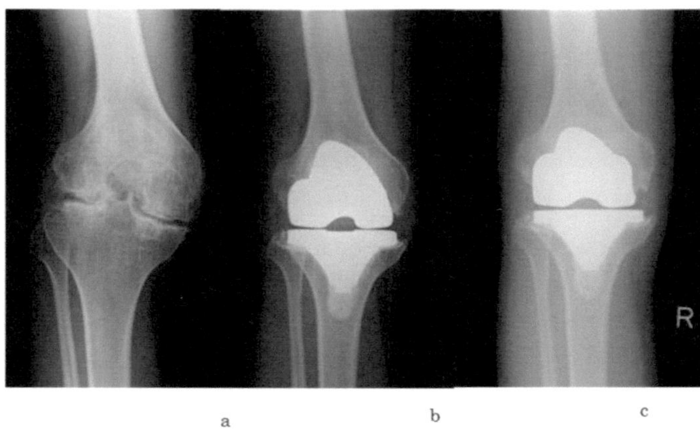

Figure 1. A 18-year-old hemophilia A patient without inhibitor. No virus infection. Severe hemophilic arthropathy of the right knee. His knee range of motion was improved at four years after surgery: extension was -30 degrees to 0 degrees and flexion was 90 degrees to 110 degrees. (a): pre-operative radiography; (b) at one month radiography (c) at four year radiography

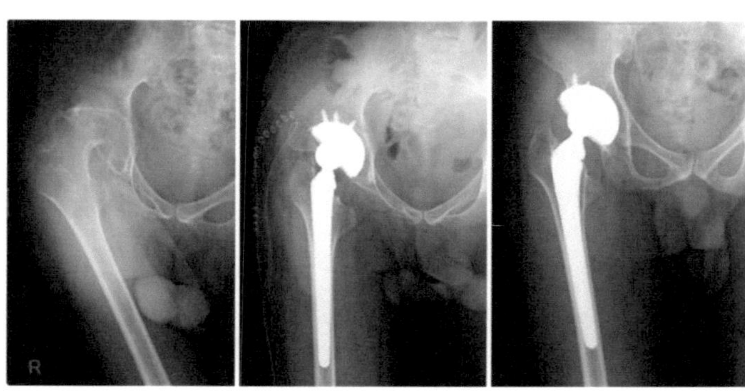

Figure 2. A 23-year-old hemophilia A patient with inhibitor. HCV is positive. Severe hemophilic arthropathy of the right hip. His back pain and tilted pelvis are improved after surgery. (a): pre-operative radiography; (b) just operative radiography (c) at five year radiography

As for surgical technique, we believe orthopedic surgeons do not need special skills when deficient factor level is kept with concentrate adequately. However, there are some careful points on TJA for hemophilia, in addition to the aforementioned surgical risks for hemophilia, which are higher infection rate, higher revision rate or shorter durability (table 1), and the occurrence of deep venous thrombosis (DVT).

Authers	Year	Number of TJA	Average of Follow-up (years)	Infection rate (%)	Aseptic loosening rate (%)
Cohen et al	2000	21 TKAs	5.6	10	0
Norian et al	2002	53 TKAs	5	13.2	9.4
Sheth et al	2004	14 TKAs	6.4	0	0
Goddard et al	2010	70 TKAs	9.2	1.5	8.6
Habermann et al	2007	15 THAs	11	6.7	6.7
Miles et al	2008	34 THAs	6.3	3	9
Yoo et al	2009	23 THAs	7.7	0	4.8
Powell et al	2005	35 TKAs 16 THAs	6.9	TKA:14.3 THA:6.3	0
Wang et al	2012	40 TKAs 18 THAs	10.7	TKA:13 THA:0	TKA:2.5 THA:5.6

Table 1. Infection and aseptic loosening rate after TJA in hemophilia including current study [35-38,40-44]

As for the infection after TJA, most reports show a deep infection rate of 10-16% [35-41], and our result shows much lower infection rate of 2.5 (2/81). However, these rates are higher than infection rate of 1-2% consistently reported in the literatures in the general population [45]. HIV infection had been important factor as major influence factor on bacterial infection, however the recent clinical results suggest there is no difference in the infection rate between HIV positive and negative. It is unclear why the ratio after TJA for hemophilia is much higher than that for non-hemophilia. The hypothesis that much frequent venous self-infusion is influenced on highly infection rate [40] is one of possibilities, but there is no evidence as yet.

As for durability, there are a few long clinical reports. When revision for aseptic mechanical failure was considered as endpoint, the survival rate for 40 TKAs at 10 years was 93%. The survival rate for 18 THAs at 8.5 years was 89% [36]. According to clinical result for 60 TKAs at a mean follow-up of 9.2 years, Kaplan-Meier analysis using infection and aseptic loosening as endpoint showed the survival rate at 20 years to be 94.0% [35]. These survival rates were similar to that in young non-hemophilia patients [46,47], however we believe it is not good enough rate for young hemophilic patients who have multi-arthropathy.

Hemophilia patients are often considered that their risk of DVT is lower by virtue of their bleeding disorder. However, they have as same risk of DVT as non-hemophilic patients, because the coagulation factor level is normalized by administration of concentrates at perioperative periods. In our hospital, all patients use compression devices and not administrate drugs such as heparin or aspirin. Thrombosis has been checked by ultrasound and not detected at pre- and post-operation. Subclinical DVT was observed in 10% of hemophilia patients undergoing major orthopedic surgery [48]. According to the simple questionnaires survey at hemophilia treatment center in the United States, 78% provided thrombo-prophylaxis to selected patients. Of those providing of thrombo-prophylaxis, 67% used compression stocking or devices, 24% used low molecular weight heparin, 1% fondaparinux, 3% unfractionated heparin. 4% warfarin and 1% aspirin [49].

Finally, the cost of hemophilia treatment is major economical concern. The concentrate cost is occupied of major part of TJA cost and it is depended on the patient body weight. And the price of concentrates and insurance situation are quite differences internationally, so that we introduced our situation in this chapter. The cost is too expensive to performed surgery without insurance coverage, however Japanese general health insurance is covered with most of the cost, fortunately. The cost of TJA at peri-operative periods about two weeks is forty to fifty thousand dollars for average Japanese hemophilic patients without inhibitor (50-70kg). The cost for inhibitor cases is about 5 to 10-folds.

Total joint arthroplasty for hemophilia is a challenging surgery and never a simple undertaking, however hemophilia patient need to improve their life style and release severe pain. We believe it is a safe and effective procedure in the management of hemophilic arthropathy at hemophilia centers.

Author details

Hideyuki Takedani*

Address all correspondence to: takedani@ims.u-tokyo.ac.jp

Department of Joint Surgery Research Hospital of the Institute of Medical Science The University of Tokyo 4-6-1 Shiroganedai, Minato-ku, Tokyo 108-8639, Japan

References

[1] Pollmann, H., Richter, H., Ringkamp, H., & Jurgens, H. (1999). When are children diagnosed as having severe haemophilia and when do they start to bleed? A 10 -year single-centre PUP study. *Eur J Pediatr.*, Dec, 158(3), S166-170.

[2] Valentino, L. A., Hakobyan, N., Enockson, C., et al. (2012). Exploring the biological basis of haemophilic joint disease: experimental studies. *Haemophilia.*, May, 18(3), 310-318.

[3] Stein, H., & Duthie, R. B. (1981). The pathogenesis of chronic haemophilic arthropathy. *J Bone Joint Surg Br*, 63B(4), 601-9.

[4] Manco-Johnson, M. J., Abshire, T. C., Shapiro, A. D., et al. (2007). Prophylaxis versus episodic treatment to prevent joint disease in boys with severe hemophilia. *N Engl J Med*, Aug 9, 357(6), 535-544.

[5] Valentino, L. A., Hakobyan, N., Rodriguez, N., & Hoots, W. K. (2007). Pathogenesis of haemophilic synovitis: experimental studies on blood-induced joint damage. *Haemophilia*, Nov, 13(3), 10-13.

[6] Roosendaal, G., & Lafeber, F. P. (2006). Pathogenesis of haemophilic arthropathy. *Haemophilia*, Jul, 12(3), 117-121.

[7] De Palma, A. F., & Cotler, J. M. (1956). Hemophilic arthropathy. *AMA Arch Surg*, Feb, 72(2), 247-250.

[8] Arnold, W. D., & Hilgartner, M. W. (1977). Hemophilic arthropathy. Current concepts of pathogenesis and management. *J Bone Joint Surg Am*, Apr, 59(3), 287-305.

[9] Pettersson, H., Ahlberg, A., & Nilsson, I. M. (1980). A radiologic classification of hemophilic arthropathy. *Clin Orthop Relat Res.* [149], Jun, 153-9.

[10] Takedani, H., Fujii, T., Kobayashi, Y., Haga, N., Tatsunami, S., & Fujii, T. (2011). Inter-observer reliability of three different radiographic scores for adult haemophilia. *Haemophilia.*, Jan, 17(1), 134-138.

[11] Nuss, R., Kilcoyne, R. F., Rivard, G. E., & Murphy, J. (2000). Late clinical, plain X-ray and magnetic resonance imaging findings in haemophilic joints treated with radiosynoviorthesis. *Haemophilia.*, Nov, 6(6), 658-663.

[12] Funk, M. B., Schmidt, H., Becker, S., et al. (2002). Modified magnetic resonance imaging score compared with orthopaedic and radiological scores for the evaluation of haemophilic arthropathy. *Haemophilia.*, Mar, 8(2), 98-103.

[13] Kilcoyne, R. F., & Nuss, R. (2003). Radiological assessment of haemophilic arthropathy with emphasis on MRI findings. *Haemophilia*, 9(1), 57-63, discussion 63-54.

[14] Lundin, B., Babyn, P., Doria, AS, et al. (2005). Compatible scales for progressive and additive MRI assessments of haemophilic arthropathy. *Haemophilia*, Mar, 11(2), 109-115.

[15] Lundin, B., Manco-Johnson, M. L., Ignas, D. M., et al. (2012). An MRI scale for assessment of haemophilic arthropathy from the International Prophylaxis Study Group. *Haemophilia*, Jul 5.

[16] Biggs, R., Douglas, AS, Macfarlane, R. G., Dacie, J. V., & Merskey, Pitney W. R. (1952). Christmas disease: a condition previously mistaken for haemophilia. *Br Med J.*, Dec 27, 2(4799), 1378-1382.

[17] Mannucci, P. M., & Tuddenham, E. G. (2001). The hemophilias--from royal genes to gene therapy. *N Engl J Med.*, Jun 7, 344(23), 1773-1779.

[18] Key, N. S., & Negrier, C. (2007). Coagulation factor concentrates: past, present, and future. *Lancet.*, Aug 4, 370(9585), 439-448.

[19] Takedani, H., Mikami, S., Abe, Y., Kin, H., & Kawasaki, N. (2000). [Total hip and knee arthroplasty for arthropathy in a hemophiliac]. *Rinsho Ketsueki.*, Feb;, 41(2), 97-102.

[20] Kasper, C. K. (2000). Protocols for the treatment of haemophilia and von Willebrand disease. *Haemophilia.*, Jul;, 6(1), 84-93.

[21] Guidelines for the management of hemophilia. (2005). Montreal: World Federation of Hemophilia.

[22] Goddard, N. (2010). Joint replacement. *In Lee CA, Berntop EE, Hoots WK. (ed.) Textbook of Hemophilia second edition.Cornwall: Wiley-Blackwell*, 176-181.

[23] Gregg-Smith, S. J., Pattison, R. M., Dodd, C. A., Giangrande, P. L., & Duthie, R. B. (1993). Septic arthritis in haemophilia. J Bone Joint Surg Br. May , 75(3), 368-370.

[24] Wiedel, J. D., Luck, J. V., & Gilbert, M. S. (1989). Total knee arthroplasty in the patient with haemophilia; evaluation and long term results. *Gilbert MS, Greene WB. (ed.) Musculo-skeltal problems in Hemophilia. New York National: Hemophilia foundation*, 152-157.

[25] Ragni, M. V., Crossett, L. S., & Herndon, J. H. (1995). Postoperative infection following orthopaedic surgery in human immunodeficiency virus-infected hemophiliacs with CD4 counts < or = 200/mm3. *J Arthroplasty.*, Dec, 10(6), 716-721.

[26] Birch, N. C., Ribbans, W. J., Goldman, E., & Lee, CA. (1994). Knee replacement in haemophilia. *J Bone Joint Surg Br.*, Jan, 76(1), 165-166.

[27] Phillips, A. M., Sabin, C. A., Ribbans, W. J., & Lee, C. A. (1997). Orthopaedic surgery in hemophilic patients with human immunodeficiency virus. *Clin Orthop Relat Res.* [343], Oct, 81-87.

[28] Hicks, J. L., Ribbans, W. J., Buzzard, B., et al. (2001). Infected joint replacements in HIV-positive patients with haemophilia. *J Bone Joint Surg Br.*, Sep, 83(7), 1050-1054.

[29] Rodriguez-Merchan, E. C., & Wiedel, J. D. (2002). Total knee arthroplasty in HIV-positive haemophilic patients. *Haemophilia.*, May, 8(3), 387-392.

[30] Valentino, L. A., Cooper, D. L., & Goldstein, B. (2011). Surgical experience with rFVIIa (NovoSeven) in congenital haemophilia A and B patients with inhibitors to factors VIII or IX. *Haemophilia*, Jul, 17(4), 579-589.

[31] Jimenez-Yuste, V., Rodriguez-Merchan, E. C., Alvarez, M. T., Quintana, M., Fernandez, I., & Hernandez-Navarro, F. (2008). Controversies and challenges in elective orthopedic surgery in patients with hemophilia and inhibitors. *Semin Hematol.*, Apr, 45(2, 1), S64-67.

[32] Takedani, H., Kawahara, H., & Kajiwara, M. (2010). Major orthopaedic surgeries for haemophilia with inhibitors using rFVIIa. *Haemophilia*, Mar, 16(2), 290-295.

[33] Gringeri, A., & Mannucci, P. M. (2005). Italian guidelines for the diagnosis and treatment of patients with haemophilia and inhibitors. *Haemophilia*, Nov, 11(6), 611-619.

[34] Monroe, D. M., Mackman, N., & Hoffman, M. (2010). Wound healing in hemophilia B mice and low tissue factor mice. *Thromb Res.*, Apr, 125(1), S74-77.

[35] Goddard, N. J., Mann, H. A., & Lee, C. A. (2010). Total knee replacement in patients with end-stage haemophilic arthropathy: 25-year results. *J Bone Joint Surg Br.*, Aug, 92(8), 1085-1089.

[36] Wang, K., Street, A., Dowrick, A., & Liew, S. (2012). Clinical outcomes and patient satisfaction following total joint replacement in haemophilia--23-year experience in knees, hips and elbows. *Haemophilia.*, Jan, 18(1), 86-93.

[37] Cohen, I., Heim, M., Martinowitz, U., & Chechick, A. (2000). Orthopaedic outcome of total knee replacement in haemophilia A. *Haemophilia.*, Mar, 6(2), 104-109.

[38] Powell, D. L., Whitener, C. J., Dye, C. E., Ballard, J. O., Shaffer, M. L., & Eyster, M. E. (2005). Knee and hip arthroplasty infection rates in persons with haemophilia: a 27 year single center experience during the HIV epidemic. *Haemophilia.*, May, 11(3), 233-239.

[39] Silva, M., & Luck, J. V. Jr. (2005). Long-term results of primary total knee replacement in patients with hemophilia. *J Bone Joint Surg Am.*, Jan, 87(1), 85-91.

[40] Sheth, DS, Oldfield, D., Ambrose, C., & Clyburn, T. (2004). Total knee arthroplasty in hemophilic arthropathy. *J Arthroplasty.*, Jan, 19(1), 56-60.

[41] Norian, J. M., Ries, MD, Karp, S., & Hambleton, J. (2002). Total knee arthroplasty in hemophilic arthropathy. *J Bone Joint Surg Am.*, Jul, 84A(7), 1138-1141.

[42] Habermann, B., Eberhardt, C., Hovy, L., Zichner, L., Scharrer, I., & Kurth, AA. (2007). Total hip replacement in patients with severe bleeding disorders A 30 years single center experience. *Int Orthop.*, Feb, 31(1), 17-21.

[43] Miles, J., Rodriguez-Merchan, E. C., & Goddard, N. J. (2008). The impact of haemophilia on the success of total hip arthroplasty. *Haemophilia*, Jan, 14(1), 81-84.

[44] Yoo, M. C., Cho, Y. J., Kim, K. I., Ramteke, A., & Chun, Y. S. (2009). The outcome of cementless total hip arthroplasty in haemophilic hip arthropathy. *Haemophilia*, May, 15(3), 766-773.

[45] Bengtson, S., & Knutson, K. (1991). The infected knee arthroplasty. A 6-year follow-up of 357 cases. *Acta Orthop Scand.*, Aug, 62(4), 301-311.

[46] Pospischill, M., & Knahr, K. (2005). Cementless total hip arthroplasty using a threaded cup and a rectangular tapered stem. Follow-up for ten to 17 years. *J Bone Joint Surg Br.*, Sep, 87(9), 1210-1215.

[47] Seyler, T. M., Bonutti, P. M., Shen, J., Naughton, M., & Kester, M. (2006). Use of an alumina-on-alumina bearing system in total hip arthroplasty for osteonecrosis of the hip. *J Bone Joint Surg Am.*, Nov, 88(3), 116-125.

[48] Hermans, C., Hammer, F., Lobet, S., & Lambert, C. (2010). Subclinical deep venous thrombosis observed in 10% of hemophilic patients undergoing major orthopedic surgery. May. *J Thromb Haemost.*, 8(5), 1138-1140.

[49] Pradhan, S. M., Key, N. S., Boggio, L., & Pruthi, R. (2009). Venous thrombosis prophylaxis in haemophilics undergoing major orthopaedic surgery: a survey of haemophilia treatment centres. *Haemophilia.*, Nov, 15(6), 1337-1338.

Chapter 15

Revision Hip Arthroplasty: Management of Bone Loss

Plamen Kinov and Peter Tivchev

Additional information is available at the end of the chapter

http://dx.doi.org/10.5772/53249

1. Introduction

Total hip arthroplasty (THA) is one of the most successful surgical procedures with well documented survivorship at up to 25 years. With ageing of the population and higher arthritis prevalence in older adults, the demand for the procedure increases worldwide [89]. In addition, over the last two decades the age range has been broadened to include younger patients. Over 270 000 hip replacements are performed annually in the US alone, and the annual volume of hip joint replacement is projected to double by the year 2030 [89]. Although very successful procedure, significant percentage of patients undergoing total hip arthroplasty require revision within 10 to 15 years after the surgery. Aseptic loosening and the associated osteolysis have been recognized as the main reason for implant failure in 71% of cases [66]. Other indications for revision include periprosthetic fracture, dislocation, and infection. New technologies in implant design and advances in surgical technique have improved the outcomes after primary total hip arthroplasty and decreased the rate of complications. However, as a consequence of increased rate of primary THA's the prevalence of revision hip surgery is increasing proportionally. The increased rate and costs of revision procedures impose high demands on both surgeon and healthcare system. Moreover, the cost of hip replacement is exponentially increasing [82].

Bone loss is the major challenge in revision setting. In 2009, Bozic et al. reviewed the most common causes for revision hip arthroplasty [8]. Aseptic loosening, instability, and infection were reported as the main reasons for revision surgery. This study underlined the need for a complex approach to evaluation and management of patients with implant failure after hip replacement. Such approach will guarantee precise diagnosis, proper selection of revision implant and surgical approach, uncomplicated surgery, and optimal clinical result.

This chapter provides an overview of aseptic loosening of revision hip arthroplasty and outlines the management strategies in the clinical scenario of a failed hip prosthesis.

2. Patient evaluation

Various signs and symptoms can occur in the clinical setting of a failed hip prosthesis. Painful hip arthroplasty is the most common complication after total hip arthroplasty reaching 18% of patients in some series [6]. Most of these painful hips will require revision. Groin pain can be referred to implant failure easily whereas occasional hip pain, pain in the buttock, knee pain or migrating pain can have different etiology. Other diseases and conditions such as disk disease, radiculopathy, inguinal or femoral hernia, pelvic infections, tumors, and trauma may have manifestations similar to that of a failed prosthesis.

The differential diagnosis of hip pain requires a careful history and examination. In simple cases, the reason could be identified with clinical examinations and standard radiographs only. Thorough examination elicits the underlying cause of hip complains such as infection, neurological injury, referred pain, wear, aseptic loosening or instability. In many cases, the diagnosis is a challenge to the surgeon. In addition to clinical history and physical examination, radiographic examination and advanced imaging techniques could help establish exact localization of pain, and its possible connection with the implant. Additional radiographic examinations as well as an algorithmic approach with special diagnostic imaging and tests help establishing precise diagnosis. Computed tomography and 3-D computed tomography is often helpful in establishing periprosthetic osteolysis and its severity. In addition to plain radiographs arthrography with contrast medium could be considered in certain cases.

Once extrinsic and periarticular diseases have been excluded as a reason for the hip pain, septic loosening should be excluded. Laboratory investigations are the initial tests that help differentiate septic from aseptic loosening. A standard set includes WBC, Erythrocyte sedimentation rate (ESR), C-reactive protein (CRP), complete chemistries and urinalysis. In addition to plain radiographs and laboratory tests joint aspiration is considered the most important diagnostic tool in ruling out periprosthetic infection. The aspirate should be sent for cell count and anaerobic and aerobic cultures. Recently, local markers such as interleukin-6 (IL-6) and other cytokines [34], synovial CRP, and leukocyte esterase (LE) [118] from joint aspirate have been proposed. All of these local markers have shown accuracy of more than 90% in predicting periprosthetic infection. Nuclear medicine scans with technetium-99m-HDP, gallium citrate, and labeled WBC have been used to diagnose the presence of infection. However, because of poor sensitivity, specificity, and accuracy, it is cost-prohibitive and remains a tertiary tool. Nuclear medicine is used only if infection could not be proven otherwise. Intraoperatively, diagnostic evaluations such as Gram stains and frozen sections have been proposed.

Guidelines and algorithms for evaluation of painful hip arthroplasty have been published in the literature and implemented in practice [119]. Such approach helps eliminate infection of the failed hip that would change treatment approach and could exclude one-stage revision.

http://dx.doi.org/10.5772/53249

3. Classification systems for bone defects

It is important to have a practical, relatively simple classification system for assessment of bone defects associated with loose hip implants. The use of a radiographic classification system helps to establish the severity and localization of bone defects, and to guide treatment decisions. It should allow the surgeon to be prepared for the possible intraoperative findings and to plan adequate treatment approach. Numerous classification systems have been described in the literature [17,23,25,32,40,58,60,99,116,137,158].

3.1. AAOS classification

The American Academy of Orthopedic Surgeons (AAOS) classification system of bone defects, described by D'Antonio et al. identifies the pattern and localization of osteolysis but does not quantify the bone loss [23-25]. It is one of the most widely used classification system in the literature.

3.2. Paprosky classification

Perhaps the most widely used classification system, the Paprosky Classification [32,116,158] (Tables 1, 2) was developed to establish bone defect type, size, and localization in order to allow selection of appropriate cementless reconstructive option for a given bone loss pattern. We base our clinical decisions on this classification system.

The key advantage of this classification is the assessment of the host bone ability to provide initial stability of a cementless implant until bone ingrowth occurs. The bone defects are usually classified on the basis of plain radiographs. However, final assessment is made intraoperatively, after removal of the failed implant and thorough debridement of the host bone. Intraoperative assessment of implant stability is made with help of trial components. The remaining host bone determines the stability of the implant and the type of the defect.

Type	Radiographic and intraoperative findings
1	Minimal metaphyseal bone loss
2	Extensive metaphyseal bone loss and an intact diaphysis
3A	Extensive metadiaphyseal bone loss and a minimum of 4 cm of intact cortical bone in the diaphysis
3B	Extensive metadiaphyseal bone loss and <4 cm of intact cortical bone in the diaphysis
4	Extensive metadiaphyseal bone loss and a nonsupportive diaphysis

Table 1. Paprosky classification systems for femoral defects.

Type	Radiographic and intraoperative findings
1	Acetabular rim, anterior-posterior column intact
2	Less than 3 cm superior migration Distorted acetabular rim. Intact anterior and posterior columns Adequate stability with Trial. Greater than 50% contact surface
2A	Superior and medial cavitation defect. Intact rim
2B	Segmental supero-lateral defect (less than 1/3 of circumference)
2C	Medial defect with cup medial to Kohler's line (Protrusio)
3	Greater than 3 cm superior migration Non-supportive acetabular rim for biological fixation
3A	Lateral to Kohler's line. Intact medial support Moderate ischial lysis (<15 mm below superior obturator line) Medial limb of teardrop is intact Superior and lateral migration "up and out" Contact of trial with bone over 40-60%
3B	Broken Kohler's line. No medial or superior support Extensive ischial osteolysis (>15 mm below superior obturator line) Complete destruction of tear drop Superior and medial migration "up and in" Under 40% contact surface. High risk of occult pelvic discontinuity

Table 2. Paprosky classification system for acetabular defects.

4. Preoperative planning

Careful preoperative planning is a prerequisite for successful revision surgery. The principle aims in revision hip arthroplasty are to achieve supportive host bone, secure implant fixation and to restore hip center and joint kinematics. The type and severity of host bone loss determine the method of reconstruction. Careful preoperative planning improves effectiveness during surgery, and helps distinguish more complex alternatives for reconstruction if needed.

Thorough clinical and radiographic examination is essential for determining the extent and severity of bone loss, quality of the host bone, exclusion of infection, additional deformities, and potentially confounding factors. Computed tomography may be needed in the presence of massive bone loss. In case of medial migration of the failed components angiography with contrast medium should be considered. Manual or digital templating helps for adequate selection (size, diameter, length) of revision implant and reduce the operative room inventory. Templating also helps determine whether stable initial fixation could be obtained and the need for additional procedures. Preoperative planning is critical for the assessment of the need of graft, tools for implant removal, and selection of proper components available at the time of surgery. Appropriate surgical exposure should be planned with an extensile approach often necessary. Classification system of bone defects based on radiographs that assesses the severity of bone loss according to the type of fixation for a given bone loss pattern is beneficial. In our practice, we find the Paprosky classification system a useful tool for guidance of clinical decisions. Any attempt should be made to identify the failed implant. The implant manufacturer should be contacted for implant-specific extraction devices if available. In case of isolated partial revision, it is advisable to have an option for partial (liner or head) exchange.

5. Surgical approaches in revision arthroplasty

The aims of revision surgery are to extract the failed prosthesis with minimal soft tissue and bone damage, to restore bone loss, and to implant prosthesis with stable and durable fixation. Ultimate goals are long-lasting and painless joint function. To obtain these goals arthroplasty surgeons may require a variety of approaches for adequate exposure of the femur and acetabulum in different revision settings. Usually arthroplasty surgeons are familiar and most comfortable with a certain approach and use it in most surgeries. However, in order to obtain reproducible results after revision of most difficult cases, surgeons should be familiar with all approaches to the hip joint. Next to standard approaches used in primary total hip arthroplasty, extensile approaches were developed in order to minimize damage to the host bone, safely remove the loose implant and provide good visualization for correct insertion of the revision components. Contained defects can be reconstructed through any conventional approach. For uncontained defects, we prefer to have wide access and, therefore, we use transtrochanteric approach or trochanteric slide osteotomy with preserved insertion of vastus lateralis. If greater exposure is needed extended trochanteric osteotomy is advisable.

5.1. Extended trochanteric osteotomy

The extended trochanteric osteotomy (ETO) is one of the significant achievements in revision surgery [9] (Figure 1).

It is safe and straightforward, saving time and minimizing risk of fracture during cement and failed implant removal. However, it limits femoral component options to those that rely on distal fixation. Advantages of the technique are: predictable healing of the osteotomy, decrease in intraoperative fractures and femoral perforations, direct access to the distal canal for cement removal and neutral reaming, and decreased surgical time [9,104]. Favorable clinical results after use of ETO have been published in the literature [9,104].

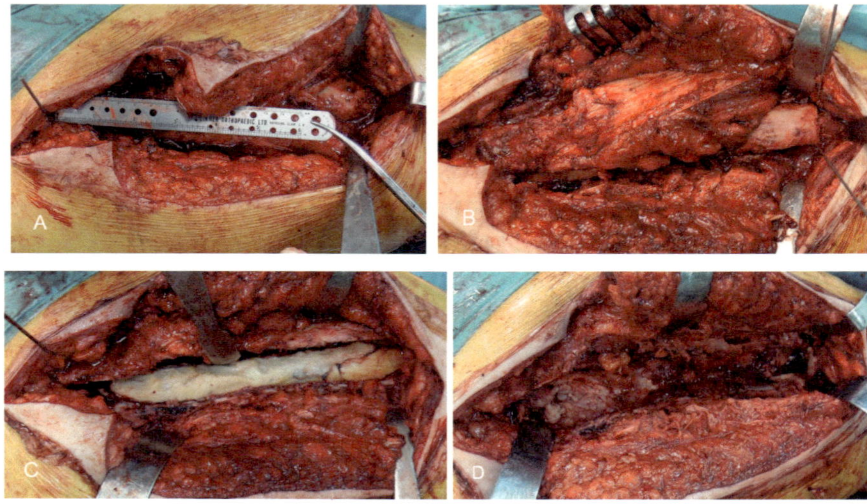

Figure 1. (A) The Extended trochanteric osteotomy is performed by cutting from the greater trochanter distally along the long axis of the femur. (B) The bone is cut with a saw. (C) The flap with the attached muscles is elevated. (D) Exposed femoral bone bed.

6. Surgical revision options

Majority of hip revisions could be performed using cementing technique. However, patients with severe bone loss and poor bone quality require complex alternatives for revision.

6.1. Options for Femoral revision

6.1.1. Cemented fixation of the femoral component

Various studies publish the outcomes after cemented femoral revision [2,13,122]. Use of the early cementing technique produced disappointing results [2,69]. Gaining more extensive experience resulted in acceptable short- to mid-term results [13,81,122]. Re-revision rates ranging from 4.3% to 6.0% and radiographic loosening ranging from 12% to 44% after mid-term follow-up of 3.4 to 4.5 years were reported (Table 3). However, long-term studies showed suboptimal outcomes after revision with an early cementing technique. At 8.1-year follow-up of the initial group of cemented revisions, Pellicci et al. found more than doubled incidence of re-revision and radiographic loosening ranging from 5.4% to 19% and from 13.6% to 29%, respectively [121]. Similar results were published by Kavanagh et al. in a 10-year follow-up study [79]. Sixty-four per cent of the stems had been revised or were radiographically loose. The incidence of revision had more than doubled from 18% at 3 years to 39% at final follow-up.

Authors	Year	Hips (No)	Follow-up (yrs)	Re-revision rate (%)	Radiographic loosening (%)
		Early technique			
Amstutz et al. [2]	1982	66	2.1	9.0	29.9
Pellicci et al. [122]	1982	110	3.4	5.4	13.6
Pellicci et al. [121]	1985	99	8.1	19.0	29.0
Kavanagh et al. [81]	1985	166	4.5	6.0	44.0
Engelbrecht et al. [39]	1990	138	7.4	8.8	38.0
		Improved technique			
Rubash and Harris [134]	1988	43	6.2	2.0	11.0
Katz et al. [78]	1997	79	11.9	5.4	16.0
Callaghan et al. [13]	1985	139	3.6	4.3	12.0
Estok and Harris [43]	1994	38	11.7	10.5	10.5
Mulroy and Harris [109]	1996	43	15.1	20.0	6.0

Table 3. Results of cemented femoral revision.

The main reason for suboptimal results with early cemented revisions was difficulty in obtaining stable and long-lasting fixation in compromised host bone stock where the rate of re-revision was very high [83]. In early studies, the reactive sclerotic bone between the fibrous membrane and the native cancellous bone was not removed [12]. Poor fixation of the revision femoral component compared to that in the primary setting may be due to inadequate excision of residual fibrous membrane, incomplete drying of bone, suboptimal cement filling technique, or insufficient cement-bone interlock on the smooth sclerotic bone surface. In such setting, even long cemented stems, are generally difficult to be inserted with adequate primary and long lasting stability. Femoral revision using so-called modern cementing techniques may yield promising results (Figure 2).

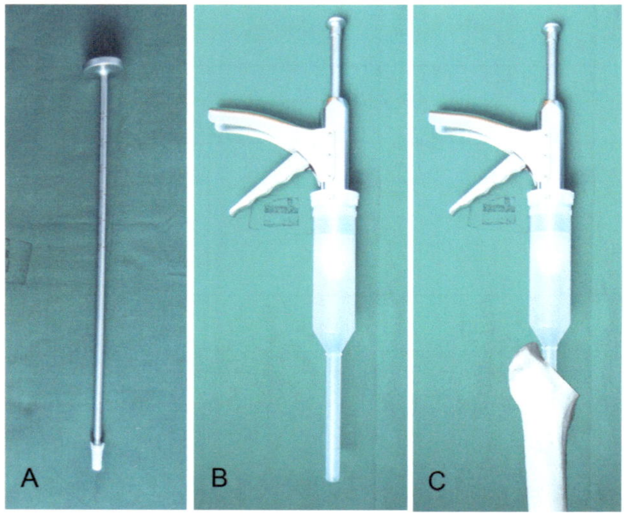

Figure 2. Modern cementing technique. (A) Distal cement plug. (B) Cement injector. (C) Delivery and pressurization of cement using cement injector.

Different studies have demonstrated that modern cementing techniques have improved implant survival and clinical outcome compared with the mid-term results after revision with use of so-called first-generation technique [71,85,109,128,134] (Figure 3).

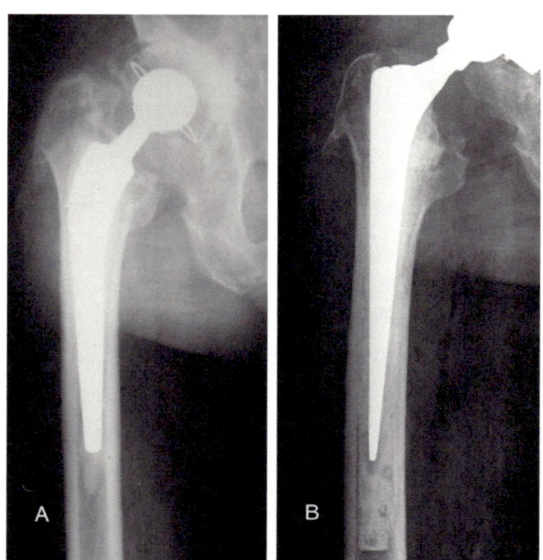

Figure 3. (A) Preoperative radiograph of a failed cemented prosthesis. (B) Grade A cemented fixation achieved with modern cementing technique.

Cemented femoral revision has several advantages in elderly patients. It allows early mobilization, a shorter operating time, and possibly less risk of a peroperative fracture. Use of modern cementing techniques seems to improve fixation of the femoral components and clinical outcomes and justifies its use. Whenever possible the failed arthroplasty should be revised before occurrence of severe bone loss and femoral enlargement.

6.1.1.1. Cement-within-cement fixation of the femoral component

Removal of the well-fixed cement mantle around the stem can be extremely difficult, time consuming, and risky procedure. A solution to the problem, cement-within-cement revision was first proposed by Eftekhar who advised on preserving the existing well cemented mantle and re-cementing the new stem into it [36]. In a biomechanical study, Greenwald et al. demonstrated that the separation strength was 94% that of a single block when the existing cement mantle was adequately prepared [56]. The technique requires that the old cement surface be dried and roughened in order to provide contact area for fixation of the new cement. The cement should be injected in the early liquid phase in order to prevent lamination and to promote polymerization within the existing cement mantle.

This technique has been questioned by other authors [96], but subsequent biomechanical and clinical studies have favored its use in properly selected cases [35,67,97]. In a cadaver study, Rosenstein et al. demonstrated that cut strength at the cement-cement interface was greater than the strength at the cement bone interface [133]. However, the cut strength of the cement bone interface was 30% weaker when cement was placed against a revised bone surface.

6.1.2. Impaction grafting technique for femoral revision

Femoral impaction grafting with a cemented stem was first performed in Exeter in 1987 [67] (Figure 4). The rationale behind this simple concept is to rebuild femoral bone stock and to provide secure fixation to the femoral stem. The biologic approach of bone restoration during revision hip arthroplasty is a highly appealing solution for restoring host bone stock a difficult procedure with usually deficient femurs.

Following the initial report of Gie and coworkers of highly successful results after 56 revisions with follow-up of 18-49 months [53] the technique received wide attention and spread rapidly [64,114,141,161]. Further studies confirmed the favorable outcomes, and it became evident that the technique resulted in restoration of femoral bone loss as the impacted allograft was incorporated and remodeled [67,161].

The technique of impaction grafting appeared to be reliable, reproducible, can be learned rapidly, and produced predictably favorable outcomes. In a series of 226 revisions, Halliday et al. reported the Exeter initial experience with femoral impaction grafting [64]. The overall rate of mechanical failure was 7% (16/221) at a minimum follow-up of five years. Ten to 11-year survivorship with removal of the stem for any reason as the end point was 90.5% and survivorship with revision for aseptic loosening as the end point was 99.1% [64]. In 2006, Schreurs et al. published their results with the technique using a cemented polished tapered stem at an average 10.4-year follow-up [140]. The average subsidence of the stem within the cement mantle was 3 mm, and seven stems migrated 5 mm. [140]. No stem was revised for aseptic loosening. Three periprosthetic fractures at the sults of 1305 femoral revisions with impaction grafting from the Swedish arthroplasty registry [114]. Survivorship at 15 years for aseptic loosening was 99.1%, for infection 98.6%, for subsidence 99.0%, and for fracture 98.7%.

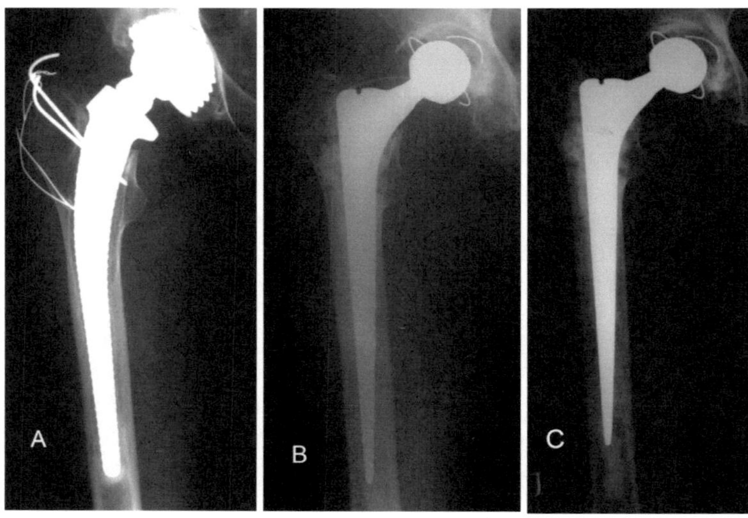

Figure 4. Femoral impaction grafting. (A) Preoperative radiograph. B) Immediate postoperative and, (C) at 8 years after revision.

However, other authors reported higher percentage of intraoperative complications, mainly femoral fractures and suboptimal cementing technique [84,86,101,123]. A high incidence of up to 12% intraoperative femoral fractures have been reported [64,140,103]. Stem subsidence of greater than 5 mm is a typical complication with this technique with a prevalence of up to 38% in some series [38,49,86,101]. Impaction grafting has certain disadvantages: it is prone to femoral fractures [103]; has a steep learning curve; and shows highly variable outcomes, probably related to the surgical technique. The causes of early subsidence of the stem might be insufficient impaction of the allograft, suboptimal cement penetration and interdigitation, use of synthetic graft substitutes, or other graft additives, loss of primary fixation of the allograft-cement composite due to soft-tissue infiltration and substitution of the allograft in the process of remodeling and revascularization, unrecognized femoral fracture, or fracture of the cement-allograft composite. However, in a study on saw femurs, Flannery et al. and Cummins et al. were unable to find a correlation between threshold force needed to achieve stable construct in impaction bone grafting without fracture and bone mineral density, canal-cortex ratio, or cortical thickness [22,48]. According to Gokhale et al. four variables (age, intramedullary canal diameter, stem design, and density of the graft at the tip of the stem) affected the subsidence of the stem [54].

The original technique of impaction grafting utilized the Exeter stem [53]. The impacted graft is subjected to continuous loading and deformation. Thus, the use of double-tapered polished stem appears suitable option as the stem could achieve secondary stability after subsidence. Arguing that the technique is more important than the type of prosthesis other authors have used different implant designs from those of Exeter wedge shaped prosthesis [49,77, 124]. Uncemented technique was also used with an equally good outcome at mid-term follow-up [100].

Femoral impaction bone grafting is a suitable indication for cases with severe bone deficiency. The technique is expensive, prone to complications, hast steep learning curve, and results depend on surgical skills. It may be a viable revision option for young patients with severe bone loss.

6.1.3. Proximal femoral allografts in revision surgery

Severe bone loss in femoral revision is increasing problem as the number of patients with multiple previous revision increases. These complex cases are further increasing as the age of patients undergoing hip replacement is diminishing.

A stable initial fixation is hardly obtainable in complex cases with circumferential proximal bone loss >5 cm in length. Severe bone loss makes femoral revision using conventional techniques difficult. Alternatives include distal fixation of the stem or use of a proximal femoral allograft. Distal fixation requires the use of a proximally femoral replacement prosthesis or megaprosthesis. This has some disadvantages such as: instability due to poor soft-tissue attachment [62,120], early loosening of the distally fixed stem [47], stress shielding [10,46,110], intraoperative fractures [110] or difficulty with fixation in an ectatic femur. Various studies of revisions using megaprosthesis reported survival rate within the range 58% to 84% at five to ten year follow-up [98,120,164].

The viable revision technique using proximal femoral allograft consists of a long-stem prosthesis cemented to the allograft but not to the host bone [59] (Figure 5). Uncemented fixation of the allograft prosthesis construct would not result in long lasting stability of the prosthesis as neither in-growth nor on-growth could be expected at the allograft-implant interface. The importance of the allograft-host bone contact is a key factor for achieving stability of the construct and ensuring long-term stability of the implant [136].

Individual studies published encouraging results after use of proximal femoral allograft-prosthesis construct in large segmental defects of the proximal femur. In a series of 44 revisions with a mean follow-up of 7.2 years Vastel et al. observed two deep infections, two aseptic loosening and two fractures bellow the tip of the prosthesis [155]. The final prosthesis survivorship rate with revision as the end point was 82.4% at 14 years of follow-up. The nonunion of the greater trochanter was considered major complication and was observed in 25 cases. In another series of 30 hips who underwent revision total hip replacement with an allograft prosthetic composite Sternheim et al. observed favorable long-term outcome [149]. The survivorship at 10, 15 and 20 years was 93%, 75.5% and 75.5%, respectively. Encouraging results were published by Blackley et al. with 78% successful results for an average of eleven-year follow-up [7]. The allograft-prosthesis construct survivorship at five years was 90% and at 10 years was 86%. A recent systematic review of 498 hips with a mean follow-up of 8.1 years reported survival rate of 82% [131]. The major complications were aseptic loosening observed in 13.7% of patients followed by dislocation in 12.8%.

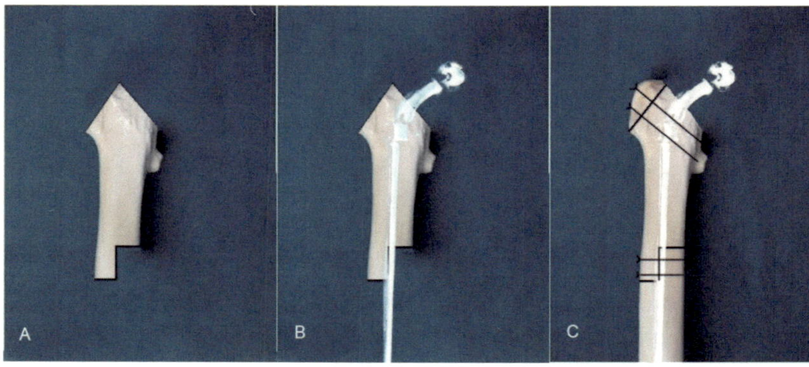

Figure 5. The technique of bone reconstruction with use of a proximal femoral allograft-prosthesis construct as described by Gross et al. [59]. (A) The proximal allograft is shaped from a proximal femoral allograft according to the preoperative planning. It should accommodate the selected stem and the step cut of approximately 2 by 2 cm of the host bone. (B) The stem is cemented in the femoral allograft. The contact surface of the allograft to the host bone should be free of cement. (C) The proximal femur-allograft construct is stabilized to the host bone by the stem of the implant. The step cut is reinforced by cerclage wires. Usually, the construct is reinforced with cortical struts prepared from the remnants of the allograft or from bone-bank allografts.

The use of a proximal femoral allograft-prosthesis construct has some inherited disadvantages characteristic for complex surgery. Allograft resorption eventually leading to failure of the revision is of major concern with longer follow-up [61]. Usually, it was observed after several years of follow-up but did not progress [7,155]. Authors that utilize uncemented distal fixation support the concept of direct loading of the host-allograft junction and argue that it minimizes allograft resorption [7,59]. On the other hand, cementing the prosthesis to the distal femur and thus stress shielding the allograft may explain the high rate of allograft resorption [61]. Nonunion of the allograft-host junction [7] or the greater trochanter [61,155] are of major concern with this technique. A step-cut osteotomy may provide rotational stability while an oblique osteotomy may provide greater surface area for bone healing compared to a transverse osteotomy. Dislocation is a frequent complication after revision with proximal femoral allograft with incidence ranging from to 7.3% to 16.7% [15, 61,131,155]. As with other cases, the high risk of dislocation may be lowered by optimal reconstruction of length, adequate version and high offset of the prosthesis-allograft construct and by maintaining the soft tissue tension and its attachment to the host femur [131]. The infection rates after revision with allograft-prosthesis construct are higher than that reported after primary hip arthroplasty. Rates of infection ranging from 0 to 10.9% were reported [15,94,132,136,155]. However, considering the high complexity of the technique these levels of infection are not unacceptable.

Femoral revision using proximal femoral allograft cemented to a long-stem prosthesis is appealing option for revision. The current data from the literature support the use of the technique as a durable solution, with available evidence reporting a long-term survivorship up to 86%. It is of a particular interest in the young patients because of its potential to improve bone stock and provide a substrate for subsequent revision. The development and refinement of this technique should be encouraged.

6.1.4. Cementless fixation of the femoral component

Obtaining stable and long lasting fixation in femoral revision in patients with severe bone deficiency is a difficult task. Long-term results after cemented revision have not been optimal [81,83,121]. High failure rates ranging between 12% to 44% at mid-term follow-up have been reported [2,81,83,121]. The main reason was difficulty in obtaining stable and long-lasting fixation in severe bone loss. Cementless fixation proved a promising alternative and was soon introduced in practice. However, for fears of stress shielding the ingrowth surface of first-generation designs was confined to the proximal part of the stem. Although highly successful in primary arthroplasty, the limited amount of porous coating with proximal fixation led to less favorable results in revision surgery (Table 4). Failure rates of 4% to 10% were reported at short- to mid-term follow-up. These results were slightly better than those obtained with an early cementing technique. The technique yielded acceptable results in less severe deformities [71]. Retrieval studies have demonstrated that less bone ingrowth occurs in revision stems compared to primary stems [21]. Porous surface extending to the diaphysis is needed to ensure stable primary fixation. In support of this, various authors have reported promising long-term results after revision with use of extensively coated uncemented stems [1,41,88,115].

Proximal femoral deficiency results from osteolysis, infection, fracture or bone damage during implant extraction. In such cases with severe bone loss, distal fixation with cylindrical, tapered or fluted stem designs is a viable option [4,14,41]. The technique requires accurate preparation of 4 cm to 7 cm of diaphyseal bone [41,92,102]. It is adaptable and can be used in situations with different severity of bone loss. Moreover, it can be used in periprosthetic fractures and is adjustable with extended trochanteric osteotomy. Distal stem fixation is the most successful strategy in terms of primary and secondary mechanical stability, bone osteointegration, and most importantly clinical results [4]. The main reason for its success is the fact that the implant is in contact with viable bone. Success rates of 90% to 95% have been reported with extensively coated monoblock stems over 10-year follow-up [105,115,158]. However, issues, such as thigh pain and proximal stress shielding, were reported frequently.

The principles of the Wagner stem are utilized in the tapered stems [156]. The cone prosthesis achieves good contact between the supportive distal diaphysis and the middle or distal third of the stem (Figure 6). The conical shape and the longitudinal splines promotes primary axial and rotational stability, which are prerequisites for osteointegration and long-lasting endurance of the cementless implant. The concept of modularity was introduced in the tapered stems with the advantages of versatile proximal fill and distal fit [76]. By modularity the sizes and shapes of the prosthesis can be increased by varying the diameter and shape of the proximal and distal part of the stem and locking them in different way. Modularity offers certain advantages such as correction and restoration of leg length, correction of offset and version, selection of optimal proximal fill, as well as compatibility with extended trochanteric osteotomy [4,92]. The potential problem of thigh pain was not associated with tapered stem design [156]. Disadvantages of modular taper stem designs include complexity, risk of stem fracture, fretting and corrosion of the junction, increased inventory, and higher cost.

Authors	Year	Hips (No)	Follow-up (yrs)	Re-revision rate (%)	Radiographic loosening (%)
Lawrence et al. [95]	1993	174	7.4	5.7	1.1
Engh et al. [42]	1988	127	4.4	1.6	2.4
Kang et al. [76]	2008	39	2 (minimum)	2.6	0
Krishnamurthy el al. [88]	1997	297	8.3	1.7	0.7
Harris et al. [65]	1988	23	2 (minimum)	0	4.3
Moreland and Bernstein [106]	1995	175	5.0	1.1	4.2*
Moreland and Moreno [105]	2001	137	9.3	4	-

* Mechanical failure

Table 4. Results of cementless femoral revision.

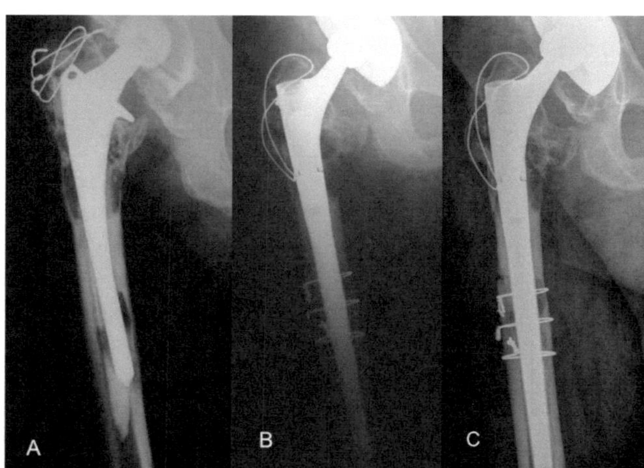

Figure 6. Cementless revision of Paprosky type 3A defect with a modular tapered stem (A) resulting in good initial (B) and mid-term stability at 2 years (C).

Various studies have reported favorable outcomes of various uncemented tapered distal fixation stems with high survival of more than 95% at 5 to 10-year follow-up [41,88,102]. The technique of cementless revision with distal fixation of the stem has been shown to be a reliable and straightforward. It ads no additional risks or complications. It can be used in all but the most severe segmental defects [4,14,41,102]. When the simple principles of the method are followed it provides stable and durable fixation of the revision implant. However, distal fixation does not restores host bone, thus making further revision surgery more difficult.

6.2. Options for acetabular revision

The goals of revision arthroplasty are to relieve pain and to improve function. In order to obtain these goals stable and durable fixation of the revision components must be achieved with restoration of hip center. Acetabular revision is the most difficult part of hip revision. Unfortunately, there is no single surgical technique to solve the problem of fixation. The achievement of stable initial and long-lasting fixation is challenged by the severity of different acetabular defects and soft tissue damage. The main acetabular reconstruction option is cementless pres-fit fixation of the cup with or without allograft [19,73]. When severe combined segmental and cavitary bone deficiencies, poor bone quality and viability or pelvic discontinuity are identified, other more complex options for acetabular reconstruction are required. These include trabecular metal (TM) cups, modular metallic augments, reconstruction cages, reinforcement rings, cup-cages, and structural or morsellized allografts that can be used to support the reconstruction.

6.2.1. Cemented fixation of the acetabular component

In cases with no or moderate bone loss revision could be performed with simple cemented exchange of the implant. Historically, early revisions were performed with the same technique that had been used for primary arthroplasty. However, difficulties in achieving consistent long-term results had prevented use of this technique. Failure to achieve adequate cement interdigitation explained poor results reported with early cementing techniques. Key factors for good cementing technique are optimal exposure of cancellous bone, adequate containment of the cup, and a clean and dry socket [130]. Sutherland and colleagues demonstrated that preservation of the subchondral bone can increase stiffness and stress concentration at the bone-cement junction [150]. Callaghan et al [13] reported 4.3% revisions and 34% radiographic loosening at 3.6-year follow-up of cemented revisions. Similar high rates of loosening were reported by Pellicci et al at 3.4-year follow-up [122]. The long-term results after cemented revision were considerably worse [121]. Even with improvement of the cementing technology, the cemented acetabular fixation has not improved (Table 5).

At longer follow-up, using modern cementing techniques failure rates ranging from 35% to 65% were reported [78,112]. Ten-year survivorship of the acetabular component with radiographical loosening as the endpoint event was 72% [78]. Consequently, cement fixation of the acetabular component has become less popular among orthopedic surgeons. In contrast, hemispherous porous-coated cups with bone ingrowth potential were developed and demonstrated consistently better results.

Authors	Year	Hips (No)	Follow-up (yrs)	Re-revision rate (%)	Radiographic loosening (%)
Raut et al. [127]	1995	387	5.5	6.2	18.8
Estok and Harris [43]	1994	32	11.7	22.0	19.0
Mulroy and Harris [109]	1996	29	15.1	38.0	44.0
Katz et al. [78]	1997	79	11.9	16.0	23.5
Eisler et al. [38]*	2000	83	3.6	8.0	22.0
Huo and Salvati [70]	1993	113	4.1	1.0	5.0

* Third generation cementing technique

Table 5. Results of acetabular revision using modern cementing technique.

6.2.2. Cementless fixation of the acetabular component

The approach to each individual case depends upon the severity and localization of host bone loss. Results after cementless revision of the acetabular component have outperformed cemented fixation [30,31,44]. With supportive and viable host bone and a reliable ingrowth surface a hemispheric metal shell supported with screws is a straightforward solution for acetabular reconstruction (Table 6). The success of the technique has been so dramatic that it is currently considered the gold standard by most arthroplasty surgeons in the USA.

Authors	Hips (No)	Follow-up (yrs)	Re-revision rate (%)	Radiographic loosening (%)
Della Valle CJ et al. [30]	138	15.0 (minimum)	4.5*	1.5
Park et al. [117]	138	20.0 (minimum)	8.0*	5.0
Wysocki et al. [162]	187	5.0 (minimum)	2.0	5.0
Lachiewicz and Hussamy [91]	60	5.0	0	0
Tanzer et al. [152]	140	3.4	0.7	4.3
Silverton et al. [145]	109	8.3	0	5.0
Templeton et al. [153]	61	12.9	0	3.0

*Combined wear and loosening

Table 6. Results of cementless cup revision.

In minor or contained defects, hemispherical cup with/without grafting produced excellent results [30,31,44]. Cementless fixation is suitable for patients with Paprosky types 1, 2A and 2B defects: without hip center migration or pelvic discontinuity. As a general rule, at least 50% of the host bone is needed to be in contact with the implant in order to support a hemispherical cup. Transfixational screws are usually used to support ingrowth of the press-fit cup. Morcellized allografts could be used to fill the cavitary defects. In a deficient acetabulum with major bone loss such as Paprosky type 3 defects a hemispherical cup could be placed against the intact supportive roof ("high hip center"). Sometimes extra large (jumbo cup) or oblong cups can bypass severe bone defects and provide stable initial fixation for bone ingrowth. Cementless fixation results in a anatomical hip center or in a high hip center [26].

6.2.2.1. High hip center

The failed acetabular components migrate in the direction of joint reaction forces creating a deficient acetabular bed with greater superoinferior dimension compared to the anteroposterior dimension. In such revision setting implantation of the cementless hemispheric press-fit cup in the anatomical hip center is not possible. A straightforward decision for treatment of such defects is to place a small hemispherical press-fit cup against the supportive bone at the roof of the acetabular defect - the so-called high hip center (Figure 7). Most authors consider arbitrary the hip center high if it is proximally greater than 35 mm to the inter-teardrop line [27].

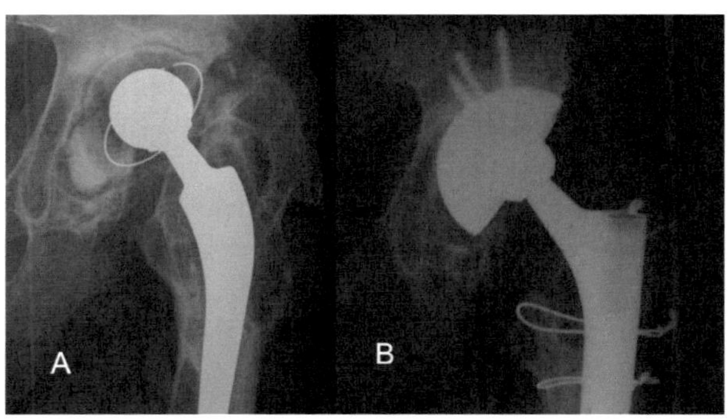

Figure 7. Type 3A defect of the acetabulum (A) resulting in high placement of the cup (B).

Results after cementless press-fit fixation of the acetabular component inserted with screws outperformed cemented revision. With use of this approach, despite extensive acetabular bone loss excellent implant fixation was consistently reported. The durability of cementless acetabular fixation was proven in long-term studies, too. In the study of Templeton et al., none of the cementless cups have been revised for aseptic loosening at 12.9-year follow-up and only 3 cups have migrated [153]. In a study with minimum follow-up of 20 years, Park et al. demonstrated 95% survivorship with revision of the cup for aseptic loosening or radiographic signs for loosening as the end point [117]. However, with longer follow-up, the problem of polyethylene wear and osteolysis emerged. In their series, re-revisions for wear and osteolysis were first performed at approximately twelve years postoperatively [117]. At last follow-up 20 years after revision, the incidence of reoperations for polyethylene wear and/or osteolysis continued to increase.

The technique saves costs, time, and eliminates the use of structural allografts or cement. However, high rate of complications was reported [27,74]. This might reflect the complexity of the procedure. Certain disadvantage of the technique is restoration of limb-length discrepancy on the femoral side whereas the defect is on the acetabular side. This would result in abnormal hip biomechanics. Increased hip joint reactive forces with high hip center and impingement might partially explain the relatively higher rate of dislocation with this technique [117,162].

Considering the excellent results reported with porous coated press-fit acetabular components in terms of implant fixation, we believe that the use of press-fit cups should be considered in every revision setting if there is sufficient host bone stock to support the cup.

6.2.2.2. Jumbo cups

Extra-large cups offer certain advantages in maximizing the contact area between the cup and host bone when revising deficient acetabulum. There is no universally-accepted definition of the jumbo cup. Extra-large cups are arbitrary defined compared to the size of the pelvis, the hip joint, and the previous implant. Whaley and coworkers defined jumbo cups as having a minimum outside diameter of 66 mm (men) or 62 mm (women) [159]. This was based upon the fact that the revision cups used at their institution were 10 mm larger than the mean implant diameters used for primary hip arthroplasty.

The method has certain advantages [126]: the acetabulum is prepared straightforward by reaming to a large hemispere; the large implant fills in the deficiencies and bone grafting is usually unnecessary; the center of rotation is transferred inferiorly and to some extent laterally restoring hip biomechanics (Figure 8); the large implant provides greater contact area and greater lever arm. Disadvantage of the technique are the limitations in restoring bone stock. Moreover, most of the defects are oblong with a greater superoinferior dimension than anteroposterior dimension. Converting an oblong defect to a hemispherical with extensive reaming may disrupt posterior wall or column which is critical for cup stability [159]. This risk of host bone compromise may result in high implantation of the socket.

Whaley et al. reported on 89 acetabular revisions using extra-large hemispherical components from the Mayo clinic [159]. The probability of survivorship of the cup at eight years was 93% with removal for any reason as the end point, and 95% with radiographical loosening or revision for aseptic loosening as the end point [159]. Wedemeyer et al., Obenaus et al., and Dearborn and Harris published similar results with cup survivorship with an end point aseptic loosening higher than 94% at mid-term follow-up [26,113,157].

The technique saves costs, time, and eliminates the use of structural allografts or cement. However, the rate of complications reported was rather high. In the series of Park et al., the most common reason for revision in 11.6% of 138 hips was infection and dislocation [117]. Similar high rates of revision were reported by Dearborn and Harris [26] and Della Valle et al. [30]. This might reflect the complexity of the procedures.

Extra large cups are a reasonable alternative in patients with moderate defects (Paprosky type 2).

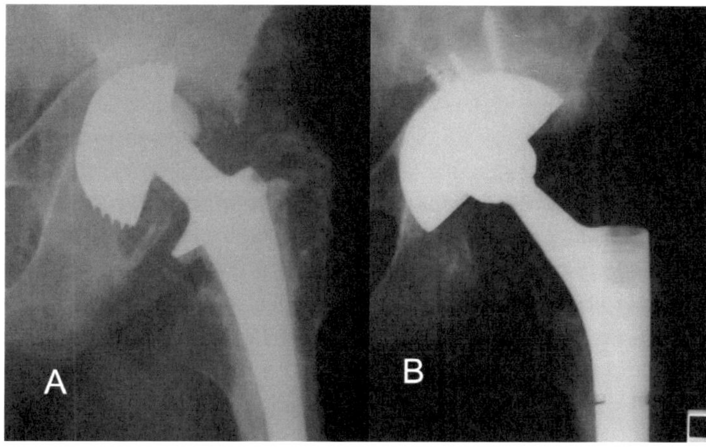

Figure 8. Correction of the center of rotation with a large oversized cup.

6.2.2.3. Oblong cups

As described earlier, large oval contained defects cannot be filled-in superoinferiorly without excessive reaming of the anterior or posterior column of the acetabulum to produce hemisphere. Another option is high placement of the cup. Attractive alternative in such cases is oblong cup. Oblong cup has smaller anteroposterior and mediolateral dimensions compared to the superiorinferior dimension. By accommodating the implant to the defect oblong cups can restore hip center and increase implant contact with host bone. Advantages of the technique are: lack of increased reaming of the anterior or posterior columns or metallization of the cup; increased contact between the device and the host bone; restoration of hip center [19,73]; and avoidance of structural allografts [5]. Disadvantages include higher cost, difficulties in cases with insufficient contact [16], possible component malpositioning, failure to restore bone [5], and excessive bone removal in order to achieve press-fit [126].

In a multicenter study on 38 hips revised with oblong press-fit cups, Berry et al. published good results at mean 3 years after surgery [5]. There was only one failure for acetabular loosening that required re-revision. Mean Harris Hip Score (HHS) increased from 50 points preoperatively to 90 points after revision. The hip center was 37 mm above the inter-teardrop line before the operation and was corrected to 25 mm above the inter-teardrop line. Civinini et al. published good mid-term results after revising with oblong cup Paprosky type 2 and 3 acetabular defects [19]. In a series of 55 hips followed-up for an average of 7.2 years only one cup was revised for loosening. Similar good results were reported by DeBoer and Christie on 18 hips revised with oblong press-fit cups [28]. At the latest follow-up, 4.5 years after revision no component was loose and the mean HHS increased from 41 points preoperatively to 91 points after revision. The authors reported near anatomic restoration of the hip center to 17 mm above the inter-teardrop line after revision. Chen and Engh reported less favorable results in 37 revisions (29 with massive type 3 defects) followed-up for an average of 41 months [16]. Eight percent of the hips were probably loose and 16% were unstable. Eight of the 14 hips that had more than two centimeters of superior migration of the component and disruption of Koehler's line on preoperative radiographs failed [16]. The authors found a correlation between loosening and average distance from the inferior edge of the cup and the interteardrop line. Five of the six unstable components initially had not reached to the level of the radiographic teardrop or distal to it [16]. In their early series, Sutherland [151] reported a 50% failure rate (3 of 6) after revision with an oblong cup of type 3 defects. Discouraging mid-term results were published by Babis et al. using a cementless oblong cup for revision of Paprosky 3A defects [3]. After a mean follow-up of 60.5 months 18 hips (29.0%) were revised and a further four hips (6.4%) were loose and awaited revision. Further analyses proved that careful patient selection is critical for the success of this revision technique.

Acetabular revision with an oblong cup is an attractive alternative, especially when the surgeon plans correction of an elevated hip center [16,108]. The technique is suitable for Paprosky type 2A, 2B and 3A defects where the acetabular defect is oval. Obtaining initial stability and supplementary fixation by screws are mandatory for the stability of the implant and are key factors for long-term success of the reconstruction. However, the medial wall should be intact and the failed component should not have migrated more than two centimeters. Pelvic discontinuity is also a contraindication for this technique. Alternative techniques such as structural allograft or cage should be considered in such revision settings.

6.2.3. Impaction grafting technique for acetabullar revision

Cemented acetabular revision yielded unacceptably high rate of loosening [13,80,81]. Possible reason is the deficient, weaken and sclerotic acetabular bone frequently found at revision. An attractive alternative for cup fixation in massive contained defects is impaction grafting where the cup is cemented on a premoulded bed of impacted morsellized cancellous bone. In such revision setting the contact with host bone is very limited if not absent. The morsellized bone has osteoinductive and osteocunductive properties and is used as a filler scaffold of contained defects. The technique of impaction bone grafting and cemented fixation of the cup was first described in 1984 by Slooff and coworkers [146], and later standardized by the same authors with minor modifications and technique-specific instrumentation [11,142]. Morsellized graft could be used with a cementless hemispherous cup if more than 50% of the cup is in contact with viable host bone [57]. Transfixing screws should be used for additional stabilization of the cup. In cases with less than 50% contact between the cup and viable host bone the cemented cup into impacted cancellous bone should be used [146].

The technique can provide stable and durable reconstruction of the hip joint. However, initial mechanical stability of the morsellized allograft-cemented cup composite is a prerequisite for a successful biological reconstruction. Subsequent remodeling and incorporation of grafts, provides long-term stability. In contrast to cementless revision, this technique could restore bone loss. The modern evolved technique consists of reconstruction of segmental and rim defects with use of a metal mesh or a solid graft. The sclerotic areas are perforated with multiple 2-mm drill-holes, and fresh-frozen morsellized bone chips are impacted layer by layer into the acetabulum. The clinical success of the of impaction grafting depends on the surgical technique and on the biological and mechanical properties of the morsellized bone graft. Various factors connected with the graft such as graft type (cancellous, cortical-cancellous, chemical composites, synthetic additives), graft processing (fresh frozen, freeze-dried, irradiated), graft particle size and grade influence the clinical result. The originators of the technique use fresh frozen allografts [11,142,143].

The technique of acetabular impaction grafting is well-established and various authors demonstrated reproducible results [20,51,143,154]. Schreurs et al. reported good results after acetabular revision with impaction allografting at 15 to 20-year follow-up [142]. With revision for aseptic loosening as the endpoint, cup survivorship was 84% at 15 years [142]. In a 20 to 28-year follow-up study, Busch et al. from the same study group evaluated 42 patients with impaction grafting younger than 50 years [11]. With revision for aseptic loosening as the end point, survivorship was 85% after twenty years and 77% after twenty-five years [11]. With end point event signs of loosening on radiographs, survival was 71% at twenty years and 62% at twenty-five years. Results declined over time, but the authors concluded that the technique is useful in younger patients with major bone defects [11].

Acetabular revision using impaction grafting is a reliable alternative for biologic restoration of hip joint mechanics. The procedure is technically demanding and exacting. Results comparable to those after revision with cementless hemispheric cups were obtained after use of correct surgical technique.

6.2.4. Reconstruction cages

Reconstruction cages and antiprotrusio rings are an established method of treatment for severe acetabular bone loss if contact with 50% host bone could not be established [57]. They have the advantage of fixation into viable host bone of the ileum and ischium with flanges while protecting allograft (Figure 9). Failure rates higher than 60% at an average of 2.9 years have been reported in cases with massive allografts not supported by cages [116]. Because of the poor results following use of unsupported structural allograft use of reconstruction cages has been advised [148]. Reinforcement rings or reconstruction cages can provide adequate support for the reconstruction with massive allografts in Paprosky type 2C and type 3 defects. Favorable results were reported after use of reconstruction cages by different authors [50,68,107,125]. Recently, this treatment approach has been questioned as TM implants provide more favorable conditions for graft incorporation and bone ingrowth [148].

The reconstruction cages and antiprotrusio rings have definite advantages: the cage and ring allow for restoration of hip center; they provide uniform load to the allograft stimulating bone remodeling and incorporation into host bone [72]; cementing allows use of local antibiotic protection; allow correct placement of the cemented cup independent of the cage or ring. The cage protects either the morsellized or structural allograft while it remodels, and if the cage fails cementless revision can be done [55,57].

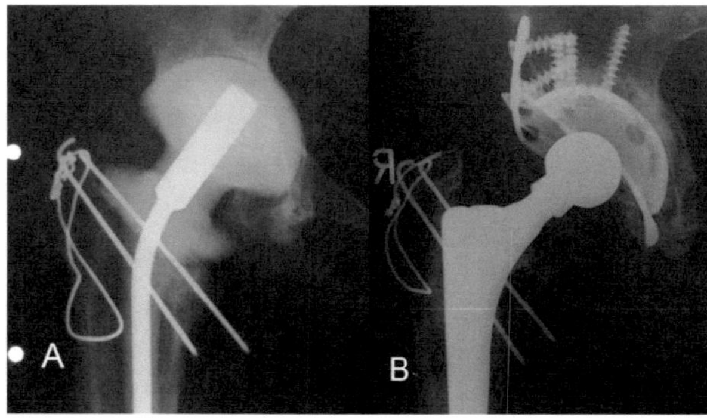

Figure 9. Reconstruction of a Paprosky type 2C defect (A) with a cage (B). Remodeling of the allograft at 2 years.

Disadvantages include higher cost, need for wide surgical exposure of the superolateral part of the ileum. The later may risk injury of the superior gluteal nerve and limping. The major concern with standard nonporous cages and rings is that they do not allow bone ingrowth. Finally, they loosen and break. However, this inability of bone ingrowth is compensated by the mechanical stability and incorporation of the graft reducing the risk of fatigue fracture of the cage. Close fit between the cage and the allograft as well as adequate fixation of the cage are a prerequisite for successful reconstruction. Cement augmentation of screws is recommended in cases with severe osteolysis or osteoporosis.

The limits of using antiprotrusio rings were demonstrated by Haentjens and coworkers and Zehntner and Ganz [63,163]. High rate of migration up to 44% (12/27) at mid-term follow-up of 7.2 years was reported [163]. Previous designs of reconstruction cages did not allow bone ingrowth and a failure rate of 16.4% due to loosening was reported on average 4.6 years after surgery [55]. Sporer et al. reported a 2- to 8-year follow-up of 45 hips where a cage was used for a type 3 defects [148]. Nine hips were revised for aseptic loosening, and an additional nine hips were radiographically loose.

In contrast, Winter et reported no loosening or revision in 38 hips followed-up at mean 7.3 years after revision with cage [160]. In a long-term study, 18 acetabular revisions for pelvic discontinuity have been reported on average 13.5 years after surgery [129]. Two cages were revised for aseptic loosening, and another two allografts showed signs of severe osteolysis. Survivorship of the acetabular component at 16.6 years with end points revision for any reason, loosening or nonunion of the allograft was 72%. The increased rate of loosening and revision is probably multifactorial and reflexes the increased case load. Frequent indication for use of reconstruction cages is pelvic discontinuity. However, designs without bone ingrowth do not have potential for biologic fixation and rely solely on mechanical fixation.

Antiprotrusio cages and rings are an effective technique for treatment of severe bone defects. However, in recent years, newer implant designs have gained popularity. In cases with more than 50% host bone support cementless cup transfixed with screws is the treatment method of choice. Trabecular metal implants, porous augments, and triflanged acetabular components are an attractive alternative for complex acetabular reconstructions,

[33,57,148]. TM cups have been proposed if contact with viable host bone is 30% to 50%. If contact with viable host bone is less than 30% a cup-cage construct was suggested [57]. Longer follow-up studies are needed to support the clinical use of these new implants.

6.2.5. Structural acetabular allografts

One of the most difficult scenarios in revision surgery is a reconstruction of a massive acetabular bone loss. Structural acetabullar allografts are a suitable revision option for uncontained bone defects (Paprosky type 2B, 3A and 3B). The size of the allograft may range from a femoral head in superolateral uncontained defects to total acetabular allograft when severe uncontained defects or pelvic discontinuity are present.

Advantages of the technique include restoration of hip center and restoration of bone stock for future revisions [50,68,90,125]. However, actual restoration of viable and mechanically competent bone is questionable. Moreover, results are unpredictable. The technique is demanding and associated with various complications.

Results after revision with structural allografts have been largely controversial. Harris initially reported successful results after reconstruction of severe acetabular defects with structural allografts [135]. However, the encouraging period of initial good functioning for 5 to 10 years was followed by later failures. In 1993, Kwong et al. reported 47% failures in 30 hips with a mean follow-up period of 10 years [90]. In 1997, the senior author reported total rate of revision or loosening 60% at an average of 16.5 years [144]. High hip center for placement of the cup was suggested in cases with severe acetabular bone loss [135].

In a series of 33 hips followed-up on average 7 years after revision with a structural allograft, Garbuz et al. reported 55% success rate [50]. Fifteen hips were revised: seven hips because of failure of the prosthesis and eight hips because of failure of both the allograft and the prosthesis. Gross et al. reported on 107 hips reconstructed with bulk allograft [58]. Thirty hips (28%) were revised and in 15.9% of cases (17 hips) the indication was aseptic loosening. The authors reported 76% successful results in the 33 hips with minimum duration of follow-up of 5 years (average, 7.1 years) after the revision. However, eight hips needed additional reoperation because of failure of the graft and another six hips were revised for loosening. Hooten et al. reported on a series of 31 revisions with structural allograft and cementless cup followed-up on average 46 months after surgery [68]. Twelve (44%) cups were radiographically loose and five of these hips were revised. In contrast, Paprosky et al. reported a failure rate of 19 per cent (6/31) at an average follow-up of 5.7 years after revision with use of a structural allograft [116]. The only failures in that series were in hips in which the allograft supported more than 50 per cent of the cup. In another study, Morsi et al. found a success rate of 86% (25/29) at mean follow-up of 7.1 years [107]. They used a minor bulk allograft that supported less than 50% of the cup.

Although results after revision with structural allograft are controversial, most authors agree that the rate of success increases if more than 50% of the cup is in contact with viable host bone [50,68,116]. According to Morsi et al. [107] and Pollock and Whiteside [125] a repeat revision does not mean failure of the reconstruction. This complex reconstruction can be considered successful if bone stock is restored for future revisions.

Revision with structural allograft is a suitable option for restoration of hip center. The role of the allograft is to support the cementless cup with partial stability until adequate ingrowth occurs. The success after the procedure is technically-related. In order to optimize result after revision with structural allograft a number of principles should be followed. Structural allografts combined with antiprotrusio cages, and a cemented cup should be considered only in cases with insufficient host bone to provide a stable fixation for a press-fit cup [26].

For an optimal result, an appropriate allograft must be selected to match the mechanical requirements of the desired reconstruction. The method of processing of the bone allografts is important for the clinical result. Greater success rate with fresh frozen bone allografts was obtained compared to freeze-dried allografts [58]. The trabecullae of the allograft should be in the direction of load for optimal stress transfer. After trimming of the allograft in order to obtain maximal contact with the host bone the allograft is fixed with 6.5 mm parallel screws in the direction of load. In case of pelvic discontinuity, the column should be fixed with a plate before fixating the allograft. Use of reinforcement cages improves results after reconstruction with structural allograft [50,138].

6.2.6. *Custom triflanged implants*

Custom triflanged prostheses have been proposed for treatment of massive acetabular defects and pelvic discontinuity, but the experience is limited and the rate of complications is high [75]. The implant is manufactured from 3-D CT data reconstruction of the degree and localization of bone loss as well as its spatial orientation.

In 2007, DeBoer et al. evaluated the outcome of revision with a custom-designed porous-coated triflanged acetabular implant in 20 hips at an average 10-year follow-up [28]. A definite healing of the pelvic discontinuity was found in 18 hips (90%). The remaining two implants were radiographically stable and did not migrate even when discontinuity persisted. However, the overall dislocation rate in the series was 25%. Christie et al. followed-up retrospectively 67 complex revisions with custom-made triflanged implant [18]. Two discontinuities persisted, but both were asymptomatic and no implant was revised. Six (7.8%) hips were revised for recurrent dislocation. Using custom triflanged acetabular components Dennis reported three failures in 24 revisions with mid-term follow-up of 4 years [33]. He questions the value of the technique in pelvic discontinuity unless supplemented with additional column plating.

The technique has high cost, it is time consuming, requires extensile exposure, and lacks modularity. It could not be used in urgent clinical situation where it is not possible to wait for manufacturing the product. With complex implant and technically challenging surgery custom-designed triflanged prosthesis should be reserved for cases where less costly and less technically demanding options could not be used. Many surgeons consider it a salvage procedure for cases where the bone loss is catastrophic.

http://dx.doi.org/10.5772/53249

6.2.7. Trabecular metal cups

Trabecular metal cups can be used in massive contained or uncontained defects. As tantalum provides favorable environment for biological fixation, TM cups have been suggested for revision of Paprosky type 3 defects [57,148] instead of an allograft-cage construct.

Early results with use of TM implants have been encouraging [111]. TM has decreased the need for at least 50% contact of the implant with viable host bone. In Paprosky 3A an 3B defects, because cages do not provide biologic fixation, Gross suggested use of a cup and cage construct (the so-called cup-cage technique) when less than 30% contact can be made with viable host bone [57]. The rationale behind the technique is that load will be taken off the cage, once bone ingrowth occurs into the trabecular metal cup. So early and mid-term failures of the cages will be prevented.

Sporer et al. reported on 13 hips with pelvic discontinuity revised with tantalum cups with or without augments [147]. At mean 2.6 years after revision 12 of the 13 cups were radiographically stable. Lakstein et al. reported on 53 revisions of contained defects with 50% or less contact with host bone using TM cups [93]. Two cups (4%) were revised, and two additional cups (4%) had radiographical evidence of probable loosening at a mean 45-month follow-up. The fact that some of the TM cups lacked contact with a viable host bone is impressive. Four hips (8%) dislocated and one (2%) sciatic nerve palsy was observed. In a large multicenter study, 263 revisions with tantalum TM cups were followed-up at an average 7 years after surgery. At the most recent follow-up, all cups were radiographically stable and no revision for loosening was reported. Eight dislocations (3%) in the series were successfully treated with closed reduction, and one sciatic palsy partially resolved at last follow-up. Kosashvili et al. reported on 26 revisions of pelvic discontinuities using cages combined with trabecular metal components and morsellized bone (cup-cage technique) [87]. At mean follow-up of 45 months 23 hips (88.5%) were radiographically stable.

Promising midterm results have been demonstrated after revision with use of these new techniques. Currently, the preference is to biological fixation whenever possible, and to alternative options when initial stability could not be obtained.

6.2.8. Modular components (metal augments)

Modular metal augments of various sizes and shape are used to decrease defect size and to restore bone defect to contained one capable of supporting a revision cup (Figure 10).

The size and placement of augments is highly dependable on the bone loss pattern. Augments are secured with multiple screws to host bone and remaining defects are filled in with morsellized bone. The hemispherical cup is impacted into the defect with the interface between the shell and the metal augment cemented.

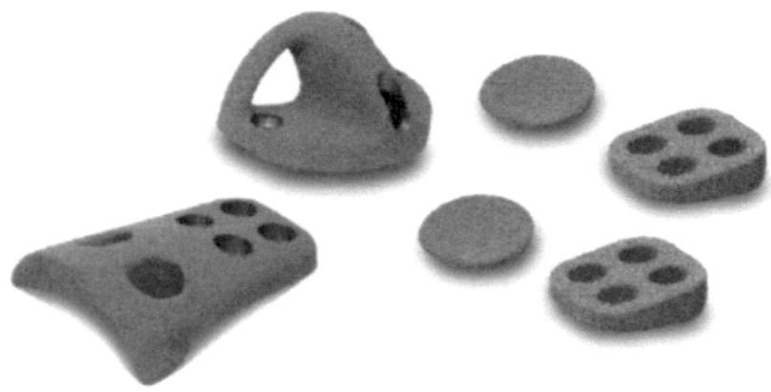

Figure 10. TM modular augments (courtesy of Zimmer, Warsaw, IN, USA).

7. Conclusion

During the last two decades, revision hip arthroplasty is constantly in the focus of orthopedic surgeons as the numbers of these difficult and risky surgeries are increasing. Up to date, he paradigms of revision surgery has been evolving constantly. From polyethylene wear, osteolysis and loosening, to complexities such as pelvic discontinuity, there is a wide range of surgical options for successful reconstruction. Analysis of clinical results from various studies outlines the preference for biological fixation of the revision implant whenever possible. It is vital for the surgeon to be familiar with different treatment approaches and to anticipate various intraoperative scenarios. Systematic approach with considerable preoperative evaluation and planning will achieve a good result. Prerequisite for a successful and durable revision include viable host bone, adequate surgical technique, and stable and endurable implant. Current improvements in surgical techniques, implant designs, as well as biomaterials and bearing surfaces are a significant contribution for obtaining favorable outcome after revision hip arthroplasty. However, we do not have complex solution. The optimal surgical approach for revision THA varies considerably among different settings. On the other hand, the economic burden of total joint replacement is increasing at a steep rate. This necessitates improved methods for evaluation of existing technology and particularly patient-derived outcomes assessment instruments. Further research and well-designed clinical studies are needed in order to provide optimal treatment to the increasing number of patients requiring revision surgery in the future.

Author details

Plamen Kinov and Peter Tivchev

Queen Giovanna – ISUL University Hospital, Department of Orthopedics and Traumatology, Medical University of Sofia, Bulgaria

References

[1] Amanatullah DF, Meehan JP, Cullen AB, Kim SH, Jamali AA. Intermediate-term radiographic and patient outcomes in revision hip arthroplasty with a modular calcar design and porous plasma coating. J Arthroplasty 2011; 26(8):1451-4.

[2] Amstutz HC, Ma SM, Jinnah RH, Mai L. Revision of aseptic loose total hip arthroplasties. Clin Orthop Relat Res 1982; 170:21-33.

[3] Babis GC, Sakellariou VI, Chatziantoniou AN, Soucacos PN, Megas P. High complication rate in reconstruction of Paprosky type IIIa acetabular defects using an oblong implant with modular side plates and a hook. J Bone Joint Surg Br 2011; 93(12): 1592-6.

[4] Barrack RL. Orthopaedic crossfire - Stem modularity is unnecessary in revision total hip arthroplasty: in the affirmative. J Arthroplasty 2003; 18(3 Suppl 1):98-100.

[5] Berry DJ, Sutherland CJ, Trousdale RT, Colwell CW Jr, Chandler HP, Ayres D, Yashar AA. Bilobed oblong porous coated acetabular components in revision total hip arthroplasty. Clin Orthop Relat Res 2000; 371:154-60.

[6] Bin Nasser A, Beaulé PE, O'Neill M, Kim PR, Fazekas A. Incidence of groin pain after metal-on-metal hip resurfacing. Clin Orthop Relat Res 2010; 468(2):392-9.

[7] Blackley HR, Davis AM, Hutchison CR, Gross AE. Proximal femoral allografts for reconstruction of bone stock in revision arthroplasty of the hip. A nine to fifteen-year follow-up. J Bone Joint Surg Am 2001; 83(3):346-54.

[8] Bozic KJ, Kurtz SM, Lau E, Ong K, Vail TP, Berry DJ. The epidemiology of revision total hip arthroplasty in the United States. J Bone Joint Surg Am 2009; 91:128-33.

[9] Bradford MS, Jablonsky WS, Paprosky WG, Younger TI. Revision of the difficult femur using the extended proximal femoral osteotomy. AAOS 1999; 48:19.

[10] Bruns J, Delling G, Gruber H, Lohmann CH, Habermann CR. Cementless fixation of megaprostheses using a conical fluted stem in the treatment of bone tumours. J Bone Joint Surg Br 2007; 89(8):1084-7.

[11] Busch VJ, Gardeniers JW, Verdonschot N, Slooff TJ, Schreurs BW. Acetabular reconstruction with impaction bone-grafting and a cemented cup in patients younger than fifty years old: a concise follow-up, at twenty to twenty-eight years, of a previous report. J Bone Joint Surg Am 2011; 93(4):367-71.

[12] Callaghan JJ. Revision of the femoral component using cement fixation. In: Bono JV, McCarthy JC, Thornhil TS, Bierbaum BE, Turner RH. (eds.) Revision total hip arthroplasty. New York: Springer-Verlag; 1999. p. 204.

[13] Callaghan JJ, Salvati EA, Pellicci PM, Wilson PD Jr, Ranawat CS. Results of revision for mechanical failure after cemented total hip replacement, 1979 to 1982. A two to five-year follow-up. J Bone Joint Surg Am 1985; 67(7):1074-85.

[14] Cameron HU. Orthopaedic crossfire - Stem modularity is unnecessary in revision total hip arthroplasty: in opposition. J Arthroplasty 2003; 18(3 Suppl 1):101-3.

[15] Chandler H, Clark J, Murphy S, McCarthy J, Penenberg B, Danylchuk K, Roehr B. Reconstruction of major segmental loss of the proximal femur in revision total hip arthroplasty. Clin Orthop Relat Res 1994; 298:67-74.

[16] Chen WM, Engh CA Jr, Hopper RH Jr, McAuley JP, Engh CA. Acetabular revision with use of a bilobed component inserted without cement in patients who have acetabular bone stock deficiency. J Bone Joint Surg Am 2000; 82(2):197-206.

[17] Chiang PP, Burke DW, Freiberg AA, Rubash HE. Osteolysis of the pelvis. Evaluation and treatment. Clin Orthop Relat Res 2003; 417:164-74.

[18] Christie MJ, Barrington SA, Brinson MF, Ruhling ME, DeBoer DK. Bridging massive acetabular defects with the triflange cup: 2- to 9-year results. Clin Orthop Relat Res 2001; 393:216-27.

[19] Civinini R, Capone A, Carulli C, Villano M, Gusso MI. Acetabular revisions using a cementless oblong cup: five to ten year results. Int Orthop 2008; 32(2):189-93.

[20] Comba F, Buttaro M, Pusso R, Piccaluga F. Acetabular reconstruction with impacted bone allografts and cemented acetabular components: a 2- to 13-year follow-up study of 142 aseptic revisions. J Bone Joint Surg Br 2006; 88(7):865-69.

[21] Cook SD, Barrack RL, Thomas KA, Haddad RJ Jr. Tissue growth into porous primary and revision femoral stems. J Arthroplasty 1991; 6(Suppl):S37-46.

[22] Cummins F, Reilly PO, Flannery O, Kelly D, Kenny P. Defining the impaction frequency and threshold force required for femoral impaction grafting in revision hip arthroplasty. A human cadaveric mechanical study. Acta Orthop 2011; 82(4):433-7.

[23] D'Antonio J, McCarthy JC, Bargar WL, Borden LS, Cappelo WN, Collis DK, Steinberg ME, Wedge JH. Classification of femoral abnormalities in total hip arthroplasty. Clin Orthop Relat Res 1993; 296:133-39.

[24] D'Antonio JA. Periprosthetic bone loss of the acetabulum. Classification and management. Orthop Clin North Am 1992; 23:279-90.

[25] D'Antonio JA, Capello WN, Borden LS, Burgar WL, Bierbaum BE, Boettcher WG, Steinberg ME, Stulberg SD, Wedge JH. Classification and management of acetabular abnormalities in total hip arthroplasty. Clin Orthop Relat Res 1989; 243:126-37.

[26] Dearborn JT, Harris WH. Acetabular revision arthroplasty using so-called jumbo cementless components: an average 7-year follow-up study. J Arthroplasty 2000; 15(1): 8-15.

[27] Dearborn JT, Harris WH. High placement of an acetabular component inserted without cement in a revision total hip arthroplasty. Results after a mean of ten years. J Bone Joint Surg Am 1999; 81(4):469-80.

[28] DeBoer DK, Christie MJ, Brinson MF, Morrison JC. Revision total hip arthroplasty for pelvic discontinuity. J Bone Joint Surg Am 2007; 89(4):835-40.

[29] DeBoer DK, Christie MJ. Reconstruction of the deficient acetabulum with an oblong prosthesis: three- to seven-year results. J Arthroplasty 1998; 13(6):674-80.

[30] Della Valle CJ, Shuaipaj T, Berger RA, Rosenberg AG, Shott S, Jacobs JJ, Galante JO. Revision of the acetabular component without cement after total hip arthroplasty. A concise followup, at fifteen to nineteen years, of a previous report. J Bone Joint Surg Am 2005; 87(8):1795-800.

[31] Della Valle CJ, Berger RA, Rosenberg AG, Galante JO. Cementless acetabular reconstruction in revision total hip arthroplasty. Clin Orthop Relat Res 2004; 420:96-100.

[32] Della Valle CJ, Paprosky WG. Classification and an algorithmic approach to the reconstruction of femoral deficiency in revision total hip arthroplasty. J Bone Joint Surg Am 2003; 85:(Suppl. 4):1-6.

[33] Dennis DA. Management of massive acetabular defects in revision total hip arthroplasty. J Arthroplasty 2003; 18(3 Suppl 1):121-5.

[34] Deirmengian C, Hallab N, Tarabishy A, et al. Synovial fluid biomarkers for periprosthetic infection. Clin Orthop Relat Res 2010; 468(8):2017-23.

[35] Duncan WW, Hubble MJW, Howell JR, Whitehouse SL, Timperley AJ, Gie GA. Revision of the femoral stem using a cement-in-cement technique: a five- to 15-year review. J Bone Joint Surg Br 2009; 91(5):577-82.

[36] Eftekhar NS. Principles of total hip arthroplastv. St Louis : CV Mosby Co; 1978.

[37] Eisler T, Svensson O, Iyer V, Wejkner B, Schmalholz A, Larsson H, Elmstedt E. Revision total hip arthroplasty using third-generation cementing technique. J Arthroplasty. 2000 Dec;15(8):974-81.

[38] Eldridge JD, Smith EJ, Hubble MJ, Whitehouse SL, Learmonth ID. Massive early subsidence following femoral impaction grafting. J Arthroplasty 1997; 12(5):535-40.

[39] Engelbrecht DJ, Weber FA, Sweet MBE, Jakim I. Long term results of revision total hip arthroplasty. J Bone Joint Surg Br 1990; 72:41-5.

[40] Engelbrecht E, Siegel A. Komplikationen nach Hüftgelenks-endoprothesen. Radiologe 1989; 29(10): 508-18.

[41] Engh CA Jr, Hopper RH Jr, Engh CA Sr. Distal ingrowth components. Clin Orthop Relat Res 2004; 420:135-41.

[42] Engh CA, Glassman AH, Griffin WL, Mayer JG. Results of cementless revision for failed cemented total hip arthroplasty. Clin Orthop Relat Res 1988; 235:91-110.

[43] Estok DM 2nd, Harris WH. Long-term results of cemented femoral revision surgery using second-generation techniques. An average 11.7-year follow-up evaluation. Clin Orthop Relat Res 1994; 299:190-202.

[44] Etienne G, Bezwada HP, Hungerford DS, Mont MA. The incorporation of morselized bone grafts in cementless acetabular revisions. Clin Orthop Relat Res 2004; 428:241-46.

[45] Farfalli GL, Buttaro MA, Piccaluga F. Femoral fractures in revision hip surgeries with impacted bone allograft. Clin Orthop Relat Res 2007; 462:130-6.

[46] Fink B, Grossmann A, Schulz MS. Bone regeneration in the proximal femur following implantation of modular revision stems with distal fixation. Arch Orthop Trauma Surg 2011; 131(4):465-70.

[47] Fink B, Grossmann A. Modified transfemoral approach to revision arthroplasty with uncemented modular revision stems. Oper Orthop Traumatol 2007; 19(1):32-55.

[48] Flannery OM, Britton JR, O'Reilly P, Mahony N, Prendergast PJ, Kenny PJ. The threshold force required for femoral impaction grafting in revision hip surgery. Acta Orthop 2010; 81(3):303-7.

[49] Franzén H, Toksvig-Larsen S, Lidgren L, Onnerfält R. Early migration of femoral components revised with impacted cancellous allografts and cement. A preliminary report of five patients. J Bone Joint Surg Br 1995; 77(6):862-4.

[50] Garbuz D, Morsi E, Gross AE. Revision of the acetabular component of a total hip arthroplasty with a massive structural allograft. Study with a minimum five-year follow-up. J Bone Joint Surg Am 1996 May;78(5):693-7.

[51] Garcia-Cimbrelo E, Cruz-Pardos A, Garcia-Rey E, Ortega-Chamarro J. The survival and fate of acetabular reconstruction with impaction grafting for large defects. Clin Orthop Relat Res 2010; 468(12):3304-13.

[52] Gerber SD, Harris WH: Femoral head autografting to augment acetabular deficiency in patients requiring total hip replacement. J Bone Joint Surg 1986; 68:1241-8.

[53] Gie GA, Linder L, Ling RS, Simon JP, Slooff TJ, Timperley AJ. Impacted cancellous allografts and cement for revision total hip arthroplasty. J Bone Joint Surg Br 1993; 75:14-21.

[54] Gokhale S, Soliman A, Dantas JP, Richardson JB, Cook F, Kuiper JH, Jones P. Variables affecting initial stability of impaction grafting for hip revision. Clin Orthop Relat Res 2005; 432:174-80.

[55] Goodman S, Saastamoinen H, Shasha N, Gross A. Complications of ilioischial reconstruction rings in revision hip surgery. J Arthroplasty 2004;19:436-46.

[56] Greenwald AS, Narten NC, Wilde AH. Points in the technique of recementing in the revision of an implant arthroplasty. J Bone Joint Surg Br 1978; 60(1):107-10.

[57] Gross AE. Restoration of acetabular bone loss 2005. J Arthroplasty 2006; 21(4 Suppl 1):117-20.

[58] Gross AE, Duncan CP, Garbuz D, Mohamed EM. Revision arthroplasty of the acetabulum in association with loss of bone stock. Instr Course Lect 1998;48:57-66.

[59] Gross AE, Hutchison CR, Alexeeff M, Mahomed N, Leitch K, Morsi E. Proximal femoral allografts for reconstruction of bone stock in revision arthroplasty of the hip. Clin Orthop Relat Res 1995; 319:151-8.

[60] Gustilo RB, Pasternak HS. Revision total hip arthroplasty with titanium ingrowth prosthesis and bone grafting for failed cemented femoral component loosening. Clin Orthop Relat Res 1988; 235:111-9.

[61] Haddad FS, Spangehl MJ, Masri BA, Garbuz DS, Duncan CP. Circumferential allograft replacement of the proximal femur. A critical analysis. Clin Orthop Relat Res 2000; 371:98-107.

[62] Haentjens P, De Boeck H, Opdecam P. Proximal femoral replacement prosthesis for salvage of failed hip arthroplasty: complications in a 2-11 year follow-up study in 19 elderly patients. Acta Orthop Scand 1996; 67(1):37-42.

[63] Haentjens P, de Boeck H, Handelberg F, Casteleyn PP, Opdecam P. Cemented acetabular reconstruction with the Müller support ring. A minimum five-year clinical and roentgenographic follow-up study. Clin Orthop Relat Res 1993; 290:225-35.

[64] Halliday BR, English HW, Timperley AJ, Gie GA, Ling RS Femoral impaction grafting with cement in revision total hip replacement. Evolution of the technique and results. J Bone Joint Surg Br 2003; 85(6):809-17.

[65] Harris WH, Krushell RJ, Galante JO. Results of cementless revisions of total hip arthroplasties using the Harris-Galante prosthesis. Clin Orthop Relat Res 1988; 235:120-6.

[66] Herberts P, Malchau H. Long-term registration has improved the quality of hip replacement: a review of the Swedish THR Register comparing 160,000 cases. Acta Orthop Scand. 2000 Apr;71(2):111-21.

[67] Holt G, Hook S, Hubble M. Revision total hip arthroplasty: the femoral side using cemented implants. Int Orthop 2011; 35(2):267-73.

[68] Hooten JP Jr, Engh CA Jr, Engh CA. Failure of structural acetabular allografts in cementless revision hip arthroplasty. J Bone Joint Surg Br 1994; 76(3):419-22.

[69] Hunter GA, Welsh RP, Cameron HU, Bailey WH. The results of revision of total hip arthroplasty. J Bone Joint Surg Br 1979; 61:419-21.

[70] Huo MH, Salvati EA. Revision total hip arthroplasty using cement. Tech Orthop1993; 7:58-64.

[71] Iorio R, Healy WL, Presutti AH. A prospective outcomes analysis of femoral component fixation in revision total hip arthroplasty. J Arthroplasty 2008; 23:662-9.

[72] Issack PS, Nousiainen M, Beksac B, Helfet DL, Sculco TP, Buly RL. Acetabular component revision in total hip arthroplasty. Part II: management of major bone loss and pelvic discontinuity. Am J Orthop 2009; 38(11):550-6.

[73] Issack PS, Nousiainen M, Beksac B, Helfet DL, Sculco TP, Buly RL. Acetabular component revision in total hip arthroplasty. Part I: cementless shells. Am J Orthop 2009; 38(10):509-14.

[74] Jamali AA, Dungy DS, Mark A, Schule S, Harris WH. Isolated acetabular revision with use of the Harris-Galante Cementless Component. Study with intermediate-term follow-up. J Bone Joint Surg Am 2004; 86(8):1690-7.

[75] Joshi AB, Lee J, Christensen C. Results for a custom acetabular component for acetabular deficiency. J Arthroplasty 2002;17:643-8.

[76] Kang MN, Huddleston JI, Hwang K, Imrie S, Goodman SB. Early outcome of a modular femoral component in revision total hip arthroplasty. J Arthroplasty 2008; 23: 220-5.

[77] Karrholm J, Hultmark P, Carlsson L, Malchau H. Subsidence of a non-polished stem in revisions of the hip using impaction allograft: evaluation with radiostereometry and dual-energy x-ray absorptiometry. J Bone Joint Surg Br 1999; 81:135-42.

[78] Katz RP, Callaghan JJ, Sullivan PM, Johnston RC. Long-term results of revision total hip arthroplasty with improved cementing technique. J Bone Joint Surg Br 1997; 79:322-6.

[79] Kavanagh BF, Wallrichs S, Ilstrup D, Berry D, Fitzgerald RH. Ten year follow up of cemented revision total hip replacement. Orthop Trans 1993; 17:943.

[80] Kavanagh BF, Fitzgerald RH Jr. Multiple revisions for failed total hip arthroplasty not associated with infection. J Bone Joint Surg Am 1987; 69(8):1144-9.

[81] Kavanagh BF, Ilstrup DM, Fitzgerald RH Jr. Revision total hip arthroplasty. J Bone Joint Surg Am 1985; 67(4):517-26.

[82] Kelly MP, Bozic KJ. Cost drivers in total hip arthroplasty: effects of procedure volume and implant selling price. Am J Orthop 2009; 38(1):E1-4.

[83] Kershaw Ci, Atkins RM, Dodd CAF, Bulstrode CJK. Revision total hip arthroplasty for aseptic failure: a review of 276 cases. J Bone Joint Surg Br 1991; 73:564-8.

[84] Kinov P. Aseptic loosening of hip arthroplasty. PhD thesis. Medical University of Sofia; 2007.

[85] Kinov P, Bukarev D, Dimov V, Kazakov K, Tivchev P. Revision total hip arthroplasty with cementing technique-five-year results. Chir Narzadow Ruchu Ortop Pol 2007; 72(4):293-6.

[86] Knight JL, Helming C. Collarless polished tapered impaction grafting of the femur during revision total hip arthroplasty: pitfalls of the surgical technique and follow-up in 31 cases. J Arthroplasty 2000; 15(2):159-65.

[87] Kosashvili Y, Backstein D, Safir O, Lakstein D, Gross AE. Krishnamurthy AB, MacDonald SJ, Paprosky WG. 5- to Acetabular revision using an anti-protrusion (ilio-ischial) cage and trabecular metal acetabular component for severe acetabular bone loss associated with pelvic discontinuity. J Bone Joint Surg Br 2009; 91(7):870-6.

[88] Krishnamurthy AB, MacDonald SJ, Paprosky WG. 5-13-year follow-up study on cementless femoral components in revision surgery. J Arthroplasty 1997; 12(8):839-47.

[89] Kurtz S, Mowat F, Ong K, Chan N, Lau E, Halpern M. Prevalence of primary and revision total hip and knee arthroplasty in the United States from 1990 through 2002. J Bone Joint Surg Am 2005; 87:1487-97.

[90] Kwong LM, Jasty M, Harris WH. High failure rate of bulk femoral head allografts in total hip acetabular reconstructions at 10 years. J Arthroplasty 1993; 8:341-6.

[91] Lachiewicz PE, Hussamy OD. Revision of the acetabulum without cement with use of the Harris-Galante porous-coated implant: two to eight-year results. J Bone Joint Surg Am 1994; 76:1834-9.

[92] Lakstein D, Kosashvili Y, Backstein D, Safir O, Lee P, Gross AE. Revision total hip arthroplasty with a modular tapered stem. Hip Int 2010; 20(2):136-42.

[93] Lakstein D, Backstein D, Safir O, Kosashvili Y, Gross AE. Trabecular Metal cups for acetabular defects with 50% or less host bone contact. Clin Orthop Relat Res 2009; 467(9):2318-24.

[94] Langlais F, J. C. Lambotte, P. Collin, and H. Thomazeau, Long-term results of allograft composite total hip prostheses for tumors. Clin Orthop Relat Res 2003; 414:197-211.

[95] Lawrence JM, Engh CA, Macalino GE. Revision total hip arthroplasty. Long-term results without cement. Orthop Clin North Am 1993; 24(4):635-44.

[96] Li PL, Ingle PJ, Dowell JK. Cement-within-cement revision hip arthroplasty: should it be done? J Bone Joint Surg Br 1996; 78(5):809-11.

[97] Lieberman JR, Moeckel BH, Evans BG, Salvati EA, Ranawat CS. Cement-within-cement revision hip arthroplasty. J Bone Joint Surg Br 1993; 75(6):869-71.

[98] Malkani AL, F. H. Sim, and E. Y. S. Chao. Custom-made segmental femoral replacement prosthesis in revision total hip arthroplasty. Orthop Clin North Am 1993; 24(4): 727-33.

[99] Mallory TH. Preparation of the proximal femur in cementless total hip revision. Clin Orthop Relat Res 1988; 235:47-60.

[100] Masterson S, Lidder S, Scott G. Impaction femoral allografting at revision hip arthroplasty: uncemented versus cemented technique using a Freeman femoral component. J Bone Joint Surg Br 2012; 94(1):51-5.

[101] Masterson EL, Masri BA, Duncan CP. The cement mantle in the Exeter impaction allografting technique. A cause for concern. J Arthroplasty 1997; 12(7):759-64.

[102] McAuley JP, Engh CA Jr. Femoral fixation in the face of considerable bone loss: cylindrical and extensively coated femoral components. Clin Orthop Relat Res 2004; 429:215-21.

[103] Meding JB, Ritter MA, Keating EM, Faris PM. Impaction bonegrafting before insertion of a femoral stem with cement in revision total hip arthroplasty: a minimum two-year follow-up study. J Bone Joint Surg Am 1997; 79:1834-41.

[104] Miner TM, Momberger NG, Chong D, Paprosky WL. The extended trochanteric osteotomy in revision hip arthroplasty: a critical review of 166 cases at mean 3-year, 9-month follow-up. J Arthroplasty 2001; 16(Suppl 1):188-94.

[105] Moreland JR, Moreno MA. Cementless femoral revision arthroplasty of the hip: minimum 5 years followup. Clin Orthop Relat Res 2001; 393:194-201.

[106] Moreland JR, Bernstein ML. Femoral revision hip arthroplasty with uncemented, porous-coated stems. Clin Orthop Relat Res 1995; 319:141-50.

[107] Morsi E, Garbuz D, Gross AE. Revision total hip arthroplasty with shelf bulk allografts. A long-term follow-up study. J Arthroplasty 1996;11(1):86-90.

[108] Moskal JT, Higgins ME, Shen J. Type III acetabular defect revision with bilobed components: five-year results. Clin Orthop Relat Res 2008; 466(3):691-5.

[109] Mulroy WF, Harris WH. Revision total hip arthroplasty with use of so-called second-generation cementing techniques for aseptic loosening of the femoral component. A fifteen-year-average follow-up study. J Bone Joint Surg Am 1996; 78:325-30.

[110] Nadaud MC, Griffin WL, Fehring TK, Mason JB, Tabor OB Jr, Odum S, Nussman DS. Cementless revision total hip arthroplasty without allograft in severe proximal femoral defects. J Arthroplasty 2005; 20(6):738-44.

[111] Nehme A, Lewallen DB, Hanssen AD. Modular porous metal augments for treatment of severe acetabular bone loss during revision hip arthroplasty. Clin Orthop Relat Res 2004; 429:201-8.

[112] Nelson CL. Cemented cup revisions. Am J Orthop 2002; 31(8):479-80.

[113] Obenaus C, Winkler H, Girtler R, Huber M, Schwägerl W. Extra-large press-fit cups without screws for acetabular revision. J Arthroplasty 2003; 18(3):271-7.

[114] Ornstein E, Linder L, Ranstam J, Lewold S, Eisler T, Torper M. Femoral impaction bone grafting with the Exeter stem - the Swedish experience: survivorship analysis of

1,305 revisions performed between 1989 and 2002. J Bone Joint Surg Br 2009; 91(4): 441-6.

[115] Paprosky W G, Greidanus N V, Antoniou J. Minimum 10-year-results of extensively porous-coated stems in revision hip arthroplasty. Clin Orthop Relat Res 1999; 369:230-42.

[116] Paprosky WG, Perona PG, Lawrence JM. Acetabular defect classification and surgical reconstruction in revision arthroplasty. A 6-year follow-up evaluation. J Arthroplasty 1994; 9(1):33-44.

[117] Park DK, Della Valle CJ, Quigley L, Moric M, Rosenberg AG, Galante JO. Revision of the acetabular component without cement. A concise follow-up, at twenty to twenty-four years, of a previous report. J Bone Joint Surg Am 2009; 91:350-5.

[118] Parvizi J, Jacovides C, Antoci V, Ghanem E. Diagnosis of periprosthetic joint infection: the utility of a simple yet unappreciated enzyme. J Bone Joint Surg Am 2011; 93(24):2242-48.

[119] Parvizi J, Della Valle CJ. AAOS Clinical Practice Guideline: diagnosis and treatment of periprosthetic joint infections of the hip and knee. J Am Acad Orthop Surg 2010; 18(12):771-2.

[120] Parvizi J, Tarity TD, Slenker N, Wade F, Trappler R, Hozack WJ, Sim FH. Proximal femoral replacement in patients with non-neoplastic conditions. J Bone Joint Surg Am 2007; 89(5):1036-43.

[121] Pellicci PM, Wilson Jr PD, Sledge CB, Salvati EA, Ranawat CS, Poss R, Callaghan JJ.. Long-term results of revision total hip replacement. A follow-up report. J Bone Joint Surg Am 1985; 67:513-6.

[122] Pellicci PM, Wilson PD Jr, Sledge CB, Salvati EA, Ranawat CS, Poss R. Revision total hip arthroplasty. Clin Orthop Relat Res 1982; 170:34-41.

[123] Pekkarinen J, Alho A, Lepistö J, Ylikoski M, Ylinen P, Paavilainen T. Impaction bone grafting in revision hip surgery. A high incidence of complications. J Bone Joint Surg Br 2000; 82(1):103-7.

[124] Piccaluga F, González Della Valle A, Encinas Fernández JC, Pusso R. Revision of the femoral prosthesis with impaction allografting and a Charnley stem. A 2- to 12-year follow-up. J Bone Joint Surg Br 2002; 84(4):544-9.

[125] Pollock FH, Whiteside LA. The fate of massive allografts in total hip acetabular revision surgery. J Arthroplasty 1992; 7:271-6.

[126] Pulido L, Rachala SR, Cabanela ME. Cementless acetabular revision: past, present, and future. Revision total hip arthroplasty: the acetabular side using cementless implants. Int Orthop 2011; 35(2):289-98.

[127] Raut VV, Siney PD, Wroblewski BM. Cemented Charnley revision arthroplasty for severe femoral osteolysis. J Bone Joint Surg Br 1995; 77(3):362-5.

[128] Raut VV, Siney PD, Wroblewski BM: Cemented revision for aseptic acetabular loosening: a review of 387 hips. J Bone Joint Surg Br 1995; 77:357-61.

[129] Regis D, Sandri A, Bonetti I, Bortolami O, Bartolozzi P. A minimum of 10-year follow-up of the Burch-Schneider cage and bulk allografts for the revision of pelvic discontinuity. J Arthroplasty 2012; 27(6):1057-63.

[130] Ritter MA, Thong AE. The role of cemented sockets in 2004: is there one? J Arthroplasty 2004; 19(4 suppl 1):92-4.

[131] Rogers BA, Sternheim A, Backstein D, Safir O, Gross AE. Proximal femoral allograft for major segmental femoral bone loss: a systematic literature review. Adv Orthop 2011; 2011:257572.

[132] Roque PJ, Mankin HJ, Malchau H. Proximal femoral allograft: prognostic indicators. J Arthroplasty 2010; 25(7):1028-33.

[133] Rosenstein A, MacDonald W, Iliadis A, McLardy-Smith P. Revision of cemented fixation and cement-bone interface strength. Proc Inst Mech Eng (H) 1992; 206(1):47-9.

[134] Rubash HE, Harris WH. Revision of nonseptic, loose, cemented femoral components using modem cementing techniques. J Arthroplasty 1988; 3:241-8.

[135] Russotti GM, Harris WH. Proximal placement of the acetabular component in total hip arthroplasty. A long-term follow-up study. J Bone Joint Surg Am 1991; 73(4): 587-92.

[136] Safir O, Kellett CF, Flint M, Backstein D, Gross AE. Revision of the deficient proximal femur with a proximal femoral allograft. Clin Orthop Relat Res 2009; 467(1):206-12.

[137] Saleh KJ, Holtzman J, Gafni A, Saleh L, Davis A, Resig S, Gross AE. Reliability and intraoperative validity of preoperative assessment of standardized plain radiographs in predicting bone loss at revision hip surgery. J Bone Joint Surg Am 2001; 83:1040-6.

[138] Saleh KJ, Jaroszynski G, Woodgate I, Saleh L, Gross AE. Revision total hip arthroplasty with the use of structural acetabular allograft and reconstruction ring: a case series with a 10-year average follow-up. J Arthroplasty 2000; 15(8):951-8.

[139] Schreurs BW, Luttjeboer J, Thien TM, de Waal Malefijt MC, Buma P, Veth RP, Slooff TJ. Acetabular revision with impacted morselized cancellous bone graft and a cemented cup in patients with rheumatoid arthritis. A concise follow-up, at eight to nineteen years, of a previous report. J Bone Joint Surg Am 2009; 91(3):646-51.

[140] Schreurs BW, Arts JJ, Verdonschot N, Buma P, Slooff TJ, Gardeniers JW. Femoral component revision with use of impaction bone-grafting and a cemented polished stem. Surgical technique. J Bone Joint Surg Am 2006; 88(Suppl 1 Pt 2):259-74.

[141] Schreurs BW, Arts JJ, Verdonschot N, Buma P, Slooff TJ, Gardeniers JW. Femoral component revision with use of impaction bone-grafting and a cemented polished stem. J Bone Joint Surg Am 2005; 87(11):2499-507.

[142] Schreurs BW, Bolder SB, Gardeniers JW, Verdonschot N, Slooff TJ, Veth RP. Acetabular revision with impacted morsellised cancellous bone grafting and a cemented cup. A 15- to 20-year follow-up. J Bone Joint Surg Br 2004; 86(4):492-7.

[143] Schreurs BW, Slooff TJ, Buma P, Gardeniers JW, Huiskes R. Acetabular reconstruction with impacted morsellised cancellous bone graft and cement. A 10- to 15-year follow-up of 60 revision arthroplasties. J Bone Joint Surg Br 1998; 80(3):391-395.

[144] Shinar AA, Harris WH. Bulk structural autogenous grafts and allografts for reconstruction of the acetabulum in total hip arthroplasty. Sixteen-year-average follow-up. J Bone Joint Surg Am 1997; 79(2):159-68.

[145] Silverton CD, Rosenberg AG, Sheinkop MB, Kull LR, Galante JO. Revision of the acetabular component without cement after total hip arthroplasty. A follow-up note regarding results at seven to eleven years. J Bone Joint Surg Am 1996; 78(9):1366-70.

[146] Slooff TJ, Huiskes R, van Horn J, Lemmens AJ. Bone grafting in total hip replacement for acetabular protrusion. Acta Orthop Scand 1984; 55: 593-6.

[147] Sporer SM, Paprosky WG. Acetabular revision using a trabecular metal acetabular component for severe acetabular bone loss associated with a pelvic discontinuity. J Arthroplasty 2006; 21(6 Suppl 2):87-90.

[148] Sporer SM, O'Rourke M, Paprosky WG. The treatment of pelvic discontinuity during acetabular revision. J Arthroplasty 2005; 20(4 Suppl 2):79-84.

[149] Sternheim A, Rogers BA, Kuzyk PR, Safir OA, Backstein D, Gross AE. Segmental proximal femoral bone loss and revision total hip replacement in patients with developmental dysplasia of the hip: the role of allograft prosthesis composite. J Bone Joint Surg Br 2012; 94(6):762-7.

[150] Sutherland AG, D'Arcy S, Smart D, Ashcroft GP. Removal of the subchondral plate in acetabular preparation. Int Orthop 2000; 24(1):19-22.

[151] Sutherland CJ. Early experience with eccentric acetabular components in revision total hip arthroplasty. Am J Orthop 1996; 25:284-9.

[152] Tanzer M, Drucker D, Jasty M, McDonald M, Harris WH. Revision of the acetabular component with an uncemented Harris-Galante porous-coated prosthesis. J Bone Joint Surg Am 1992; 74(7):987-94.

[153] Templeton JE, Callaghan JJ, Goetz DD, Sullivan PM, Johnston RC. Revision of a cemented acetabular component to a cementless acetabular component. A ten to fourteen-year follow-up study. J Bone Joint Surg Am 2001; 83(11):1706-11.

[154] van Egmond N, De Kam DC, Gardeniers JW, Schreurs BW. Revisions of extensive acetabular defects with impaction grafting and a cement cup. Clin Orthop Relat Res 2011; 469(2):562-73.

[155] Vastel L, Lemoine CT, Kerboull M, Courpied JP. Structural allograft and cemented long-stem prosthesis for complex revision hip arthroplasty: use of a trochanteric claw plate improves final hip function. Int Orthop 2007; 31(6):851-7.

[156] Wagner H, Wagner M. Cone prosthesis for the hip joint. Arch Orthop Trauma Surg 2000; 120(1-2):88-95.

[157] Wedemeyer C, Neuerburg C, Heep H, von Knoch F, von Knoch M, Löer F, Saxler G. Jumbo cups for revision of acetabular defects after total hip arthroplasty: a retrospective review of a case series. Arch Orthop Trauma Surg 2008; 128:545-50.

[158] Weeden SH, Paprosky WG. Minimum 11-year follow up of extensively porous coated stems in femoral revision total hip arthroplasty. J Arthroplasty 2002; 17(Suppl 1): 134-7.

[159] Whaley AL, Berry DJ, Harmsen WS. Extra-large uncemented hemispherical acetabular components for revision total hip arthroplasty. J Bone Joint Surg Am 2001; 83(9): 1352-7.

[160] Winter E, Piert M, Volkmann R, Maurer F, Eingartner C, Weise K, Weller S. Allogeneic cancellous bone graft and a Burch-Schneider ring for acetabular reconstruction in revision hip arthroplasty. J Bone Joint Surg Am. 2001 Jun;83-A(6):862-7.

[161] Wraighte PJ, Howard PW. Femoral impaction bone allografting with an Exeter cemented collarless, polished, tapered stem in revision hip replacement: a mean follow-up of 10.5 years. J Bone Joint Surg Br 2008; 90(8):1000-4.

[162] Wysocki RW, Della Valle CJ, Shott S, Rosenberg AG, Berger RA, Galante JO. Revision of the acetabulum with a contemporary cementless component. J Arthroplasty 2009; 24(6 Suppl):58-63.

[163] Zehntner MK, Ganz R. Midterm results (5.5-10 years) of acetabular allograft reconstruction with the acetabular reinforcement ring during total hip revision. J Arthroplasty 1994; 9:469-79.

[164] Zehr RJ, Enneking WF, Scarborough MT. Allograft-prosthesis composite versus megaprosthesis in proximal femoral reconstruction. Clin Orthop Relat Res 1996; 322:207-23.

Chapter 16

Ankle Osteoarthritis and Arthroplasty

Nadr M. Jomha, Angela Scharfenberger, Gordon Goplen and M. Elizabeth Pedersen

Additional information is available at the end of the chapter

http://dx.doi.org/10.5772/54224

1. Introduction

The World Health Organization estimates that 10% of the world's population over the age of 60 suffers from osteoarthritis (OA) [1]. The majority of these cases involve the hip and knee. Symptomatic osteoarthritis of the ankle with radiographic changes is seen in approximately 11% of patients seeking treatment for "arthritis" [1]. Idiopathic arthritis, as seen in the hip and knee, is rare in the ankle joint. The majority of ankle arthritis is secondary to trauma (70%), with a smaller percentage being attributed to inflammatory arthropathies such as RA (12%) and only 7% attributed to primary OA [2]. Ankle arthritis can be a debilitating disease. In fact, the mental and physical disability associated with end-stage arthritis of the ankle is at least as severe as that associated with end stage hip arthritis [3].

1.1. Anatomy

The ankle joint consists of the tibio-talar joint incorporating articular surfaces between the talar dome with the tibial plafond, and the medial talus with the medial malleolus. In addition, there is an articulation between the lateral talus with the lateral malleolus. It is mainly a rolling joint with congruent surfaces at high loads, allowing it to withstand large pressures [1]. The ankle carries 5 times body weight during normal walking activities [4]. The majority of the load (75%) is distributed across the tibio-talar joint but some force is transmitted through the medial and lateral sides [5]. Pathological conditions such as a mal-united ankle fracture results in changes in the contact stresses and the overall contact area [5].

1.2. History

Patients with arthritic changes to the ankle have the typical "arthritic" complaints as seen in other affected joints. Patients often present with pain, swelling and stiffness. The pain may be worse with weight bearing/impact activities, with weather changes, and may wake them at night. Painful symptoms may be worse with initiation of activities (especially first thing in the morning) but may improve during the activity. The pain usually intensifies with prolonged activity and after the activity is completed. Stiffness can be present, usually worse first thing in the morning or after a prolonged rest. Swelling can be particularly bothersome and is usually intermittent. Patients complain of pain in the anterior talo-crural area and have difficulty with reciprocal stair climbing and hills. Subfibular or lateral foot pain is not common and is more typical for patients with subtalar arthritis which may be seen in combination with ankle arthritis. Patients with subtalar arthritis complain of difficulties with walking on uneven ground.

Given that most ankle arthritis is post-traumatic, a history of previous trauma should be determined including a history of severe or repetitive ankle sprains [6]. History of previous infection is important to ascertain as it can be a contraindication to joint arthroplasty and current infection should be treated immediately with antibiotics and possibly debridement. Systemic illness such as rheumatoid arthritis, gout, and hemophilia should be noted. Patients with diabetes mellitus can present with Charcot deformity including arthritis.

1.3. Physical exam

Patients should be inspected for general lower limb alignment, including the knees, ankle, hindfoot, midfoot and forefoot, paying particular attention to varus/valgus mal-alignment of the hindfoot and dorsiflexion/plantarflexion mal-alignment of the ankle. Inspection should note any swelling about the ankle, wasting of the calf musculature and previous surgical incisions. Gait should be observed. Patients generally have a foreshortened stance phase, and may walk with their foot externally rotated. Patients with ankle arthritis walk with a shorter stride length, reduced walking speed, and a shorter stance phase of the affected limb [4, 5, 7, 8]. Active and passive range of motion should be compared to the other side for ankle dorsi/plantar flexion and subtalar eversion/inversion. In severe ankle arthritis, it is important to differentiate range of motion coming from the ankle joint as opposed to the hindfoot and midfoot joints. Heel eversion and inversion may also show restrictions of movement. Palpation should include all bone prominences and the anterior margin of the ankle joint looking for areas of tenderness or synovitis. Sensory changes or motor dysfunction should be noted for possible neurological abnormalities. Both dorsalis pedis and posterior tibial pulses should be assessed along with capillary refill and any abnormalities may require further vascular investigations with ABI and/or CT angiogram.

1.4. Imaging

Standard radiographs should include WEIGHTBEARING AP/Lateral and mortise views of both ankles, and AP and lateral views of the foot. Radiographs can be reviewed for the classic signs of OA including loss of joint space, subchondral sclerosis, cyst formation and osteophyte formation. CT scan can be useful to determine arthritic changes in adjacent joints, or to look at the surrounding bone stock when considering arthroplasty but this technique is compromised for diagnosing early OA with cartilage loss because it is not done in the

http://dx.doi.org/10.5772/54224

weightbearing position; therefore it can be misleading regarding joint space maintenance and overall joint alignment. MRI is not required when assessing ankle arthritis. If there is a past history of infection, quiescent infection should be ruled out with a bone/gallium scan combination or a white blood cell scan.

2. Conservative treatment

2.1. Medications

Non-steroidal anti-inflammatories drugs (NSAIDs) have long been the mainstay for symptomatic treatment of arthritic joint pain. These drugs control the pain of arthritis but are not disease modifying agents. Current classes of drugs include standard NSAIDs (eg. Ibuprofen, Naproxen, Indomethacin). The newer Cox 2 inhibitors [eg. Celecoxib (Celebrex) and Rofecoxib (Vioxx)] have less gastrointestinal side effects [9, 10]; however, concern about higher risks of myocardial infarction, thrombosis and stroke lead to withdrawl of Rofecoxib (Vioxx) from the market in 2004 Patients with long term NSAID use are counseled to have blood pressure and kidney function checked regularly with their family physicians as all NSAIDS still put patients at risk for renal-related complications.

Nutraceuticals such as glucosamine sulphate and chondroitin sulphate are popular non-prescription remedies. There have been a multiple studies on these products, the vast majority done in the arthritic knee population. Findings include pain modification similar to NSAIDS with a similar side effect profile, although the onset is slower [11, 12]. Other studies suggest actual disease modification with long term glucosamine use, as seen by NON progression of joint space narrowing [13, 14]. More recent authors have found no difference between glucosamine and placebo [15] and no evidence of disease modification or pain relief [16]. Popular dosing for glucosamine is 1.5 grams per day.

2.2. Injections

Corticosteroids demonstrate both anti-inflammatory response and immunosuppressive effect. After intra-articular administration, there is a decrease in erythema, swelling, heat and tenderness. This may be secondary to altered movement and function of leucocytes, reduced micro vascular dilation and permeability, and reduced prostaglandin synthesis. Side effects can include septic arthritis, tendon rupture, post injection wheal and flare, facial flushing, atrophic skin changes, toxic effect on cartilage (at large doses) and possible systemic absorption. Standard limit of injections in weight bearing joints is 3-4 injections per year [17].

Hyaluronic acid (HA) is a major component of synovial fluid, and comprises part of the structure of hyaline cartilage. Viscosupplementation by injection of HA derivatives (as available in pharmaceutical components) has multiple proposed mechanisms of action. Biologic effects include an anti-inflammatory as well as anti-oxidant effect, and restoration of endogenous synthesis via positive feedback loop. Viscoelastic properties include a "mechanical spongy" trapping of immune complexes and inflammatory cells and restoration of synovial fluid viscosity and elasticity. Multiple versions of HA exist from multiple pharmaceutical companies. Not all are available in all countries [18]. Some examples of currently available products include Hyalgan (sodium hyaluronate; Sanofi-Aventis, Bridgewater, NJ, USA), Synvisc (hylan GF-20; Genzyme Corportation, Cambridge, MA, USA), Supartz (sodium hyaluronate; Smith & Nephew, London, UK), Orthovisc (high molecular weight hyaluronan; Anika Therapeutics, Inc., Bedford, MA, USA), Euflexxa (1% sodium hyaluronate; Ferring Pharmaceuticals, Inc., Saint-Prex, Switzerland), and Durolane (stabilize hyaluronic acid; Smith & Nephew, York, UK). Most require multiple injections although newer ones (eg Durolane) are coming to market that require only one injection. Side effect of HA injections are rare but include anaphylaxis, pseudogout type reaction, and Severe Acute Inflammatory Reaction (SAIR) which presents like septic arthritis.

The effectiveness of hyaluronic acid derivatives in the ankle joint has not been determined due to poorly conducted studies with mixed results from the few good studies performed [19, 20] although a recent randomized control trial article comparing HA to saline in the ankle showed no therapeutic benefit from the HA injection. Both HA and Saline injection resulted in similar changes in VAS, AOS and AOFAS scores [21]. Further high quality studies need to be completed before a definitive recommendation for HA derivatives in the ankle can be given.

2.3. Bracing

There is a paucity of any literature on bracing and shoe modifications. Practically, bracing progresses from a simple lace-up ankle brace to a more elaborate rigid Ankle Foot Orthosis (AFO) (Figure 1). A rigid AFO works by restricting painful ankle range of motion.

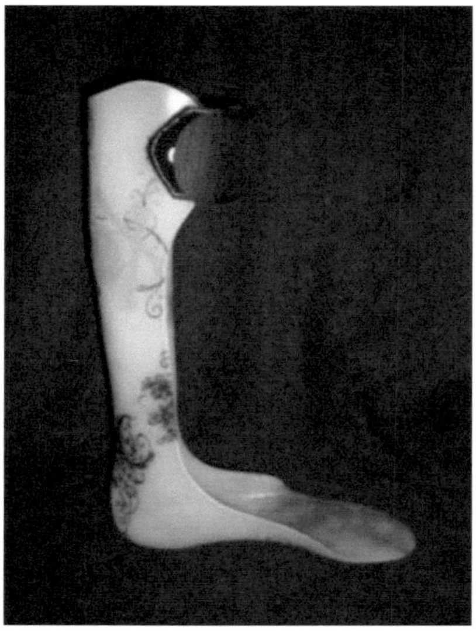

Figure 1. Photograph of a rigid AFO.

http://dx.doi.org/10.5772/54224

More severely affected joints may be helped by a clamshell AFO (offloading AFO) (Figure 2). This type of orthosis works by transferring weight from the ankle to the calf using the clamshell portion that wraps around the calf (similar in principle to a patellar-tendon brace). This type of AFO can have a hinge to maintain ankle range of motion or can be rigid to restrict motion as well as off-load the joint.

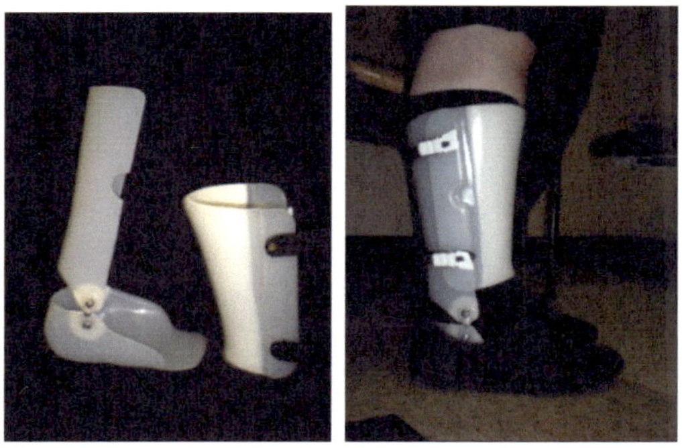

Figure 2. Offloading AFO with a hinge. Picture on the left demonstrates the AFO in a separated condition while the right picture shows it applied to the patient.

Some patients may benefit from shoe modifications such as a rocker bottom shoe (Figure 3). This provides increased toe-off, thereby stressing the ankle joint less.

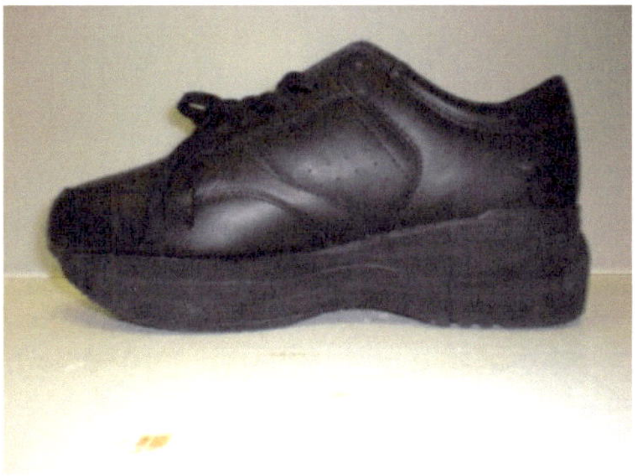

Figure 3. Forefoot rocker bottom shoe.

3. Surgical options

After non-operative treatments have been exhausted, surgical treatments can be considered. These options will depend on the location and extent of the arthritis.

3.1. Focal joint abnormalities

Localized lesions within the ankle joint can progress to generalized osteoarthritis. As documented in the knee, larger lesions have a worse prognosis than smaller lesions [22, 23]. Smaller lesions (usually considered 1cm^2 or less can be asymptomatic or often are dealt with by arthroscopic debridement of loose cartilage with or without microfracture technique. If there is underlying bone necrosis, removal of this bone and overlying damaged cartilage can provide symptomatic relief. For larger lesions, the surgical options become more complicated and less predictable. There are a variety of techniques that can be used but no specific technique has been shown to superior to the rest. The most basic and economical procedure is microfacture. This technique can be used to induce local mesenchymal stem cells to influx to the defect and produce a fibrocartilage repair surface that can function well, particularly in the short to medium term [24, 25],. Although most research has been performed in the knee, this can be successful in the ankle as well [26, 27]. Of the more complicated procedures, perhaps the most publicized is autologous chondrocyte implantation (ACI) first described in 1994 in the knee [28]. It is also performed in the ankle [29]. Although there is a lot of literature published on this technique in the knee, the inability to reproduce the complex nature of the articular matrix has led to further investigation into variations of the technique including matrix-associated chondrocyte implantation (MACI) [30, 31] and characterized chondrocyte implantation (CCI) [32]. Both of these techniques attempt to improve on the quality of matrix formed during the procedure. Other techniques utilize intact matrix to replace damaged matrix. This ensures the complex structure of the matrix is maintained. These techniques include osteochondral autograft transplantation (OATS) [33, 34] and mosaicplasty [35]) [36, 37], and bulk osteochondral allografts [38-41]. Finally, other more experimental techniques such as synthetic scaffolds and mesenchymal stem cells have been tried with variable success [42-45].

3.1.1. Cell-based techniques

Microfracture – Microfracture is a well-established technique for full thickness cartilage defects with an intact subchondral bone plate. The cartilage is debrided to form a well-contained defect with stable margins. The underlying bone is perforated with a sharp awl or pick at 3-4mm intervals while ensuring a stable subchondral plate remains intact to support the incoming cells. The perforations should penetrate deep enough to allow mesenchymal stem cells from the underlying spongy bone to enter the defect. The blood that emerges from the bone forms a clot and the stem cells differentiate into chondrocytes and fibrochondrocytes to produce a fibrocartilage that fills the defects.

Post-operatively, the patient is allowed early ROM but should be non-weight bearing for a period of time to allow some tissue formation. The length of time depends on the size and location of the lesion. Advantages of this technique include that it is one operation with low cost. Disadvantages include that fibrocartilage instead of hyaline cartilage is formed, filling of the defect is unpredictable and often incomplete [46]. That said, if good results can be obtained, the results in the ankle may not deteriorate over time [27]. This is considered a first line treatment by many surgeons, especially those that do not have access to the more complicated and expensive exogenous cell- or tissue-based therapies.

Autologous Chondrocyte Implantation (ACI and its analogues) – ACI is the most publicized technique for repairing/regenerating pure cartilage defects in the knee joint. First popularized by Brittberg in 1994 [28], thousands of patients have been treated using this technique in the knee joint but far fewer in the ankle joint. Studies in the ankle have reported good intermediate- and long-term results [47, 48]. Despite the historical background and extensive use, the technique has been modified to incorporate a matrix (MACI) or utilizing specific chondrocytes from the harvest (CCI) in an attempt to improve results. This suggests that the results from ACI are not optimal. ACI is a complicated technique that entails removing a portion of cartilage from a relative non-weight bearing portion of the joint and sending it to a lab for processing. Typically the donor cartilage is harvested from the ipsilateral knee joint [47, 48]. The ankle joint is typically not used as no specific safe area has been clearly defined [49]. During processing, the cells are removed from the matrix and expanded up to 20 million cells over a period of 3-4 weeks. The cells are then re-implanted at a second surgical procedure. This entails opening the joint, preparing the defect by making sure it has well-defined margins with an intact subchondral plate to prevent the intrusion of mesenchymal stem cells from the bone. A periosteal flap is harvested from a nearby area and sutured over the defect leaving a small area for injection of the expanded cells. The cells are injected under that flap that is then closed and sealed with fibrin glue. Often, a malleolar osteotomy is required to gain access to areas of the talar dome.

MACI is the next generation of ACI that incorporates the use of a scaffold [50-52]. The procedure is similar to that of ACI except that a matrix is used instead of a periosteal flap. The matrix is impregnated with the cells and shaped to the size of the defect. It is inserted and fixed by different mechanisms. Advantages of this technique include that it can be done arthroscopically in some cases and does not require the extra step of harvesting and suturing the periosteal flap. Thus it is less invasive. It has not been shown to be conclusively better than ACI. CCI (characterized chondrocyte implantation) is almost exactly the same as ACI except that the laboratory preselects specific cells that the company believes are predisposed to form articular cartilage out of all those that are harvested. These are the cells that are then expanded and re-implanted with the theory that the identified subpopulation of chondrocytes will produce a more physiologically intact matrix. The disadvantage of this technique is some patients do not have sufficient cells that meet the criteria for an enhanced population and, therefore, are not candidates for this procedure.

The results for these procedures have generally been good. Concerns with these procedures include that two separate surgical procedures are required and the cell processing can be prohibitively expensive. These major concerns limit their availability, especially when they have not been conclusively shown to be superior to other techniques [53]. The uncertainties of these techniques have led some researchers to investigate the use of mesenchymal stem cells instead of chondrocytes. This would allow the surgery to be completed at one time and may produce young chondrocytes that could potentially produce a more robust cartilage. These techniques are in the more experimental stage and more commonly used in the knee joint.

3.1.2. Tissue-based techniques

Osteochondral autograft transplantation is a technique developed for small to medium sized defects. It consists of harvesting osteochondral plugs from less weight bearing portions of the same joint (or a different joint such as the knee when dealing with the ankle) and implanting them into the defect. This is accomplished by using 6mm diameter reamers to a depth of 10-15mm into the subchondal bone. A corresponding osteochondral core is harvested from another area and gently impacted into the newly formed defect attempting to achieve a press-fit while maintaining the contour of the articular surface. With lesions larger than 6mm diameter (ie most lesions that require treatment), multiple cores are required and press-fit with an interdigitating method and termed mosaicplasty. Once again, there are some reported good results using this technique [33, 36, 37, 54] but this is a complicated technique with multiple drawbacks. Harvesting cores from the ankle is usually not possible, therefore another joint must be violated and the harvest sites are not without possible complications such as knee pain and instability [35, 55]. Typically an osteotomy is required to gain access to the talar dome because the plugs must be inserted perpendicular to the surface of the joint. Alignment of the multiple plugs is difficult to ensure a smooth surface and the cartilage from the harvest often is of different thickness compared to the insertion site resulting in a variable underlying subchondral bone. Obtaining precise contour matching for lesions on the "shoulder" of the talus can be extremely difficult. Bone plugs of only 6mm diameter are susceptible to fracture resulting in unstable fixation and the boundary between the transplanted cartilage and native cartilage heals with fibrocartilage.

Osteochondral allografts can be done orthotopically and can be used for partial or whole joint replacement procedures. Popularized by Gross in the 1970's, these allografts were typically fresh and used for all types of defects in many joints including those defects due to tumours and trauma. Historically, these grafts were used in defects that consisted of bone and cartilage but can be used for cartilage-only defects as well. Good to excellent medium- and long-term results have been reported [38-41, 56] but the use of this technique became restricted as concerns regarding transmission of infectious diseases became more prevalent. Considering that this is not a life threatening disorder, the risk of transmission of infectious diseases does not seem warranted (although disease transmission has been very rarely reported) and this method is rarely used. To decrease the risk by allowing more time for testing, hypothermic storage at 4°C was developed and allows the tissues to be stored for 28-42 days prior to transplantation. Unfortunately, cellular deterioration tends to begin after 7-14 days [57, 58]. Given that regulatory clearance takes about 14 days, the viability of the cells within the tissue may not be as healthy as those in fresh allograft or in autograft. Investigations have been ongoing to develop storage techniques that eliminate the possibility of infectious disease transmission and tissue deterioration over time while enabling the creation of a large tissue bank for ready access. Recently we have developed a cryopreservation technique that can store the tissue indefinitely without deterioration and this may improve access to the tissue required for this technique [59]. Despite the limitations of hypothermic storage, there has been a resurgence of osteochondral allografting in recent years. This is the only biologic technique that can resurface whole joints [60, 61] and has been quite successful for partial joint replacements [40, 62]. Bugbee et al [60] have published promising results in total ankle arthroplasty using osteochondral allografts and similar procedures have been performed in Europe [61] but further improvements are required.

3.2. Early osteoarthritic changes

Once osteoarthritic changes become evident, cell based cartilage resurfacing techniques become less relevant due to the generalized nature of the process. There are some surgical techniques that can be used to palliate symptoms depending on the location and severity of the arthritis.

Exostectomies – Occasionally impingement symptoms can be a significant component of arthritis pain. This usually occurs with anterior osteophytes off the distal tibia or talar neck. Occasionally these osteophytes can form around the malleoli. When impingement pain is a prominent feature, removal of the osteophytes, either open or arthroscopically, can be performed with significant improvement of symptoms. The exostectomy can include only the osteophytes itself or also part of the arthritic articular surface leaving only healthier cartilage tissue (Figure 4).

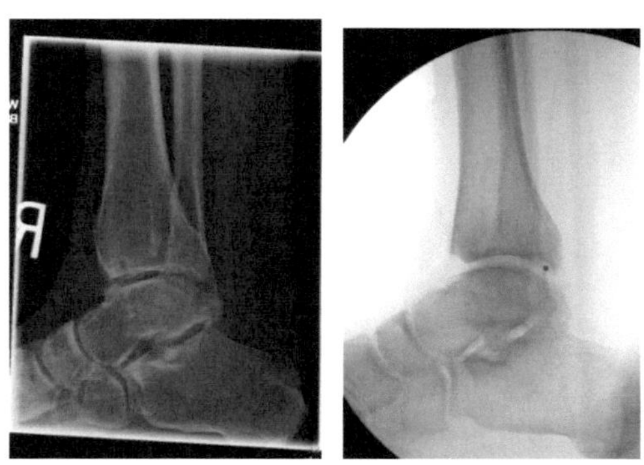

Figure 4. Left image shows preoperative lateral radiograph demonstrating anterior tibial and talar neck osteophytes. Right image shows intraoperative fluoroscopic image after anterior tibial and talar neck exostectomies.

Osteotomies – Occasionally the osteoarthritis is more severe in one portion of the joint. This is often medial or lateral. Offloading the arthritic portion of the joint with a closing (Figure 5), opening wedge osteotomy (Figure 6) or a dome osteotomy (Figure 7) can also provide some symptomatic relief [63-65].

Distraction arthroplasty – Recently, some investigation has gone into determining the effect of distraction arthroplasty. Joint distraction using an external fixator can alter the internal joint environment and possibly improve joint function. Early results are promising, even with more advanced osteoarthritis, but much more work needs to be completed [66].

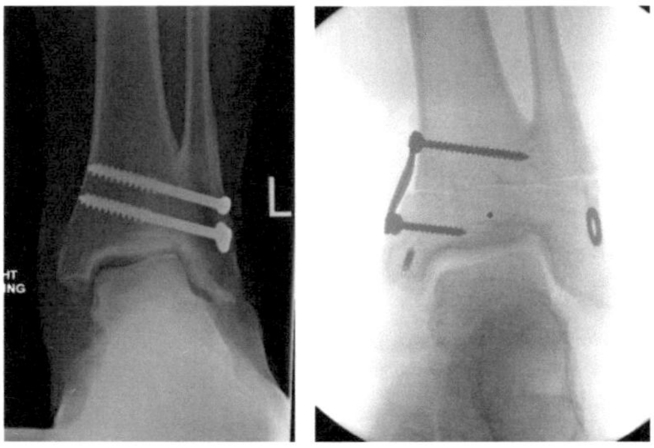

Figure 5. Radiographic images of medial closing wedge osteotomy after a distal tibial-fibular fusion resulted in lateral joint overload. Right image is an intraoperative fluoroscopic view after fixation with a compression staple.

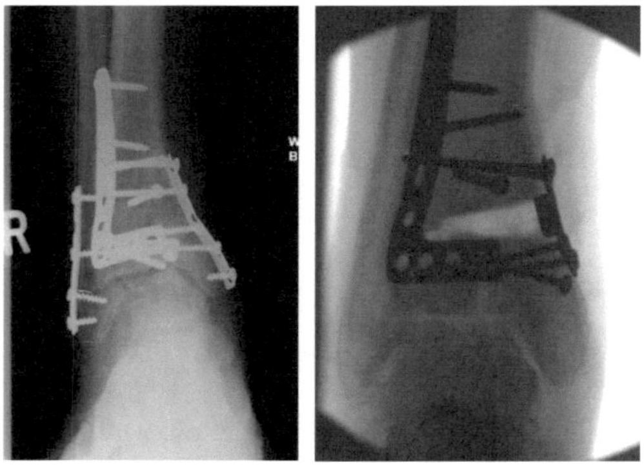

Figure 6. Radiographic images of a medial opening wedge osteotomy after open reduction and internal fixation resulted in a varus malunion. The distal screws were removed from the original plate and an opening wedge osteotomy was performed using an interposition plate.

http://dx.doi.org/10.5772/54224

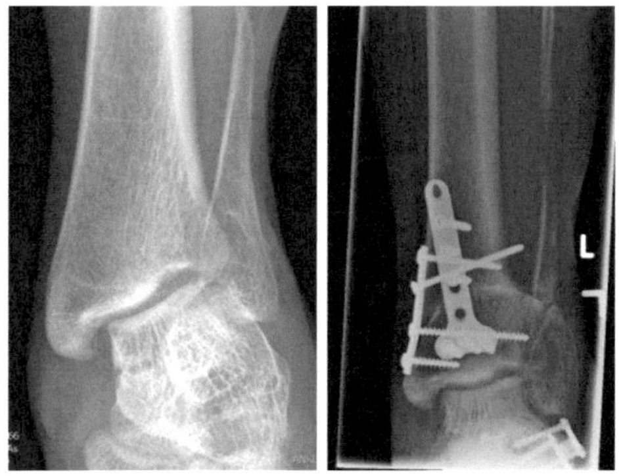

Figure 7. Dome osteotomy of the distal tibia. Original radiograph show severe valgus malunion due to a growth arrest after an open fracture as a child. The dome osteotomy was performed to incorporate the tibia and fibula and rotate the joint as a whole. Medial joint has been fully corrected while the lateral joint remains elevated due to intra-articular incongruity.

3.3. Global osteoarthritis

Once the osteoarthritis becomes global and more severe, the treatment options become more limited. The mainstay of treatment for end-stage ankle arthritis is ankle fusion although synthetic total joint arthroplasty is becoming more common as will be discussed. In addition, total ankle arthroplasty allografting is an experimental technique that has recently been developed that may be used in select cases.

Ankle fusion is the mainstay treatment for end-stage ankle arthritis. It has been performed for over 130 years [67] and there are research stucies that demonstrate the long-term effectiveness [68, 69]. Complications of ankle fusion include nonunion, malunion, infection, nerve injury, persisting pain, loss of ankle range of motion, limp, and arthritis of surrounding joints due to overload [70, 71]. Ankle fusion entails removing all of the remaining articular cartilage from the joint as well as the underlying subchondral bone leaving exposed cancellous bone. The surfaces are shaped so that there is excellent contact between the talar dome and the tibial plafond. Most techniques incorporate the medial malleolus as a medial buttress while some also include the lateral malleolus. Once the surfaces are prepared, internal fixation (occasionally external fixation) is applied. Postoperative splinting in either an aircast or plaster cast is employed for 6-12 weeks with non-weight bearing from 1-12 weeks depending on bone quality and rigidity of fixation and progression of fusion radiographically.

Over the years, many techniques have been described with increasing success with regards to fusion rates. Successful fusion rates can be expected to range from 86-100% depending on patient characteristics and surgical techniques [68, 72-83]. The most commonly used techniques utilize internal fixation. This can be completed using anterior, lateral or posterior approaches. Fixation can be achieved using crossed screws, plate and screws or an intramedullary nail. Another more recent method includes the joint debridement achieved arthroscopically with percutaneous screw fixation. Alternatively, external fixation using standard external fixation techniques or Ilizarov can be used after open joint debridement.

Traditionally, open techniques using an anterior approach going either medial or just lateral to the tibialis anterior tendon have been used. This approach typically provides access to the medial and superior aspects of the joint [75, 77]. This technique can be employed in ankles that do not have much structural deformity. Once the articular surfaces are properly prepared, the talus is compressed into the medial axilla and fixed by a variety of measures including crossed screws [76] (Figure 8), plate and screws [75, 77] or external fixation/Ilizarov [79, 80] (Figure 9). Less commonly, an intramedullary ankle arthrodesis nail can be used for fixation but this must also cross the subtalar joint [78, 83] (Figure 10).

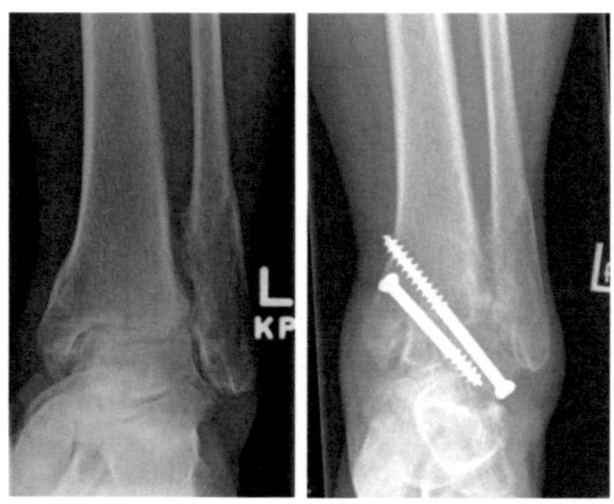

Figure 8. Left image showing severe OA changes but relatively normal structureal anatomy. Right image show fusion using crossed screws with the second screw entering the lateral process of the talus and crossing the joint pushing the talus into the medial axillay of the ankle mortice to achieve extra stability.

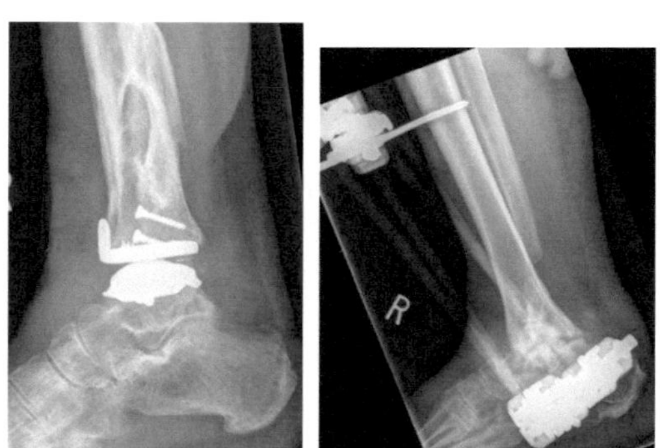

Figure 9. Total ankle replacement complicated by infection. Right image shows ankle replacement removed and attempt fusion using spanning external fixator.

http://dx.doi.org/10.5772/54224

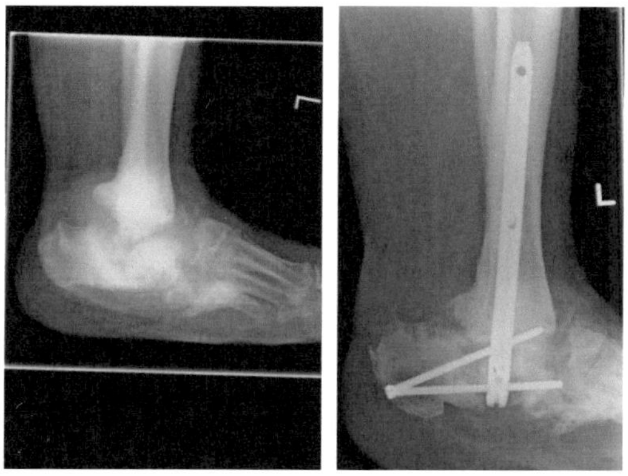

Figure 10. Severe Charcot arthropathy in an obese diabetic patient. Limb salvage ankle fusion using an ankle arthrodesis nail.

In ankles with more significant deformation, especially with bone loss, a more extensive approach may be considered. This entails a lateral approach and employs a fibular osteotomy approximately 5-6cm above the syndesmosis [72, 82] (Figure 11). The fibula is osteotomized obliquely over a 1cm distance and displaced from the tibia using anterior dissection while leaving an intact posterior hinge. The distal fibular segment is split sagitally and the inner ½ removed so that the other ½ (still attached by the posterior soft tissue hinge) can be used as a lateral buttress plate across the joint. Through this lateral incision, the surfaces of the talus and tibial plafond can be prepared for the fusion. This can be supplemented by a small anterior medial incision over the medial gutter for that surface preparation. This approach allows contouring of the fusion surfaces to achieve good bone apposition and to correct mal-alignment. Often supplemental bone graft is required to fill eroded defects. Fixation can be carried out by screws including two screws from the fibular strut into either the tibia and the talus or the tibia alone (to allow talar compression during weightbearing postoperatively).

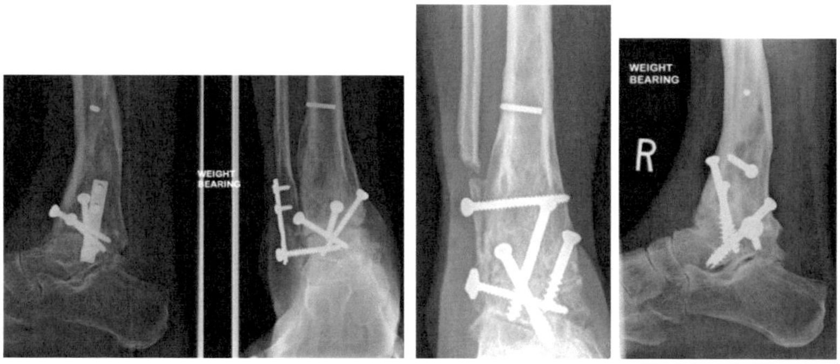

Figure 11. First 2 images on the left show attempted fusion using inadequate screw fixation with screws barely crossing the fusion site while the fibula was left intact despite screws inserted across it. Revision fusion demonstrating the use of the distal fibula as a strut plate graft with proper screw placement to achieve fusion.

Some surgeons prefer the posterior approach to the ankle for fusion [84-86]. This approach can be through or beside the Achilles tendon and can provide good exposure while minimizing risk to compromised anterior soft tissues when present. This approach can be extended to incorporate the subtalar joint in the fusion mass and a blade plate is often used for fixation.

In the circumstances of infection or soft tissue compromise, alternative approaches should be considered. The ankle joint can be adequately debrided with minimal invasiveness using arthroscopy [79, 87, 88] potentially decreasing soft tissue complications. Alternative fixation such as external fixators [78] or the Ilzarov [83] can be used to limit the issues of hardware insertion during ongoing infection. These devices may also be able to correct deformity over time.

As noted, ankle fusion can provide excellent relief of pain with significant improvement of function [89]. Surgical techniques have advanced such that it should be expected to have a 90-100% fusion rate in uncomplicated cases. Meticulous soft tissue handling and intraoperative care can mitigate complications. Despite these results, ongoing concerns of limitations of ankle motion and the increased stress on surrounding joints resulting in increased incidence of arthritis has led to the development of the total ankle arthroplasty as will be discussed in the next section.

4. Arthroplasty implants

4.1. Historical perspective

Total ankle arthroplasties were first introduced in the 1970s [90]. The first prosthesis, created by Lord and Marotte, was designed as an inverted total hip replacement [91]. Although Lord and Marotte's primary results were failures, over the next 20 years, more than 23 designs were developed using that generation's technology from hip and knee replacements characterized by cemented, two component, constrained implants [92]. Despite good initial results using this technology, there were problems with component loosening, severe osteolysis, infection, impingement and soft tissue breakdown [93, 94]. Kitaoka reviewed results of the first generation TAR that included three studies with greater than 5 year follow-up and found a 41% revision rate [95]. The high rate of failure for these first generation implants and difficult salvage procedures tempered enthusiasm and led to questions as to whether the ankle joint could be replaced successfully [92, 95-97]. Hintermann accurately stated, "in an era of joint replacement surgery, ankle procedures have failed to achieve what has been accomplished with other joints" [98].

The first generation implants were designed without proper understanding of ankle biomechanics [99, 100]. The ankle was assumed to be a hinge joint and the rotational and translational motions were not recreated which lead to loosening [97, 101]. These implants were either highly constrained or unconstrained. The highly constrained implants led to large shear and rotational forces that were distributed through a small joint surface and even smaller prosthesis interface [94, 102, 103]. The unconstrained implants were unstable due to lack of attention to soft tissue balancing and failure to address soft tissue impingement [94, 104, 105].

In general, ankle arthroplasties were implanted through an anterior approach to the ankle but the importance of the soft tissue envelope was underestimated and excess traction on the skin led to wound complications [92, 93]. The guides, jigs and instruments were not well designed and sizing was inaccurate so implants were mal-positioned and malleolar fractures were common [92]. Patients were left with mal-aligned implants either because the angular deformity was not corrected at the time of surgery [5] or because the ligaments were ignored leading to problems with functional mal-alignment despite good intraoperative positioning [94, 102]. Finally, most implants were cemented and required large bone resection including up to 17mm on the tibial side and 7mm on the talar side. This caused the implant to be cemented into soft cancellous bone which was unable to support the bone cement interface [92, 106]. Subsidence was further exacerbated by non-anatomically shaped, undersized implants [5, 92, 93, 107]. The aggressive bone resection of the tibia also changed the level of the ankle axis causing alterations in the ankle biomechanics [5]. When function was assessed via gait analysis, there was not as much improvement as had been anticipated. Gait analyses of the first generation implants revealed that patients were subconsciously protecting the joint by not bearing weight normally across the ankle despite denying pain and were not using normal ankle dorsiflexion in the stance phase despite adequate passive dorsiflexion on physical exam [4, 5, 106].

4.2. Biomechanical considerations

In order to understand the reasons for failure and to design a better total ankle arthroplasty, it was important to understand the biomechanics of the foot and ankle. The ankle is a highly constrained joint that does not function as a simple hinge joint because the axis is oblique extending further plantar and posterior on the lateral side. This creates eversion with dorsiflexion and inversion with plantarflexion [108]. Further, the axis of rotation changes throughout the range of motion so that when the ankle moves from a plantarflexed to a dorsiflexed position there is a combination of distraction, sliding and compression [108, 109]. Finally, there are rotational and translational movements that also need to be recreated with a replacement arthroplasty [94, 110].

The most important concepts in the design of an ankle arthroplasty are constraint and congruency. Constraint can be defined as the resistance of an implant to a particular degree of freedom of motion such as anterior-posterior translation or axial rotation [94]. In highly constrained implants such as a hinged ankle replacement, all axial torque forces are translated through the bone-prosthesis interface as shear forces that can lead to component loosening [92, 111]. Congruency or conformity can be defined as the closeness of fit of the various components of the implant [92, 94]. In a fully conforming implant, the articular surface of the tibia has the same radius of curvature as the articulating surface of the talus in both anterior-posterior and medial-lateral directions. This decreases the wear rate because the polyethylene contact stress remains below the fatigue threshold for delamination and pitting [92]. In a partially conforming or incongruent implant the round talus articulates with a flat tibia or there are differences in the radius of curvature of the 2 surfaces [92]. The optimal design for a total ankle replacement is with bearing surfaces that are not only highly conforming to ensure contact throughout the bearing surface thus reducing wear but also sufficiently constrained to give the implant sufficient inherent stability to minimize shear stresses at the prosthesis-bone interface [94, 112].

Second generation implants used these two concepts to improve the design of total ankle arthroplasties. In general, the two primary alternatives were 1) a two component, partially conforming ankle replacement which replaced all three articulations by changing the ankle into a two bone joint by fusing the distal tibia-fibular joint [5, 92] or 2) a three component design which resurfaced the tibio-talar joint and the talar side of the lateral and medial gutters [5, 92]. Third generation implants are more anatomically designed and rely on ligament support as well as hindfoot "balancing" to allow the components to recreate the ankle biomechanics [113].

Gait studies of the newer implants show a satisfactory recovery of the natural overall mobility of the ankle joint in all three planes of motion [114]. Further, in three component designs, there may be some movement of the polyethylene separate from the other components which helps to restore normal biomechanics [114]. Functional motion and muscle-generated moments during walking improved at the ankle joint after arthroplasty – especially plantar flexor muscle function. This function is important because it restrains the forward movement of the tibia during the first half of the gait cycle and brings about plantarflexion of the ankle during the propulsive phase of gait [99]. Brodsky has shown significant improvement in velocity, step length for operated side, total ankle ROM during gait, and maximum sagittal ankle joint power at push-off [115].

4.3. Current implants

Lewis has described key aspects for a successful ankle joint arthroplasty based on careful review of the first and second generation implants [97]. It is important that implant size be designed to balance the need for minimal bone resection with the requirement for sufficient implant to distribute stresses over a large area to decrease the risk of subsidence [97]. The anatomical axis needs to be recreated while also understanding that there is large variability in the axis between individuals [97, 116]. It is also important to recreate all the motions at the ankle joint instead of just plantar flexion and dorsiflexion [97]. This includes talar tilt as the ankle is coupled to the subtalar joint to accommodate to uneven ground, and the rotational motion of internal rotation coupled to plantar flexion and external rotation coupled to dorsiflexion. Failure to understand and recreate these motions will place abnormal stress through the implant-bone interface [97]. It is critical to understand the necessity of ligament support for ankle stability [5]. An implant designed to be sufficiently stable to negate the need for ligament support will transfer abnormal stress to the bone-implant interface leading to loosening [94, 102, 103]. In contrast, an implant designed with low stability that is implanted into an ankle without sufficient ligamentous support will fail due to component mal-alignment or dislocation of the polyethylene [94, 97, 104, 105]. The requirement to withstand high loads means that ultra-high molecular weight polyethylene is generally recommended [97, 117].

Third generation ankle arthroplasties are now in use. The new designs show better understanding of ankle biomechanics and allow for sliding and rotational movements [92]. There are many different third generation implants used across the world and the following discussion provides a representative sample of those commonly used in the Western world but is not inclusive of all implants. The implants will be discussed in relation to design rationale.

The common surgical approach, as will be discussed in further detail later, is an anterior approach in the interval between tibialis anterior tendon and extensor hallucis longus tendon. The neurovascular bundle is carefully protected under the extensor hallucis longus tendon. The major disadvantage of this approach is the high rate of wound healing complications [92, 118, 119]. The BOX ankle replacement (Finsbury Orthopaedics, Leatherhead, Surrey, UK) uses an anterolateral approach between the extensor digitorum longus tendon and the peroneal tertius tendon [112]. The Eclipse (Integra LifeSciences, Plaisboro, NJ) is inserted through either a medial (preferred) or lateral approach [112]. The disadvantage of this approach is the need for fixation of the disrupted medial or lateral malleolus.

The current implants are either mobile (3 component design) or fixed (2 component design) bearing [101]. Mobile bearing designs allow for greater congruence, which can increase the risk of dislocation, but they share the stress through 2 articular surfaces, which may increase weardue to "back side wear" [101, 120]. There is also the potential for "overstuffing" the joint with three component designs in an attempt to reduce the chance of polyethylene dislocation [121]). Overstuffing tightens the joint, increases ligament strain, decreases range of motion and increases the shear stress at the bone-prothesis interface [5, 121]. Fixed bearing designs increase the constraint so they may have higher rates of loosening but have decreased back side wear if the locking mechanism is intact [94, 101]. Current mobile bearing designs include the STAR (Waldemar Link, Hamburg, Germany; 1978)(Figure 12), Buechel-Pappas (Endotec, South Orange, NJ; 1989), Salto (Tornier, Saint Ismier, France; 1997), Hintegra (Integra LifeSciences/Newdeal, Lyon, France; 2002)(Figure 12), Mobility (DePuy International, Leeds, UK; 2005)(Figure 12), BOX (Finsbury Orthopaedics, Leatherhead, Surrey, UK; 2005), CCI Evolution (Van Straten Medical, The Netherlands, 2007), and Zenith (Corin, Cirencester, UK; 2009). Two component designs include the Agility (DePuy/Ace, Warsaw, IN; 1985)(Figure 13), TNK (Kyocera, Kyoto, Japan; 1996), INBONE (Wright Medical Technologies, Arlington, TN; 2005)(Figure 13), Salto Talaris (Tornier, Saint Ismier, France; 2006), and Eclipse (Integra LifeSciences, Plainsboro, NJ; 2007).

Most ankle arthroplasty implants are constructed from cobalt-chromium alloys which are hard, corrosion resistant and biocompatible (Hintegra, Agility, Mobility, Inbone talus, BOX, Salto and Salto-Talaris, and Buechel-Pappas). The CCI Evolution adds molybdenum to the alloy to increase strength (Van Straten Medical, The Netherlands, 2007). The STAR and Inbone (tibia only) use titanium implants which are softer but can be more porous to allow for better ingrowth. The TNK is a ceramic implant (Kyocera, Kyoto, Japan; 1996).

Initial implants were cemented; however, due to the high rate of failure, most implants today are uncemented relying on bone ingrowth stimulated by hydroxyapatite coating, sintered metal beads, plasma spray metals or fiber metals [101]. The different methods to encourage bony ingrowth include ensuring the metal is porous such as the Hintegra which is 20% porous [92]. Some implants, like the STAR, use a single or dual plasma spray. Others use a thin film ceramic coating. The Buechel-Pappas and CCI Evolution use a porous coating covered by a titanium nitride thin-film ceramic [92] which also improves the smoothness of the surface. The Zenith uses the trademarked "BONIT" coating which is the application of a thin calcium phosphate layer to the titanium plasma spray. The last common technique is the use of hydroxyapatite incorporated in the Hintegra [92].

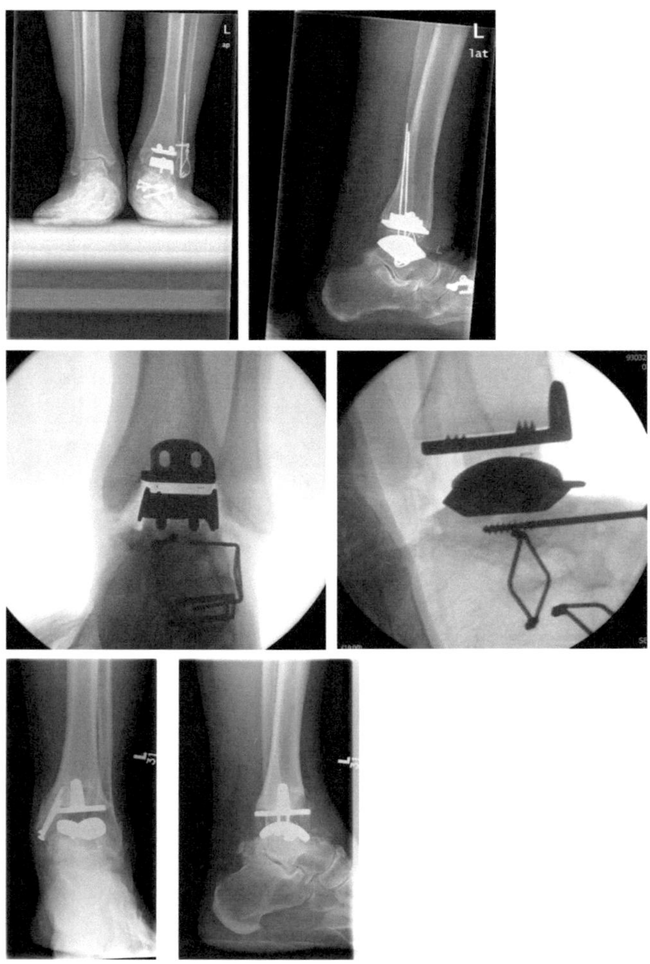

Figure 12. Radiographic images of three currently used mobile bearing total ankle arthroplasty designs. The top two images are STAR, middle two images are Hintegra and the bottom two images are Mobility.

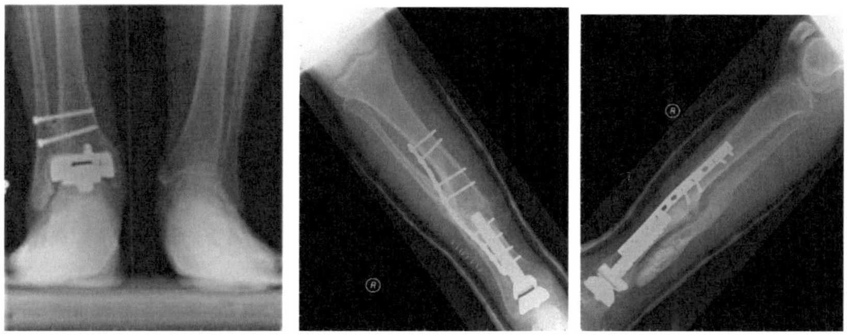

Figure 13. Radiographic images of two currently used fixed bearing total ankle arthroplasty designs. The left image is Agility while the right two images are Inbone.

In most implants the tibial cut is made first. Unlike the knee, the ankle cannot be dislocated sufficiently to allow for intramedullary guides to make the tibial cuts so all ankle arthroplasties, with the exception of the Inbone, use extramedully tibial guides with or without a foot holder. The Inbone uses an external guide and radiographs to guide the insertion of an intramedullary reamer and combines it with a foot holder to place the tibial cutting guide [112]. After the tibial cut has been completed and the intramedullary canal has been reamed, the tibial stem and plate components are inserted one at a time into the joint and built inside the ankle and tibia. The downside of using this intramedullary technique is that the subtalar joint is violated as the tibial canal is reamed retrograde through the calcaneus, talus and then tibia.

Other implants, such as the Buechel-Pappas, Mobility and Agility use intramedullary posts on the tibia to provide fixation by creating an anterior cortical window to insert the tibial component which is then replaced and generally heals without incident. If the tibial component does not have an intramedullary stem, the fixation can be with a fin (CCI Evolution), a fin with a cylinder (Salto), double cylinders (STAR), bars (BOX) or an anterior shield which may or may not be augmented with screws (Hintegra).

Tibial components can either rely on support from the intramedullary stem (Inbone) or cortical bone anteriorly and posteriorly (Hintegra). Some tibial components are rectangular and others are trapezoidal designed to be larger anterior than posterior (STARand CCI Evolution). Finally, while most are flat, they can be designed with a curve (BOX).

The design of the talus implant can be with a symmetrical curve (STAR, Buechel-Pappas, INBONE, Mobility) or asymmetrical so that the radius of curvature for the medial side is less than that for the lateral side (Salto, Hintegra, BOX, CCI Evolution). Most implants resurface the talus (STAR, Buechel-Pappas, Salto, Hintegra, Mobility, BOX, CCI Evolution, and Zenith), but the Inbone and Agility use a flat talar cut. Some designs replace the medial and lateral talar articulations (STAR, Buechel-Pappas, TNK, Salto, and Hintegra) while others do not (Agility, BOX, Mobility, CCI Evolution, and Zenith,). Finally, the polyethylene is ultra-high molecular weight polyethylene in the STAR, Buechel-Pappas, Salto, Hintegra and Inbone.

In summary, the third generation implants have been designed using the knowledge gained from more indepth study of the anatomy and biomechanics of the ankle joint as well as the causes of the failures of the first and second generation implants. When choosing an implant, the surgeon should consider the approach, the need for intramedullary guides and fixation of the tibial component, the relative importance of preserving talar bone stock by resurfacing the talus as opposed to a flat cut, the need for replacing the medial and lateral articulations of the talus, and the role for ultra-high molecular weight polyethylene.

5. Surgical considerations

Clinical indications for total ankle arthroplasty include end stage ankle arthritis that has exhausted all non-operative and joint-sparing operative treatments in a patient willing to undertake the risks of a major surgical procedure. Contraindications to this procedure include:

- Active infection
- Compromised soft tissues
- Inadequate blood supply
- Peripheral neuropathy (including Charcot arthropathy)
- Significant lower extremity neuromuscular impairment
- Severe ligamentous laxity
- Excessive malalignment
- Avascular necrosis of a significant portion of the tibia or talus
- Severe osteoporosis
- Inadequate bone stock
- Skeletal immaturity
- High demand lifestyle
- Pertinent metal allergy
- Sensory or motor dysfunction

Age is not explicitly mentioned as a contraindication in the literature. The safe zone appears to be somewhere after skeletal maturity and in conjunction with the assumption of a low demand lifestyle. Excessive malalignment is a nebulous term. The commonly accepted range is from 15-20 degrees of varus or valgus to not surgically correctable. It would appear that excessive malalignment is relative to the surgeon's skill and experience. Obesity as a contraindication to total ankle arthroplasty is controversial and was not correlated to aseptic loosening in a recent article [122].

5.1. Surgical approach

There are several different types of ankle arthroplasty systems currently on the market as discussed. Each system has unique features best explained by the surgical technique manual provided by the company marketing that system. There are, however, certain common aspects and principles of all of the systems which we will outline in this section.

5.2. Preoperative planning

The condition of the soft tissue envelope including locations of scars and documentation of neurovascular status are important when planning a total ankle arthroplsty. Ankle arthroplasty may be contraindicated in some cases due to an impaired soft tissue envelope or inadequate blood supply to the foot.

Long leg weight-bearing views will help identify concurrent ipsilateral limb deformities which may affect ankle alignment. Anteroposterior and lateral views of the tibia are also important because intraoperative alignment is usually referenced off of the tibia. Weightbearing anteroposterior and lateral views of the ankle and foot are important to assess the joint being replaced but also to identify coexisting deformities and/or arthritis affecting the rest of the foot which may affect the surgical plan resulting in additional procedures that can be performed in a staged manner or concurrently depending on surgeon skill and preference.

5.3. Positioning

The patient is positioned supine on a radiolucent table to allow fluoroscopic guidance of the procedure. The ipsilateral hip is supported to prop the foot perpendicular to the floor to allow easy access to both the medial and lateral aspects of the joint and enable evaluation of alignment intraoperatively. Rotation of the foot relative to the leg on the contralateral side should be noted before prepping and draping to determine what is normal for that patient.

5.4. Prepping and draping

A thigh tourniquet is utilized to provide hemostasis during the procedure. The leg is prepped and draped as a free extremity right up to the tourniquet to provide access to the knee. Many total ankle arthroplasty systems use the length of the tibia and an external alignment device as a guide to proper alignment.

5.5. Surgical exposure

The most common surgical approach to the ankle for insertion of a total ankle arthroplasty is the anterior approach. Some systems that involve tibiofibular fusion as part of the procedure may require and an additional lateral incision but still utilize the anterior approach as well. An incision is made over the anterior aspect of the ankle midway between the malleoli (Figure 14). The incision needs to be long enough to allow placement of the distal tibial cutting block and visualization of the talar neck. Care is taken to minimize injury to the branches of the superficial and deep peroneal nerves. The retinaculum is then split to expose the underlying tendons. The extensor hallucis longus tendon will be retracted laterally to protect the underlying neurovascular structures which should be located deep and lateral to the extensor hallucis longus tendon (Figures 14 and 15). If possible, the sheath of the tibialis anterior should be left intact to prevent undue pressure on the wound post-operatively (Figure 16). The anterior capsule is incised vertically and then peeled away in a subperiosteal plane medially and laterally to expose the joint (Figure 17). One should be able to see the medial malleolus clearly but the lateral malleolus is more posterior and often is not as easily seen.

Distal tibial osteophytes are now removed taking note of a commonly occurring large osteophyte anterior to the fibula. Care should be taken to differentiate the osteophyte from the fibula itself. There will also be osteophytes on the neck of the talus which can be removed with a curette, rongeur or burr to reestablish its normal contour. This will help with cutting block placement and ankle positioning when cuts are made (Figure 18).

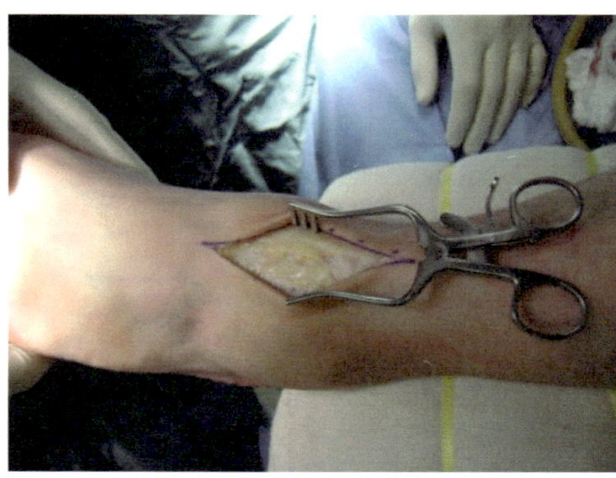

Figure 14. Anterior incision midway between the malleoli. Toes are to the left and knee is to the right. Blunt retractors and extreme soft tissue care are required.

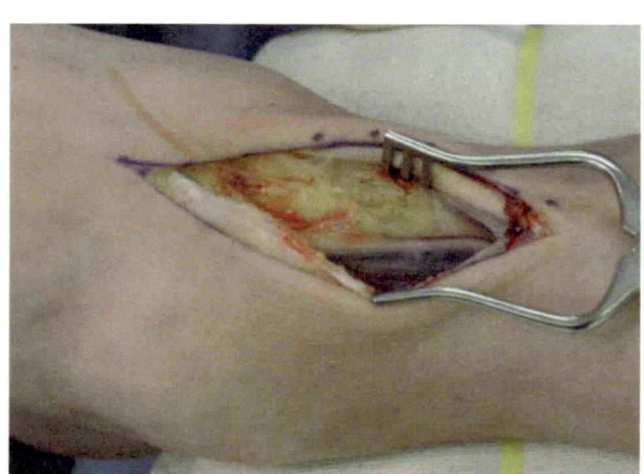

Figure 15. Exposure of the neurovascular bundle by retraction of the extensor hallucis longus tendon.

http://dx.doi.org/10.5772/54224

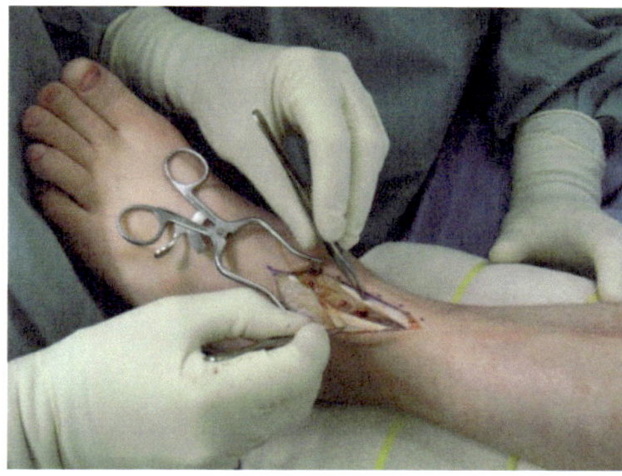

Figure 16. Tibialis anterior sheath.

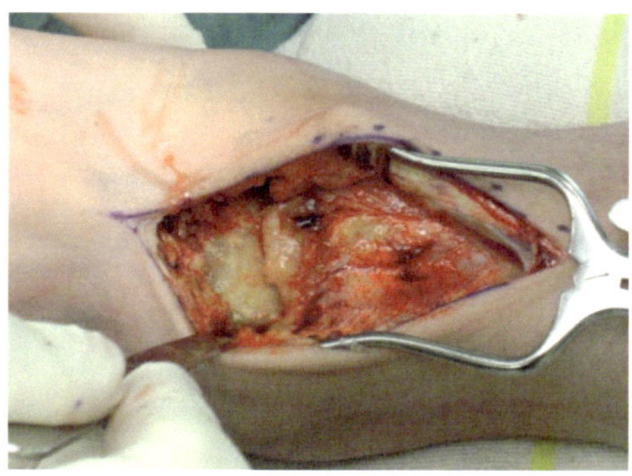

Figure 17. Exposure of the joint.

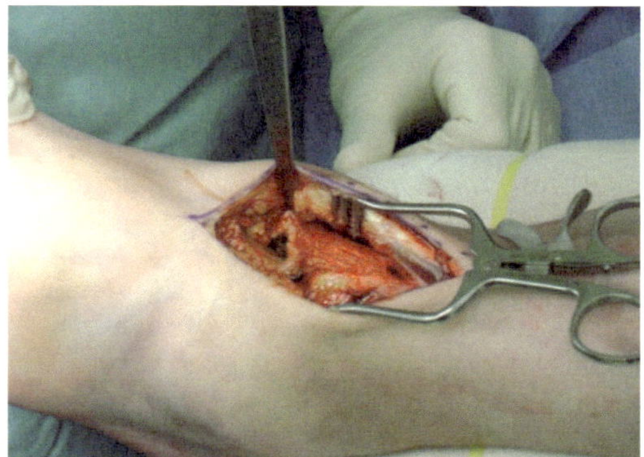

Figure 18. Anterior tibial osteophyte requires removal.

The soft tissues should be handled with extreme caution. Blunt self-retaining retractors should be repositioned periodically to prevent prolonged pressure on the soft tisse. Care should be taken with the bone as well. Levering on the medial malleolus may result in fracture. Notching the fibula during the distal tibial resection can result in fracture as well. Exposure can be facilitated by instruments such as laminar spreaders, distractors and various retractors. Performing the talar cuts can also facilitate removal of posterior malleolar fragments in systems that require this.

5.6. Alignment

The tibia is used to guide placement of the cutting blocks either with an external rod placed parallel to the shaft of the tibia by direct visualization or overlapped with the tibial canal fluoroscopically. The distal tibia is cut perpendicular to the anatomical axis of the tibia in the coronal plane. Most systems build in a posterior slope to the distal tibial cut in the sagittal plane and this can be adjusted in certain cases to allow more or less slope depending on the patient's needs. Longitudinal alignment of the talar component is usually in line with the second ray of the foot.

5.7. Ligamentous balancing

Ligamentous balancing is not yet as sophisticated as for total knee arthroplasty. The posterior capsule is resected during the removal of the posterior malleolus. Medially, the deltoid ligament can be released in a subperiosteal plane from the medial malleolus and/or talus, pie-crusted, released mid-substance or relatively lengthened through a medial malleolar osteotomy [123-126]. Laterally, the talofibular ligaments should be treated with care. Aggressive release from the talus can result in iatrogenic lateral instability. If there is a preexisting lateral instability, consent should be obtained for a lateral ligament reconstruction if required. Generally, stability is assessed after the bony cuts are made. A gastrocsoleus slide or Achilles tendon lengthening may be required if the ankle does dorsiflex past neutral after the ankle arthroplasty has been performed.

5.8. Closure

Repair of the extensor retinaculum during closure is very important. If left uncovered, the tibialis anterior may erode through the incision putting the arthroplasty and possibly even the leg at risk.

5.9. Post-op care

In the case of an uncomplicated ankle arthroplasty with no extra ligament reconstruction or fusion the patient has a short period of non-weight-bearing activity in a splint or cast followed by weight-bearing activity in a cast until the six week post-operative visit. Subsequently, physiotherapy to work on dorsiflexion and plantar flexion, gait retraining and leg strengthening is initiated.

There are no guidelines in regards to deep venous thrombosis (DVT) prophylaxis after total ankle arthroplasty but it would prudent to use propylaxis in patients with significant risk factors. Obesity, previous venous thromboembolism, and absence of full postoperative weightbearing were identified as risk factors for the development of DVT in a study on total ankle arthroplasty in the obese [122]. The importance of these risk factors was echoed by Barg et al in their article looking at risk factors for DVT in total ankle arthroplasty patients who were give thromboprophylaxis [127]. Other factors associated with increased incidence of DVTs include cancer, use of high dose estrogen replacement, and smoking.

5.10. Radiological follow-up

Ankle replacements should be followed radiologically as well as clinically in the post-operative period including weightbearing anteroposterior and lateral x-rays. One should look for changes in position which would indicate loosening of the components. Persistent periprosthetic lucencies should be followed for progression. There are a variety of angular measurements based on anatomical axes and component position as well as standardized distances from anatomical landmarks to component landmarks that can be used to assess technical success of prostheses implantation or subsequent subsidence [128].

5.11. Complications

The complications associated with total ankle arthroplasty would be familiar to any shoulder, hip or knee arthroplasty surgeon. and can be classified in different ways. Glazebrook et al recently published an evidence-based classification system that groups complications according to their correlation with failure of the prosthesis [3]. The goal of this classification system is to provide prognostic information to help surgeons deal with complications more effectively. To develop this classification system, the current literature on second and third generation prosthetic ankle arthroplasty outcomes were reviewed. Based on this information they were able to provide a summary of total ankle arthroplasty implant survival and complication rates. Twenty studies met their inclusion criteria with follow-up periods ranging from two to twelve years. In total 2,386 ankle arthroplasties were reviewed. They reported nine main complications including:

- Subsidence – 10.7%
- Aseptic loosening – 8.7%
- Intra-op fracture – 8.1%
- Wound healing problem – 6.6%
- Technical error – 6.0%
- Implant failure – 5.0%
- Non-union – 4.4%
- Post-op bone fracture – 2.0%

- Deep infection – 1.7%

These complications were compiled into three groups depending on how likely the complication would lead to failure of the arthroplasty. The three complications that lead to arthroplasty failure greater than 50% of the time were deep infection, aseptic loosening and implant failure. Other complications not included in this review that should be noted include tendon laceration, nerve injury, and instability (due to ligamentous imbalance). Impingement is another complication that is minor in terms of prosthesis survival but can have a significant effect in terms of patient satisfaction. It is usually medial and can be caused by osteophytes, scar tissue or tibialis posterior tendon degeneration.

5.12. Outcomes

In order to evaluate the outcomes of contemproary total ankle arthroplasty, it is instructive to look at the results published by joint registries from around the world. While not as common as registries for total hip and knee arthroplasty, there are at least four registries reported in the literature.

In 2007 the Norwegian registry reported on their experiences with total ankle arthroplasty [129]. This registry looked at 257 joints implanted between 1994 and 2005. This included a small number of cemented implants. The average age at the time of implantation was 58 for women and 60 for men. The The 5-year survival rate was 89% and the 10-year survival rate was 76%. There was no difference in the survival rates of the cemented and cementless prostheses.

The New Zealand registry reported on 202 joints in total also in 2007 [130]. This included both second and third generation prostheses. The average age of the patients at the time of implantation was 65. The most common diagnosis was primary osteoarthritis. The 5-year survival rate was 86%.

In 2010 the Finnish registry published their results on 573 total ankle arthroplasties [131]. These were all third-generation mobile-bearing designs. The average age of the patients was 55. The 5-year survival was 83%.

The Swedish Registry reported on the ten year survival of 780 third-generation total ankle arthoplasties in 2011 [132]. The registry included a variety of uncemented, three component implants. Revision rate was used as the primary outcome variable. The overall 10 year survival rate was 69% although this increased to 78% of the STAR prostheses were excluded. It is interesting to note that the other registries did include the STAR prostheses in their results.

Overall, age, sex, and diangosis did not affect survival in the Norwegian, New Zealand or Finnish registries. The Swedish registry, however, found that the risk for revision was higher in female patients under 60 years of age with a diagnosis of primary osteoarthritis or posttraumatic arthritis.

There have been a lot of outcome studies published in recent years but a disproportionate number have been published by the prostheses designers themselves according to Labek et al [133]. Approximately 50% of the publications reporting on total ankle arthroplasty outcomes have been produced by implant developers. Furthermore, the revision rates from the national registries (Swedish, Norwegian and New Zealand) have a much higher revision rate than those published in peer-reviewed scientific journals that include the manufacturers' reports [133].

That said, it is still worthwhile to look at all of the published data. There have been three relatively recent reviews of total ankle arthroplasty outcome study data [69, 134, 135]. The most recent one was published by Gougoulias et al in 2010 [134]. They included thirteen Level IV studies looking at 1105 total ankle arthroplasties. The most common diagnosis was posttraumatic arthritis. The overall failure rate was approximately 10% at 5 years. Range of motion did not change in one study and improved by 4-14 degrees in four others. In the studies reporting them, there were superficial wound complications in 0-14%, and deep infections in 0-4.6%. In seven studies, rates of residual pain in the hindfoot ranged from 23 to 60%. Interestingly, the most common sporting activities after total ankle arthroplasty were identified as swimming, cycling and fitness/weight training.

In an older review published in 2007 by Haddad et al, the intermediate outcomes of total ankle arthroplasty and ankle fusion were compared [69]. They looked at ten papers which evaluated total ankle arthroplasty and thirty-nine which looked at ankle fusion. The mean American Orthopaedic Foot and Ankle Society Ankle Hindfoot score was 78.2 for the arthroplasty group and 75.6 for the fusion group. The average age of patients undergoing arthroplasty was 58 and fusion 50. The majority of the fusion patients were male, while the major of the arthroplasty patients were female. Rheumatoid arthritis was the primary indication for total ankle arthroplasty, posttraumatic arthritis for fusion. The 5-year implant survival rate for the arthroplasty group was 90%, while the 10-year survival rate was 77%. They noted that a weakness of their review was that there were no direct comparisons of total ankle arthroplasty to ankle fusion.

Stengel et al's review in 2005 identified 10 adequate studies with a total of 497 ankle arthroplasties [135]. The total ankle arthroplasty patients showed a mean improvement in hindfoot scores of 45.2 points. Range of motion improved an average of 6.3%. Complications ranged from a 1.6% deep infection rate to a 14.7% impingement rate. The five year prosthesis survival rate was 90.6%.

Since the publication of the most recent of the above reviews, there have been some other publications of note. The long-term results of the United States STAR trial were published in 2011 [136]. They prospectively followed 80 patients treated with 84 STAR prostheses. The average age at implantation was 61 years. Their American Orthopaedic Foot and Ankle Society ankle-hindoot scores improved from an average of 42.7 to 81.9 points. Average range of motion was 39.5 degrees. Implant survival was 96% at 5 years and 90% at 10 years.

Bonnin et al recently published the long term follow-up of patients they had implanted with the SALTO total ankle arthroplasty and reported on previously [137]. They analyzed 98 prostheses with and average followup of 8.9 years. The mean American Foot and Ankle Society ankle-hindfoot score was 79. Range of motion was 27 degrees. The survival rate was

85% with an end point being the revision of a component. Limitations of this study included the series of patients being operated on by the implant designers and the implants and technique changed during the course of the study.

Wood et al compared the STAR implant to the Buechel-Pappas implant in a randomised trial [138]. The study involved 200 joint replacements. They were followed out for 6 years. The STAR survivorship was 95% and the Buechel-Pappas 79% with the end point being revision. The difference was not found to be statistically different.

Total ankle arthroplasty has been shown to improve ankle joint mechanics. Hahn et al demonstrated that both arthroplasty and fusion impoved gait function and reduced pain but that arthroplasty patients gained a more natural ankle joint function with increased range of motion [139]. Piriou et al were also interested in how gait was affected by total ankle arthroplasty [140]. They compared 12 arthroplasty patients to 12 fusion and 12 control patients. Neither the arthroplasty patients nor the fusion patients regained normal movement or walking speed, but the arthroplasty group had greater movement at the ankle, more symmetrical timing of gait and better restored ground reaction force patterns than the fusion group. The fusion group had a faster gait and longer step length than the arthroplasty group. Schuh et al compared 21 ankle fusion patients to 20 total ankle arthroplasty patients in regards to sport and recreational activities as well as functional outcome directly [89]. They found no signifcant difference between the groups concerning activity levels, participation in sports activities.

Finally, despite improved motion and decreased pain, total ankle arthroplasty does not result in weight loss. Penner at al investigated weight loss after total ankle arthroplasty and found that although pain and disability were reduced in overweight and obese patients after both ankle arthroplasty and fusion, the mean body mass index (BMI) remained unchanged [141].

6. Conclusion

Ankle arthritis can be a debilitating disorder as disabling mentally and physically as hip arthritis. There are a myriad of nonoperative and joint sparing operative treatments that can improved symptoms but do not arrest the disease process. When end-stage osteoarthritis develops, the gold standard has been ankle fusion. Some limitations to a successful ankle fusion such as stiffness and arthritic progression of surrounding joints as well as the successful replacements of the hip and knee joint led to the development of total ankle arthroplasty. Second and third generation prostheses have markedly improved function and long-term results compared to first generation prostheses. Although the procedure can be technically demanding and is associated with numerous potential complications, patients generally experience improved function and decreased pain. Based on current literature, it seems reasonable to expect an 80% prosthesis survival after 10 years. Further investigations into ankle joint mechanics, risk factors for implant failure and methods to minimize complications should lead to additional improvements in long-term outcomes. Finally, prospective, long-

http://dx.doi.org/10.5772/54224

term direct comparison studies of ankle fusion versus total ankle arthroplasty are required to determine which procedure is best for which patient.

Acknowledgements

Orthotic photographs provided by Orthotic Solutions, Edmonton, Alberta, Canada.

Author details

Nadr M. Jomha, Angela Scharfenberger, Gordon Goplen and M. Elizabeth Pedersen

*Address all correspondence to: njomha@ualberta.ca

Division of Orthopaedic Surgery, Department of Surgery, University of Alberta, Edmonton, Alberta, Canada

References

[1] Buckwalter JA, Saltzman C, Brown T. The impact of osteoarthritis: implications for research. Clin Orthop Relat Res. 2004 Oct(427 Suppl):S6-15.

[2] Saltzman CL. Ankle Arthritis. In: Coughlin M, Mann R, Saltzman C, eds. *Surgery of the foot and ankle*. 8th ed. Philadelphia, PA: Mosby Elselvier 2007:928.

[3] Glazebrook M, Daniels T, Younger A, Foote CJ, Penner M, Wing K, et al. Comparison of health-related quality of life between patients with end-stage ankle and hip arthrosis. J Bone Joint Surg Am. 2008 Mar;90(3):499-505.

[4] Stauffer RN, Chao EY, Brewster RC. Force and motion analysis of the normal, diseased, and prosthetic ankle joint. Clin Orthop Relat Res. 1977(127):189-96.

[5] Thomas RH, Daniels TR. Ankle arthritis. J Bone Joint Surg Am. 2003 May;85-A(5): 923-36.

[6] Valderrabano V, Horisberger M, Russell I, Dougall H, Hintermann B. Etiology of ankle osteoarthritis. Clin Orthop Relat Res. 2009 Jul;467(7):1800-6.

[7] Khazzam M, Long JT, Marks RM, Harris GF. Preoperative gait characterization of patients with ankle arthrosis. Gait & posture. 2006 Aug;24(1):85-93.

[8] Valderrabano V, Hintermann B, Dick W. Scandinavian total ankle replacement: a 3.7-year average followup of 65 patients. Clin Orthop Relat Res. 2004 Jul(424):47-56.

[9] Bombardier C, Laine L, Reicin A, Shapiro D, Burgos-Vargas R, Davis B, et al. Comparison of upper gastrointestinal toxicity of rofecoxib and naproxen in patients with

rheumatoid arthritis. VIGOR Study Group. The New England journal of medicine. 2000 Nov 23;343(21):1520-8, 2 p following 8.

[10] Silverstein FE, Faich G, Goldstein JL, Simon LS, Pincus T, Whelton A, et al. Gastrointestinal toxicity with celecoxib vs nonsteroidal anti-inflammatory drugs for osteoarthritis and rheumatoid arthritis: the CLASS study: A randomized controlled trial. Celecoxib Long-term Arthritis Safety Study. Jama. 2000 Sep 13;284(10):1247-55.

[11] Muller-Fassbender H, Bach GL, Haase W, Rovati LC, Setnikar I. Glucosamine sulfate compared to ibuprofen in osteoarthritis of the knee. Osteoarthritis Cartilage. 1994 Mar;2(1):61-9.

[12] Lopes Vaz A. Double-blind clinical evaluation of the relative efficacy of ibuprofen and glucosamine sulphate in the management of osteoarthrosis of the knee in out-patients. Current medical research and opinion. 1982;8(3):145-9.

[13] Reginster JY, Deroisy R, Rovati LC, Lee RL, Lejeune E, Bruyere O, et al. Long-term effects of glucosamine sulphate on osteoarthritis progression: a randomised, placebo-controlled clinical trial. Lancet. 2001 Jan 27;357(9252):251-6.

[14] Lee YH, Woo JH, Choi SJ, Ji JD, Song GG. Effect of glucosamine or chondroitin sulfate on the osteoarthritis progression: a meta-analysis. Rheumatology international. 2010 Jan;30(3):357-63.

[15] Hughes R, Carr A. A randomized, double-blind, placebo-controlled trial of glucosamine sulphate as an analgesic in osteoarthritis of the knee. Rheumatology (Oxford). 2002 Mar;41(3):279-84.

[16] Wandel S, Juni P, Tendal B, Nuesch E, Villiger PM, Welton NJ, et al. Effects of glucosamine, chondroitin, or placebo in patients with osteoarthritis of hip or knee: network meta-analysis. BMJ (Clinical research ed. 2010;341:c4675.

[17] Pekarek B, Osher L, Buck S, Bowen M. Intra-articular corticosteroid injections: a critical literature review with up-to-date findings. Foot (Edinburgh, Scotland). 2011 Jun; 21(2):66-70.

[18] Stitek T, Jong K, Gazzilo G, Lee C. *Injection procedures: Osteoarthritis and related conditions*. Newark, NJ: Springer Science and Business Media 2011:67-89.

[19] Abate M, Schiavone C, Salini V. Hyaluronic acid in ankle osteoarthritis: why evidence of efficacy is still lacking? Clin Exp Rheumatol. 2012 Mar-Apr;30(2):277-81.

[20] Migliore A, Giovannangeli F, Bizzi E, Massafra U, Alimonti A, Lagana B, et al. Viscosupplementation in the management of ankle osteoarthritis: a review. Arch Orthop Trauma Surg. 2011 Jan;131(1):139-47.

[21] DeGroot H, 3rd, Uzunishvili S, Weir R, Al-omari A, Gomes B. Intra-articular injection of hyaluronic acid is not superior to saline solution injection for ankle arthritis: a randomized, double-blind, placebo-controlled study. J Bone Joint Surg Am. 2012 Jan 4;94(1):2-8.

[22] De Smet AA, Ilahi OA, Graf BK. Untreated osteochondritis dissecans of the femoral condyles: prediction of patient outcome using radiographic and MR findings. Skeletal Radiol. 1997;26(8):463-7.

[23] Hughston JC, Hergenroeder PT, Courtenay BG. Osteochondritis dissecans of the femoral condyles. J Bone Joint Surg [Am]. 1984;66(9):1340-8.

[24] Apprich S, Trattnig S, Welsch GH, Noebauer-Huhmann IM, Sokolwski M, Hirschfeld C, et al. Assessment of articular cartilage repair tissue after matrix-associated autologous chondrocyte transplantation or the microfracture technique in the ankle joint using diffusion-weighted imaging at 3 Tesla. Osteoarthritis Cartilage. 2012 Jul;20(7): 703-11.

[25] Saxena A, Eakin C. Articular talar injuries in athletes: results of microfracture and autogenous bone graft. Am J Sports Med. 2007 Oct;35(10):1680-7.

[26] Doral MN, Bilge O, Batmaz G, Donmez G, Turhan E, Demirel M, et al. Treatment of osteochondral lesions of the talus with microfracture technique and postoperative hyaluronan injection. Knee Surg Sports Traumatol Arthrosc. 2012;20:1298-403.

[27] Becher C, Driessen A, Hess T, Longo UG, Maffulli N, Thermann H. Microfracture for chondral defects of the talus: maintenance of early results at midterm follow-up. Knee Surg Sports Traumatol Arthrosc. 2010 May;18(5):656-63.

[28] Brittberg M, Lindahl A, Nilsson A, Ohlsson C, Isaksson O, Peterson L. Treatment of deep cartilage defects in the knee with autologous chondrocyte transplantation. The New England journal of medicine. 1994;331(14):889-95.

[29] Battaglia M, Vannini F, Buda R, Cavallo M, Ruffilli A, Monti C, et al. Arthroscopic autologous chondrocyte implantation in osteochondral lesions of the talus: mid-term T2-mapping MRI evaluation. Knee Surg Sports Traumatol Arthrosc. 2011 Aug;19(8): 1376-84.

[30] Dixon S, Harvey L, Baddour E, Janes G, Hardisty G. Functional outcome of matrix-associated autologous chondrocyte implantation in the ankle. Foot Ankle Int. 2011 Apr;32(4):368-74.

[31] Giza E, Sullivan M, Ocel D, Lundeen G, Mitchell ME, Veris L, et al. Matrix-induced autologous chondrocyte implantation of talus articular defects. Foot Ankle Int. 2010 Sep;31(9):747-53.

[32] Saris DB, Vanlauwe J, Victor J, Haspl M, Bohnsack M, Fortems Y, et al. Characterized chondrocyte implantation results in better structural repair when treating symptomatic cartilage defects of the knee in a randomized controlled trial versus microfracture. Am J Sports Med. 2008 Feb;36(2):235-46.

[33] Liu W, Liu F, Zhao W, Kim JM, Wang Z, Vrahas MS. Osteochondral autograft transplantation for acute osteochondral fractures associated with an ankle fracture. Foot Ankle Int. 2011 Apr;32(4):437-42.

[34] Gobbi A, Francisco RA, Lubowitz JH, Allegra F, Canata G. Osteochondral lesions of the talus: randomized controlled trial comparing chondroplasty, microfracture, and osteochondral autograft transplantation. Arthroscopy. 2006 Oct;22(10):1085-92.

[35] Valderrabano V, Leumann A, Rasch H, Egelhof T, Hintermann B, Pagenstert G. Knee-to-ankle mosaicplasty for the treatment of osteochondral lesions of the ankle joint. Am J Sports Med. 2009 Nov;37 Suppl 1:105S-11S.

[36] Hangody L, Dobos J, Balo E, Panics G, Hangody LR, Berkes I. Clinical experiences with autologous osteochondral mosaicplasty in an athletic population: a 17-year prospective multicenter study. Am J Sports Med. 2010 Jun;38(6):1125-33.

[37] Hangody L, Kish G, Modis L, Szerb I, Gaspar L, Dioszegi Z, et al. Mosaicplasty for the treatment of osteochondritis dissecans of the talus: two to seven year results in 36 patients. Foot Ankle Int. 2001;22(7):552-8.

[38] El-Rashidy H, Villacis D, Omar I, Kelikian AS. Fresh osteochondral allograft for the treatment of cartilage defects of the talus: a retrospective review. J Bone Joint Surg Am. 2011 Sep 7;93(17):1634-40.

[39] Adams SB, Jr., Viens NA, Easley ME, Stinnett SS, Nunley JA, 2nd. Midterm results of osteochondral lesions of the talar shoulder treated with fresh osteochondral allograft transplantation. J Bone Joint Surg Am. 2011 Apr 6;93(7):648-54.

[40] Aubin PP, Cheah HK, Davis AM, Gross AE. Long-term followup of fresh femoral osteochondral allografts for posttraumatic knee defects. Clin Orthop. 2001(391 Suppl):S318-27.

[41] Tontz WL, Jr., Bugbee WD, Brage ME. Use of allografts in the management of ankle arthritis. Foot Ankle Clin. 2003 Jun;8(2):361-73, xi.

[42] Garcia EJ, Bear RR, Schoenfeld AJ, Owens BD. Treatment of osteochondral lesions of the talus with a biosynthetic scaffold: a report of four cases. J Bone Joint Surg Am. 2010 Jul 21;92(8):1774-9.

[43] Giannini S, Buda R, Vannini F, Cavallo M, Grigolo B. One-step bone marrow-derived cell transplantation in talar osteochondral lesions. Clin Orthop Relat Res. 2009 Dec; 467(12):3307-20.

[44] Barnewitz D, Endres M, Kruger I, Becker A, Zimmermann J, Wilke I, et al. Treatment of articular cartilage defects in horses with polymer-based cartilage tissue engineering grafts. Biomaterials. 2006 May;27(14):2882-9.

[45] Candrian C, Barbero A, Bonacina E, Francioli S, Hirschmann MT, Milz S, et al. A novel implantation technique for engineered osteo-chondral grafts. Knee Surg Sports Traumatol Arthrosc. 2009 Nov;17(11):1377-83.

[46] Lee KB, Bai LB, Yoon TR, Jung ST, Seon JK. Second-look arthroscopic findings and clinical outcomes after microfracture for osteochondral lesions of the talus. Am J Sports Med. 2009 Nov;37 Suppl 1:63S-70S.

[47] Nam EK, Ferkel RD, Applegate GR. Autologous chondrocyte implantation of the ankle: a 2- to 5-year follow-up. Am J Sports Med. 2009 Feb;37(2):274-84.

[48] Giannini S, Battaglia M, Buda R, Cavallo M, Ruffilli A, Vannini F. Surgical treatment of osteochondral lesions of the talus by open-field autologous chondrocyte implantation: a 10-year follow-up clinical and magnetic resonance imaging T2-mapping evaluation. Am J Sports Med. 2009 Nov;37 Suppl 1:112S-8S.

[49] Matricali GA, Bartels W, Labey L, Dereymaeker GP, Luyten FP, Vander Sloten J. Changes in contact area characteristics of the ankle after a cartilage biopsy at the postero-medial rim of the talar dome. Osteoarthritis Cartilage. 2009 Nov;17(11):1477-84.

[50] Giannini S, Buda R, Vannini F, Di Caprio F, Grigolo B. Arthroscopic autologous chondrocyte implantation in osteochondral lesions of the talus: surgical technique and results. Am J Sports Med. 2008 May;36(5):873-80.

[51] Schneider TE, Karaikudi S. Matrix-Induced Autologous Chondrocyte Implantation (MACI) grafting for osteochondral lesions of the talus. Foot Ankle Int. 2009 Sep;30(9):810-4.

[52] Thermann H, Driessen A, Becher C. [Autologous chondrocyte transplantation in the treatment of articular cartilage lesions of the talus]. Der Orthopade. 2008 Mar;37(3):232-9.

[53] Lim HC, Bae JH, Song SH, Park YE, Kim SJ. Current treatments of isolated articular cartilage lesions of the knee achieve similar outcomes. Clin Orthop Relat Res. 2012 Aug;470(8):2261-7.

[54] Kilic A, Kabukcuoglu Y, Gul M, Ozkaya U, Sokucu S. [Early results of open mosaicplasty in osteochondral lesions of the talus]. Acta orthopaedica et traumatologica turcica. 2009 May-Jul;43(3):235-42.

[55] Reddy S, Pedowitz DI, Parekh SG, Sennett BJ, Okereke E. The morbidity associated with osteochondral harvest from asymptomatic knees for the treatment of osteochondral lesions of the talus. Am J Sports Med. 2007 Jan;35(1):80-5.

[56] Hahn DB, Aanstoos ME, Wilkins RM. Osteochondral lesions of the talus treated with fresh talar allografts. Foot Ankle Int. 2010 Apr;31(4):277-82.

[57] Williams SK, Amiel D, Ball ST, Allen RT, Wong VW, Chen AC, et al. Prolonged storage effects on the articular cartilage of fresh human osteochondral allografts. J Bone Joint Surg Am. 2003 Nov;85-A(11):2111-20.

[58] Ball ST, Amiel D, Williams SK, Tontz W, Chen AC, Sah RL, et al. The effects of storage on fresh human osteochondral allografts. Clin Orthop Relat Res. 2004 Jan(418):246-52.

[59] Jomha NM, Elliott JA, Law GK, Maghdoori B, Fraser Forbes J, Abazari A, et al. Vitrification of intact human articular cartilage. Biomaterials. 2012 Sep;33(26):6061-8.

[60] Meehan R, McFarlin S, Bugbee W, Brage M. Fresh ankle osteochondral allograft transplantation for tibiotalar joint arthritis. Foot Ankle Int. 2005 Oct;26(10):793-802.

[61] Giannini S, Buda R, Grigolo B, Bevoni R, Di Caprio F, Ruffilli A, et al. Bipolar fresh osteochondral allograft of the ankle. Foot Ankle Int. 2010 Jan;31(1):38-46.

[62] Bugbee WD, Convery FR. Osteochondral allograft transplantation. Clinics in sports medicine. 1999;18(1):67-75.

[63] Mann HA, Filippi J, Myerson MS. Intra-articular opening medial tibial wedge osteotomy (plafond-plasty) for the treatment of intra-articular varus ankle arthritis and instability. Foot Ankle Int. 2012 Apr;33(4):255-61.

[64] Knupp M, Stufkens SA, van Bergen CJ, Blankevoort L, Bolliger L, van Dijk CN, et al. Effect of supramalleolar varus and valgus deformities on the tibiotalar joint: a cadaveric study. Foot Ankle Int. 2011 Jun;32(6):609-15.

[65] Lee WC, Moon JS, Lee K, Byun WJ, Lee SH. Indications for supramalleolar osteotomy in patients with ankle osteoarthritis and varus deformity. J Bone Joint Surg Am. 2011 Jul 6;93(13):1243-8.

[66] Saltzman CL, Hillis SL, Stolley MP, Anderson DD, Amendola A. Motion versus fixed distraction of the joint in the treatment of ankle osteoarthritis: a prospective randomized controlled trial. J Bone Joint Surg Am. 2012 Jun 6;94(11):961-70.

[67] Albert E. Zur resection des Kniegelenkes. Wein Med Press. 1879;20:705-8.

[68] Hendrickx RP, Stufkens SA, de Bruijn EE, Sierevelt IN, van Dijk CN, Kerkhoffs GM. Medium- to long-term outcome of ankle arthrodesis. Foot Ankle Int. 2011 Oct;32(10): 940-7.

[69] Haddad SL, Coetzee JC, Estok R, Fahrbach K, Banel D, Nalysnyk L. Intermediate and long-term outcomes of total ankle arthroplasty and ankle arthrodesis. A systematic review of the literature. J Bone Joint Surg Am. 2007 Sep;89(9):1899-905.

[70] Crosby LA, Yee TC, Formanek TS, Fitzgibbons TC. Complications following arthroscopic ankle arthrodesis. Foot Ankle Int. 1996 Jun;17(6):340-2.

[71] Cooper PS. Complications of ankle and tibiotalocalcaneal arthrodesis. Clin Orthop Relat Res. 2001 Oct(391):33-44.

[72] Akra GA, Middleton A, Adedapo AO, Port A, Finn P. Outcome of ankle arthrodesis using a transfibular approach. J Foot Ankle Surg. 2010 Nov-Dec;49(6):508-12.

[73] Gessmann J, Ozokyay L, Fehmer T, Muhr G, Seybold D. [Arthrodesis of the infected ankle joint: results with the Ilizarov external fixator]. Zeitschrift fur Orthopadie und Unfallchirurgie. 2011 Apr;149(2):212-8.

[74] Hollawell SM. Allograft cellular bone matrix as an alternative to autograft in hindfoot and ankle fusion procedures. J Foot Ankle Surg. 2012 Mar-Apr;51(2):222-5.

[75] Guo C, Yan Z, Barfield WR, Hartsock LA. Ankle arthrodesis using anatomically contoured anterior plate. Foot Ankle Int. 2010 Jun;31(6):492-8.

[76] Zwipp H, Rammelt S, Endres T, Heineck J. High union rates and function scores at midterm followup with ankle arthrodesis using a four screw technique. Clin Orthop Relat Res. 2010 Apr;468(4):958-68.

[77] Mohamedean A, Said HG, El-Sharkawi M, El-Adly W, Said GZ. Technique and short-term results of ankle arthrodesis using anterior plating. International orthopaedics. 2010 Aug;34(6):833-7.

[78] Boer R, Mader K, Pennig D, Verheyen CC. Tibiotalocalcaneal arthrodesis using a reamed retrograde locking nail. Clin Orthop Relat Res. 2007 Oct;463:151-6.

[79] Tang KL, Li QH, Chen GX, Guo L, Dai G, Yang L. Arthroscopically assisted ankle fusion in patients with end-stage tuberculosis. Arthroscopy. 2007 Sep;23(9):919-22.

[80] Eylon S, Porat S, Bor N, Leibner ED. Outcome of Ilizarov ankle arthrodesis. Foot Ankle Int. 2007 Aug;28(8):873-9.

[81] Gougoulias NE, Agathangelidis FG, Parsons SW. Arthroscopic ankle arthrodesis. Foot Ankle Int. 2007 Jun;28(6):695-706.

[82] Colman AB, Pomeroy GC. Transfibular ankle arthrodesis with rigid internal fixation: an assessment of outcome. Foot Ankle Int. 2007 Mar;28(3):303-7.

[83] Pelton K, Hofer JK, Thordarson DB. Tibiotalocalcaneal arthrodesis using a dynamically locked retrograde intramedullary nail. Foot Ankle Int. 2006 Oct;27(10):759-63.

[84] Didomenico LA, Sann P. Posterior approach using anterior ankle arthrodesis locking plate for tibiotalocalcaneal arthrodesis. J Foot Ankle Surg. 2011 Sep-Oct;50(5):626-9.

[85] Hanson TW, Cracchiolo A, 3rd. The use of a 95 degree blade plate and a posterior approach to achieve tibiotalocalcaneal arthrodesis. Foot Ankle Int. 2002 Aug;23(8):704-10.

[86] Nickisch F, Avilucea FR, Beals T, Saltzman C. Open posterior approach for tibiotalar arthrodesis. Foot Ankle Clin. 2011 Mar;16(1):103-14.

[87] Collman DR, Kaas MH, Schuberth JM. Arthroscopic ankle arthrodesis: factors influencing union in 39 consecutive patients. Foot Ankle Int. 2006 Dec;27(12):1079-85.

[88] Cameron SE, Ullrich P. Arthroscopic arthrodesis of the ankle joint. Arthroscopy. 2000 Jan-Feb;16(1):21-6.

[89] Schuh R, Hofstaetter J, Krismer M, Bevoni R, Windhager R, Trnka HJ. Total ankle arthroplasty versus ankle arthrodesis. Comparison of sports, recreational activities and functional outcome. International orthopaedics. 2012 Jun;36(6):1207-14.

[90] Goldberg AJ, Sharp RJ, Cooke P. Ankle replacement: current practice of foot & ankle surgeons in the United kingdom. Foot Ankle Int. 2009 Oct;30(10):950-4.

[91] Lord G, Marotte JH. [Total ankle replacement (author's transl)]. Revue de chirurgie orthopedique et reparatrice de l'appareil moteur. 1980 Nov-Dec;66(8):527-30.

[92] Hintermann B, Valderrabano V. Total ankle replacement. Foot Ankle Clin. 2003 Jun; 8(2):375-405.

[93] Bolton-Maggs BG, Sudlow RA, Freeman MA. Total ankle arthroplasty. A long-term review of the London Hospital experience. J Bone Joint Surg Br. 1985 Nov;67(5): 785-90.

[94] Easley ME, Vertullo CJ, Urban WC, Nunley JA. Total ankle arthroplasty. The Journal of the American Academy of Orthopaedic Surgeons. 2002 May-Jun;10(3):157-67.

[95] Kitaoka HB, Patzer GL. Clinical results of the Mayo total ankle arthroplasty. J Bone Joint Surg Am. 1996 Nov;78(11):1658-64.

[96] Hamblen DL. Can the ankle joint be replaced? J Bone Joint Surg Br. 1985 Nov;67(5): 689-90.

[97] Lewis G. Biomechanics of and research challenges in uncemented total ankle replacement. Clin Orthop Relat Res. 2004 Jul(424):89-97.

[98] Hintermann B. Total ankle arthroplasty. St. Stefan, Austria: Springer Wein New York 2005.

[99] Dyrby C, Chou LB, Andriacchi TP, Mann RA. Functional evaluation of the Scandinavian Total Ankle Replacement. Foot Ankle Int. 2004 Jun;25(6):377-81.

[100] Michelson JD, Schmidt GR, Mizel MS. Kinematics of a total arthroplasty of the ankle: comparison to normal ankle motion. Foot Ankle Int. 2000 Apr;21(4):278-84.

[101] Yalamanchili P, Neufeld S, Lin S. Total ankle arthroplasty: A modern perspective. Curr Orthop Prac. 2009;20(2):106-11-.

[102] Neufeld SK, Lee TH. Total ankle arthroplasty: indications, results, and biomechanical rationale. American journal of orthopedics (Belle Mead, NJ. 2000 Aug;29(8):593-602.

[103] Pyevich MT, Saltzman CL, Callaghan JJ, Alvine FG. Total ankle arthroplasty: a unique design. Two to twelve-year follow-up. J Bone Joint Surg Am. 1998 Oct;80(10): 1410-20.

[104] Gould JS, Alvine FG, Mann RA, Sanders RW, Walling AK. Total ankle replacement: a surgical discussion. Part II. The clinical and surgical experience. American journal of orthopedics (Belle Mead, NJ. 2000 Sep;29(9):675-82.

[105] Gould JS, Alvine FG, Mann RA, Sanders RW, Walling AK. Total ankle replacement: a surgical discussion. Part I. Replacement systems, indications, and contraindications. American journal of orthopedics (Belle Mead, NJ. 2000 Aug;29(8):604-9.

[106] Demottaz JD, Mazur JM, Thomas WH, Sledge CB, Simon SR. Clinical study of total ankle replacement with gait analysis. A preliminary report. J Bone Joint Surg Am. 1979 Oct;61(7):976-88.

[107] Gill LH. Challenges in total ankle arthroplasty. Foot Ankle Int. 2004 Apr;25(4): 195-207.

[108] Inman VT. Inman's joints of the ankle. Baltimore, MD: Williams & Wilkins 1976.

[109] Sammarco J. Biomechanics of the ankle. I. Surface velocity and instant center of rotation in the sagittal plane. Am J Sports Med. 1977 Nov-Dec;5(6):231-4.

[110] Komistek RD, Stiehl JB, Buechel FF, Northcut EJ, Hajner ME. A determination of ankle kinematics using fluoroscopy. Foot Ankle Int. 2000 Apr;21(4):343-50.

[111] Saltzman CL. Perspective on total ankle replacement. Foot Ankle Clin. 2000 Dec;5(4): 761-75.

[112] Cracchiolo A, 3rd, Deorio JK. Design features of current total ankle replacements: implants and instrumentation. The Journal of the American Academy of Orthopaedic Surgeons. 2008 Sep;16(9):530-40.

[113] Chou LB, Coughlin MT, Hansen S, Jr., Haskell A, Lundeen G, Saltzman CL, et al. Osteoarthritis of the ankle: the role of arthroplasty. The Journal of the American Academy of Orthopaedic Surgeons. 2008 May;16(5):249-59.

[114] Cenni F, Leardini A, Belvedere C, Bugane F, Cremonini K, Miscione MT, et al. Kinematics of the three components of a total ankle replacement: in vivo fluoroscopic analysis. Foot Ankle Int. 2012 Apr;33(4):290-300.

[115] Brodsky JW, Polo FE, Coleman SC, Bruck N. Changes in gait following the Scandinavian Total Ankle Replacement. J Bone Joint Surg Am. 2011 Oct 19;93(20):1890-6.

[116] Barnett CH, Napier JR. The axis of rotation at the ankle joint in man; its influence upon the form of the talus and the mobility of the fibula. Journal of anatomy. 1952 Jan;86(1):1-9.

[117] Newton SE, 3rd. Total ankle arthroplasty. Clinical study of fifty cases. J Bone Joint Surg Am. 1982 Jan;64(1):104-11.

[118] Conti SF, Wong YS. Complications of total ankle replacement. Foot Ankle Clin. 2002 Dec;7(4):791-807, vii.

[119] Raikin SM, Kane J, Ciminiello ME. Risk factors for incision-healing complications following total ankle arthroplasty. J Bone Joint Surg Am. 2010 Sep 15;92(12):2150-5.

[120] Kobayashi A, Minoda Y, Kadoya Y, Ohashi H, Takaoka K, Saltzman CL. Ankle arthroplasties generate wear particles similar to knee arthroplasties. Clin Orthop Relat Res. 2004 Jul(424):69-72.

[121] Conti S, Lalonde KA, Martin R. Kinematic analysis of the agility total ankle during gait. Foot Ankle Int. 2006 Nov;27(11):980-4.

[122] Barg A, Knupp M, Anderson AE, Hintermann B. Total ankle replacement in obese patients: component stability, weight change, and functional outcome in 118 consecutive patients. Foot Ankle Int. 2011 Oct;32(10):925-32.

[123] Cornelis Doets H, van der Plaat LW, Klein JP. Medial malleolar osteotomy for the correction of varus deformity during total ankle arthroplasty: results in 15 ankles. Foot Ankle Int. 2008 Feb;29(2):171-7.

[124] Reddy SC, Mann JA, Mann RA, Mangold DR. Correction of moderate to severe coronal plane deformity with the STAR ankle prosthesis. Foot Ankle Int. 2011 Jul;32(7): 659-64.

[125] Shock RP, Christensen JC, Schuberth JM. Total ankle replacement in the varus ankle. J Foot Ankle Surg. 2011 Jan-Feb;50(1):5-10.

[126] Ryssman DB, Myerson MS. Total ankle arthroplasty: management of varus deformity at the ankle. Foot Ankle Int. 2012 Apr;33(4):347-54.

[127] Barg A, Henninger HB, Hintermann B. Risk factors for symptomatic deep-vein thrombosis in patients after total ankle replacement who received routine chemical thromboprophylaxis. J Bone Joint Surg Br. 2011 Jul;93(7):921-7.

[128] Bestic JM, Peterson JJ, DeOrio JK, Bancroft LW, Berquist TH, Kransdorf MJ. Postoperative evaluation of the total ankle arthroplasty. Ajr. 2008 Apr;190(4):1112-23.

[129] Fevang BT, Lie SA, Havelin LI, Brun JG, Skredderstuen A, Furnes O. 257 ankle arthroplasties performed in Norway between 1994 and 2005. Acta orthopaedica. 2007 Oct;78(5):575-83.

[130] Hosman AH, Mason RB, Hobbs T, Rothwell AG. A New Zealand national joint registry review of 202 total ankle replacements followed for up to 6 years. Acta orthopaedica. 2007 Oct;78(5):584-91.

[131] Skytta ET, Koivu H, Eskelinen A, Ikavalko M, Paavolainen P, Remes V. Total ankle replacement: a population-based study of 515 cases from the Finnish Arthroplasty Register. Acta orthopaedica. 2010 Feb;81(1):114-8.

[132] Henricson A, Nilsson JA, Carlsson A. 10-year survival of total ankle arthroplasties: a report on 780 cases from the Swedish Ankle Register. Acta orthopaedica. 2011 Dec; 82(6):655-9.

[133] Labek G, Klaus H, Schlichtherle R, Williams A, Agreiter M. Revision rates after total ankle arthroplasty in sample-based clinical studies and national registries. Foot Ankle Int. 2011 Aug;32(8):740-5.

[134] Gougoulias N, Khanna A, Maffulli N. How successful are current ankle replacements?: a systematic review of the literature. Clin Orthop Relat Res. 2010 Jan;468(1): 199-208.

[135] Stengel D, Bauwens K, Ekkernkamp A, Cramer J. Efficacy of total ankle replacement with meniscal-bearing devices: a systematic review and meta-analysis. Arch Orthop Trauma Surg. 2005 Mar;125(2):109-19.

[136] Mann JA, Mann RA, Horton E. STAR ankle: long-term results. Foot Ankle Int. 2011 May;32(5):S473-84.

[137] Bonnin M, Gaudot F, Laurent JR, Ellis S, Colombier JA, Judet T. The Salto total ankle arthroplasty: survivorship and analysis of failures at 7 to 11 years. Clin Orthop Relat Res. 2011 Jan;469(1):225-36.

[138] Wood PL, Sutton C, Mishra V, Suneja R. A randomised, controlled trial of two mobile-bearing total ankle replacements. J Bone Joint Surg Br. 2009 Jan;91(1):69-74.

[139] Hahn ME, Wright ES, Segal AD, Orendurff MS, Ledoux WR, Sangeorzan BJ. Comparative gait analysis of ankle arthrodesis and arthroplasty: initial findings of a prospective study. Foot Ankle Int. 2012 Apr;33(4):282-9.

[140] Piriou P, Culpan P, Mullins M, Cardon JN, Pozzi D, Judet T. Ankle replacement versus arthrodesis: a comparative gait analysis study. Foot Ankle Int. 2008 Jan;29(1):3-9.

[141] Penner MJ, Pakzad H, Younger A, Wing KJ. Mean BMI of overweight and obese patients does not decrease after successful ankle reconstruction. J Bone Joint Surg Am. 2012 May 2;94(9):e57.

Section 5

Complications After Arthroplasty

Chapter 17

Complications Following Total Hip Arthroplasty

Asim Rajpura and Tim Board

Additional information is available at the end of the chapter

http://dx.doi.org/10.5772/53030

1. Introduction

Total hip arthroplasty (THA) is an increasingly common and successful operation, with 76,759 procedures logged in the National Joint Registry for England and Wales in 2010 [1]. Overall satisfaction rates rank amongst the highest of any joint replacement procedure, with over 90% reporting a good to excellent overall outcome [2, 3].

Complications related to THA can be classified as either procedure specific or systemic. Advances in technology, anaesthesiology and surgical technique have resulted in an overall temporal decrease in complication rates despite the increasing incidence of co-morbidities in the patient population [4]. Table 1 highlights rates of complications most commonly encountered after THA.

2. Systemic / non-surgical

2.1. Thromboembolic complications

Deep Vein Thrombosis

Distal deep vein thrombosis (DVT) can range from being asymptomatic, to resulting in long term valvular damage resulting in chronic venous insufficiency. Proximal propagation can result in more serious pulmonary embolism. The overall incidence of DVT, including both radiologically diagnosed asymptomatic DVT and symptomatic DVT, post THA in early studies was reported to be as high as 70% without any form of prophylaxis [15]. Recent systematic review of several randomised control trials concerned with DVT prophylaxis has estimated this figure to be around 44% [16]. The recent FOTO study has shown a symptomatic DVT rate of 1.3% in THA patients with extended duration [36 day) chemical prophylaxis [8].

The overall combined incidence of asymptomatic and symptomatic DVT with prophylaxis has not declined with time, converse to the findings with knee arthroplasty in which the incidence has declined significantly [17]. This may be due to the increasing frequency of co morbidities within patients undergoing THA which act as risk factors for DVT.

Systemic		Procedure Specific	
Complication	**Rate**	**Complication**	**Rate**
Subclinical Fat Embolism	90%[5]	Dislocation (Posterior approach with repair)	0.49%[6]
Symptomatic Fat Embolism	Unknown	Leg length discrepancy (patient perceived)	30%[7]
Symptomatic Deep Vein Thrombosis with prophylaxis	1.3%[8]	Infection	1.08%[9]
Symptomatic Pulmonary Embolism with prophylaxis	0.5 – 0.6%[10]	Aseptic Loosening	2% failure rate at 15 years (Corail uncemented stem) [11] 3.2% failure rate at 30 years (Exeter Cemented Stem)[12]
Mortality	0.29 – 0.6%[4]	Periprosthetic Fracture (Postoperative femoral)	1.1%[13]
Myocardial Infarction	0.5%[10]	Heterotopic Ossification (Grade III/IV)	3 – 7%[14]

Table 1. Complication rates for Total Hip Arthroplasty

THA is thought to mainly affect 2 limbs of Virchow's triad, namely hypercoagulability and venous stasis. Activation of the coagulation cascade begins during surgery, primarily during preparation and insertion of the femoral prosthesis, with cemented prostheses providing a greater stimulus than uncemented implants [18]. Whether this increases the incidence of DVT with cemented fixation is unclear as the evidence is inconclusive [15, 19]. Venous haemodynamics are also altered not only during surgery, but also for up to 6 weeks post operatively [20]. Significant reductions in venous capacitance and outflow are seen in both legs, with greater changes seen in the operated leg, and this has been shown to correlate directly with the incidence of postoperative DVT [20]. Complete femoral vein occlusion has also been noted during THA, particularly during the posterior approach when the limb is internally rotated and flexed for operation on the femur [18].

Numerous risk factors for postoperative DVT have been identified. Major risk factors in approximate order of importance include: hip fracture, malignancy, antiphospholipid syndrome, immobility, previous history of DVT, use of selective oestrogen receptor modulators, oral contraceptives, morbid obesity, stroke, atherosclerosis and a ASA greater than 3 [21]. However 50% of patients who develop DVT have no identifiable clinical risk factor [21]. Genetic predispositions include antithrombin III and protein C deficiency and prothrombin gene mutation [21]. In order to aid recognition of 'at risk' patients, the National Institute for Health and Clinical Excellence (NICE) has published a table of relevant patient related risk factors as shown in Table 2 [16].

Active cancer or cancer treatment	Active heart or respiratory failure
Acute medical illness	Age over 60 years
Antiphospholipid syndrome	Behcet's disease
Central venous catheter in situ	Continuous travel of more than 3hours approximately 4weeks before or after surgery
Immobility (for example, paralysis or limb in plaster)	Inflammatory bowel disease
Myeloproliferative diseases	Nephrotic syndrome
Obesity (body mass index > 30kg/m2]	Paraproteinaemia
Paroxysmal nocturnal haemoglobinuria	Personal or family history of VTE
Pregnancy or puerperium	Recent myocardial infarction or stroke
Severe infection	Use of oral contraceptives or hormonal replacement therapy
Varicose veins with associated phlebitis	
Inherited Thrombophilias for example:	
High levels of coagulation factors (for example, Factor VIII)	Hyperhomocysteinaemia
Low activated protein C resistance (for example, Factor V Leiden)	Protein C, S and antithrombin deficiencies
Prothrombin 2021A gene mutation	

Table 2. Patient related risk factors for Venous Thromboembolism [16]

Prophylaxis against DVT begins with the type of anaesthesia used. Regional compared to general anaesthesia has been shown to reduce the risk of DVT post THA by over 50% [22, 23]. This is thought to be due to the relative hyperkinetic blood flow seen in the lower limbs during regional anaesthesia compared to general anaesthesia, and the stabilising effect of local anaesthetics on the cell membranes of vascular endothelium and platelets [24]. Mechanical and chemical prophylaxis remains a somewhat contentious issue, with various differing opinions existing regarding prophylaxis regimes. Numerous randomised controlled trials exist supporting the use of mechanical methods such as pneumatic compression devices (figure 1) and chemical methods such as low molecular weight heparins and fondaparinux, a factor Xa inhibitor [25-34].

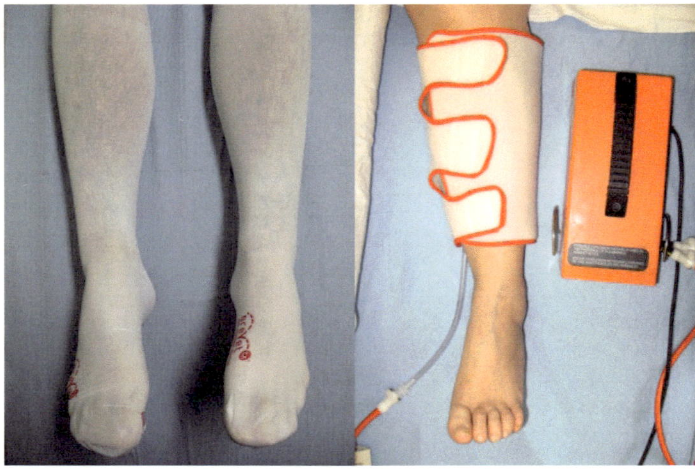

Figure 1. Left: Thrombo-Embolic Deterrent Stockings, Right: Flotron pumps (Huntleigh Healthcare Ltd, Luton, UK)

There has been recent increasing interest in oral factor Xa inhibitors such as Rivaroxaban and Apixaban. The RECORD trial has demonstrated greater effectiveness for oral Rivaroxaban compared to subcutaneous Enoxaparin with equal side effect profiles [35, 36]. Pooled analysis of the ADVANCE-2 and ADVANCE-3 trials has also demonstrated greater efficacy for oral Apixaban compared to subcutaneous Enoxaparin [37]. There has been some recent concern however regarding the increased rate of wound complications, specifically with the use of Rivaroxaban [38]. A retrospective analysis by Jensen et al. demonstrated a greater return to theatre rate for wound complications such as prolonged drainage and haematoma associated with the use of Rivaroxaban compared to Tinzaparin [38]. The authors suggest that trial data to date has not fully evaluated the complications profile of Rivaroxaban, as only major bleeding was used as a primary outcome measure, and further randomised trials are necessary to examine rates of surgical complications.

Current recommendations by National Institute for Health and Clinical Excellence (NICE) in England state that, THA patients should be offered mechanical prophylaxis in the form of intermittent pneumatic compression devices or compression stockings, and chemical prophylaxis with either low molecular weight heparin, Fondaparinux, Rivaroxaban or Dabigatran. This should be continued for 28-35 days post operatively [39].

2.2. Pulmonary embolism

DVTs that propagate proximally have the potential embolise to the lungs resulting in pulmonary emboli (PE). Mild emboli can be asymptomatic, whereas massive embolism can be fatal, and PE is one of the leading causes of mortality post THA. Rates for symptomatic pulmonary embolism in recent large case series of primary THA in which chemical prophylaxis was used, has been between 0.51-0.6% [10, 40]. In the absence of prophylaxis this is estimated to be around 3%, with approximately 6% of symptomatic PEs post THA result in fatality [16].

As with DVT, both mechanical and chemical methods such as pneumatic compression pumps and low molecular weight heparins have been shown to provide effective prophylaxis against symptomatic PE [25, 41-44]. However due to the low rate of fatal PE, trials and even meta-analyses have failed to demonstrate statistically significant effects on the rate of fatal PE by using thromboembolic prophylaxis [45]. Power analysis indicates a trial involving 67,000 patients would be needed to demonstrate a statistically significant difference [46].

Vena Caval filters as shown in figure 2 can also be used to prevent migration of venous emboli into the pulmonary circulation. However no RCTs exist supporting their use in surgical patients and significant complications such as pneumothorax, air embolism and arteriovenous fistulae can develop either during their placement or post procedure [47]. UK NICE guidelines therefore recommend their use in patients with recent or existing thromboembolic disease in whom anticoagulation is contraindicated [39].

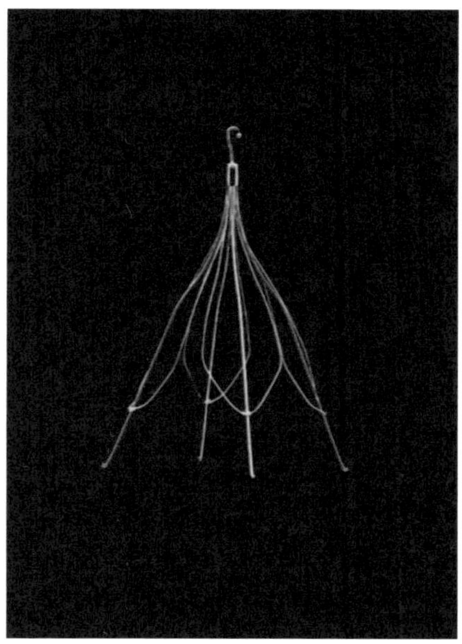

Figure 2. Retrievable Inferior Vena Caval Filter, courtesy of Cook Medical

2.3. Fat embolism

During insertion of the femoral component, rises in intramedullary pressure can force medullary fat and marrow contents into the venous circulation via the metaphyseal vessels [48-50]. Fat and marrow embolus can then pass into and through the pulmonary circulation depending on the size of the emboli [51, 52]. Large emboli can lodge within the pulmonary circulation leading to pulmonary hypertension and haemodynamic instability. Trans-pulmonary passage of micro-emboli can result in cerebral embolism potentially causing neurological complications [51, 53].

Subclinical fat embolisation can been detected in up to 90% of patients undergoing THA [5]. However the exact incidence of fat embolism syndrome characterised by the classic triad of respiratory insufficiency, neurolgic symptoms and upper body petechiae is unknown [54].

Measures to reduce the risk of fat embolism include medullary lavage to reduce the fat load during cement pressurisation [55]. Vacuum cementation techniques using drainage cannulae have also been shown to be effective in reducing the intramedullary pressure rises during cementation therefore reducing the risk of emboli [56]. Treatment of established fat embolism syndrome is essentially supportive, frequently requiring intensive care unit admission for respiratory support.

3. Mortality and cardiorespiratory complications

Published rates for mortality following primary THA are low, ranging from between 0.29% to 0.6% [4, 10]. Mortality rates have declined slightly with time despite the increasing incidence of relevant co-morbidities [4]. Cardiovascular complications account for the most common cause of death [57].

Age has been identified as one of the strongest predictors of post operative mortality after joint arthroplasty [10]. Octegenarians have been shown to have a mortality rate 3.4 times higher than patients between 65-79 years of age and were 2.4 times more likely to suffer a post operative myocardial infarction [58]. Other significant risk factors for post operative mortality and morbidity include male sex, smoking and higher American Society of Anesthesiologists' (ASA) grade which is representative of relevant significant co-morbidities such as artherosclerosis, diabetes, renal impairment and valvular disease [10, 59, 60]. Greenfield et al. found that the incidence of morbidity after THA varied from 3% to 41% when comparing those with the lowest and highest incidence of co-morbidities [61]. The role of anaesthesia is somewhat controversial. Some studies suggest regional compared to general anaesthesia may reduce the risk of thromboembolic and cardiorespiratory complications and short term mortality [62, 63]. Others have shown no difference between the 2 groups in terms of morbidity and mortality [64]. Therefore no conclusive evidence exists supporting one form of anaesthesia, but the overall consensus would appear to favour regional techniques [54].

4. Procedure specific / surgical complications

4.1. Dislocation

Dislocation is the 3rd most common cause for revision after THA [65]. Published rates for dislocation after primary THA vary widely between 0.2% to 7% [66]. Up to 70% of dislocations occur early within 6 weeks [67]. Early dislocation carries a better prognosis compared to late dislocation which is defined as occurring after 3 months, as late dislocation usually has a multifactiorial aetiology including component wear and soft tissue laxity [68, 69]. Approximately a third of dislocating THAs managed conservatively after the first episode will go on to become recurrent dislocators [67]. Risk factors for dislocation can be classified as either patient, surgery or implant related.

4.2. Patient related risk factors

Patients with neuromuscular and cognitive disorders such as cerebral palsy, muscular dystrophy and dementia, have been shown to have higher rates of dislocation [70]. Fracture as the primary indication for surgery is the indication most strongly linked with dislocation [71]. This is thought to be due to the lack of capsular hypertrophy normally seen with osteoarthritis which provides additional stability. Previous hip surgery of any sort has also been shown to double the risk of dislocation [68]. Factors such as height, weight, age and sex of the patient have not been conclusively shown to affect the rates of dislocation [67].

4.3. Surgical risk factors

Surgical factors include surgical approach, soft tissue tension, component design and orientation, and surgeon experience. The majority of dislocations occur in a posterior direction and therefore the posterior approach has been deemed to be the approach with the highest risk of dislocation. Early data supported this theory with Woo et al reporting a rate of 5.8% for posterior approach compared to 2.3% for an antero-lateral approach [68]. However recent research investigating the role of posterior capsular and external rotator repair has shown comparable rates to other approaches [72, 73]. A recent meta-analysis has shown a reduction of the dislocation rate from 4.46% to 0.49% by carrying out a posterior soft tissue repair [6]. Therefore with meticulous soft tissue repair, surgical approach should have little effect on dislocation rates. Besides the posterior structures, the glutei and joint capsule also provide soft tissue tension reducing dislocation risk. Therefore following a transtrochanteric approach, trochanteric non union greater than 1cm can result in abductor insufficiency increasing the rates of dislocation by over 6 fold [68]. Inadequate offset is another factor affecting soft tissue tension and has been shown to increase dislocation risk [74].

4.4. Implant related factors

Component positioning and design both play key roles in reducing dislocation risk. "Safe zones" for acetabular cup position are defined as an abduction angle of 40° ± 10° and anteversion of 20° ± 10° [75, 76]. With a posterior approach reduced cup anteversion has been shown to be a major risk factor for dislocation [77]. Archbold et al. have suggested the use of the transverse acetabular ligament as a landmark to judge cup anteversion [78]. Using this technique they reported a 0.6% dislocation rate using a posterior approach with soft tissue repair. How this relates to the traditionally defined safe zones is currently being examined. Femoral component positioning has been less well studied. Recent studies have suggested the use of a 'combined anteversion' technique in which the acetabular and stem combined anteversion should be 35° ± 10° [79, 80].

Femoral head size also affects stability. Larger heads provide more favourable head-neck ratios, reducing possible impingement, and seat deeper within the acetabulum requiring a greater 'jump distance' to cause dislocation as illustrated in figure 3. Such advantages have been validated using cadaveric and computer modelling [81-83]. Clinical data from both the Norwegian and Australian joint registries has also shown a reduction in rates of revision for dislocation with increasing head size [84, 85].

Surgeon experience is another factor that has been identified in influencing dislocation rates. Hedlundh et al. found that surgeons who had performed less than 30 THAs had a double rate of dislocation compared to more experienced surgeons [86]. A recent systematic review has also demonstrated reduced dislocation rates with increased surgical volume [87].

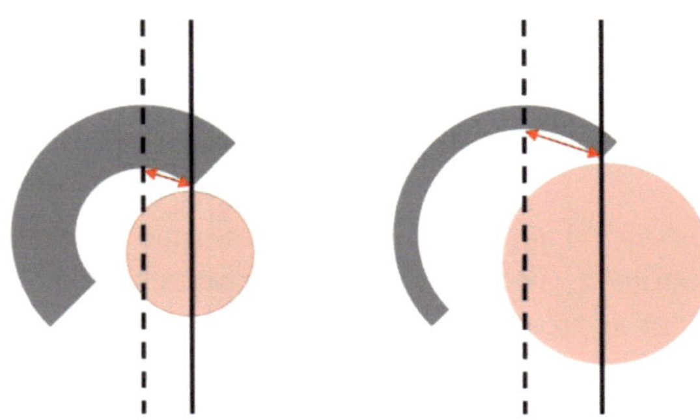

Figure 3. Jumping Distance highlighted by red arrow demonstrates distance the head needs to travel before dislocation occurs. Increasing head size increases this distance

5. Management

Management of dislocation initially involves closed reduction which is usually successful in the majority of cases. This should be performed ideally under anaesthesia with muscle relaxation to reduce the chance of damage to the femoral head [88, 89]. Some surgeons advocate the use of an abduction brace after reduction but little evidence exists supporting their use.

Indications for operative intervention include recurrent or irreducible dislocation, component malposition, soft tissue laxity and dislocation due to impingement. Strategies during revision include component realignment, removal of osteophytes causing impingement, modular component exchange to increase head size and improve head-neck ratio, liner exchange if worn and addressing soft tissue laxity using capsulorrhaphy, trochanteric advancement or tendon allografts.

Selected patients unsuitable for major revision surgery can be treated with posterior lip augmentation devices (PLAD) as shown in figure 4. These consist of a C shaped piece of UHMWPE and a steel backing plate, and are applied to the posterior lip of the acetabulum and held in place with up to 5 screws. This constrains the head within the augmented sock-

http://dx.doi.org/10.5772/53030

et. Contraindications to its use include gross component malalignment and loosening. McConway et al. reviewed 307 recurrently dislocating THAs treated with PLADs [90]. Persistent instability occurred in only 5 patients [1.6%) and there was no evidence of accelerated loosening affecting the acetabular component.

Salvage procedures for failed revision or uncorrectable aetiology include the use of constrained cups or conversion to bipolar hemiarthroplasty. However both of these procedures are associated with poor functional outcome and constrained cups can result in premature loosening [70]. Therefore their use is usually reserved for low demand patients. The final salvage option is Girdlestone resection for the unreconstructable hip.

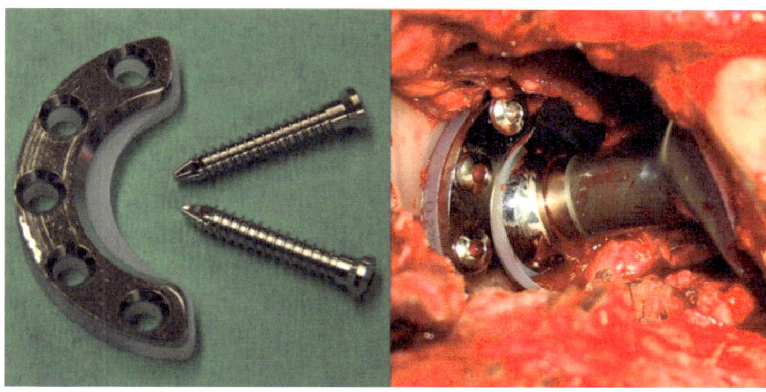

Figure 4. Posterior Lip Augementation Device (PLAD, Depuy, UK)

5.1. Leg length discrepancy

Leg length discrepancy (LLD) is the most common cause of patient dissatisfaction and subsequent litigation after THA [91]. LLD can result in nerve palsies, abnormal gait, lower back pain and reduced functional outcome [92]. Wylde et al. showed up to 30% of patients after primary THA can have a perceived LLD, but only 36% of these had an anatomic LLD greater than 5mm [7].

Nerve palsies are potentially the most serious complications of LLD. Sciatic and peroneal nerve palsies have both been associated with limb lengthening. Edwards et al suggested sciatic and peroneal nerve palsies are associated with lengthening greater than 4 and 3.8cm respectively [93]. Farrell et al however found an average lengthening of only 1.7cm was a significant risk factor for nerve palsies [94]. Therefore safe limits for limb lengthening before traction nerve palsies develop are yet to be defined, and it may be that any minor degree of lengthening may make the nerve more susceptible to other trauma [94].

Minor LLD less than 1cm is usually well tolerated by patients. However LLD greater than 2cm has been shown to significantly affect the gait cycle, increasing physiological demand [95]. LLD greater than 3cm in the elderly was shown to cause significant increases in heart rate and quadriceps activity in the lengthened limb, which may be especially relevant in patients with cardio-respiratory co-morbidities [95].

Avoiding potential problems with LLD begins with patient history and examination. It is crucial to determine patient perceived leg length in order to counsel the patient effectively regarding likely outcomes. True leg length can then be determined, measuring from the ipsilateral anterior superior iliac spine to the medial malleolus, followed by apparent leg length by measuring from the umbilicus to the medial malleolus. Apparent leg length can be affected by pelvic obliquity secondary to either lumbar spine pathology or contractures about the hip. Significant LLD due to fixed pelvic obliquity secondary to chronic lumbar spine pathology cannot usually be corrected as it may involve significant shortening or lengthening. With pelvic obliquity secondary to contractures, the true length only needs to be corrected as after the THA the pelvis will balance with time [96].

Radiographs can also be used to determine leg length by referencing the position of the lesser trochanter in relation to a line drawn across the inferior aspect of the pelvis as shown in figure 5. Templating can then be carried out to determine the correct level of the neck cut for the femoral prosthesis and the position of the acetabular component in order to determine the new hip centre. Both of these directly affect leg length.

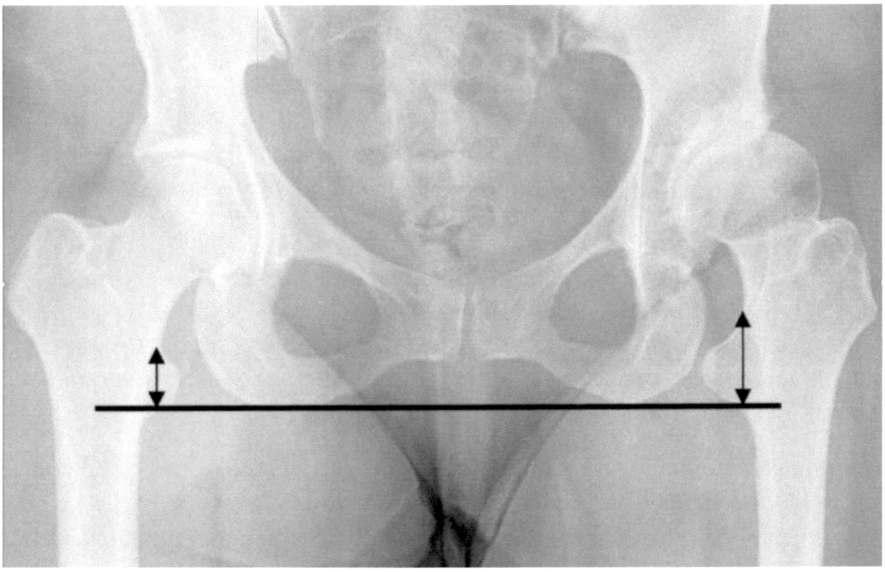

Figure 5. Radiographic estimation of LLD can be made by measuring vertically from the top of the lesser trochanter to a line drawn across the inferior margin of the pelvis

Intraoperative methods include the use of measurements taken from reference pins placed in the pelvis to a mark on the greater trochanter [97-99]. Mihalko et al described using a large fragment screw placed above the superior rim of the acetabulum and marking a point on the greater trochanter a fixed distance from this prior to dislocation. After insertion of the prostheses this distance was rechecked giving an indication of leg length changes [98]. Shiramizu et al used a similar method but with a steimann pin in the ilium and a custom calliper to measure the distances [99]. They found a mean LLD of only 2.1mm with this method.

Minor LLD postoperatively can be treated using a shoe raise. Prescription of such devices should be delayed for 3-6 months to allow any residual pelvic tilt secondary to contractures to resolve as the soft tissues can progressively relax. Failure of conservative measures and symptoms such as severe pain, nerve palsies and instability can necessitate surgical intervention. Shortening can be treated using soft tissue release and exchange of modular heads to give modest changes in leg length or more extensive surgery such as exchange of the femoral component to give greater neck length or offset. Lengthening can also be treated with component exchange but secondary procedures such as trochanteric advancement or the use of larger heads or stems with increased offset may be needed to maintain stability [100].

5.2. Infection

Infection post THA is potentially one of the most catastrophic and challenging to treat complications. During the early development of THA, Charnley reported a deep infection rate of 9.4% in unventilated operating theatres [101]. This initial unacceptably high deep infection rate stimulated the development of several prophylactic measures including ultraclean laminar air flow ventilation and peri-operative antibiotics. With the aid of such measures, infection rates in the UK between 1993 and 1996 fell to 1.08% [9].

5.3. Prophylaxis

Bacterial contamination of theatre air was initially recognized as a risk factor for post operative sepsis by Lister in 1867 [102]. Charnley later introduced the concept of ultraclean air flow ventilation that produces less than 10 colony forming units per cubic meter [103]. His reported infection rates in THA fell to 1% with the use of such enclosures. A MRC trial published in 1982 demonstrated a deep sepsis rate of 0.6% with ultraclean ventilation compared to 1.5% with conventional ventilation [104]. The use of ultraclean air ventilation during joint arthroplasty has subsequently become universally adopted practice within the UK [105].

The use of peri-operative antibiotics during THA is also a common prophylactic measure. Early trials using cloxacillin in THA found a 12% infection rate without prophylaxis compared to 0% with [106]. Currently cephalosporins are commonly used prophylaxis for THA. There is however a gradual move away from these due to the emergence of MRSA and problems with Clostridium difficile infection. Alternative regimens include flucloxacillin and gentamicin, or vancomycin and gentamicin. There is no conclusive evidence with regards to the optimal antibiotic regimen or duration of administration. However no benefit of extended prophylaxis beyond 24 hours has been demonstrated [107]. Therefore antibiotic regimes should be ideally guided by local microbiological knowledge so locally prevalent organisms can be targeted. Other measures shown to reduce rates of infection or bacterial load include the use of occlusive clothing, exhaust suits, pulsed wound lavage, preoperative showering and reducing theatre traffic [105].

5.4. Pathogenesis

Infection can arise by direct bacterial contamination at the time of surgery or later haematogenous spread. Staphylococcus aureus was the most common causative organism in an early series published by Charnley [108]. Coagulase negative staphylococci have become increasingly prevalent over the years with a recent series showing such organisms responsible for 58% of infections [109]. This is thought to be due to the effect of antibiotic use on bacterial flora [105]. Risk factors for periprosthetic infection include obesity, revision surgery, inflammatory arthritis, open skin lesions on the affected limb, blood transfusion, urinary infections and high ASA score [110].

Pathogenesis begins with bacterial adhesion. Primary adhesion occurs due to physical interactions (hydrophobic/electrostatic) between the bacteria and prosthetic surface. This is followed by bacterial aggregation through membrane adhesion molecules and generation of exopolysaccharides which form a glyocalyx or biofilm surrounding the bacteria [111]. This biofilm is thought to protect the bacteria from antibiotics and host defences [112].

5.5. Classification

Periprosthetic infections can be classified into 4 main catogeries [113]. Early postoperative infection is one that becomes apparent within one month of the procedure. Late chronic infection presents later than 1 month after operation and has an insidious course of gradual onset of pain and swelling with minimal systemic symptoms. Acute haematogenous spread results in an acute onset of symptoms associated with a documented or suspected bacteraemia. The final type is positive intra-operative culture, this is an occult infection diagnosed by positive cultures taken at time of revision surgery.

5.6. Diagnosis

Diagnosis of peri-prosthetic infection can be extremely challenging. Hip pain is the most consistent symptom. Presence of systemic symptoms such as fevers or rigors can be very variable. Examination may reveal local wound tenderness, signs of inflammation, discharge, sinuses and a painful range of movement.

Plain radiographs may show evidence of osteopenia or osteolysis, periostiitis and endosteal scalloping. However none of these can reliably differentiate between infection and aseptic loosening. Radionucleotide scanning using technetium or gallium can also been used. Technetium uptake reflects active bone turnover and gallium binds to transferrin, accumulating in inflammatory foci. Technetium scanning has a greater sensitivity than gallium for infection but their inability to differentiate infection and aseptic loosening limits their application [114, 115]. However its relatively high negative predictive value can make technetium bone scanning a useful initial screening test [116]. 18F-Fluoro-deoxyglucose [18-FDG) PET scanning is a newer technique that has increased sensitivity and specificity for infection. Pooled data from recent studies demonstrate a sensitivity of 85.5% and a specificity of 92.6% for periprosthetic infection [117]. Availability of PET scanners however still remains poor. Using radio-labelled white cells or immunoglobulins is another technique which has shown improved sensitivity and specificity relative to traditional three phase bone scans. Their widespread availability combined with the lack of established diagnostic criteria for 18-FDG PET scans, makes labelled white cell scans the current nuclear medicine investigation of choice for periprosthetic infection [118].

Blood investigations include ESR, CRP and Interleukin-6. ESR and CRP are non specific inflammatory markers and therefore can be elevated by concurrent illnesses. In the absence of such conditions an ESR greater than 30 mm/hr has a sensitivity and specificity of 82 and 85% respectively for peri-prosthetic infection, and the values for a CRP greater than 10mg/l are 96% and 92% [119]. Elevated levels of interleukin-6 have also been associated with periprosthetic infection with a sensitivity and specificity of 100% and 95% in one study [120]. However other chronic inflammatory conditions such as rheumatoid arthritis and other illnesses such as AIDS and Multiple Sclerosis can also cause elevated levels.

Cytological and microbiological analysis of hip aspirate taken under sterile conditions can give useful information regarding not only the presence of infection but also the potential offending organism. Ali et al. have shown a sensitivity and specificity of 0.82 and 0.91 for radiologically guided guided hip aspiration. However recent antibiotics can affect cultures and therefore antibiotics must be stopped for at least 2 weeks prior to aspiration.

5.7. Treatment

The aims of treatment of an infected prosthesis are eradication of infection and restoration of function. The classification by Tsukyama et al. can be used to help guide treatment [113]. Acute infections either presenting as early infection or acute haematogenous spread can be treated by component retention and thorough debridement, irrigation and intravenous antibiotics. However such treatment must be undertaken within 2 weeks of onset of symptoms [121]. Success rates between 50-74% have been reported with such a strategy [113].

Late chronic infection is best treated with full revision. This can be performed as a single stage exchange arthroplasty or a 2 stage exchange procedure. Originally described by Bucholz, a single stage procedure involves prosthesis removal, soft tissue debridement and lavage, followed by re-implantation of a new prosthesis if a clean uninfected bed is achieved, followed by appropriate antibiotic therapy [122]. Review of 1299 cases treated with single stage revision showed an 83% success rate at an average follow up of 4.8 years [123]. Factors associated with successful outcome were good general health of the patient, absence of wound complications after the primary procedure, methicillin sensitive organisms and infection with organisms sensitive to antibiotics within the cement [123]. Advantages of a single stage procedure include lower patient morbidity and lower incidence of complications such as fracture and dislocation. However 2 stage procedures have consistently demonstrated higher success rates compared to single stage procedures [124-128]. Thus 2 stage exchange still remains the most common strategy.

2 stage procedures involve initial prosthesis removal, soft tissue debridement and insertion of an antibiotic loaded cement spacer. This can be in the form of an articulating spacer allowing some range of movement and reducing soft tissue contracture. This is followed by

appropriate antibiotic therapy and a usual interval of 6 weeks prior to reimplantation of the definite new prosthesis. Success rates of between 87 to 94% have been reported with cemented 2 stage revision [124, 125, 128].

6. Nerve and vessel injury

The overall incidence of nerve injury after THA is estimated to be around 1% [129]. Sciatic nerve palsies account for 79% of all cases, followed by femoral nerve palsies (13%), combined femoral and sciatic nerve palsy (5.8%) and obturator nerve palsy (1.6%) [129]. In the majority of cases (47%) the aetiology is unknown. Other causes include traction (20%), contusion (19%), haematoma (11%) and dislocation (2%), with laceration only accounting for 1% of all nerve palsies [130]. Risk factors for nerve injury include female sex, revision surgery and developmental dysplasia of the acetabulum [129].

When the sciatic nerve is affected, it most commonly involves the common peroneal division. This is thought to be due to the lower amount of connective tissue present between the funiculi and its relatively tethered position at the sciatic notch compared to the tibial branch [129, 131]. These factors are thought to make the peroneal branch more susceptible to trauma and traction. The use of the posterior approach has traditionally been associated with increased risk of sciatic nerve damage. However a Cochrane review in 2006 found no difference in the incidence of nerve palsy between the posterior and direct lateral approaches [132]. Femoral nerve palsy is less common and is usually secondary to direct compression, usually due to a malpositioned retractor [130].

Indications for surgical intervention in a patient with nerve palsy include haematoma causing compression, palsy associated with excessive lengthening and palsy that can be definitely attributed to implanted metalwork. Electrodiagnostic studies can be helpful in determining the level of the lesion. Outcomes of nerve palsies are variable, with 40% of patients showing a good recovery, 45% of patients having mild residual motor or sensory symptoms and 15% left with a dense motor or sensory deficit [129]. Partial nerve lesions and maintenance of some motor function are good prognostic indicators, with recovery possible for up to 3 years after the initial insult [133].

Vascular injury during THA is extremely rare. Published incidence varies between 0.04 to 0.08% [134, 135]. As opposed to knee arthroplasty, vascular injury in THA is usually the result of direct trauma either during component insertion or removal [136]. Risk factors include revision surgery, previous vascular injury or surgery and pre-existing atherosclerosis [137]. The majority of vascular injuries are arterial but venous injury has been described [138]. Venous injuries however may be under diagnosed as they may run a relatively benign course remaining undetected.

The majority of vascular injuries are either the result direct trauma from acetabular retractors or acetabular screw insertion [130]. Wasielewski et al. have described an acetabular quadrant system to help guide safe screw insertion [139]. The postero-superior and poster-inferior quadrants are the safest zones for screw insertion as they have they areas of greatest bone stock [139].

6.1. Wear and aseptic loosening

Aseptic loosening is the most common cause for revision surgery, accounting for 75% of revision cases [140]. Aseptic failure occurs as a result of a chronic inflammatory reaction secondary to particulate wear debris eventually resulting in osteoclast activation, osteolysis and loosening [141].

The pathogenesis begins with the generation of wear particles from the bearing surface, and also non bearing surfaces such as the interface between acetabular shell and the liner insert, known as backside wear. The morphology of the wear debris is dependent on the type of implant used. Particles from polyethylene bearing surfaces can vary from submicron in size to several millimetres. The average size of polyethylene debris has been shown to be around 0.5 μm and it is this submicron sized particle that has been shown to have the most bio-reactivity [142, 143]. The rate of generation of the wear particles has also been shown to correlate with the degree of osteolysis [142]. Inadequate initial fixation can also contribute to loosening by generating micromotion and increasing the rate of generation of particulate debris [144]. This highlights the importance of good cementation techniques in reducing the risk of aseptic failure. Pressure within the joint fluid has also been suggested to contribute to osteolysis. Increased joint fluid pressure in animal models has been shown to induce bone loss at the prosthesis bone interface possibly by interfering with bone perfusion causing osteocyte death [145, 146]. Increased joint fluid pressures have been noted in THAs undergoing revision and pressure waves generated by load bearing have been demonstrated in retroacetabular lytic lesions [147, 148]. Thus increased fluid pressures may directly contribute to osteolysis and also perpetuate the dissemination of the wear debris throughout the prosthesis bone interface, enhancing the biological response.

The primary response to wear debris is predominantly macrophage mediated. The exact mechanism of macrophage activation is still unclear. Macrophages can be activated as a result of either phagocytosis of particulate matter and also possibly through cell membrane interactions with particulate matter [149]. Macrophage activation causes the release of pro-inflammatory cytokines and growth factors including TNF-α, Interleukin-1, TGF-β and RANKL [150]. This results in the production of a pseudomembrane at the bone cement prosthesis interface consisting of macrophages, fibroblasts and lymphocytes within a connective tissue matrix [151]. TNF-α and Interleukin-1 both promote osteoclastic differentiation and activation, but it is the up regulation of the RANK/RANKL pathway that is the key to activating osteoclastogenesis and subsequent osteolysis [143]. Recent studies have suggested individual genetic susceptibility to osteolysis may exist via single nucleotide polymorphisms in the implicated cytokine genes, possibly by altering the magnitude of the biological response [152-155].

Alternative bearing surfaces can be used to reduce wear rates, debris generation and subsequent osteolysis. Highly crosslinked polyethylene, ceramic on ceramic and metal on metal bearings have all been shown to have reduced wear rates compared to standard ultra-high molecular weight polyethylene (UHWPE) [156-164]. However there are concerns regarding the increased bioreactivity of crosslinked polyethylene debris compared to standard UHWPE which may offset the benefits of reduced volumetric wear [165, 166]. Volumetric wear is also lower with metal on metal bearings. However as the particle size is much smaller, usually between 20-90nm, the overall surface area is much larger compared to UHWPE raising concerns of possible increased bioreactivity.

Pain is usually the primary presenting symptom of aseptic failure. Gross acetabular loosening can cause groin pain whereas thigh pain can indicate femoral loosening [167]. Early loosening however may also be asymptomatic merely detected on routine follow up radiographs. Clinical signs may include inability to straight leg raise, shortening of the leg due to subsidence and increasing external rotation of the leg if the femoral stem twists into retroversion. Investigations for aseptic loosening are similar to those for infection discussed earlier. Blood inflammatory markers such as CRP are usually normal with aseptic loosening [168]. Radiological tests include plain radiography, subtraction and nuclear arthrography and bone scintigraphy. Meta-analysis has shown similar diagnostic performance for all of these tests and therefore suggests plain radiographs and bone scintigraphy as the tests of choice due to their lower risk of patient morbidity [169]. CT 3D imaging is also useful for the evaluation of lytic lesions as plain 2 dimensional radiographs can underestimate the size of the lesion as demonstrated in figure 1 [170, 171].

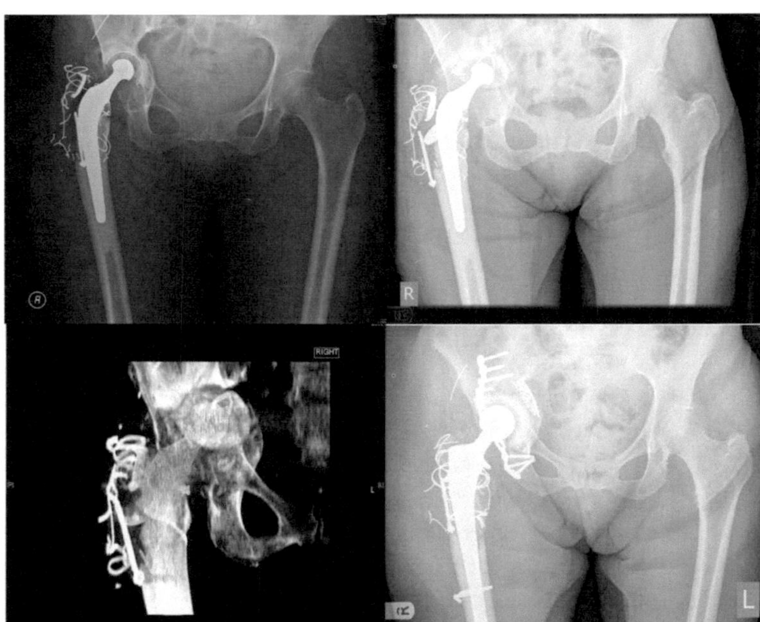

Figure 6. Top left & right, Progressive acetabular osteolysis over 1.5 years, **Bottom left,** 3D CT reconstruction demonstrating lesion and pelvic discontinuity, **Bottom right,** defect reconstructed with mesh and bone graft and plate to posterior column to address discontinuity

Treatment of aseptic loosening is guided by the severity of the patient's symptoms and the rate and volume of osteolysis. Indications for surgical treatment in asymptomatic patients are progressive osteolysis and risk of catastrophic mechanical failure such as periprosthetic fracture. Nonsurgical treatment using bisphosphonates and anti cytokine therapy such as anti-TNF-α to prevent progression of osteolysis has been suggested. However their efficacy is yet to be determined [172]. Goals of surgical treatment include removal of wear debris and also the wear generator, reconstruction of the osseous lesion and restoration of mechanical stability [173]. This can involve exchange of bearing surfaces, bone grafting of lytic lesions and revision of loose components.

7. Bearing specific complications

7.1. Ceramic on ceramic bearings

Ceramic articulations have become increasingly popular due to their low wear profile and good biocompatibility. However potential complications of ceramic bearings include chipping and incomplete seating of ceramic liners during insertion, fracture and bearing generated noise.

Currently all ceramic acetabular bearings consist of a modular ceramic liner which is inserted into a metal shell implanted into the acetabulum. Incomplete seating of the liner due to soft tissue interposition or deformation of the metal shell has been reported [174, 175]. Thus extra care and good visualisation of the acetabulum is imperative when inserting a modular ceramic liner. Chipping during impaction has also been reported and this can also be secondary to deformation of the metal shell [176]. Using titanium sleeved or recessed ceramic liners has been shown to reduce such risks [177].

Risk of fracture for modern 3rd generation ceramic bearings is extremely low. Willman et al. found a fracture rate of 0.004% for femoral heads manufactured after 1994 [178]. Fracture of both the liner and femoral head have however been reported [179, 180]. Head fracture has been associated with improper handling during implantation. Contamination of the stem-ball interface with blood or soft tissue has been shown to significantly reduce the load required for inducing fracture [181]. Impingement of the femoral neck on the edge of ceramics liner is thought to be a major risk factor for liner fracture [179, 182]. Therefore correct positioning of the acetabular component is especially important for ceramic bearings.

Noise generated from ceramic bearings is a recently described phenomenon. Published rates of "squeaky" ceramic bearings range from 2.7% to 20.9% [183, 184]. Component malposition has been implicated [185]. However recent studies have found no association between cup inclination and version and the incidence of squeaking [183, 184]. Short neck length is the only factor that has been associated with squeaking, possibly due to impingement or micro-seperation to due increased joint laxity [184]. Revision of squeaking hips has revealed evidence of stripe wear but there is currently no evidence to suggest squeaking is a precursor for ceramic fracture [186, 187].

7.2. Metal on metal bearings

Metal on metal bearings also have superior wear rates compared to standard UHMWPE [161, 163, 164]. However there is increasing concern regarding metal ion toxicity and hypersensitivity type reactions. Volumetric wear is considerably lower for metal bearings compared to UHMWPE, but the absolute number of particles generated is estimated to be 13500 times higher [188]. Therefore the total surface area is considerably higher. Thus the bioreactivity of metal wear particles may be higher than polyethylene or ceramic debris, and the nanometre scale of the particles and dissolution of metal ions allows distant transport, raising concerns of systemic toxicity.

The possibility of systemic toxicity has raised interest in serum metal ion levels in patients with modern metal on metal bearings. Recent studies using standardised measurement techniques have reported mean serum chromium levels of between 0.86 – 17.7 μg/L [189-192]. Safe levels of serum metal ion levels have however yet to be determined [193]. Concerns regarding carcinogenesis and immune suppression secondary to raised blood metal ion levels have been raised [194, 195]. Teratogenicity is also another potential concern as transplacental crossage of metal ions has been demonstrated [196]. However, currently no conclusive evidence exists supporting these theories [197, 198]. A positive correlation between cup inclination and blood metal ion levels has been demonstrated with metal on metal bearings [191, 199]. This is probably due to increased edge loading with increasing cup inclination and serum metal ion levels have been suggested as a tool to monitor the performance of metal on metal bearings [190]. Therefore metal ion exposure can be minimised with proper cup orientation.

Local tissue reactions to metal on metal articulations have also been reported [200-202]. Metal ions are thought to induce an immune reaction leading to tissue necrosis and osteolysis. This is in contrast to UHMWPE which induces a macrophage reaction to particulate wear debris. Willert et al. has called this unique reaction, aseptic lymphocytic vasculitic associated lesions (ALVAL) [200]. Histologically this reaction is characterised by perivascular lymphocytic infiltration and plasma cells. Clinical presentation can vary between chronic groin pain to extensive tissue necrosis forming pseudotumours [201]. Exact incidence of such tissue reactions is unknown but is estimated to be around 1% [201]. Risk factors associated with the development of these adverse reactions include small component size and component malposition [203]. Stemmed metal on metal hip replacements also appear to have a higher rate of revision and their use has now been discouraged [204].

8. Periprosthetic fracture

Periprosthetic fractures can occur either intraoperatively or in the postoperative period. Overall, periprosthetic fractures more commonly affect the femoral component of the THA. Data from the largest published series by Berry et al. reports the incidence of intra- and postoperative femoral fracture as 1% and 1.1% respectively [13]. Rates of intraoperative fracture after cementless fixation are higher, 5.4% for primary THAs and 21% for revision surgery [13].

http://dx.doi.org/10.5772/53030

The treatment of unstable postoperative periprosthetic femoral fractures is now almost always operative. Loosening, non-union, varus malunion and morbidity associated with prolonged immobility have made conservative management unpopular [205]. Treatment can be guided by using the Vancouver classification which is the most widely accepted system for classifying such fractures [206]. This system takes into account three main factors, site of the fracture, stability of the implant and quality of the surrounding bone. Type A fractures occur in the trochanteric region and are subdivided into type A_G and A_L fractures. A_G fractures involve the greater trochanter and usually stable and can therefore be treated conservatively with protected weightbearing. A_L fractures involve the lesser trochanter, and are also usually insignificant unless a large portion of the calcar is involved potentially affecting implant stability, in which case revision THA may be necessary. Type B fractures occur around or just distal to the stem and are subdivided into type B_1, B_2 and B_3 fractures. B_1 fractures have a well fixed stem and can be treated with open reduction and internal fixation. Combined plate and cerclage wire systems are commonly used for such fractures. Type B_2 fractures have a loose stem but good bone stock. These are usually revised with long stem implants bypassing the fracture, and can be augmented by plates, cables and strut allografts to improve stability. Type B_3 fractures have a loose stem and poor stock stock. These are the most difficult to treat and require either revision THA with structural allografts to reconstitute the proximal femur, distally fixed long stemmed implants of custom proximal femoral replacement. Type C fractures occur distal to the stem. The stem can therefore essentially be ignored and the fracture treated with standard open reduction and internal fixation.

Acetabular fractures are somewhat less common with reported intraoperative rates ranging between 0.02-0.4% [207, 208]. Data regarding postoperative fractures is currently not available [13]. The majority of intraoperative acetabular fractures occur during acetabular insertion especially during impaction of pressfit cementless components [209]. Underreaming by greater than 2mm has been suggested to significantly increase fracture risk [210].

The aims of treatment of intraoperative acetabular fractures include stabilizing the fracture and preventing further propagation and maintaining component stability [209]. Techniques include plating the anterior and posterior columns and using bone graft and jumbo revision cups if there is marked bone loss. Treatment of postoperative fractures follows similar principles. Early postoperative fractures with stable cups and minimally displaced fractures, especially around uncemented implants with supplemental screw fixation, can be treated conservatively. Unstable cups require revision with fixation of the fracture. Late presenting fractures are frequently associated with osteolysis and therefore usually require revision with bone grafting [211].

9. Heterotopic ossification

Heterotopic ossification (HO) is the abnormal formation of mature lamellar bone within extraskeletal soft tissues. HO is most commonly asymptomatic, merely detected on follow up radiology. When symptomatic, stiffness is the most common presentation. Pain and soft tissue signs such as localised warmth, mild oedema and erythema are uncommon but can cause confusion raising concerns over infection [212].

Early changes of HO within the soft tissues can be detected after 3 weeks on bone scan and plain radiographic changes can take 6 weeks to become apparent [212]. Extensive bone deposition can occur within 3 months, but full maturation takes up to one year [213]. The abductor compartment is most commonly affected. HO is most commonly classified using the Brooker classification [214]. This is based upon plain anteroposterior radiographs of the pelvis and is outlined in figure 7.

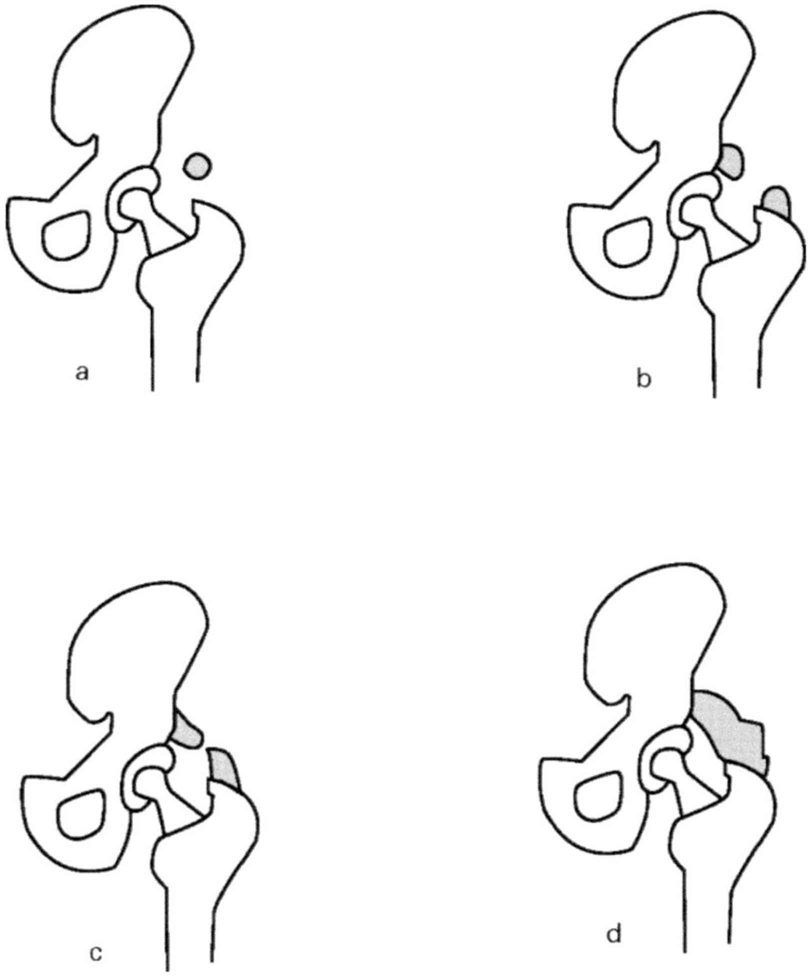

Figure 7. Brooker classification showing a) grade 1: islands of bone within the soft tissues about the hip, b) grade 2: bony spurs from either the femur or the pelvis, with a gap of more than 1 cm between opposing bony ends, c) grade 3: the gaps between the spurs are less than 1 cm and d) grade 4: apparent ankylosis of the hip due to the heterotopic ossification.

The pathophysiology is believed to involve inappropriate differentiation of pluripotent mesenchymal stem cells into osteoblasts, causing the excess bone formation [215]. Overexpression of bone morphogenetic protein-4 has been implicated [216, 217].

Incidence of clinically significant HO is reported to be between 3 – 7% [218, 219]. Risk factors include male gender, previous history of HO, pre-existing hip fusion, hypertrophic osteoarthritis, ankylosing spondylitis, diffuse idiopathic skeletal hyperostosis, Paget's disease, post traumatic osteoarthritis, osteonecrosis and rheumatoid arthritis [14]. Surgical factors include extensive soft tissue dissection, haematoma and persistence of bone debris. Evidence implicating the role of surgical approach is debatable [14].

Treatment of symptomatic patients can initially involve intensive physiotherapy during the maturation phase. The efficacy of this treatment is however yet to be determined. Surgical management involves excision of the HO after maturation of the bone is allowed, followed by appropriate prophylaxis. Improvements in range of motion in all planes has been reported with surgical excision [220].

Patients at high risk of HO should be given prophylaxis either in the form of non steroidal anti-inflammatory medication (NSAIDs) or radiotherapy. Preoperative radiotherapy, 4 hours before, or post operative radiotherapy within 72 hours has been shown to be the most effective method of prophylaxis [221-223]. This involves a single dose of between 7 – 8 Gy. Combination therapy with NSAIDs and radiotherapy can be considered in patients at highest risk of HO such as patients undergoing excision of symptomatic HO [14].

10. Conclusion

- Complications following total hip arthroplasty can be classified into procedure specific or systemic. On the whole complication rates have fallen with time due to improved surgical and anaesthetic technique.
- The most common symptomatic systemic complication is DVT and data suggests that DVT rates post THA have not fallen with time.
- The most common cause for revision is aseptic loosening. Registry data suggests up to 75% of revision surgery may be due to aseptic loosening.
- Infection is one of the most feared complications. Rates with prophylactic measures such as antibiotics and clean air enclosures have however dropped significantly to below 1%.
- Leg length discrepancy is one of the most common causes of patient dissatisfaction and is the most common cause of litigation in the USA.

Despite the potential wide range of complication that can occur after THA, it remains one of the most successful orthopaedic interventions

List of abbreviations used

THA: Total Hip Arthroplasty

DVT: Deep Vein Thrombosis

PE: Pulmonary Embolism

THA: Total Hip Arthroplasty

PLAD: Posterior Lip Augmentation Device

UHMWPE: Ultra High Molecular Weight Polyehtylene

LLD: Limb Length Discrepancy

TGF-β: Transforming Growth Factor – Beta

RANKL: Receptor activator of nuclear factor kappa-B ligand

UHMWPE: Ultra High Molecular Weight Polyethylene

TNF-α: Tumour Necrosis Factor – Alpha

ALVAL: aseptic lymphocytic vasculitic associated lesions

HO: Heterotopic Ossification

Author details

Asim Rajpura and Tim Board*

*Address all correspondence to: tim@timboard.co.uk

Wrightington Hospital, Hall Lane, Appley Bridge, Wigan, Lancashire, UK

References

[1] Registry NJ. Summary of annual statistics (England and Wales). National Joint Registry 2009 [cited 2009 04/02/2009].

[2] Jones CA, Voaklander DC, Johnston DW, Suarez-Almazor ME. Health related quality of life outcomes after total hip and knee arthroplasties in a community based population. J Rheumatol. 2000 Jul;27(7):1745-52.

[3] Mancuso CA, Salvati EA, Johanson NA, Peterson MG, Charlson ME. Patients' expectations and satisfaction with total hip arthroplasty. J Arthroplasty. 1997 Jun;12(4): 387-96.

[4] Liu SS, Gonzalez Della Valle A, Besculides MC, Gaber LK, Memtsoudis SG. Trends in mortality, complications, and demographics for primary hip arthroplasty in the United States. Int Orthop. 2008 May 7.

[5] Pitto RP, Koessler M. The risk of fat embolism during cemented total hip replacement in the elderly patient. Chir Organi Mov. 1999 Apr-Jun;84(2):119-28.

[6] Kwon MS, Kuskowski M, Mulhall KJ, Macaulay W, Brown TE, Saleh KJ. Does surgical approach affect total hip arthroplasty dislocation rates? Clin Orthop Relat Res. 2006 Jun;447:34-8.

[7] Wylde V, Whitehouse SL, Taylor AH, Pattison GT, Bannister GC, Blom AW. Prevalence and functional impact of patient-perceived leg length discrepancy after hip replacement. Int Orthop. 2008 Apr 25.

[8] Samama CM, Ravaud P, Parent F, Barre J, Mertl P, Mismetti P. Epidemiology of venous thromboembolism after lower limb arthroplasty: the FOTO study. J Thromb Haemost. 2007 Dec;5(12):2360-7.

[9] Blom AW, Taylor AH, Pattison G, Whitehouse S, Bannister GC. Infection after total hip arthroplasty. The Avon experience. J Bone Joint Surg Br. 2003 Sep;85(7):956-9.

[10] Mantilla CB, Horlocker TT, Schroeder DR, Berry DJ, Brown DL. Frequency of myocardial infarction, pulmonary embolism, deep venous thrombosis, and death following primary hip or knee arthroplasty. Anesthesiology. 2002 May;96(5):1140-6.

[11] Hallan G, Lie SA, Furnes O, Engesaeter LB, Vollset SE, Havelin LI. Medium- and long-term performance of 11,516 uncemented primary femoral stems from the Norwegian arthroplasty register. J Bone Joint Surg Br. 2007 Dec;89(12):1574-80.

[12] Ling RS, Charity J, Lee AJ, Whitehouse SL, Timperley AJ, Gie GA. The long-term results of the original exeter polished cemented femoral component a follow-up report. J Arthroplasty. 2009 Jun;24(4):511-7.

[13] Berry DJ. Epidemiology: hip and knee. Orthop Clin North Am. 1999 Apr;30(2): 183-90.

[14] Board TN, Karva A, Board RE, Gambhir AK, Porter ML. The prophylaxis and treatment of heterotopic ossification following lower limb arthroplasty. J Bone Joint Surg Br. 2007 Apr;89(4):434-40.

[15] Kim YH, Oh SH, Kim JS. Incidence and natural history of deep-vein thrombosis after total hip arthroplasty. A prospective and randomised clinical study. J Bone Joint Surg Br. 2003 Jul;85(5):661-5.

[16] NICE. Venous thromboembolism: reducing the risk of venous thromboembolism (deep vein thrombosis and pulmonary embolism) in inpatients undergoing surgery: National Collaborating Centre for Acute Care; 2007.

[17] Xing KH, Morrison G, Lim W, Douketis J, Odueyungbo A, Crowther M. Has the incidence of deep vein thrombosis in patients undergoing total hip/knee arthroplasty

changed over time? A systematic review of randomized controlled trials. Thromb Res. 2008;123(1):24-34.

[18] Sharrock NE, Go G, Harpel PC, Ranawat CS, Sculco TP, Salvati EA. The John Charnley Award. Thrombogenesis during total hip arthroplasty. Clin Orthop Relat Res. 1995 Oct(319):16-27.

[19] Borghi B, Casati A. Thromboembolic complications after total hip replacement. Int Orthop. 2002;26(1):44-7.

[20] McNally MA, Mollan RA. Total hip replacement, lower limb blood flow and venous thrombogenesis. J Bone Joint Surg Br. 1993 Jul;75(4):640-4.

[21] Beksac B, Gonzalez Della Valle A, Salvati EA. Thromboembolic disease after total hip arthroplasty: who is at risk? Clin Orthop Relat Res. 2006 Dec;453:211-24.

[22] Modig J, Hjelmstedt A, Sahlstedt B, Maripuu E. Comparative influences of epidural and general anaesthesia on deep venous thrombosis and pulmonary embolism after total hip replacement. Acta Chir Scand. 1981;147(2):125-30.

[23] Davis FM, Laurenson VG, Gillespie WJ, Wells JE, Foate J, Newman E. Deep vein thrombosis after total hip replacement. A comparison between spinal and general anaesthesia. J Bone Joint Surg Br. 1989 Mar;71(2):181-5.

[24] Davis FM, Laurenson VG, Gillespie WJ, Foate J, Seagar AD. Leg blood flow during total hip replacement under spinal or general anaesthesia. Anaesth Intensive Care. 1989 May;17(2):136-43.

[25] Stannard JP, Harris RM, Bucknell AL, Cossi A, Ward J, Arrington ED. Prophylaxis of deep venous thrombosis after total hip arthroplasty by using intermittent compression of the plantar venous plexus. Am J Orthop. 1996 Feb;25(2):127-34.

[26] Ryan MG, Westrich GH, Potter HG, Sharrock N, Maun LM, Macaulay W, et al. Effect of mechanical compression on the prevalence of proximal deep venous thrombosis as assessed by magnetic resonance venography. J Bone Joint Surg Am. 2002 Nov;84-A(11):1998-2004.

[27] Zufferey P, Laporte S, Quenet S, Molliex S, Auboyer C, Decousus H, et al. Optimal low-molecular-weight heparin regimen in major orthopaedic surgery. A meta-analysis of randomised trials. Thromb Haemost. 2003 Oct;90(4):654-61.

[28] Lassen MR, Borris LC, Anderson BS, Jensen HP, Skejo Bro HP, Andersen G, et al. Efficacy and safety of prolonged thromboprophylaxis with a low molecular weight heparin (dalteparin) after total hip arthroplasty--the Danish Prolonged Prophylaxis (DaPP) Study. Thromb Res. 1998 Mar 15;89(6):281-7.

[29] Turpie AG, Bauer KA, Eriksson BI, Lassen MR. Fondaparinux vs enoxaparin for the prevention of venous thromboembolism in major orthopedic surgery: a meta-analysis of 4 randomized double-blind studies. Arch Intern Med. 2002 Sep 9;162(16): 1833-40.

[30] Lassen MR, Bauer KA, Eriksson BI, Turpie AG. Postoperative fondaparinux versus preoperative enoxaparin for prevention of venous thromboembolism in elective hip-replacement surgery: a randomised double-blind comparison. Lancet. 2002 May 18;359(9319):1715-20.

[31] Pitto RP, Hamer H, Heiss-Dunlop W, Kuehle J. Mechanical prophylaxis of deep-vein thrombosis after total hip replacement a randomised clinical trial. J Bone Joint Surg Br. 2004 Jul;86(5):639-42.

[32] Kakkar VV, Howes J, Sharma V, Kadziola Z. A comparative double-blind, randomised trial of a new second generation LMWH (bemiparin) and UFH in the prevention of post-operative venous thromboembolism. The Bemiparin Assessment group. Thromb Haemost. 2000 Apr;83(4):523-9.

[33] Dahl OE, Andreassen G, Aspelin T, Muller C, Mathiesen P, Nyhus S, et al. Prolonged thromboprophylaxis following hip replacement surgery--results of a double-blind, prospective, randomised, placebo-controlled study with dalteparin (Fragmin). Thromb Haemost. 1997 Jan;77(1):26-31.

[34] Turpie AG, Eriksson BI, Lassen MR, Bauer KA. A meta-analysis of fondaparinux versus enoxaparin in the prevention of venous thromboembolism after major orthopaedic surgery. J South Orthop Assoc. 2002 Winter;11(4):182-8.

[35] Eriksson BI, Borris LC, Friedman RJ, Haas S, Huisman MV, Kakkar AK, et al. Rivaroxaban versus enoxaparin for thromboprophylaxis after hip arthroplasty. N Engl J Med. 2008 Jun 26;358(26):2765-75.

[36] Kakkar AK, Brenner B, Dahl OE, Eriksson BI, Mouret P, Muntz J, et al. Extended duration rivaroxaban versus short-term enoxaparin for the prevention of venous thromboembolism after total hip arthroplasty: a double-blind, randomised controlled trial. Lancet. 2008 Jul 5;372(9632):31-9.

[37] Raskob GE, Gallus AS, Pineo GF, Chen D, Ramirez LM, Wright RT, et al. Apixaban versus enoxaparin for thromboprophylaxis after hip or knee replacement: pooled analysis of major venous thromboembolism and bleeding in 8464 patients from the ADVANCE-2 and ADVANCE-3 trials. J Bone Joint Surg Br. 2012 Feb;94(2):257-64.

[38] Jensen CD, Steval A, Partington PF, Reed MR, Muller SD. Return to theatre following total hip and knee replacement, before and after the introduction of rivaroxaban: a retrospective cohort study. J Bone Joint Surg Br. 2011 Jan;93(1):91-5.

[39] NICE. Venous thromboembolism, reducing the risk of venous thromboembolism (deep vein thrombosis and pulmonary embolism) in patients admitted to hospital. London: National Clinical Guideline Centre; 2010.

[40] Pulido L, Parvizi J, Macgibeny M, Sharkey PF, Purtill JJ, Rothman RH, et al. In hospital complications after total joint arthroplasty. J Arthroplasty. 2008 Sep;23(6 Suppl 1): 139-45.

[41] Roderick P, Ferris G, Wilson K, Halls H, Jackson D, Collins R, et al. Towards evidence-based guidelines for the prevention of venous thromboembolism: systematic reviews of mechanical methods, oral anticoagulation, dextran and regional anaesthesia as thromboprophylaxis. Health Technol Assess. 2005 Dec;9(49):iii-iv, ix-x, 1-78.

[42] Haas S, Breyer HG, Bacher HP, Fareed J, Misselwitz F, Victor N, et al. Prevention of major venous thromboembolism following total hip or knee replacement: a randomized comparison of low-molecular-weight heparin with unfractionated heparin (ECHOS Trial). Int Angiol. 2006 Dec;25(4):335-42.

[43] Hooker JA, Lachiewicz PF, Kelley SS. Efficacy of prophylaxis against thromboembolism with intermittent pneumatic compression after primary and revision total hip arthroplasty. J Bone Joint Surg Am. 1999 May;81(5):690-6.

[44] Eriksson BI, Kalebo P, Anthymyr BA, Wadenvik H, Tengborn L, Risberg B. Prevention of deep-vein thrombosis and pulmonary embolism after total hip replacement. Comparison of low-molecular-weight heparin and unfractionated heparin. J Bone Joint Surg Am. 1991 Apr;73(4):484-93.

[45] Handoll HH, Farrar MJ, McBirnie J, Tytherleigh-Strong G, Milne AA, Gillespie WJ. Heparin, low molecular weight heparin and physical methods for preventing deep vein thrombosis and pulmonary embolism following surgery for hip fractures. Cochrane Database Syst Rev. 2002(4):CD000305.

[46] Fender D, Harper WM, Thompson JR, Gregg PJ. Mortality and fatal pulmonary embolism after primary total hip replacement. Results from a regional hip register. J Bone Joint Surg Br. 1997 Nov;79(6):896-9.

[47] Joels CS, Sing RF, Heniford BT. Complications of inferior vena cava filters. Am Surg. 2003 Aug;69(8):654-9.

[48] Kallos T, Enis JE, Gollan F, Davis JH. Intramedullary pressure and pulmonary embolism of femoral medullary contents in dogs during insertion of bone cement and a prosthesis. J Bone Joint Surg Am. 1974 Oct;56(7):1363-7.

[49] Tronzo RG, Kallos T, Wyche MQ. Elevation of intramedullary pressure when methylmethacrylate is inserted in total hip arthroplasty. J Bone Joint Surg Am. 1974 Jun; 56(4):714-8.

[50] Wenda K, Degreif J, Runkel M, Ritter G. Pathogenesis and prophylaxis of circulatory reactions during total hip replacement. Arch Orthop Trauma Surg. 1993;112(6):260-5.

[51] Colonna DM, Kilgus D, Brown W, Challa V, Stump DA, Moody DM. Acute brain fat embolization occurring after total hip arthroplasty in the absence of a patent foramen ovale. Anesthesiology. 2002 Apr;96(4):1027-9.

[52] Forteza AM, Koch S, Romano JG, Zych G, Bustillo IC, Duncan RC, et al. Transcranial doppler detection of fat emboli. Stroke. 1999 Dec;30(12):2687-91.

[53] Edmonds CR, Barbut D, Hager D, Sharrock NE. Intraoperative cerebral arterial embolization during total hip arthroplasty. Anesthesiology. 2000 Aug;93(2):315-8.

[54] Memtsoudis SG, Rosenberger P, Walz JM. Critical care issues in the patient after major joint replacement. J Intensive Care Med. 2007 Mar-Apr;22(2):92-104.

[55] Christie J, Robinson CM, Singer B, Ray DC. Medullary lavage reduces embolic phenomena and cardiopulmonary changes during cemented hemiarthroplasty. J Bone Joint Surg Br. 1995 May;77(3):456-9.

[56] Pitto RP, Kossler M, Draenert K. [Prevention of fat and bone marrow embolism in cemented total hip endoprosthesis with vacuum cement technique]. Z Orthop Ihre Grenzgeb. 1998 Jul-Aug;136(4):Oa24.

[57] Aynardi M, Pulido L, Parvizi J, Sharkey PF, Rothman RH. Early mortality after modern total hip arthroplasty. Clin Orthop Relat Res. 2009 Jan;467(1):213-8.

[58] Kreder HJ, Berry GK, McMurtry IA, Halman SI. Arthroplasty in the octogenarian: quantifying the risks. J Arthroplasty. 2005 Apr;20(3):289-93.

[59] Eagle KA, Berger PB, Calkins H, Chaitman BR, Ewy GA, Fleischmann KE, et al. ACC/AHA Guideline Update for Perioperative Cardiovascular Evaluation for Noncardiac Surgery--Executive Summary. A report of the American College of Cardiology/American Heart Association Task Force on Practice Guidelines (Committee to Update the 1996 Guidelines on Perioperative Cardiovascular Evaluation for Noncardiac Surgery). Anesth Analg. 2002 May;94(5):1052-64.

[60] Moller AM, Pedersen T, Villebro N, Munksgaard A. Effect of smoking on early complications after elective orthopaedic surgery. J Bone Joint Surg Br. 2003 Mar;85(2):178-81.

[61] Greenfield S, Apolone G, McNeil BJ, Cleary PD. The importance of co-existent disease in the occurrence of postoperative complications and one-year recovery in patients undergoing total hip replacement. Comorbidity and outcomes after hip replacement. Med Care. 1993 Feb;31(2):141-54.

[62] Parker MJ, Handoll HH, Griffiths R. Anaesthesia for hip fracture surgery in adults. Cochrane Database Syst Rev. 2001(4):CD000521.

[63] Sculco TP, Ranawat C. The use of spinal anesthesia for total hip-replacement arthroplasty. J Bone Joint Surg Am. 1975 Mar;57(2):173-7.

[64] O'Hara DA, Duff A, Berlin JA, Poses RM, Lawrence VA, Huber EC, et al. The effect of anesthetic technique on postoperative outcomes in hip fracture repair. Anesthesiology. 2000 Apr;92(4):947-57.

[65] Skutek M, Bourne RB, MacDonald SJ. (i) International epidemiology of revision THR. Current Orthopaedics. 2006;20(3):157-61.

[66] Patel PD, Potts A, Froimson MI. The dislocating hip arthroplasty: prevention and treatment. J Arthroplasty. 2007 Jun;22(4 Suppl 1):86-90.

[67] Sanchez-Sotelo J, Berry DJ. Epidemiology of instability after total hip replacement. Orthop Clin North Am. 2001 Oct;32(4):543-52, vii.

[68] Woo RY, Morrey BF. Dislocations after total hip arthroplasty. J Bone Joint Surg Am. 1982 Dec;64(9):1295-306.

[69] von Knoch M, Berry DJ, Harmsen WS, Morrey BF. Late dislocation after total hip arthroplasty. J Bone Joint Surg Am. 2002 Nov;84-A(11):1949-53.

[70] Soong M, Rubash HE, Macaulay W. Dislocation after total hip arthroplasty. J Am Acad Orthop Surg. 2004 Sep-Oct;12(5):314-21.

[71] Lee BP, Berry DJ, Harmsen WS, Sim FH. Total hip arthroplasty for the treatment of an acute fracture of the femoral neck: long-term results. J Bone Joint Surg Am. 1998 Jan;80(1):70-5.

[72] Goldstein WM, Gleason TF, Kopplin M, Branson JJ. Prevalence of dislocation after total hip arthroplasty through a posterolateral approach with partial capsulotomy and capsulorrhaphy. J Bone Joint Surg Am. 2001;83-A Suppl 2(Pt 1):2-7.

[73] White RE, Jr., Forness TJ, Allman JK, Junick DW. Effect of posterior capsular repair on early dislocation in primary total hip replacement. Clin Orthop Relat Res. 2001 Dec(393):163-7.

[74] Fackler CD, Poss R. Dislocation in total hip arthroplasties. Clin Orthop Relat Res. 1980 Sep(151):169-78.

[75] Lewinnek GE, Lewis JL, Tarr R, Compere CL, Zimmerman JR. Dislocations after total hip-replacement arthroplasties. J Bone Joint Surg Am. 1978 Mar;60(2):217-20.

[76] Barrack RL, Lavernia C, Ries M, Thornberry R, Tozakoglou E. Virtual reality computer animation of the effect of component position and design on stability after total hip arthroplasty. Orthop Clin North Am. 2001 Oct;32(4):569-77, vii.

[77] Nishii T, Sugano N, Miki H, Koyama T, Takao M, Yoshikawa H. Influence of component positions on dislocation: computed tomographic evaluations in a consecutive series of total hip arthroplasty. J Arthroplasty. 2004 Feb;19(2):162-6.

[78] Archbold HA, Mockford B, Molloy D, McConway J, Ogonda L, Beverland D. The transverse acetabular ligament: an aid to orientation of the acetabular component during primary total hip replacement: a preliminary study of 1000 cases investigating postoperative stability. J Bone Joint Surg Br. 2006 Jul;88(7):883-6.

[79] Amuwa C, Dorr LD. The combined anteversion technique for acetabular component anteversion. J Arthroplasty. 2008 Oct;23(7):1068-70.

[80] Barsoum WK, Patterson RW, Higuera C, Klika AK, Krebs VE, Molloy R. A computer model of the position of the combined component in the prevention of impingement in total hip replacement. J Bone Joint Surg Br. 2007 Jun;89(6):839-45.

[81] Kluess D, Martin H, Mittelmeier W, Schmitz KP, Bader R. Influence of femoral head size on impingement, dislocation and stress distribution in total hip replacement. Med Eng Phys. 2007 May;29(4):465-71.

[82] Burroughs BR, Hallstrom B, Golladay GJ, Hoeffel D, Harris WH. Range of motion and stability in total hip arthroplasty with 28-, 32-, 38-, and 44-mm femoral head sizes. J Arthroplasty. 2005 Jan;20(1):11-9.

[83] Bartz RL, Nobel PC, Kadakia NR, Tullos HS. The effect of femoral component head size on posterior dislocation of the artificial hip joint. J Bone Joint Surg Am. 2000 Sep; 82(9):1300-7.

[84] Bystrom S, Espehaug B, Furnes O, Havelin LI. Femoral head size is a risk factor for total hip luxation: a study of 42,987 primary hip arthroplasties from the Norwegian Arthroplasty Register. Acta Orthop Scand. 2003 Oct;74(5):514-24.

[85] Conroy JL, Whitehouse SL, Graves SE, Pratt NL, Ryan P, Crawford RW. Risk factors for revision for early dislocation in total hip arthroplasty. J Arthroplasty. 2008 Sep; 23(6):867-72.

[86] Hedlundh U, Ahnfelt L, Hybbinette CH, Wallinder L, Weckstrom J, Fredin H. Dislocations and the femoral head size in primary total hip arthroplasty. Clin Orthop Relat Res. 1996 Dec(333):226-33.

[87] Battaglia TC, Mulhall KJ, Brown TE, Saleh KJ. Increased surgical volume is associated with lower THA dislocation rates. Clin Orthop Relat Res. 2006 Jun;447:28-33.

[88] Schuh A, Mittelmeier W, Zeiler G, Behrend D, Kircher J, Bader R. Severe damage of the femoral head after dislocation and difficult reduction maneuvers after total hip arthroplasty. Arch Orthop Trauma Surg. 2006 Mar;126(2):134-7.

[89] Kop AM, Whitewood C, Johnston DJ. Damage of oxinium femoral heads subsequent to hip arthroplasty dislocation three retrieval case studies. J Arthroplasty. 2007 Aug; 22(5):775-9.

[90] McConway J, O'Brien S, Doran E, Archbold P, Beverland D. The use of a posterior lip augmentation device for a revision of recurrent dislocation after primary cemented Charnley/Charnley Elite total hip replacement: results at a mean follow-up of six years and nine months. J Bone Joint Surg Br. 2007 Dec;89(12):1581-5.

[91] Hofmann AA, Skrzynski MC. Leg-length inequality and nerve palsy in total hip arthroplasty: a lawyer awaits! Orthopedics. 2000 Sep;23(9):943-4.

[92] Konyves A, Bannister GC. The importance of leg length discrepancy after total hip arthroplasty. J Bone Joint Surg Br. 2005 Feb;87(2):155-7.

[93] Edwards BN, Tullos HS, Noble PC. Contributory factors and etiology of sciatic nerve palsy in total hip arthroplasty. Clin Orthop Relat Res. 1987 May(218):136-41.

[94] Farrell CM, Springer BD, Haidukewych GJ, Morrey BF. Motor nerve palsy following primary total hip arthroplasty. J Bone Joint Surg Am. 2005 Dec;87(12):2619-25.

[95] Gurney B, Mermier C, Robergs R, Gibson A, Rivero D. Effects of limb-length discrepancy on gait economy and lower-extremity muscle activity in older adults. J Bone Joint Surg Am. 2001 Jun;83-A(6):907-15.

[96] Maloney WJ, Keeney JA. Leg length discrepancy after total hip arthroplasty. J Arthroplasty. 2004 Jun;19(4 Suppl 1):108-10.

[97] Desai AS, Connors L, Board TN. Functional and radiological evaluation of a simple intra operative technique to avoid limb length discrepancy in total hip arthroplasty. Hip Int. 2011 Apr 5;21(2):192-8.

[98] Mihalko WM, Phillips MJ, Krackow KA. Acute sciatic and femoral neuritis following total hip arthroplasty. A case report. J Bone Joint Surg Am. 2001 Apr;83-A(4):589-92.

[99] Shiramizu K, Naito M, Shitama T, Nakamura Y, Shitama H. L-shaped caliper for limb length measurement during total hip arthroplasty. J Bone Joint Surg Br. 2004 Sep;86(7):966-9.

[100] Clark CR, Huddleston HD, Schoch EP, 3rd, Thomas BJ. Leg-length discrepancy after total hip arthroplasty. J Am Acad Orthop Surg. 2006 Jan;14(1):38-45.

[101] Charnley J. A Clean-Air Operating Enclosure. Br J Surg. 1964 Mar;51:202-5.

[102] Lister J. Antiseptic principle in the practice of surgery. Br Med J. 1967 Apr 1;2(5543): 9-12.

[103] Charnley J. Low Friction Arthroplasty of the Hip Theory and Practice. Berlin/Heidelberg: Springer-Verlag; 1979.

[104] Lidwell OM, Lowbury EJ, Whyte W, Blowers R, Stanley SJ, Lowe D. Effect of ultraclean air in operating rooms on deep sepsis in the joint after total hip or knee replacement: a randomised study. Br Med J (Clin Res Ed). 1982 Jul 3;285(6334):10-4.

[105] Bannister G. (v) Prevention of infection in joint replacement. Current Orthopaedics. 2002;16(6):426-33.

[106] Ericson C, Lidgren L, Lindberg L. Cloxacillin in the prophylaxis of postoperative infections of the hip. J Bone Joint Surg Am. 1973 Jun;55(4):808-13, 43.

[107] Nelson CL, Green TG, Porter RA, Warren RD. One day versus seven days of preventive antibiotic therapy in orthopedic surgery. Clin Orthop Relat Res. 1983 Jun(176): 258-63.

[108] Charnley J, Eftekhar N. Postoperative infection in total prosthetic replacement arthroplasty of the hip-joint. With special reference to the bacterial content of the air of the operating room. Br J Surg. 1969 Sep;56(9):641-9.

[109] Gambhir AK, Wroblewski BM, Kay PR. (iii) The infected total hip replacement. Current Orthopaedics. 2000;14(4):257-61.

[110] Pulido L, Ghanem E, Joshi A, Purtill JJ, Parvizi J. Periprosthetic joint infection: the incidence, timing, and predisposing factors. Clin Orthop Relat Res. 2008 Jul;466(7): 1710-5.

[111] Dunne WM, Jr. Bacterial adhesion: seen any good biofilms lately? Clin Microbiol Rev. 2002 Apr;15(2):155-66.

[112] Gristina AG, Shibata Y, Giridhar G, Kreger A, Myrvik QN. The glycocalyx, biofilm, microbes, and resistant infection. Semin Arthroplasty. 1994 Oct;5(4):160-70.

[113] Tsukayama DT, Estrada R, Gustilo RB. Infection after total hip arthroplasty. A study of the treatment of one hundred and six infections. J Bone Joint Surg Am. 1996 Apr; 78(4):512-23.

[114] Levitsky KA, Hozack WJ, Balderston RA, Rothman RH, Gluckman SJ, Maslack MM, et al. Evaluation of the painful prosthetic joint. Relative value of bone scan, sedimentation rate, and joint aspiration. J Arthroplasty. 1991 Sep;6(3):237-44.

[115] Kraemer WJ, Saplys R, Waddell JP, Morton J. Bone scan, gallium scan, and hip aspiration in the diagnosis of infected total hip arthroplasty. J Arthroplasty. 1993 Dec; 8(6):611-6.

[116] Bauer TW, Parvizi J, Kobayashi N, Krebs V. Diagnosis of periprosthetic infection. J Bone Joint Surg Am. 2006 Apr;88(4):869-82.

[117] Zhuang H, Yang H, Alavi A. Critical role of 18F-labeled fluorodeoxyglucose PET in the management of patients with arthroplasty. Radiol Clin North Am. 2007 Jul;45(4): 711-8, vii.

[118] Love C, Marwin SE, Palestro CJ. Nuclear medicine and the infected joint replacement. Semin Nucl Med. 2009 Jan;39(1):66-78.

[119] Spangehl MJ, Masri BA, O'Connell JX, Duncan CP. Prospective analysis of preoperative and intraoperative investigations for the diagnosis of infection at the sites of two hundred and two revision total hip arthroplasties. J Bone Joint Surg Am. 1999 May; 81(5):672-83.

[120] Di Cesare PE, Chang E, Preston CF, Liu CJ. Serum interleukin-6 as a marker of periprosthetic infection following total hip and knee arthroplasty. J Bone Joint Surg Am. 2005 Sep;87(9):1921-7.

[121] Crockarell JR, Hanssen AD, Osmon DR, Morrey BF. Treatment of infection with debridement and retention of the components following hip arthroplasty. J Bone Joint Surg Am. 1998 Sep;80(9):1306-13.

[122] Buchholz HW, Elson RA, Engelbrecht E, Lodenkamper H, Rottger J, Siegel A. Management of deep infection of total hip replacement. J Bone Joint Surg Br. 1981;63-B(3): 342-53.

[123] Jackson WO, Schmalzried TP. Limited role of direct exchange arthroplasty in the treatment of infected total hip replacements. Clin Orthop Relat Res. 2000 Dec(381): 101-5.

[124] Younger AS, Duncan CP, Masri BA, McGraw RW. The outcome of two-stage arthroplasty using a custom-made interval spacer to treat the infected hip. J Arthroplasty. 1997 Sep;12(6):615-23.

[125] Stockley I, Mockford BJ, Hoad-Reddick A, Norman P. The use of two-stage exchange arthroplasty with depot antibiotics in the absence of long-term antibiotic therapy in infected total hip replacement. J Bone Joint Surg Br. 2008 Feb;90(2):145-8.

[126] Sanchez-Sotelo J, Berry DJ, Hanssen AD, Cabanela ME. Midterm to long-term follow-up of staged reimplantation for infected hip arthroplasty. Clin Orthop Relat Res. 2009 Jan;467(1):219-24.

[127] Haddad FS, Masri BA, Garbuz DS, Duncan CP. The treatment of the infected hip replacement. The complex case. Clin Orthop Relat Res. 1999 Dec(369):144-56.

[128] McDonald DJ, Fitzgerald RH, Jr., Ilstrup DM. Two-stage reconstruction of a total hip arthroplasty because of infection. J Bone Joint Surg Am. 1989 Jul;71(6):828-34.

[129] Schmalzried TP, Noordin S, Amstutz HC. Update on nerve palsy associated with total hip replacement. Clin Orthop Relat Res. 1997 Nov(344):188-206.

[130] Barrack RL. Neurovascular injury: avoiding catastrophe. J Arthroplasty. 2004 Jun; 19(4 Suppl 1):104-7.

[131] Schmalzried T, Amstutz H, Dorey F. Nerve palsy associated with total hip replacement. Risk factors and prognosis. J Bone Joint Surg Am. 1991 August 1, 1991;73(7): 1074-80.

[132] Jolles BM, Bogoch ER. Posterior versus lateral surgical approach for total hip arthroplasty in adults with osteoarthritis. Cochrane Database Syst Rev. 2006;3:CD003828.

[133] Yuen EC, Olney RK, So YT. Sciatic neuropathy: clinical and prognostic features in 73 patients. Neurology. 1994 Sep;44(9):1669-74.

[134] Calligaro KD, Dougherty MJ, Ryan S, Booth RE. Acute arterial complications associated with total hip and knee arthroplasty. J Vasc Surg. 2003 Dec;38(6):1170-7.

[135] Abularrage CJ, Weiswasser JM, Dezee KJ, Slidell MB, Henderson WG, Sidawy AN. Predictors of lower extremity arterial injury after total knee or total hip arthroplasty. J Vasc Surg. 2008 Apr;47(4):803-7; discussion 7-8.

[136] Parvizi J, Pulido L, Slenker N, Macgibeny M, Purtill JJ, Rothman RH. Vascular injuries after total joint arthroplasty. J Arthroplasty. 2008 Dec;23(8):1115-21.

[137] Wilson JS, Miranda A, Johnson BL, Shames ML, Back MR, Bandyk DF. Vascular injuries associated with elective orthopedic procedures. Ann Vasc Surg. 2003 Nov;17(6): 641-4.

[138] Doi S, Motoyama Y, Itoh H. External iliac vein injury during total hip arthroplasty resulting in delayed shock. Br J Anaesth. 2005 Jun;94(6):866.

[139] Wasielewski RC, Crossett LS, Rubash HE. Neural and vascular injury in total hip arthroplasty. Orthop Clin North Am. 1992 Apr;23(2):219-35.

[140] Malchau H, Herberts P, Eisler T, Garellick G, Soderman P. The Swedish Total Hip Replacement Register. J Bone Joint Surg Am. 2002;84-A Suppl 2:2-20.

[141] Willert HG. Reactions of the articular capsule to wear products of artificial joint prostheses. J Biomed Mater Res. 1977 Mar;11(2):157-64.

[142] Maloney WJ, Smith RL. Periprosthetic osteolysis in total hip arthroplasty: the role of particulate wear debris. Instr Course Lect. 1996;45:171-82.

[143] Holt G, Murnaghan C, Reilly J, Meek RM. The biology of aseptic osteolysis. Clin Orthop Relat Res. 2007 Jul;460:240-52.

[144] Hirakawa K, Jacobs JJ, Urban R, Saito T. Mechanisms of failure of total hip replacements: lessons learned from retrieval studies. Clin Orthop Relat Res. 2004 Mar(420): 10-7.

[145] Aspenberg P, Van der Vis H. Migration, particles, and fluid pressure. A discussion of causes of prosthetic loosening. Clin Orthop Relat Res. 1998 Jul(352):75-80.

[146] van der Vis H, Aspenberg P, de Kleine R, Tigchelaar W, van Noorden CJ. Short periods of oscillating fluid pressure directed at a titanium-bone interface in rabbits lead to bone lysis. Acta Orthop Scand. 1998 Feb;69(1):5-10.

[147] Walter WL, Walter WK, O'Sullivan M. The pumping of fluid in cementless cups with holes. J Arthroplasty. 2004 Feb;19(2):230-4.

[148] Robertsson O, Wingstrand H, Kesteris U, Jonsson K, Onnerfalt R. Intracapsular pressure and loosening of hip prostheses. Preoperative measurements in 18 hips. Acta Orthop Scand. 1997 Jun;68(3):231-4.

[149] Abu-Amer Y, Darwech I, Clohisy JC. Aseptic loosening of total joint replacements: mechanisms underlying osteolysis and potential therapies. Arthritis Res Ther. 2007;9 Suppl 1:S6.

[150] Purdue PE, Koulouvaris P, Potter HG, Nestor BJ, Sculco TP. The cellular and molecular biology of periprosthetic osteolysis. Clin Orthop Relat Res. 2007 Jan;454:251-61.

[151] Goldring S, Schiller A, Roelke M, Rourke C, O'Neil D, Harris W. The synovial-like membrane at the bone-cement interface in loose total hip replacements and its proposed role in bone lysis. J Bone Joint Surg Am. 1983 June 1, 1983;65(5):575-84.

[152] Malik MH, Bayat A, Jury F, Ollier WE, Kay PR. Genetic susceptibility to hip arthroplasty failure--association with the RANK/OPG pathway. Int Orthop. 2006 Jun;30(3): 177-81.

[153] Malik MH, Jury F, Bayat A, Ollier WE, Kay PR. Genetic susceptibility to total hip arthroplasty failure: a preliminary study on the influence of matrix metalloproteinase 1, interleukin 6 polymorphisms and vitamin D receptor. Ann Rheum Dis. 2007 Aug; 66(8):1116-20.

[154] Gordon A, Kiss-Toth E, Stockley I, Eastell R, Wilkinson JM. Polymorphisms in the interleukin-1 receptor antagonist and interleukin-6 genes affect risk of osteolysis in patients with total hip arthroplasty. Arthritis Rheum. 2008 Oct;58(10):3157-65.

[155] Wilkinson JM, Wilson AG, Stockley I, Scott IR, Macdonald DA, Hamer AJ, et al. Variation in the TNF gene promoter and risk of osteolysis after total hip arthroplasty. J Bone Miner Res. 2003 Nov;18(11):1995-2001.

[156] Engh CA, Jr., Stepniewski AS, Ginn SD, Beykirch SE, Sychterz-Terefenko CJ, Hopper RH, Jr., et al. A randomized prospective evaluation of outcomes after total hip arthroplasty using cross-linked marathon and non-cross-linked Enduron polyethylene liners. J Arthroplasty. 2006 Sep;21(6 Suppl 2):17-25.

[157] Muratoglu OK, Bragdon CR, O'Connor DO, Jasty M, Harris WH. A novel method of cross-linking ultra-high-molecular-weight polyethylene to improve wear, reduce oxidation, and retain mechanical properties. Recipient of the 1999 HAP Paul Award. J Arthroplasty. 2001 Feb;16(2):149-60.

[158] Lusty PJ, Tai CC, Sew-Hoy RP, Walter WL, Walter WK, Zicat BA. Third-generation alumina-on-alumina ceramic bearings in cementless total hip arthroplasty. J Bone Joint Surg Am. 2007 Dec;89(12):2676-83.

[159] Lusty PJ, Watson A, Tuke MA, Walter WL, Walter WK, Zicat B. Wear and acetabular component orientation in third generation alumina-on-alumina ceramic bearings: an analysis of 33 retrievals [corrected]. J Bone Joint Surg Br. 2007 Sep;89(9):1158-64.

[160] Smith SL, Unsworth A. An in vitro wear study of alumina-alumina total hip prostheses. Proc Inst Mech Eng [H]. 2001;215(5):443-6.

[161] Clarke IC, Good V, Williams P, Schroeder D, Anissian L, Stark A, et al. Ultra-low wear rates for rigid-on-rigid bearings in total hip replacements. Proc Inst Mech Eng [H]. 2000;214(4):331-47.

[162] Fisher J, Jin Z, Tipper J, Stone M, Ingham E. Tribology of alternative bearings. Clin Orthop Relat Res. 2006 Dec;453:25-34.

[163] McKellop H, Park SH, Chiesa R, Doorn P, Lu B, Normand P, et al. In vivo wear of three types of metal on metal hip prostheses during two decades of use. Clin Orthop Relat Res. 1996 Aug(329 Suppl):S128-40.

[164] Streicher RM, Semlitsch M, Schon R, Weber H, Rieker C. Metal-on-metal articulation for artificial hip joints: laboratory study and clinical results. Proc Inst Mech Eng [H]. 1996;210(3):223-32.

[165] Illgen RL, 2nd, Bauer LM, Hotujec BT, Kolpin SE, Bakhtiar A, Forsythe TM. Highly crosslinked vs conventional polyethylene particles: relative in vivo inflammatory response. J Arthroplasty. 2009 Jan;24(1):117-24.

[166] Illgen RL, 2nd, Forsythe TM, Pike JW, Laurent MP, Blanchard CR. Highly crosslinked vs conventional polyethylene particles--an in vitro comparison of biologic activities. J Arthroplasty. 2008 Aug;23(5):721-31.

[167] Khan NQ, Woolson ST. Referral patterns of hip pain in patients undergoing total hip replacement. Orthopedics. 1998 Feb;21(2):123-6.

[168] Shih LY, Wu JJ, Yang DJ. Erythrocyte sedimentation rate and C-reactive protein values in patients with total hip arthroplasty. Clin Orthop Relat Res. 1987 Dec(225): 238-46.

[169] Temmerman OP, Raijmakers PG, Berkhof J, Hoekstra OS, Teule GJ, Heyligers IC. Accuracy of diagnostic imaging techniques in the diagnosis of aseptic loosening of the femoral component of a hip prosthesis: a meta-analysis. J Bone Joint Surg Br. 2005 Jun;87(6):781-5.

[170] Walde TA, Weiland DE, Leung SB, Kitamura N, Sychterz CJ, Engh CA, Jr., et al. Comparison of CT, MRI, and radiographs in assessing pelvic osteolysis: a cadaveric study. Clin Orthop Relat Res. 2005 Aug(437):138-44.

[171] Leung S, Naudie D, Kitamura N, Walde T, Engh CA. Computed tomography in the assessment of periacetabular osteolysis. J Bone Joint Surg Am. 2005 Mar;87(3):592-7.

[172] Talmo CT, Shanbhag AS, Rubash HE. Nonsurgical management of osteolysis: challenges and opportunities. Clin Orthop Relat Res. 2006 Dec;453:254-64.

[173] Stulberg BN, Della Valle AG. What are the guidelines for the surgical and nonsurgical treatment of periprosthetic osteolysis? J Am Acad Orthop Surg. 2008;16 Suppl 1:S20-5.

[174] Squire M, Griffin WL, Mason JB, Peindl RD, Odum S. Acetabular component deformation with press-fit fixation. J Arthroplasty. 2006 Sep;21(6 Suppl 2):72-7.

[175] Langdown AJ, Pickard RJ, Hobbs CM, Clarke HJ, Dalton DJ, Grover ML. Incomplete seating of the liner with the Trident acetabular system: a cause for concern? J Bone Joint Surg Br. 2007 Mar;89(3):291-5.

[176] Tateiwa T, Clarke IC, Williams PA, Garino J, Manaka M, Shishido T, et al. Ceramic total hip arthroplasty in the United States: safety and risk issues revisited. Am J Orthop. 2008 Feb;37(2):E26-31.

[177] D'Antonio JA, Capello WN, Manley MT, Naughton M, Sutton K. A titanium-encased alumina ceramic bearing for total hip arthroplasty: 3- to 5-year results. Clin Orthop Relat Res. 2005 Dec;441:151-8.

[178] Willmann G. Ceramic femoral head retrieval data. Clin Orthop Relat Res. 2000 Oct(379):22-8.

[179] Ha YC, Kim SY, Kim HJ, Yoo JJ, Koo KH. Ceramic liner fracture after cementless alumina-on-alumina total hip arthroplasty. Clin Orthop Relat Res. 2007 May;458:106-10.

[180] Koo KH, Ha YC, Jung WH, Kim SR, Yoo JJ, Kim HJ. Isolated fracture of the ceramic head after third-generation alumina-on-alumina total hip arthroplasty. J Bone Joint Surg Am. 2008 Feb;90(2):329-36.

[181] Weisse B, Affolter C, Stutz A, Terrasi GP, Kobel S, Weber W. Influence of contaminants in the stem-ball interface on the static fracture load of ceramic hip joint ball heads. Proc Inst Mech Eng [H]. 2008 Jul;222(5):829-35.

[182] Min BW, Song KS, Kang CH, Bae KC, Won YY, Lee KY. Delayed fracture of a ceramic insert with modern ceramic total hip replacement. J Arthroplasty. 2007 Jan;22(1): 136-9.

[183] Restrepo C, Parvizi J, Kurtz SM, Sharkey PF, Hozack WJ, Rothman RH. The noisy ceramic hip: is component malpositioning the cause? J Arthroplasty. 2008 Aug;23(5): 643-9.

[184] Keurentjes JC, Kuipers RM, Wever DJ, Schreurs BW. High incidence of squeaking in THAs with alumina ceramic-on-ceramic bearings. Clin Orthop Relat Res. 2008 Jun; 466(6):1438-43.

[185] Walter WL, Insley GM, Walter WK, Tuke MA. Edge loading in third generation alumina ceramic-on-ceramic bearings: stripe wear. J Arthroplasty. 2004 Jun;19(4):402-13.

[186] Taylor S, Manley MT, Sutton K. The role of stripe wear in causing acoustic emissions from alumina ceramic-on-ceramic bearings. J Arthroplasty. 2007 Oct;22(7 Suppl 3): 47-51.

[187] Manley MT, Sutton K. Bearings of the future for total hip arthroplasty. J Arthroplasty. 2008 Oct;23(7 Suppl):47-50.

[188] Doorn PF, Campbell PA, Worrall J, Benya PD, McKellop HA, Amstutz HC. Metal wear particle characterization from metal on metal total hip replacements: transmission electron microscopy study of periprosthetic tissues and isolated particles. J Biomed Mater Res. 1998 Oct;42(1):103-11.

[189] Daniel J, Ziaee H, Pradhan C, McMinn DJ. Six-year results of a prospective study of metal ion levels in young patients with metal-on-metal hip resurfacings. J Bone Joint Surg Br. 2009 Feb;91(2):176-9.

[190] De Smet K, De Haan R, Calistri A, Campbell PA, Ebramzadeh E, Pattyn C, et al. Metal ion measurement as a diagnostic tool to identify problems with metal-on-metal hip resurfacing. J Bone Joint Surg Am. 2008 Nov;90 Suppl 4:202-8.

[191] De Haan R, Pattyn C, Gill HS, Murray DW, Campbell PA, De Smet K. Correlation between inclination of the acetabular component and metal ion levels in metal-on-metal hip resurfacing replacement. J Bone Joint Surg Br. 2008 Oct;90(10):1291-7.

http://dx.doi.org/10.5772/53030

[192] Savarino L, Padovani G, Ferretti M, Greco M, Cenni E, Perrone G, et al. Serum ion levels after ceramic-on-ceramic and metal-on-metal total hip arthroplasty: 8-year minimum follow-up. J Orthop Res. 2008 Dec;26(12):1569-76.

[193] MacDonald SJ. Can a safe level for metal ions in patients with metal-on-metal total hip arthroplasties be determined? J Arthroplasty. 2004 Dec;19(8 Suppl 3):71-7.

[194] Keegan GM, Learmonth ID, Case CP. Orthopaedic metals and their potential toxicity in the arthroplasty patient: A review of current knowledge and future strategies. J Bone Joint Surg Br. 2007 May;89(5):567-73.

[195] Hart AJ, Hester T, Sinclair K, Powell JJ, Goodship AE, Pele L, et al. The association between metal ions from hip resurfacing and reduced T-cell counts. J Bone Joint Surg Br. 2006 Apr;88(4):449-54.

[196] Ziaee H, Daniel J, Datta AK, Blunt S, McMinn DJ. Transplacental transfer of cobalt and chromium in patients with metal-on-metal hip arthroplasty: a controlled study. J Bone Joint Surg Br. 2007 Mar;89(3):301-5.

[197] Keegan GM, Learmonth ID, Case CP. A systematic comparison of the actual, potential, and theoretical health effects of cobalt and chromium exposures from industry and surgical implants. Crit Rev Toxicol. 2008;38(8):645-74.

[198] Smith AJ, Dieppe P, Porter M, Blom AW. Risk of cancer in first seven years after metal-on-metal hip replacement compared with other bearings and general population: linkage study between the National Joint Registry of England and Wales and hospital episode statistics. BMJ. 2012;344:e2383.

[199] Hart AJ, Buddhdev P, Winship P, Faria N, Powell JJ, Skinner JA. Cup inclination angle of greater than 50 degrees increases whole blood concentrations of cobalt and chromium ions after metal-on-metal hip resurfacing. Hip Int. 2008 Jul-Sep;18(3): 212-9.

[200] Willert HG, Buchhorn GH, Fayyazi A, Flury R, Windler M, Koster G, et al. Metal-on-metal bearings and hypersensitivity in patients with artificial hip joints. A clinical and histomorphological study. J Bone Joint Surg Am. 2005 Jan;87(1):28-36.

[201] Pandit H, Glyn-Jones S, McLardy-Smith P, Gundle R, Whitwell D, Gibbons CL, et al. Pseudotumours associated with metal-on-metal hip resurfacings. J Bone Joint Surg Br. 2008 Jul;90(7):847-51.

[202] Pandit H, Vlychou M, Whitwell D, Crook D, Luqmani R, Ostlere S, et al. Necrotic granulomatous pseudotumours in bilateral resurfacing hip arthoplasties: evidence for a type IV immune response. Virchows Arch. 2008 Nov;453(5):529-34.

[203] Haddad FS, Thakrar RR, Hart AJ, Skinner JA, Nargol AV, Nolan JF, et al. Metal-on-metal bearings: the evidence so far. J Bone Joint Surg Br. 2011 May;93(5):572-9.

[204] Smith AJ, Dieppe P, Vernon K, Porter M, Blom AW. Failure rates of stemmed metal-on-metal hip replacements: analysis of data from the National Joint Registry of England and Wales. Lancet. 2012 Mar 31;379(9822):1199-204.

[205] Fink B, Fuerst M, Singer J. Periprosthetic fractures of the femur associated with hip arthroplasty. Arch Orthop Trauma Surg. 2005 Sep;125(7):433-42.

[206] Duncan CP, Masri BA. Fractures of the femur after hip replacement. Instr Course Lect. 1995;44:293-304.

[207] McElfresh EC, Coventry MB. Femoral and pelvic fractures after total hip arthroplasty. J Bone Joint Surg Am. 1974 Apr;56(3):483-92.

[208] Haidukewych GJ, Jacofsky DJ, Hanssen AD, Lewallen DG. Intraoperative fractures of the acetabulum during primary total hip arthroplasty. J Bone Joint Surg Am. 2006 Sep;88(9):1952-6.

[209] Davidson D, Pike J, Garbuz D, Duncan CP, Masri BA. Intraoperative periprosthetic fractures during total hip arthroplasty. Evaluation and management. J Bone Joint Surg Am. 2008 Sep;90(9):2000-12.

[210] Sharkey PF, Hozack WJ, Callaghan JJ, Kim YS, Berry DJ, Hanssen AD, et al. Acetabular fracture associated with cementless acetabular component insertion: a report of 13 cases. J Arthroplasty. 1999 Jun;14(4):426-31.

[211] Masri BA, Meek RM, Duncan CP. Periprosthetic fractures evaluation and treatment. Clin Orthop Relat Res. 2004 Mar(420):80-95.

[212] Orzel JA, Rudd TG, Nelp WB. Heterotopic bone formation (myositis ossificans) and lower-extremity swelling mimicking deep-venous disease. J Nucl Med. 1984 Oct; 25(10):1105-7.

[213] owsey J CM, Robins PR. Heterotopic ossification: theoretical consideration possible etiological factors, and a clinical review of total hip arthroplasty patients exhibiting this phenomenon. The hip: procs 5th Open Scientific Meeting of the Hip Society. 1977:201-21.

[214] Brooker AF, Bowerman JW, Robinson RA, Riley LH, Jr. Ectopic ossification following total hip replacement. Incidence and a method of classification. J Bone Joint Surg Am. 1973 Dec;55(8):1629-32.

[215] Naraghi FF, DeCoster TA, Moneim MS, Miller RA, Rivero D. Heterotopic ossification. Orthopedics. 1996 Feb;19(2):145-51.

[216] Shafritz AB, Shore EM, Gannon FH, Zasloff MA, Taub R, Muenke M, et al. Overexpression of an osteogenic morphogen in fibrodysplasia ossificans progressiva. N Engl J Med. 1996 Aug 22;335(8):555-61.

[217] Hannallah D, Peng H, Young B, Usas A, Gearhart B, Huard J. Retroviral delivery of Noggin inhibits the formation of heterotopic ossification induced by BMP-4, demin-

eralized bone matrix, and trauma in an animal model. J Bone Joint Surg Am. 2004 Jan;86-A(1):80-91.

[218] Harris WH. Clinical results using the Mueller-Charnley total hip prosthesis. Clin Orthop Relat Res. 1972 Jul-Aug;86:95-101.

[219] Chao ST, Lee SY, Borden LS, Joyce MJ, Krebs VE, Suh JH. External beam radiation helps prevent heterotopic bone formation in patients with a history of heterotopic ossification. J Arthroplasty. 2006 Aug;21(5):731-6.

[220] Cobb TK, Berry DJ, Wallrichs SL, Ilstrup DM, Morrey BF. Functional outcome of excision of heterotopic ossification after total hip arthroplasty. Clin Orthop Relat Res. 1999 Apr(361):131-9.

[221] Pellegrini VD, Jr., Evarts CM. Radiation prophylaxis of heterotopic bone formation following total hip arthroplasty: current status. Semin Arthroplasty. 1992 Jul;3(3): 156-66.

[222] Gregoritch SJ, Chadha M, Pelligrini VD, Rubin P, Kantorowitz DA. Randomized trial comparing preoperative versus postoperative irradiation for prevention of heterotopic ossification following prosthetic total hip replacement: preliminary results. Int J Radiat Oncol Biol Phys. 1994 Aug 30;30(1):55-62.

[223] Lo TC, Healy WL, Covall DJ, Dotter WE, Pfeifer BA, Torgerson WR, et al. Heterotopic bone formation after hip surgery: prevention with single-dose postoperative hip irradiation. Radiology. 1988 Sep;168(3):851-4.

Chapter 18

Periprosthetic Femoral Fractures in Total Knee Arthroplasty

Vladan Stevanović, Zoran Vukašinović,
Zoran Baščarević, Branislav Starčević,
Dragana Matanović and Duško Spasovski

Additional information is available at the end of the chapter

http://dx.doi.org/10.5772/55226

1. Introduction

Total joint arthroplasty has greatly improved the treatment of knee arthrosis, but still is not without complications. Supracondylar fractures above total knee replacements are an uncommon complication (incidence 0,3% to 2.5%), occuring more frequently in patients older than 60 years with osteoporotic bone. The rate of these fractures is expected to increase in the future because of the growing number of total knee replacements and greater level of acitivity among elderly patients. The timing of such fractures has been reported to range from early in the postoperative period to more than a decade after surgery, with a mean of 2 to 4 years. During the past two decades authors were not agreed in the definition of periprosthetic supracondylar region: the lower 3 inches (7cm) of the femur [1]; 9 cm proximal to the knee joint line [2]; all fractures within 15 cm proximal to the knee joint line [3]. Generally, based on the older literature, supracondylar periprosthetic fractures were those within 15 cm of the joint line, or in the case of stemmed component, within 5 cm of the proximal end of the implant. Nevertheless, the most important is understanding that these fractures occur in regions of stress concentration adjacent to a prosthetic component, and that the presence of the prosthesis has a significant effect on fracture treatment. So, we suggest that fractures above total knee replacement should be considered supracondylar fractures if they extend within 7 cm of the prosthetic joint line or if they are within 2 cm of the femoral prosthetic flange.

The most commonly suggested predisposing factors for a periprosthetic femoral fracture after total knee arthroplasty are osteopenia, revision arthroplasty, rheumatoid arthritis, use of steroids, existing neurological disorders, misalignment of the components, and notching of the anterior femoral cortex. Different factors were found in the pathogenesis of the fracture: stress-shielding from the anterior flange of the femoral component, inadequate osseous remodeling due to postoperative hypovascularity, relative difference in elastic modulus between the implant-covered distal part of the femur and femoral cortex, endosteal ischemia from metal or bone cement, and osteolysis of the distal part of the femur secondary to polyethylene wear debris. The majority of these fractures results from a combination of axial and torsion loads. Most of them occur following minimal falls, while the rest of them are secondary to motor-vehicle accidents, seizers or closed manipulation of a stiff knee after total knee arthroplasty

2. Prevalence and pathogenesis

The prevalence of supracondylar femoral fracture in patients with total knee replacement ranges from 0.3 to 4.2%. Most of the patients who sustain fractures about a total knee arthroplasty are women, usually in their seventh decade of life. As with other supracondylar fractures in the elderly, periprosthetic fractures usually occurs after low energy trauma. Osteoporosis is often present as well, due to a number of factors including stress shielding because of a rigid implant, pharmacologic causes, hormonal influences and senility. An association with rheumatoid arthritis, especially when the patient is receiving oral corticosteroid treatment, has been noted. Neurologic disorders have also been involved in the occurrence of these fractures, due to either medication induced osteoporosis or gait disturbance. In addition, revision arthroplasty has been associated with an increased incidence of periprosthetic fractures, more commonly when constrained implants are used, as they transfer applied torque more directly to bone that is potentially already deficient. Notching of the anterior femoral cortex during total knee arthroplasty has been indicated as one factor contributing to these periprosthetic femoral fractures. The prevalence of inadvertent cortical notching of the femur during total knee arthroplasty has been reported to be as high as 27% and there are several studies performed to quantify the reduction in bending and torsion strength resulting from femoral notching in attempt to provide the clinician with useful information related to the postoperative management [5, 6]. Clearly, notching of the anterior femoral cortex is neither the only risk factor nor the principal risk factor for supracondylar femoral fracture after knee replacement. Of a total of 6470 total knee arthroplasties included in reports on this subject, only seventeen (0.26%) were complicated by a supracondylar femoral fracture associated with anterior notching compared with nearly three times as many fractures that occurred in the absence of notching [5]; biomechanical effects of femoral notching following total knee arthroplasty showed mean decrease in bending strength of 18% (8-31%) and mean reduction in torsion strength of 39.2% (19-73%) in cadaveric specimens [6]. Based on Wolff's law, distal part of the femur would strengthen after the operation as result of remodeling, thus reduction in femoral bone strength should primarily be expected in the immediate postoperative period. Therefore a clear recommendation should be given to the patients who sustain inadvertent notching that they should have additional protection in the early postoperative period, and to consider the use a femoral component with stem as a means to bypass the stress riser of the anterior cortical notch. Most important, authors believe that an anterior cortical notch should be considered as a contraindication for manipulation of the knee prosthesis in the early postoperative period [7, 8].

Anterior defects may be present without notching, such as in cases of cystic lesions of degenerative or rheumatoid origin near the proximal aspect of the anterior femoral flange. Adequate remodeling may not be possible after those cysts are filled with cement at the time of arthroplasty. These defects remain as permanent stress risers, which may predispose to fracture. Large anterior effects might be better managed during primary knee arthroplasty with bone grafting and protection of the distal femur with an intramedullary stem [9].

Another recently recognized factor leading to late supracondylar femoral fracture is the presence of a massive debris-related osteolytic defect in the distal femur; such defects have been reported in association with asymptomatic well-fixed cementless femoral component. Ankylosis of a total knee arthroplasty may also predispose a fracture by producing increased stress in the distal femoral metaphysis [10, 11].

3. Risk factors / etiology

Literature data show that patients with osteopenia are at greater risk to acquire supracondylar femoral fracture after total knee arthroplasty, followed by rheumatoid arthritis, corticosteroid treatment, female gender and older age [12,13,14]. Additional risk factors are: neurological disorders, a revision total knee replacement (TKR) and rotationally constrained implants that create increased torsion load transfer to bone [15] (Table1).

Osteopenia
Rheumatoid arthritis
Steroid use
Neurologic disorders
Revision TKR
Female gender
Seventh decade of life
Distal femoral osteolysis
Anterior femoral notching +/-

Table 1. Risk factors for supracondylar femoral fractures, in decreasing order

Clinical and biomechanical data on anterior notching of the distal femoral cortex confirm the increase of fracture risk, and theoretical mathematical analysis calculated that a three-millimeter notch results in a 30% reduction in torsion bone strength [9]. On the other hand, a series of 670 total knee prosthesis with 20% femurs with anterior notching of at 3 mm at least, and found only two supracondylar fractures [11]. Different fracture patterns are associated with notched and no notched femurs: notched femurs tend to have short oblique fractures originating from the notched cortex, whereas no notched femurs tend to have diaphyseal fractures.

Furthermore, there is a general feeling that the most significant risk factor causing supracondylar fracture is the increase in activity that elderly patients achieve after knee replacement, exposing them to a greater risk of slipping and falling.

4. Diagnostic algorithm

Patients with this type of injury usually provide a history of minor trauma, such as fall during ambulation. They usually present with pain and inability to bear weight. Since these are typically low energy injuries, major tissue swelling is uncommon. Unless marked displacement is present, deformity may not be apparent on examination.

A thorough evaluation includes careful physical examination, a review of the patient's medical history and adequate radiographic studies. The injured limb should be assessed for soft tissue integrity and neurovascular status. The location of previous skin incisions must also be noted.

A complete radiographic examination of a fracture about a total knee arthroplasty includes standard anteroposterior and lateral radiographs as well as long leg views of the involved limb; oblique images and tomography are also often useful (Table 2). The diagnostic evaluation must include a direct lateral view of the distal femur in order to guide subsequent treatment: the direct lateral view facilitates assessment of fracture displacement, while also revealing the bone available for fixation devices, the location of femoral lugs of posterior cruciate retaining components and the proximal extent of the central femoral recess in cases with posterior stabilized components. Radiographically, nondisplaced or minimally displaced fractures may be obscured by the femoral flange; it is important to identify nondisplaced fractures since displacement may occur later.

Fracture displacement and comminution
Axial limb alignment
Quality of bone stock
Location of the fracture relative to the prosthesis
Stability of the prosthesis

Table 2. Characteristics of radiography assessment

Review of prefracture radiographs can provide important data regarding baseline limb alignment, implant fixation and the presence of regions of osteolysis or polyethylene wear. The type and technical specifications of the implant and templates in place will influence the selection of fixation device if open reduction is necessary [16, 17].

The first step is to establish whether the implant is loose; if so even if the fracture is well aligned and heals, treatment that does not include revision will lead to poor result. Prefracture misalignment, osteolysis and polyethylene wear are important factors in the decision making process.

The second step in the treatment is to identify fracture displacement and to decide whether reduction is needed. Any alteration in limb axis resulting from fracture can result in altered loading of the prosthesis, which may in turn lead to enhanced wear and/or accelerated implant loosening.

The third step is to determine the appropriate treatment for displaced fracture (Figure 1).

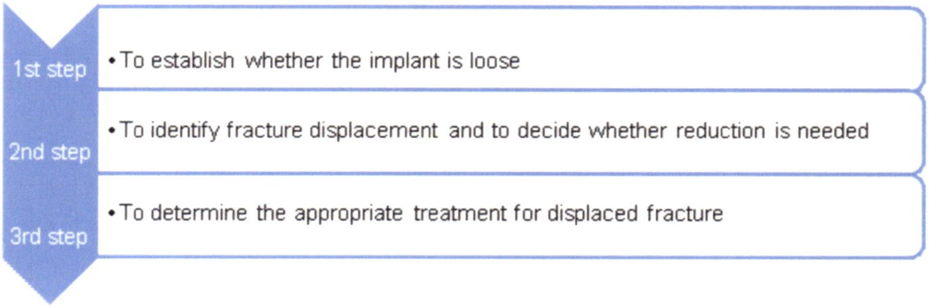

Figure 1. Diagnostic algorithm for periprosthetic supracondylar femoral fracture above total knee arthroplasty

5. Classification

Numerous systems of classification of supracondylar femoral fractures after total knee arthroplasty have been developed. Most of the classifications were based on supracondylar fractures without knee arthroplasty *(Neer et al, DiGioia and Rubash, Chen et al.)* (Table 3).

Neer et al.	Type I	Undisplaced (<5mm displacement or <5^0 angulation)*
	Type II	Displaced >1cm
	Type IIa	With lateral femoral shaft displacement
	Type IIb	With medial femoral shaft displacement
	Type III	Displaced and comminuted
DiGioia and Rubash	Group I	Extraarticular, undisplaced*
	Group II	Extraarticular, displaced*
	Group III	Severely displaced (loss of cortical contact) or angulated
Chen et al	Type I	Nondisplaced(Neer I)
	Type II	Displaced or comminuted (Neer I or II)

Table 3. Classification of supracondylar femoral fractures above total knee arthroplasty reprinted from Su ET, De Wal H, Di Cesare P. Periprosthetic Femoral Fractures Above Total Knee Replacements J Am Acad Orthop Surg, 2004; 12:12 – 20. - with permission (personal communication)

For identifying fracture displacement and deciding whether reduction is needed *Rorabeck et al.* [18] created classification that takes into account both the status of the prosthesis (intact or failing) and the displacement of the fracture:

Type I: fracture is undisplaced and the prosthesis is intact; Type II: fracture is displaced and the prosthesis is intact; Type III: fracture is displaced or undisplaced and the prosthesis is loose or failing

Summarizing above mentioned classifications, we strongly support suggested and explained in article by *Su et al.*[4] which is transcripted (Figure 2)

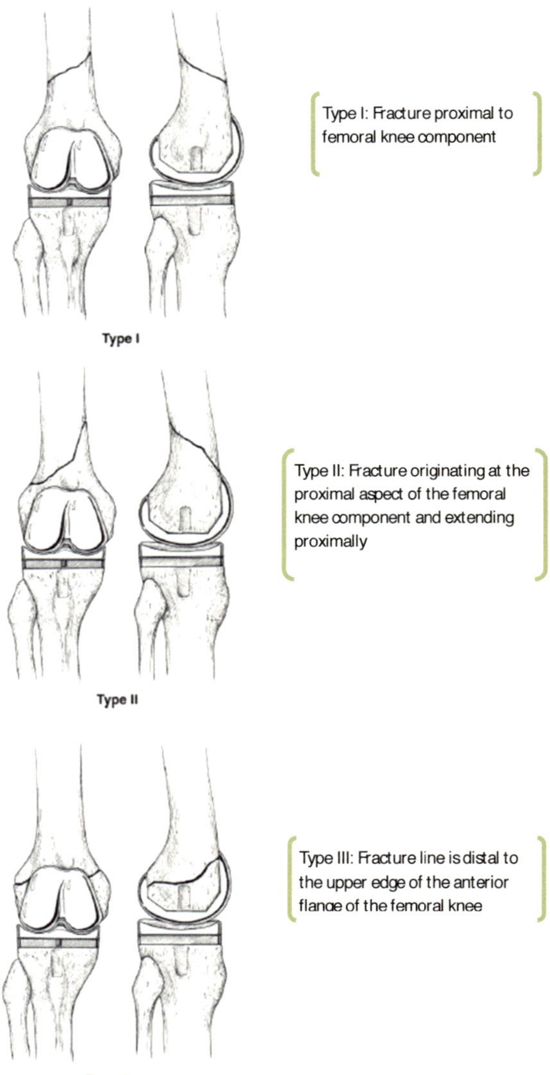

Figure 2. Reprinted from Su ET, De Wal H, Di Cesare P. Periprosthetic Femoral Fractures Above Total Knee Replacements J Am Acad Orthop Surg, 2004; 12:12 – 20. - with permission (personal communication)

http://dx.doi.org/10.5772/55226

6. Treatment options

The treatment of supracondylar fractures of the femur following total knee replacement has been a challenge for the orthopaedic surgeon, regardless the fracture and type of fixation [19, 20, 21, 22]. The major goal of treatment should be the restoration of the prefracture functional status of the patient which is characterized by: fracture union, preservation of prosthetic components without loosening, infection and other complications, maintenance of appropriate prosthetic alignment, restoration of joint range of motion. The need to meet all of these objectives makes these fractures difficult to treat: if even single goal is not achieved, the results of treatment will be suboptimal and may lead to failure of the prosthesis. There are two main treatment options: closed (without implant revision) or open (with implant revision), each with various modalities (Tables 4,5) [23, 24, 25, 26].

Skeletal traction
Application of a cast
Pins and plaster
Cast bracing

Table 4. Options for closed treatment of periprosthetic supracondylar femoral fractures

Use of condylar plate
Intramedullary fixation (flexible or rigid, interlocking)
Revision total knee arthroplasty
External fixation
Cerclage wiring with strut allograft fixation
Arthrodesis

Table 5. Options for open treatment of periprosthetic supracondylar femoral fractures

While fracture configuration influences the choice of open versus closed treatment method, fracture displacement, the degree of osteopenia, and the type and technical specifications of the prosthetic components are most valuable determinants of the operative fracture management. Treatment results are closely associated with postfracture alignment and stability [27]. Fracture displacement, intercondylar extension and comminution are negative prognostic factors. High malunion rates are common in association with varus, flexion and internal rotation deformities typically seen as a result of forces exerted by the adductor and gastrocnemius muscle group. Varus femoral malunion is associated with a risk of premature failure of the total knee arthroplasty. The choice of operative treatment method should be based on the patient's health, fracture configuration and displacement, presence of comminution, severity of osteopenia and status of the prosthetic components (loose, unstable or malaligned)[28, 29].

7. Nonoperative treatment

The advantages of nonoperative treatment are: noninvasiveness and negligible infection rate. Since fracture union is likely in nondisplaced fractures, nonoperative treatment is uniformly recommended as the initial management in these cases. Disadvantages include: a relatively high malunion rate and functional loss, particularly in patients with displaced fracture through osteopenic bone in whom maintance of reduction is difficult. Nonoperative treatment is best reserved for nondisplaced fractures that do not demonstrate intercondylar extension. Non-surgical management does eliminate surgical risks such as bleeding, infection, loss of fixation and anesthetic complications. On the other hands, prolonged recumbency in elderly patients carries the significant risk of decubitus ulcers, pneumonia, pulmonary embolia, deep venous thrombosis and diffuse muscle atrophy [30].

8. Operative treatment

Management of periprosthetic fractures of the femur above total knee arthroplasty depends on displacement at the fracture site, bone quality, size of distal fragment and condition of implants (Table 6) [31, 32, 33, 34].

Fracture type	Description of fracture	Treatment recommendation
I	Undisplaced fracture and well fixed prosthesis	Bracing, nonweightbearing
II	Displaced fracture and well fixed prosthesis Good quality bone	Internal fixation using conventional plate, intramedullary nail or locking plate
	Poor quality bone with osteopenia and comminution	Intramedullary nail or locking plate
	Decent size distal fragment Extremely distal fracture	Locking plate or buttress plate with strut allograft
III	Displaced fracture, loose prosthesis No metahyseal bone loss	Revision knee arthroplasty using a long stemmed femoral implant
	Metaphyseal bone loss or nonunion following previous surgery	Structural allograft prosthesis composite or distal femoral replacement prosthesis

Table 6. Operative guidelines for the treatment of periprosthetic supracondylar fractures above total knee arthroplasty

Open reduction and fixation with a *condylar plate* provides the potential advantages of anatomical reconstruction, rigid fixation and an early range of motion exercise. Maintenance of reduction can be a problem, particularly when a patient has a comminuted fracture through osteopenic bone, and malunion is commonly observed. Use of condylar plate is best reserved for less comminuted, displaced fractures with satisfactory bone stock. Using the *buttress condylar plate* include the ability to place the multiple screws distally in many directions and excellent visualization of the fracture to obtain an anatomic reduction. Disadvantages include extensive soft tissue stripping and less rigid fixation than with a nail or fixed angle condylar plate.

Use of *flexible intramedullary rods* is an efficient and less invasive treatment option, although shortening and rotational malunion occasionally occur as a result of the reduced axial and rotational stability. This technique should be considered for mildly displaced fractures patients with unstable general condition. It is minimally invasive procedure with limited morbidity.

New *locking plates* offer advantages over conventional plates for the treatment of periprosthetic fracture associated with total knee arthroplasty. These devices provide stable fixation in osteopenic bone, they are adaptable to different types of fracture and prosthesis and can be inserted using a minimally invasive approach. These plates are particularly useful in presence of an implant in proximal femur as it allows unicortical screw fixation if there is overlapping the distal part of the proximal implant, thus avoiding a stress riser between the two implants.

Rigid supracondylar interlocking rod fixation offers the advantage of being minimally invasive while providing good axial, angular and rotational stability. It can be performed with use of minimal patellar tendon splitting approach with percutaneous placement of interlocking screws in cases with lesser comminution with maintenance of the fracture hematoma and osseous blood supply. Contraindications include loose total knee components, severe comminution, extremely distal fracture and a presence of long total hip intramedullary stem,. This technique has several advantages over traditional open reduction with plate fixation: intramedullary implants are biomechanically superior to subperiostally placed fixation devices, who have significantly larger bending moments; there is no need for periosteal stripping, which can compromise blood supply to the fracture site and increase the risk of nonunion; plate fixation can be technically demanding and often requires the use of supplemental bone grafting.

Revision total knee arthroplasty provides the advantage of stable fixation with a dyaphisis engaging intramedullary femoral stem, allowing early range of motion and weight bearing. This technique is selected for extremely distal or comminuted fractures when stable fixation is difficult to secure with other methods, or for any fracture associated with loose, unstable, or substantially malaligned total knee components. Revision total knee arthroplasty is frequently required in cases where other methods, nonoperative or operative, have failed.

The most difficult cases involve a loose prosthesis coupled with deficient metaphyseal bone stock, rendering a basic revision procedure impossible. Such cases require excision of distal fracture fragment and replacement with either a *distal femoral replacement prosthesis* or a *structural allograft*. These treatment methods may also be required for nonunion resulting from failed osteosynthesis. Distal femoral replacement implants should be considered as a limb salvage option when other surgical options are not feasible. The use of stemmed constrained revision component with structural distal femoral allograft composite has been described as the effective means of providing both implant and fracture stability.

Periprosthetic fractures have a higher rate of nonunion than other supracondylar femoral fractures in the elderly. This has been attributed to alterations in vascularity at the fracture site due to primary surgery, the presence of metal implant and intramedullary polymethyl methacrylate (PMMA), or long term oral corticosteroid administration.

The goals of treatment, whether surgical or nonsurgical, are fracture healing, restoration and maintenance of knee range of motion, and pain free ambulation. A good result is a minimum of 90 degrees of knee motion, with femoral shortening less then 2 cm, varus/valgus malalignment less than 5 degrees, and flexion/extension malalignment less than 10 degrees. Fulfillment of these criteria enables satisfactory knee function, which is of paramout importance to the patient.

9. Complications

Major early complications include nonunion and malunion, which often lead to prosthetic loosening, pain and revision. The treatment of delayed unions with bone grafting is possible and is advocated if appropriate limb alignment and fracture fixation are maintained. In cases of deformity, early signs of prosthetic failure or inability to secure rigid fixation, revision may be the most appropriate. The most devastating complication of operative care of these fractures is infection. Incidence of periprosthetic fracture following total knee arthroplasty is gradually increasing, and management of these fractures can be challenging with complications that severely influence both the patient and surgeon. Furthermore, treatment complication rate range from 20 to 75 percent according to literature data [35]: in a review of 415 cases, there were reported a nonunion rate of 9%, fixation failure in 4%, an infection rate of 3% and revision surgery rate of 13%. Following case will demonstrate some of these problems in treating supracondylar periprosthetic femoral fractures.

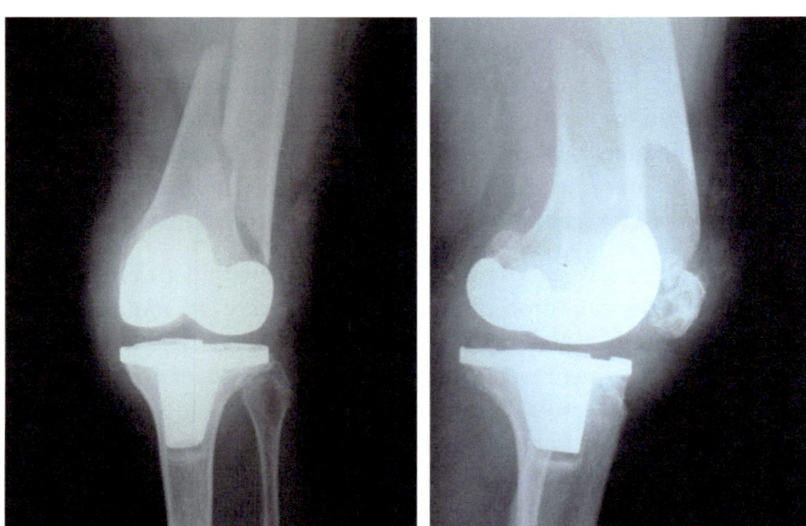

Figure 3. Anteroposterior and lateral view of type II supracondylar femoral fracture

http://dx.doi.org/10.5772/55226

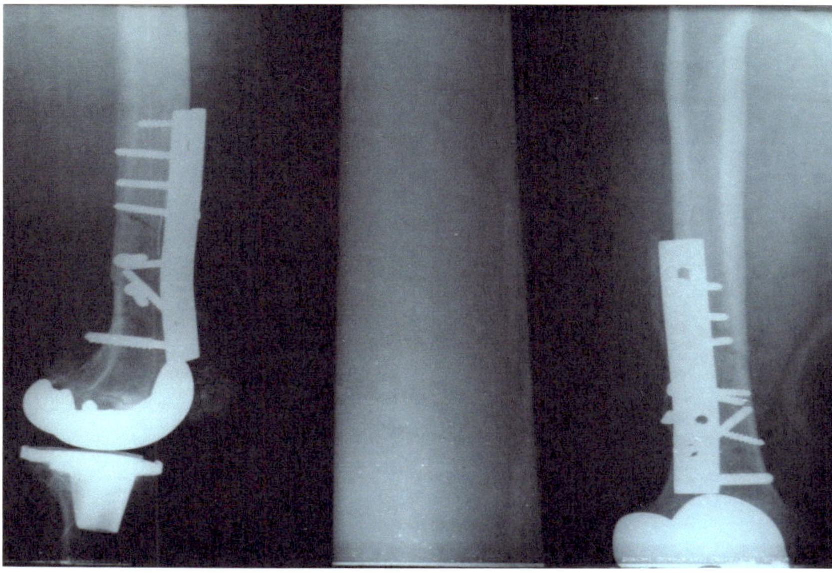

Figure 4. Operative treatment with DCP (anatomic reduction with rigid fixation)

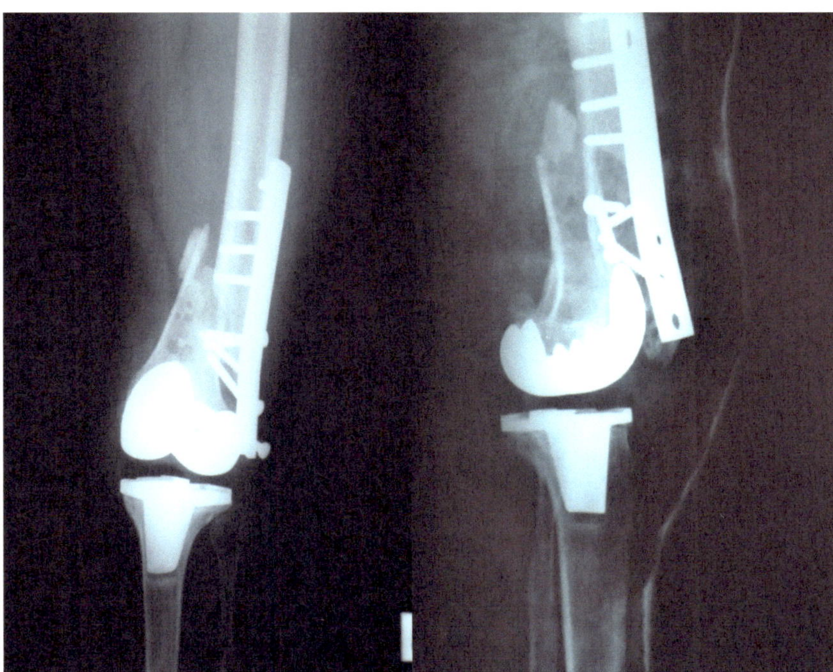

Figure 5. Loss of reduction and fixation two months following surgery

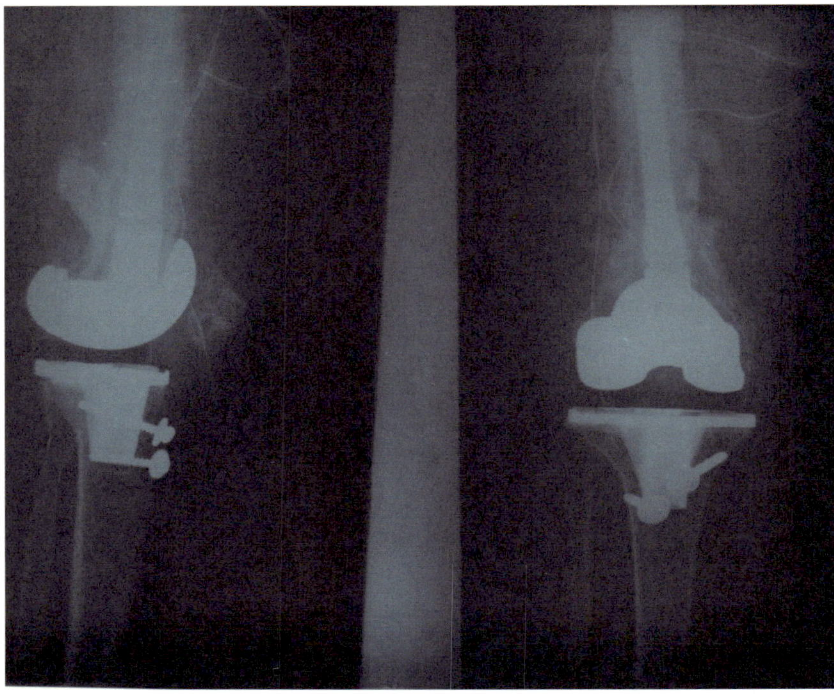

Figure 6. Revision total knee arthroplasty for loose femoral component and fracture treatment

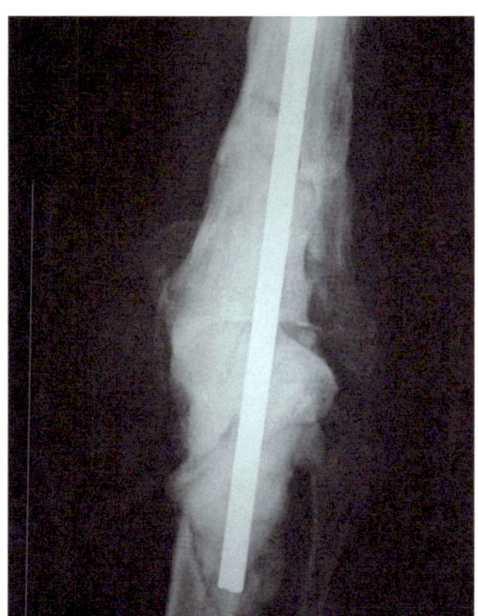

Figure 7. Devastating complication, infection, and limb salvage procedure with antibiotic cement spacer

http://dx.doi.org/10.5772/55226

10. Aftertreatment, rehabilitation

Rehabilitation process is generally guided by the characteristics of the fracture and chosen treatmen methods. As previously said, non-operative treatment is reserved for nondisplaced supracondylar fractures with stable implant and includes longer rehabilitation period to achieve patient's preambulatory status, if it is possible at all. Since surgery and more stable implants including intramedullary nails and angular locking plates allow for faster after-treatment program, rehabilitation protocol is similar to post fracture treatment in cases without knee arthroplasty. Main goals are fracture healing, implant stability and prefracture functional status.

11. Prevention

Since supracondylar femoral fractures above total knee arthroplasty are mostly seen in osteoporotic patients, prevention of osteopenia and osteoporosis including treatment with bis-phosphonate and regular exercise will be good for the well-being of the patient and implant. Surgical factors, such as anterior femoral notching, bone cement hypovascularisation and termal necrosis, and uncontrolled soft tissue manipulation should be kept in mind on regular basis in order to minimize surgeon's impact on development of potential complications including supracondylar fracture.

12. Conclusion

Periprosthetic femoral fractures above total knee prosthesis are increasing complication with constantly growing incidence since the number of total knee replacements and population agings are convergating factors. Risk factors analysis and prevention should be in surgeon and patient focus on this topic. Treatment options include first step to establish whether the implant is loose and, if so even if the fracture is well aligned and heals, treatment that does not include revision will lead to poor result. Prefracture misalignment, osteolysis and polyethylene wear are important factors in the decision making process. The second step in the treatment is to identify fracture displacement and to decide whether reduction is needed. The most appro-priate criteria of acceptable fracture alignment are for supracondylar fractures without knee prosthesis: less than 5 mm of translation; less than 5 to10 degrees of angulation; less than 10 mm of shortening and less than 10 degrees of rotational displacement. Any alteration in limb axis resulting from fracture can result in altered loading of the prosthesis, which may in turn lead to enhanced wear and/or accelerated implant loosening. The goals of treatment, whether surgical or nonsurgical, are fracture healing, restoration and maintenance of knee range of motion, and pain free ambulation. A good result is a minimum of 90 degrees of knee motion, with femoral shortening less then 2 cm, varus/valgus malalignment less than 5 degrees, and flexion/extension malalignment less than 10 degrees. Fulfillment of these criteria enables satisfactory knee function, which is of paramout importance to the patient.

Acknowledgements

This work is supported by grant number III 41004, Ministry of Education and Science Republic of Serbia.

Author details

Vladan Stevanović[1*], Zoran Vukašinović[1,2], Zoran Baščarević[1,2], Branislav Starčević[2,3], Dragana Matanović[2,4] and Duško Spasovski[1,2]

*Address all correspondence to: vladanstevanovi90@gmail.com

1 Institute for Orthopaedic Surgery „Banjica“, Belgrade, Serbia

2 Faculty of Medicine, University of Belgrade, Belgrade, Serbia

3 Clinic for Orthopaedic Surgery and Traumatology, Clinical Center of Serbia, Belgrade, Serbia

4 Clinic for Physical Therapy and Rehabilitation, Clinical Center of Serbia, Belgrade, Serbia

References

[1] Neer, C. S I. I, Grantham, S. A, & Shelton, M. L. Supracondylar fracture of the adult femur: A study of one hundred and ten cases. J Bone Joint Surge Am (1967). , 49, 591-613.

[2] Culp, R. W, Schmidt, R. G, Hanks, G, & Mak, A. Esterhai JL Jr, Heppenstall RB. Supracondylar fracture of the femur following prosthetic knee arthroplasty. Clin Orthop (1987). , 222, 212-22.

[3] Sisto, D. J, Lachiewicz, P. F, & Insall, J. N. Treatment of supracondylar fractures following prosthetic arthroplasty of the knee. Clin Orthop (1985). , 196, 265-72.

[4] Su, E. T, & De Wal, H. Di Cesare P. Periprosthetic Femoral Fractures Above Total Knee Replacements. J Am Acad Orthop Surg (2004). , 12, 12-20.

[5] Hirsch, D. M, Bhalla, S, & Roffman, M. Supracondylar fracture of the femur following total knee replacement. Report of four cases. J Bone Joint Surg Am (1981). , 63, 162-3.

[6] Lesh, M. L, Schneider, D. J, Deol, G, Davis, B, Jacobs, C. R, & Pellegrini, V. D. The consequences of anterior femoral notching in total knee arthroplasty: a biomechanical study. J Bone Joint Surg Am (2000). , 82, 1096-101.

[7] Dennis, D. A. Periprosthetic fractures following total knee arthroplasty: the good, bad and ugly. Orthopedics (1998). , 21, 1048-50.

[8] Scott, R. D. Anterior femoral notching and ipsilateral supracondylar femur fracture in total knee arthroplasty. J Arthroplasty (1988).

[9] Shawen, S. B. Belmont PJ Jr, Klemme WR, Topoleski LDT, Xenos JS, Orchowski JR. Osteoporosis and anterior femoral notching in periprosthetic supracondylar fractures. A biomechanical study. J Bone Joint Surg Am (2003). , 85, 115-21.

[10] Dennis, A. D. Periprosthetic fractures following total knee arthroplasty. J Bone Joint Surg Am (2001). , 83, 120-4.

[11] Ritter, M. A, Faris, P. M, & Keating, E. M. Anterior femoral notching and ipsilateral supracondylar femur fracture in total knee arthroplasty. J Arthroplasty (1988). , 3, 185-7.

[12] Henry, S. L. Booth RE Jr. Management of supracondylar fractures above total knee prosthesis. Tech Orthop (1995). , 9, 243-52.

[13] Merkel, K. D. Johnson EW Jr. Supracondylar fracture of the femur after total knee arthroplasty. J Bone Joint Surg Am (1986). , 68, 29-43.

[14] Aaron, R. K, & Scott, R. Supracondylar fracture of the femur after total knee arthroplasty. Clin Orthop (1987). , 219, 136-9.

[15] Dennis, D. A. Periprosthetis fractures following total knee arthroplasty. Tech Orthop (1999). , 14, 138-43.

[16] DiGioia AM 3d, Rubash HE. Periprosthetic fractures of the femur after total knee arthroplasty. A literature review and treatment algorithm. Clin Orthop (1991). , 271, 135-42.

[17] Rorabeck, C. H, Angliss, R. D, & Lewis, P. L. Fractures of the femur, tibia and patella after total knee arthroplasty: decision making and principles of management. Instr Course Lect (1998). , 47, 449-60.

[18] Rorabeck, C. H, & Taylor, J. W. Classification of periprosthetic fractures complicating total knee arthroplasty. Orthop Clin North Am (1999). , 30, 209-14.

[19] Shatzker, J, & Lambert, D. C. Supracondylar fractures of the femur. Clin Orthop (1979). , 138, 77-83.

[20] Insall, J. M. Fractures in the distal femur. In: Insall JM, editor. Surgery of the knee. New York: Churchill Livingstone, (1984). , 413-48.

[21] Hohl, M. Fractures about the knee. In: Rockwood CA, Green DP, editors. Fractures in adults.. Philadelphia: JB Lippincott,(1984). , 1478-9.

[22] Rorabeck, C. H, & Taylor, J. W. Periprosthetic fractures of the femur complicating total knee arthroplasty. Orthop Clin North Am (1999). , 30, 265-77.

[23] Harloww, M. L, & Hofmann, A. A. Periprosthetic fractures. In: Scot WN, editor. The knee. St Louis: CV Mosby, (1994). , 1405-17.

[24] Sochart, D. H, & Hardinge, K. Nonsurgical management of supracondylar fracture above total knee arthroplasty. Still the nineties option. J Arthroplasty (1997). , 12, 830-4.

[25] Ayers, D. C. Supracondylar fracture of the distal femur proximal to a total knee replacement. Instr Course Lect (1997). , 46, 197-203.

[26] Chmell, M. J, Moran, M. C, & Scott, R. D. Periarticular fractures after total knee arthroplasty: principles of management. J Am Acad Orthop Surg (1996). , 4, 109-16.

[27] Figgie, M. P, & Goldberg, V. M. Figgie HE III. The results of treatment of supracondylar fracture above total knee arthroplasty. J Arthroplasty (1990). , 5, 267-76.

[28] Kang Il KimEgol KA, Hozack WJ, Parvizi J. Periprosthetic fractures after total knee arthroplasties. Clin Orthop (2006). , 446, 167-75.

[29] Chen, F, Mont, M. A, & Bachner, R. S. Management of ipsilateral supracondylar femuir fractures following total knee arthroplasty. J Arthroplasty (1994). , 9, 521-6.

[30] Sochart, D. H, & Hardinge, K. Nonsurgical management of supracondylar fracture above total knee arthroplasty. Still the nineties option. J Arthroplasty (1997). , 12, 830-4.

[31] Engh, G. A, & Ammeen, D. J. Periprosthetic fractures adjacent to total knee implants. Treatment and clinical results. J Bone Joint Surg Am (1997). , 79, 1100-13.

[32] Cusick, R. P, Lucas, G. L, Mcqueen, D. A, & Graber, C. D. Construct stiffness of different fixation methods for supracondylar femoral fractures above total knee prosthesis. Am J Orthop (2000). , 29, 695-9.

[33] Lewis, P. L, & Rorabeck, C. H. Periprosthetic fractures. In: Engh GA, Rorabeck CH, editors. Revision total knee arthroplasty. Baltimore MD: Williams & Willkins; (1997). , 275-295.

[34] Kolb, K, Grützner, P. A, Marx, F, & Kolb, W. Fixation of Periprosthetic Supracondylar Femur Fractures Above Total Knee Arthroplasty- The Indirect Reduction Technique with the Condylar Blade Plate and the Minimally Invasive Technique with the LISS. In: Fokter S, editor. Recent Advances in Hip and Knee Arthroplasty. Rijeka: InTech, (2012). , 315-42.

[35] Herrera, D. A, Kregor, P. J, Cole, P. A, Levy, B. A, Jonssos, A, & Zlowodzki, M. Treatment of acute distal femur fractures above a total knee arthroplasty: systematic revew of 415 cases (1981-2006). Acta Orthop (2008). , 79, 22-7.

Chapter 19

Imaging Patellar Complications After Knee Arthroplasty

Pietro Melloni, Maite Veintemillas, Anna Marin and Rafael Valls

Additional information is available at the end of the chapter

http://dx.doi.org/10.5772/53666

1. Introduction

Knee arthroplasty, like hip replacement, is becoming increasingly common as the overall population begins to age. The survival rate of the knee implant is also increasing and is now similar to that of hip prostheses (85%-90% at 15 years).

Although complications in knee replacements have been widely reported and discussed, the literature contains few studies about patellar complications after total or partial knee arthroplasty.

Patellar complications after knee arthroplasty are infrequent but they can lead to unsatisfactory clinical outcome. Complications are often underestimated because the femoral component makes visualization of these lesions difficult. Evaluation must begin with a thorough history and physical examination. Laboratory tests and imaging studies can provide additional evidence to support a particular diagnosis.

The aim of this chapter is to describe and analyze complications affecting the patella in patients with total or partial knee arthroplasty and to illustrate some representative examples of the spectrum of findings on different imaging techniques, such as plain-film radiography and ultrasound (US), with the emphasis on plain-film findings.

Together with the clinical examination and follow-up, thorough plain-film and computed tomography (CT) studies should be done before and after the surgery. Later follow-up is directed toward identifying complications such as instability/dislocation, fracture, osteonecrosis, infection, erosion, impingement on the prosthesis, patellar or quadriceps tendon tear, and loosening or rupture of the patellar prosthetic button. One large study demonstrated that obtaining plain-film radiographs immediately after knee arthroplasty is not cost-effective. [1]

In the follow-up, plain-film radiographs usually suffice for the assessment of patellar complications and are helpful for guiding treatment. Some authors recommend a weight-bearing axial radiograph to better assess patellofemoral kinematics. [2-3] Although radiographs are the mainstay in evaluating loosening or infection, they are limited by their less than optimal sensitivity and specificity. [4]

In one study, the sensitivity and specificity of plain-film radiography compared to the findings at surgery were 77% and 90%, respectively, for detecting femoral component loosening, and 83% and 72%, respectively, for detecting tibial component loosening. [5] However, no specific studies about patellar prosthetic button complications are found in the literature.

In the past, the roles of CT and magnetic resonance imaging (MRI) in the assessment of joint prostheses were inconsequential due to image degradation by artifact. However, improvements in techniques and instrumentation have greatly improved the usefulness of CT and MRI in patients with joint replacements. Although no studies have addressed the routine use of these techniques for the follow-up of asymptomatic patients, some authors recommend CT to look for osteolysis in patients with painful knee prostheses with normal or equivocal radiographs and increased uptake on all three phases of a bone scan. [6] Another group of researchers [7]- [8] recommend multidetector CT in cases where osteolysis is likely, such as those with aseptic loosening and gross polyethylene wear. In patients with loosening, CT examination may also be useful to show the extent and width of lucent zones that may be less apparent on radiographs; in these cases, CT makes it possible to assess rotational alignment of components and to detect subtle or occult periprosthetic fractures of the patella. [9-10]

We use CT to assess component alignment and position as well as rotation of the patella with respect to the femur in patients with knee arthroplasty.

In patients with metallic knee prostheses, we use MRI for very specific indications, such as to evaluate the soft tissues surrounding the patella like the patellar and quadriceps tendons, Hoffa's fat pad, prepatellar subcutaneous tissue, and others. Although MRI is the technique of choice to evaluate the soft tissues [11], its use is seriously limited by drawbacks such as the high cost of acquiring, installing, and maintaining the equipment; magnetic susceptibility; the difficulties of working in a magnetic field; the large number of artifacts; long examination times that may require sedation; discomfort due to the noise inside the scanner; and possible claustrophobia. However, now nearly all implants are non-magnetizable and modern scanners allow images to be manipulated, so magnetic artifacts are no longer a problem. Thus, it could be argued that MRI will eventually supplant US; [12]; for example, MR may be helpful in detecting extracapsular spread of infection and abscess formation. [13]

2. Material and methods

Every year between 1998 and 2011, our hospital carried out more than 200 total knee replacements and 10 to 15 implantations of unicompartmental prostheses of the knee. In some knee replacement procedures, the patella was left intact, but in others patellar resurfacing

http://dx.doi.org/10.5772/53666

was performed or a prosthetic button was implanted. When the patella is intervened, it is often resurfaced with high-density polyethylene, which may be metal backed.

We retrospectively reviewed 1400 consecutive examinations in patients treated with total or partial knee arthroplasty in the last two years; 54 (3.7%) patients (35 women and 19 men) presented patellar complications. Mean patient age was 74 years (range, 55-90 years). In some cases, patients had prostheses in both knees.

All patients were followed up immediately after surgery, at 6 months, and then yearly or when necessary, using anteroposterior, lateral, and axial (Merchant view) radiographs. Lateral and axial projections are better for visualizing and evaluating the evolution of the patella after knee replacement.

In certain cases according to the clinical symptoms, patients underwent US, especially to evaluate the morphological integrity of the patellar and quadriceps tendons and other soft-tissue structures around the patella.

3. Results

The patellar complications that we observed following total knee arthroplasty include instability/dislocation, fracture, osteonecrosis, infection, erosion, impingement on the prosthesis, patellar or quadriceps tendon tear, and loosening or rupture of the patellar prosthetic button. The mean interval from total knee replacement to patellar complication was 5 years and 9 months (range, 5 months-15 years).

3.1. Instability/dislocation (n=21)

Patellar instability (n=15) is the commonest complication after knee arthroplasty. In total knee arthroplasty, most complications related to the extensor mechanism are caused by patellar maltracking instability. [14] Patellar maltracking may result from component malpositioning and limb malalignment, excessive femoral component size, prosthetic design, inadequate patellar resection, or soft-tissue imbalance. [15] Patellofemoral instability likely results most frequently from internal malrotation of the femoral or tibial components. [16]

Malpositioning of femoral and tibial components may affect patellar alignment. Although the axial rotation of the femoral component can be determined using plain-film radiographs or MRI, CT is most commonly used for this purpose. [17] Excessive combined internal rotation of tibial and femoral components is associated with patellar complications. [18] Furthermore, one study [19] found the amount of excessive combined internal rotation was directly proportional to the severity of patellofemoral complications. The rotation of the femoral component can be assessed with relation to the transepicondylar axis, the Whiteside line, or the posterior femoral condyles. The femoral component should be parallel to the transepicondylar axis and the tibial component should be in about 18 degrees of internal rotation with relation to the tibial tubercle.

Careful radiographic follow-up should be considered when deep flexion is achieved in a knee with a patella baja after total knee arthroplasty (Figure 1). Patellar dislocation (n=6) is mainly due to direct trauma to the patella or to extensor mechanism rupture [20] (Figure 2).

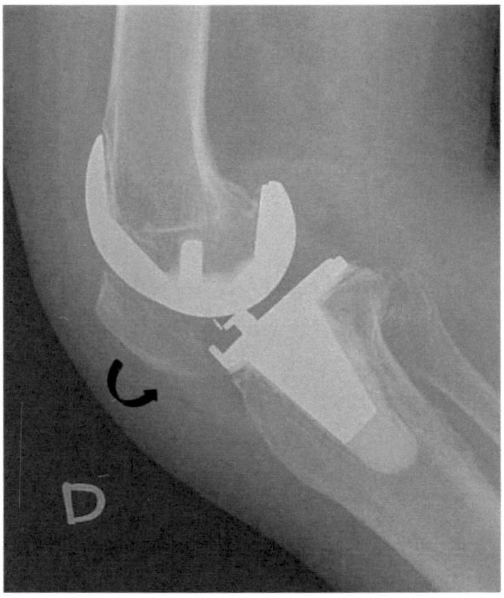

Figure 1. Patellar Instability. A 60-year-old man, five years after total knee replacement. Lateral radiograph reveals caudal displacement of the patella (curved arrow).

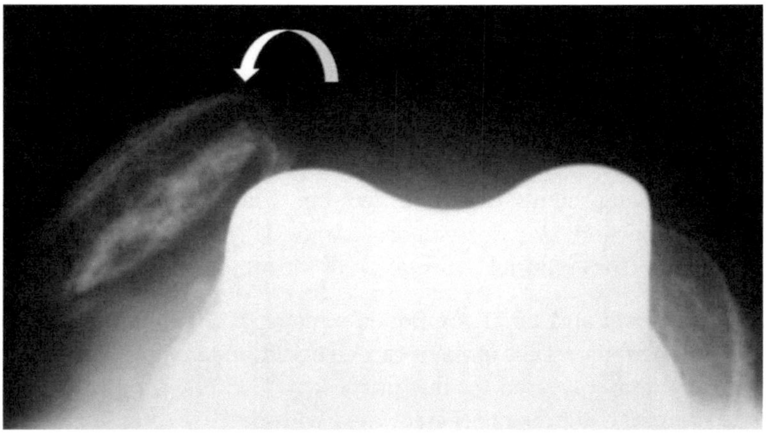

Figure 2. Patellar Dislocation. A 71-year-old woman, five years after total knee replacement. Axial radiograph (Merchant view) of the knee prosthesis with cemented prosthetic button of the patella demonstrates lateral patellar displacement on flexion (curved arrow).

Alterations in the patellotibial distance can occur during total knee arthroplasty due to excessive soft-tissue release that requires elevation of the joint to regain stability and place-

http://dx.doi.org/10.5772/53666

ment of the polyethylene patellar component distally on the patella. Another cause of acquired patella baja seen commonly in total knee arthroplasty is elevation of the joint line, referred to as pseudo-patella baja. [21]

Radiographic evaluation of the patella primarily uses the lateral view and the sunrise or Merchant's view. This projection should show the central ridge of the patella lying at or medial to the bisector of the trochlear angle. This approach is also helpful for evaluating patellar tilt, but not it is very sensitive for determining the cause of patellofemoral pain.

The lateral view reveals the patellar thickness, inferior or superior positioning, as well as adequate fixation and position of the components. The positioning of the patellar component (centralized or tilted in relation to the trochlear sulcus or subluxated/dislocated) is clearly seen and may reveal the cause of instability. Tilt can be defined as medial or lateral, depending on its relation to the femoral condyles. Subluxation can be measured as displacement from the center of the prosthetic femoral intercondylar groove. [22]

3.2. Osteonecrosis (n=5)

Patellar resurfacing during total knee arthroplasty remains controversial. Several patellar complications such as fracture, avascular necrosis, and instability are related to resurfacing. On the other hand, some authors report lower re-operation rates and postoperative pain when the patella is resurfaced. Attention should be directed to the ultimate patellar thickness. Whether or not to resurface should be determined based on the exact initial thickness. A thicker patella is prone to instability, whereas a thinner patella is associated with higher complication rates. Patellar fragmentation and sclerosis of the fragments are presumed to represent osteonecrosis (Figure 3). The osteonecrosis may be due to disruption of the vascular network of the patella during total knee replacement surgery. [23] Medial parapatellar arthrotomy, fat pad removal, and lateral release all contribute to patellar devascularization. Evolutional osteonecrosis may lead to patellar fracture.

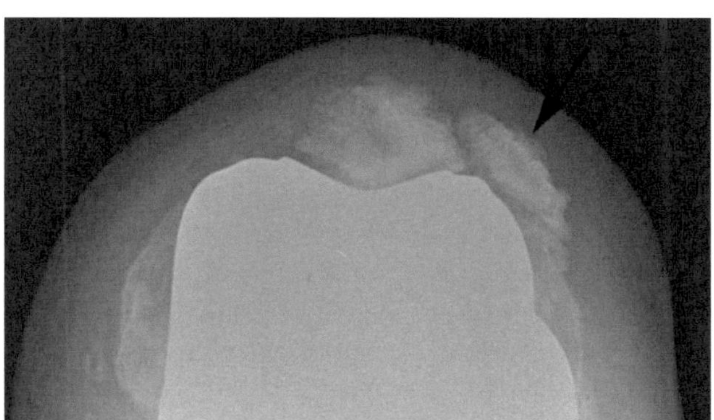

Figure 3. Patellar Necrosis. A 68-year-old man, seven years after total knee replacement. Axial radiograph of the knee prosthesis shows bony sclerosis with fragmentation of the patella (arrow).

3.3. Fracture (n=9)

Patellar fractures in association with total knee replacement are uncommon and occur predominantly in patients with resurfaced patellae. [24] Most fractures appear to occur in the first few years after total knee replacement.

Patient, implant, and technical factors are important predisposing causes of these patellar fractures. Avascularity, trauma, fatigue, and stress also play an etiologic role in some patellar fractures.

Trauma to the patella, either direct or indirect, and increased patellofemoral stress are other causes of fracture. Indirect causes might include an eccentric quadriceps muscle contraction associated with a stumble, resulting in an avulsion fracture (Figure 4).

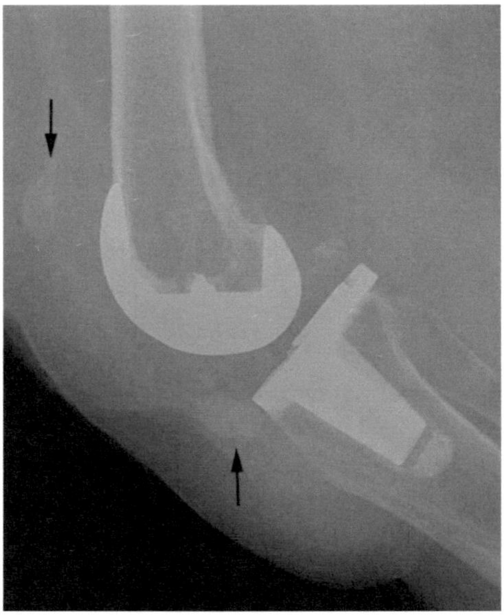

Figure 4. Patellar Avulsion Fracture. A 73-year-old woman, seven years after total knee replacement. Lateral radiograph shows a transverse avulsion fracture in the mid-portion of the patella with displacement of its poles in the cranial-caudal direction (arrows).

Patellar fractures are not associated with prior injury. Because patellar fractures are often asymptomatic and discovered incidentally, follow-up radiographs are essential for their detection. Transverse fractures seem to be related to patellar maltracking, and vertical fractures often occur through a fixation hole. CT or MRI can detect some fractures that go undetected on plain-film radiographs.

Prevention is the best treatment. Important outcome criteria include the integrity of the extensor mechanism, patellar implant fixation, and anatomic location. Surgery on patients with patella fractures has a high complication rate and should be avoided if possible. [25-26]

http://dx.doi.org/10.5772/53666

3.4. Infection (n=2)

Although rare, infection can appear in the patella after total or partial replacement of the knee. [27] Unspecific radiological signs of infection include a lytic lesion or osseous sclerosis in the patella or in the joint facet of the femur in the femoropatellar joint (Figure 5). Clinical symptoms may orient the diagnosis of infection.

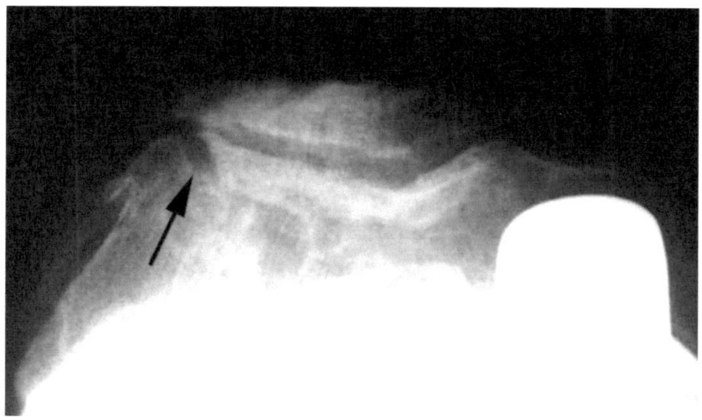

Figure 5. Patellar Infection. A 70-year-old man, nine years after partial knee replacement. Axial radiograph (Merchant view) of the knee prosthesis shows osteolysis on the lateral facet of the femur (arrow) with a non-cemented hemiarthroplasty of the knee, corresponding to a focus of infection, with sclerosis in the patella, suspected of infective infiltration. These findings were confirmed during surgery, and excisional debridement of the infection and total patellectomy were performed. Cultures were positive for *Pseudomonas aeruginosa*.

Plain-film radiographs are usually negative in the first ten days, even when clinical signs raise suspicion of infection. The radiological presentation varies, sometimes including localized rarefaction in the patella with or without sequestrum, or osseous destruction of the patella with or without an irregular bony fragment adjacent.

Surgical biopsy would provide the definitive diagnosis. The treatment of osteolytic lesions of the patella should be surgical.

3.5. Erosion/Impingement (n=6)

Patellar instability can cause erosion (n=2) in the joint facet of the patella due to friction with the femoral component of the knee arthroplasty (Figure 6). The erosion may appear as a lytic lesion that can simulate a subchondral cyst due to any arthritic process or small particle disease. Careful comparison with the pre-arthroplasty plain-films is essential. The erosion should not be confused with a dorsal defect in the posterior surface of the patella that occasionally persists into later life. The dorsal patellar defect is usually well delineated.

Patellar impingement (n=4), the so-called patellar clunk syndrome, results from the formation of a fibrous nodule over the proximal pole of the patella and reportedly occurs in cases of total kneed arthroplasty in which a posterior stabilized design is utilized. [28] Arthroscopic or open resection of the fibrous nodule can eliminate this syndrome.

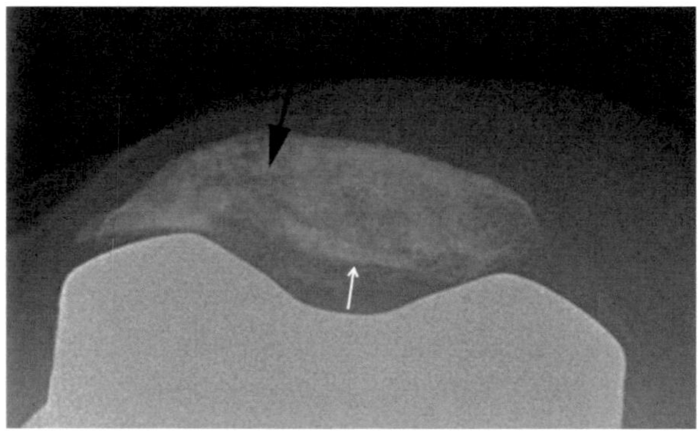

Figure 6. Patellar Osteolysis. A 75-year-old man, three years after total knee replacement. Axial radiograph (Merchant view) shows osteolysis of the lateral facet of the patella (black arrow) due to the loosening of both the total knee prosthesis and the patellar prosthetic button (white arrow). There was clinical suspicion of infection but cultures were negative.

Patellar impingement also is seen when patella baja develops after posterior stabilized total knee arthroplasty and when the patella becomes impinged against the femoral component (Figure 7). [29] Patellofemoral complications (osteoarthritis and impingement) are rarely seen after total replacement and even more rarely after unicompartmental arthroplasty [30], so their long-term consequences are not well known.

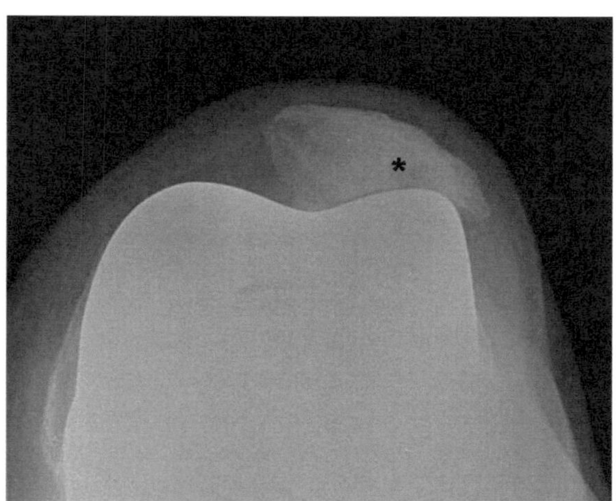

Figure 7. Patellar Impingement. A 71-year-old man, four years after total knee replacement. Axial radiograph (Merchant view) shows a reduction in the space between the knee arthroplasty and the patella, with consequent reactive patellar sclerosis (asterisk).

http://dx.doi.org/10.5772/53666

However, in our study the symptoms in knees with patellar impingement were usually more severe than in knees with degenerative changes.

3.7. Loosening or rupture of the patellar prosthetic button (n=7)

A patellar prosthetic button (patellar component) is added to total knee replacement in certain cases. Like all joint prostheses (such as hip, knee, and small joints), the patellar button may loosen or rupture with the same or similar characteristic radiological signs as in the other joints. Loosening of the patellar button (Figure 8) may cause significant anterior pain. Thin fixation pegs, maltracking, and trauma frequently induce component loosening. Revision of a failed patellar component is typically associated with a relatively high complication rate.

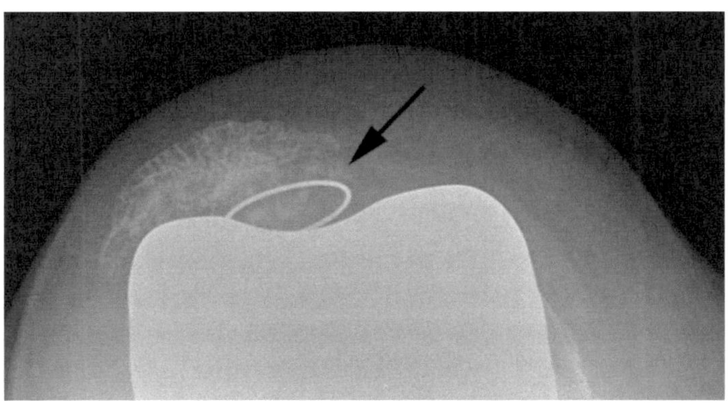

Figure 8. Prosthetic Button Loosening. A 71-year-old woman, two years after total knee replacement. Axial radiograph (Merchant view) shows patellar subluxation with prosthetic button loosening (arrow).

Osseous changes that may be observed in the patellar prosthetic button following total or partial knee arthroplasty include radiolucent lines, osteolysis, change in prosthesis position, and polyethylene wear. Radiolucent lines superimposed on the femoral component can often be obscured by the metal tray if the view is not perfectly tangential to the component surface. Nonprogressive focal radiolucent areas less than 2 mm in size are often insignificant; however, progressive, circumferential, radiolucent areas larger than 2 mm are often indicative of prosthesis loosening.

Rupture of the patellar prosthetic button (Figure 9) is rare but can occur due to polyethylene wear, fusion defects in the polyethylene structure [31], or trauma to the patella. [32] The incidence of wear in patients with all-polyethylene and metal-backed components ranges from 5% to 11%. Congruity, maltracking, and contact force are associated with polyethylene wear. Decreased polyethylene thickness in metal-backed designs is the determining factor for mechanism failure.

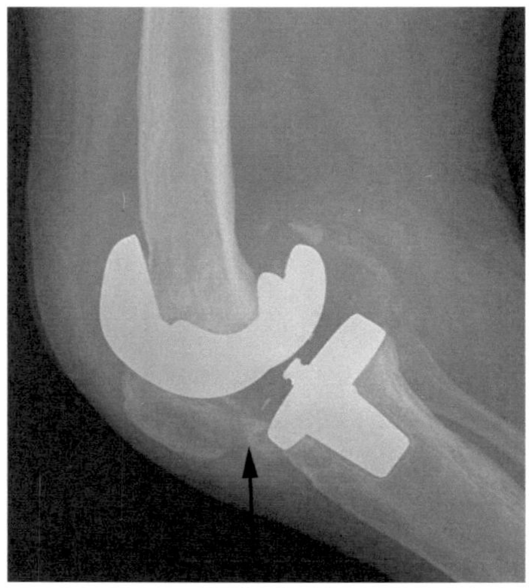

Figure 9. Prosthetic Button Rupture. A 68-year-old woman, four years after total knee replacement. Lateral radiograph shows a rupture of the patellar prosthetic button (arrow) with caudal displacement.

Prosthetic loosening, small particle disease, and infection are the most frequent causes of osteolysis of the patellar component. A change in position of components on serial images is indicative of prosthesis loosening. [33]

3.8. Patellar or quadriceps tendon tear (n=4)

Rupture of patellar or quadriceps ligaments occurs infrequently. However, the complications of an untreated rupture to the extensor mechanism can be extremely disabling. Contributing factors are excessive dissection and knee manipulation, and trauma. The same mechanical causes that produce patellar fractures can produce patellar [34] or quadriceps [35] tendon tear. US is the method of choice for studying the patellar or quadriceps tendons to confirm or rule out tendon tears (Figures 10 &11). An abrupt high patella is seen on lateral radiographs in some patients with clinical suspicion of tendon rupture after total knee replacement, but US is necessary to confirm the diagnosis. Although MRI can also be useful in this context, it is not widely used. Other diagnostic possibilities are chronic tendonitis or tendon laxness. Treatment outcomes for ruptured patellar ligaments are not good.

http://dx.doi.org/10.5772/53666

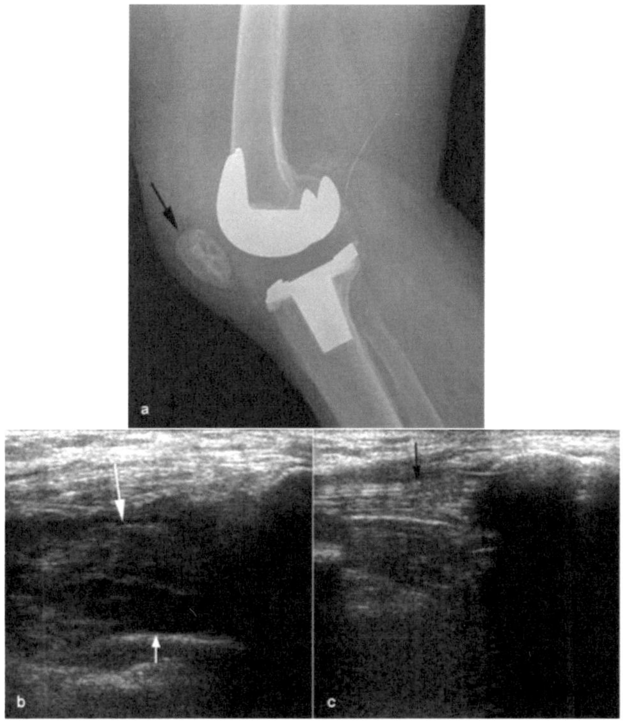

Figure 10. a-c).- **QuadricepsTendon Rupture.** A 73-year-old woman, ten years after total knee replacement. Lateral radiograph (a) shows patellar displacement and rotation with clinical suspicion of quadriceps tendon tear (black arrow). US (b) confirms a disrupted quadriceps tendon (long white arrow) with a suprapatellar fluid collection (short white arrow) and a 5 cm gap between the end of the tendon and the patella. Compare with the sonogram of the contralateral knee showing a normal quadriceps tendon (fine black arrow) with total knee replacement (c) in the same patient, who had rheumatoid arthritis.

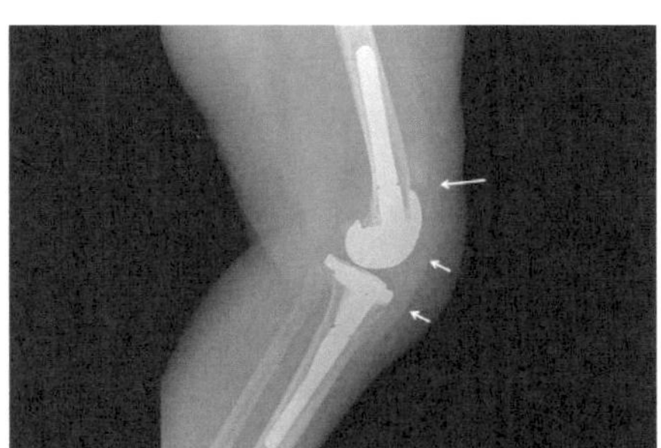

Figure 11. Patellar Tendon Rupture with Patellar Avulsion Fracture. A 69-year-old woman, twelve years after total knee replacement and two years after revision knee replacement with long femoral and tibial stems. Lateral radiograph shows cranial displacement with transverse avulsion fracture in the mid-portion of the patella (long arrow). Note the extensive soft-tissue edema in the patellar area (short arrows), leading to suspected patellar tendon rupture, which was confirmed at ultrasonography (not shown).

4. Conclusion

Patellar complications following knee arthroplasty are generally uncommon but often of potential clinical significance. Plain-film radiographs are essential for the evaluation of patellar complications after surgery and should be the initial imaging study performed. Careful attention to initial prosthesis placement and comparison of follow-up images will allow subtle abnormalities to be detected in patellar complications. US may have a special role in the evaluation of soft-tissue structures around the patella.

Author details

Pietro Melloni, Maite Veintemillas, Anna Marin and Rafael Valls

UDIAT Diagnostic Center, Corporació Sanitària i Universitària Parc Taulí, Sabadell, Spain

References

[1] Mendel E. Singer, PhD and Kimberly E. Applegate, MD. Cost-Effectiveness Analysis in Radiology. Departments of Epidemiology and Biostatistics, Metro Health Medical Center (M.E.S.), and the Department of Radiology, Rainbow Babies and Children's Hospital (K.E.A.), Case Western Reserve University School of Medicine, 10900 Euclid Ave, Cleveland, OH 44106 (M.E.S.)

[2] Nobuyuki Yoshino, Nobuyoshi Watanabe, Yukihisa Fukuda, Yoshinobu Watanabe, Shinro Takai. The influence of patellar dislocation on the femoro-tibial loading during total knee arthroplasty. Knee Surgery, Sports Traumatology, Arthroscopy. November 2011, Volume 19, Issue 11, pp 1817-1822.

[3] Shinro Takai, Nobuyuki Yoshino, Nobuyoshi Watanabe and Yukihisa Fukuda. The effect of patellar eversion to the extension and flexion gaps in total knee arthroplasty. J Bone Joint Surg Br 2010 vol. 92-b no. supp i 160-161.

[4] ACR Appropriateness Criteria® imaging after total knee arthroplasty. Weissman BN, Shah N, Daffner RH, Bancroft L, Bennett DL, Blebea JS, Bruno MA, Fries IB, Hayes CW, Kransdorf MJ, Luchs JS, Morrison WB, Palestro CJ, Roberts CC, Stoller DW, Taljanovic MS, Tuite MJ, Ward RJ, Wise JN, Zoga AC, Expert Panel on Musculoskeletal Imaging. ACR Appropriateness Criteria® imaging after total knee arthroplasty. [online publication]. Reston (VA): American College of Radiology (ACR).

[5] Jonathan Baré, MD, Steven J. MacDonald, Robert B. Bourne, MD. Preoperative Evaluations in Revision Total Knee Arthroplasty. Clinical Orthopaedics and Related Research. Number 446, pp. 40–44© 2006 Lippincott Williams & Wilkins.

[6] Use of multi-detector computed tomography for the detection of periprosthetic osteolysis in total knee arthroplasty. Reish TG, Clarke HD, Scuderi GR, Math KR, Scott WN. J Knee Surg. 2006 Oct;19(4):259-64.

[7] Imaging of total knee arthroplasty. Math KR, Zaidi SF, Petchprapa C, Harwin SF. Semin Musculoskelet Radiol. 2006 Mar;10(1):47-63. Review.

[8] Imaging of knee arthroplasty. Miller TT. Eur J Radiol. 2005 May;54(2):164-77. Review.

[9] Can CT-based patient-matched instrumentation achieve consistent rotational alignment in knee arthroplasty? Tibesku CO, Innocenti B, Wong P, Salehi A, Labey L. Arch Orthop Trauma Surg. 2012 Feb;132(2):171-7. Epub 2011 Oct 18.

[10] Rotational positioning of the tibial tray in total knee arthroplasty: a CT evaluation. Berhouet J, Beaufils P, Boisrenoult P, Frasca D, Pujol N. Orthop Traumatol Surg Res. 2011 Nov;97(7):699-704. Epub 2011 Oct 10.

[11] Magnetic resonance imaging of joint arthroplasty. Potter HG, Foo LF. Orthop Clin North Am. 2006 Jul;37(3):361-73, vi-vii. Review.

[12] Magnetic resonance imaging with metal suppression for evaluation of periprosthetic osteolysis after total knee arthroplasty. Vessely MB, Frick MA, Oakes D, Wenger DE, Berry DJ. J Arthroplasty. 2006 Sep;21(6):826-31.

[13] New MR imaging methods for metallic implants in the knee: artifact correction and clinical impact. Chen CA, Chen W, Goodman SB, Hargreaves BA, Koch KM, Lu W, Brau AC, Draper CE, Delp SL, Gold GE. J Magn Reson Imaging. 2011 May;33(5): 1121-7.

[14] Malo M, Vince KG. The unstable patella after total knee arthroplasty: etiology, prevention, and management. J Am Acad Orthop Surg. 2003 Sep-Oct;11(5):364-71.

[15] Robert Wen-Wei Hsu. The management of the patella in total knee arthroplasty. Chang Gung Med J. 2006 September-October. Vol. 29 No. 5.

[16] Efstathios K Motsis, Nikolaos Paschos, Emilios E Pakos, Anastasios D Georgoulis. Review article: Patellar instability after total knee arthroplasty. Journal of Orthopaedic Surgery 2009;17(3):351-7.

[17] Berger RA, Crossett LS, Jacobs JJ, Rubash HE; Malrotation causing patellofemoral complications after total knee arthroplasty. Clinical Orthopedics and Related Research. 1998 Nov;(356):144-53.

[18] Vanbiervliet J, Bellemans J, Innocenti B, et al. The influence of malrotation and femoral component material on patellofemoral wear during gait. Journal Of Bone & Joint Surgery, British Volume [serial online]. October 2011;93(10):1348-1354.

[19] Blisard R. Component internal rotation malrotation a factor in pain after TKA. Orthopedics Today [serial online]. September 2011;31(9):24.

[20] Rand JA. Extensor mechanism complications following total knee arthroplasty. J Knee Surg 2003;16:224–8.

[21] Chonko DJ, Lombardi AV Jr, Berend KR. Patella baja and total knee arthroplasty (TKA): etiology, diagnosis, and management. Surg Technol Int. 2004;12:231-8.

[22] Healy WL, Wasilewski SA, Takei R, Oberlander M. Patellofemoral complications following total knee arthroplasty. Correlation with implant design and patient risk factors. J Arthroplasty 1995;10:197–201.

[23] Kyung Ah, Chun Kenjirou, Ohashi D, Lee Bennett, Georges Y, El-Khoury. Patellar Fractures After Total Knee Replacement. AJR AM J Roent. 2005; sept, 185:655–660.

[24] Aglietti P, Baldini A, Buzzi R, Indelli PF. Patella resurfacing in total knee replacement: functional evaluation and complications. J Bone Joint Surg Am. 2002 Jul;84-A(7):1132-7.

[25] Bourne RB. Fractures of the patella after total knee replacement. Orthop Clin North AM. 1999 Apr; 30(2):287-91.

[26] Ortiguera CJ, Berry DJ. Patellar fracture after total knee arthroplasty. J Bone Joint Surg Am. 2002 Apr;84-A(4):532-40.

[27] Keating EM, Haas G, Meding JB. Patella fracture after total knee replacements. Clin Orthop. 2003 Nov;(416):93-7.

[28] Beight JL, Yao B, Hozack WJ, Hearn SL, Booth RE Jr. The patellar "clunk" syndrome after posterior stabilized total knee arthroplasty. Clin Orthop Relat Res. 1994 Feb; (299):139-42.

[29] Maeno S, Kondo M, Niki Y, Matsumoto H. Patellar impingement against the tibial component after total knee arthroplasty. Clin Orthop Relat Res. 2006. Nov; 452: 265.

[30] Matthew B. Collier, MS, et al. Osteolysis After Total Knee Arthroplasty: Influence of Tibial Baseplate Surface Finish and Sterilation of Polyethylene Insert. In The Journal of Bone and Joint Surgery. December 2005. Vol. 87-A. No. 12. Pp. 2702-2708.

[31] Hernigou P, Deschamps G. Patellar impingement following unicompartmental arthroplasty. J Bone Joint Surg Am. 2002 Jul;84-A(7):1132-7.

[32] MacCollum MS 3rd, Karpman RR. Complications of the PCA anatomic patella. Orthopedics. 1989 Nov;12(11):1423-8.

[33] William H Harris. Osteolysis and particle disease in hip replacement. A review. Acta Ortho~Scand 1994:65 113-123.

[34] Rand JA, Morrey BF, Bryan RS. Patellar tendon rupture after total knee arthroplasty. Clin Orthop Relat Res. 1989 Jul;(244):233-8.

[35] Dobbs RE, Hanssen AD, Lewallen DG, Pagnano MW. Quadriceps tendon rupture after total knee arthroplasty. Prevalence, complications, and outcomes. Bone Joint Surg Am. 2005 Jan;87(1):37-45.

Chapter 20

Extensor Mechanism Complications After Patellar Resurfacing in Knee Replacement – Can They Justify Non-Patellar Resurfacing?

Antonio Silvestre, Raúl Lopez, Fernando Almeida,
Pablo Renovell, Francisco Argüelles and
Oscar Vaamonde

Additional information is available at the end of the chapter

http://dx.doi.org/10.5772/53382

1. Introduction

Patellar resurfacing is still nowadays a controversial matter in articles, cross fires and meetings. We know that this is not a new subject as the issue of whether or not to resurface the patella when performing a TKA has been a debatable topic for more than two decades [1]. We can find three philosophies around what to do with the patella in TKA and there is still no best conclusion about benefits from one or another procedure.

Many randomised trials provide inconclusive evidence in relation to resurface or not the patella after TKA and these trials fail mainly because short sample sizes. Some meta-analysis have been reported last years in order to clarify this issue and though no great differences have been found between both procedures, patellar resurfacing shows better functional results and less anterior knee pain [2-4]. Nevertheless, what is cleared stated in literature is that treatment of the patellofemoral joint in knee replacement and its ultimate results are multifactorial.

Surgeons around the world can be classified into three groups according to their preference in the topic of resurfacing or not the patella: universal resurfacers, non-resurfacers and selective resurfacers. One of the reasons that non-resurfacers use as justification for their performance is that patellar resurfacing implies complications related to extensor mechanism of the knee. Moreover complications related to extensor mechanism are a common basis for

TKA revisions and these problems have less favourable outcome than patients who undergo revision for other reasons.

The use of computer-aid navigation systems in knee replacement have allowed to accurate some of the mistakes in coronal, sagittal and axial alignment of femoral and tibial implant that are related to patellar maltracking. In the near future it should be possible to navigate the patellofemoral joint, so problems linked to this compartment will diminish. Until now, there is a report of a surgical navigation system that let to assess intraoperatively patellar tracking, one of the main reasons of TKAs' failure, with the aid of a computer. The system is quite complex and it is not available for all the knee prosthesis designs. However, the method could be a valuable support to analyze patellar tracking at the time of the surgery and a real help to decide whether or not patellar replacement [5].

In this study we have reviewed our extensor mechanism complications relate to knee replacement for the last 6 years in order to analyze if they have a high rate that could justify non-patellar resurfacing. We believe that a careful and meticulous technique during patellar resurfacing can avoid most of the problems found after knee replacement. It is not reasonable that in these days in which many surgeons are worried about accurate alignment of knee components and most of them use computer-aid navigation systems to be more precise in prosthesis placement we are not as careful as in other steps of the procedure when resurfacing the patella.

2. Material and method

We have retrospectively revised all the TKA's performed in our Institution from January 2005 until December 2011. For this period of time, the two fellowship-trained surgeons (AS and FA) performed 860 TKA using a standard technique for knee replacement and similar rehabilitation protocol. Postero-stabilized cemented total knee arthroplasties were used in all cases (Performance® Biomet Warsaw, IN and Vanguard® Biomet Warsaw, IN). Patella was resurfaced in all cases according to the philosophy of our Department. Demographic data are shown in table I.

A single dose of intravenous antibiotic (cefazolin 2 gr or vancomycin 1gr in allergic patients according to the protocol of our Hospital Infection Control Committee) was given ½ hour before incision. After general o regional anaesthesia depending on patient and physician's preference, tourniquet was routinely applied as proximal as possible in the thigh. Longitudinal incision along the knee and medial para-patellar arthrotomy were performed to gain access to the joint. Surgery was performed according to the standard procedure and femur and tibial implants were cemented to the bone. Careful alignment of both components was checked before implantation. Posterior-condyle plus 3° of external rotation and trans-epicondylar axis were used without distinction to get an adequate femoral rotation. On the other hand tibial component was aligned to the medial third of the tibial tubercle. We don't usually evert the patella during this time of the procedure. Once femoral and tibial trials were in place, we arrange for the patellar resurfacing step.

http://dx.doi.org/10.5772/53382

Sex	Female: 536/ Male: 324
Side	Right: 492/ Left: 368
Age (years)	73.15±6.06
BMI (kg/m²)	27.76±3.12
Previous surgery (%)	38.3%
Radiological valgus (%)	9.7%
Pre-operative diagnoses	
Osteoarthritis	593
Osteonecrosis medial condyle	137
Metabolic arthritis	78
RA	35
Fracture sequela	17

Table 1. Demographic data and preoperative parameters

In our experience it is crucial to be as thorough as possible in patellar resurfacing step to achieve good results and avoid extensor mechanism complications. Most of these problems should be avoid with a more methodical procedure. We employ the instruments provide by the manufacturer to afford patellar resurfacing though we accept they are not always useful. However, more precise instruments in recent systems allow more accuracy placing the patella. The Vanguard System Knee® provides specifically devices (cutting guide) to improve the results. It offers a calliper or vernier to estimate patella thickness before and after the cut, a guide with a magnetize gauge to determine the deep of the cut after guide positioning and it is possible to choose single or three-peg configuration at the time of the surgery. Devices availability in theatre make the surgeons more self-assured when dealing with patello-femoral joint. Albeit these devices can't be employed in 100% of cases as patellar morphology, size or wear difficult its use. The fact that surgical instrumental can't be employed, doesn't mean patellar resurfacing is a trivial step in knee surgery.

For this series we have used all-polyethylene patellar component design with single or three-peg configuration. The prostheses employed in our cases just provide onlay patellar implants. We usually make peripheral electrocautery around the patella and remove soft-tissue synovium in the upper part of the patella to avoid patellar clunk syndrome as we perform posterior stabilized designs.

Patients received intravenous antibiotics (cefazolin 1g/8h) for 48 h after surgery according to the protocol of our Institution. Post-operative bandage was removed at the second day after surgery to check incision and vascular condition of the leg. Output drainage was removed 36-48 h after surgery. They started physiotherapy of the operated knee the second day after surgery when drains were removed if proper laboratory values were obtained. Full weight bearing on the operated limb was allowed immediately except in those cases the surgeon contraindicated the pre-established protocol because of surgical difficulties. Physiotherapists instructed the patients to walk either with walker or crutches depending on their ability. They go up stairs with the help of the banister the fourth-fifth day after surgery before leaving the Hospital.

Prophylactic low molecular weight heparin (enoxaparin) was used for the next 28 days after surgery. Patients stay at our Institution depends on his/her ability to keep up with daily activities (range 4-8 days), obviously after their haematological values were as best as possible.

Outpatient follow-up was done at 6, 12 weeks and the annually for clinical and radiological evaluation of the operated knee. We assessed clinical evaluation including gait, need for assistance devices, ROM, joint stability, knee score (KSS) and visual analog scale (VAS). Routine A-P and lateral views were done to evaluate mechanical axis and proper alignment of the implant. In those cases with extensor mechanism complications axial views and other techniques such as US, CT or MR were used to analyze the problem.

Intra-operative and post-operative complications were captured and collected for descriptive study. Arthroscopic technique was indicated in case internal injuries of the knee (patellar clunk syndrome); on the other hand open surgery was used for management of instabilities, tendon ruptures, patellar fracture…

3. Results

There were 860 primary total knee arthroplasties performed with the use of the "Performance System" (Biomet®, Warsaw, IN) and the "Vanguard System" (Biomet®, Warsaw, IN) in this series, done through a longitudinal incision with medial para-patellar arthrotomy. Underlying diagnosis was osteoarthritis and osteonecrosis of the medial condyle in more than 80% of cases. Mean follow-up was 48 months (ranging from 6 to 78 months).

Thirteen patients (1.51%) showed wound infection and developed an acute infection and eleven cases (1.27%) suffered haematogenous infection more than a year after surgery so these patients were excluded from this series as they required revision surgery (836 patients were included in this series). Co-morbidities in these patients were diabetes mellitus, rheumatoid arthritis and obesity. During follow-up elevated ESR (>20) and CRP (>5) values and clinical signs of infection were detected. Aspiration culture was positive 19 cases (79.16%) and the most frequent microorganisms identified were staphylococcus spp, meticillin-resistant staphylococcus aureus, streptococcus spp and pseudomona aeuruginosa.

In our series required time to walk by a walker or two crutches was 2.25±1.45 days and patients were able to go up and down stairs with the help of the banister at 5.03±2.67 days (range 4-15 days). More than sixty percent of patients were capable to walk without the help of any assistive aids at four weeks postoperatively. However, we advise the use of at least one cane for the first six weeks after the operation, to avoid stumbling as many patients in this series are elderly. Clinical results are shown in table II.

Knee Society Score improved from 53.48±6.21 (range 39-67) to 92.037± 7.23 (range 85-94) a year after surgery. Visual analog pain score after surgery improved to 1.891±0.31 in more than 90% of cases three months after surgical procedure. This can be judge as a satisfactory score as painful knee arthroplasty is a non-desired state after joint reconstruction.

		Preoperative	6 weeks	12 weeks	1 year
Pain (VAS)	<2 (%)	2.39	83.61	92.19	94.49
	2 to <5 (%)	35.52	13.63	5.75	3.96
	5 to <8 (%)	45.09	2.51	1.91	1.31
	>8%	17	0.24	0.24	0.24
KSS (knee score)		53.48±6.21	79.437±8.32	89.065±5.87	92.037±7.23
Average ROM		-5 /85°	0 /95°	0 / 115°	0 / 115°
Walking capability	>2 h (%)	1.91	50.35	60.04	61.96
	>1 h (%)	22	27.63	29.06	29.06
	>30' (%)	75	31.31	10.43	8.51
	Not walk (%)	1.09	0.71	0.47	0.47
Walking support	No support (%)	57.05	62.53	86.12	90.55
	1 cane or crutch (%)	42	35.81	12.58	8.27
	2 crutches (%)	0.95	0.95	0.83	0.71
Stairs	Normal (%)	63.03	77.25	85.16	85.52
	Banister (%)	35.88	21.54	14.37	14.01

Table 2. Clinical results

Mechanical axis (180º±3º) was restored in 95.04% of cases. Alignments of the femoral and tibial implants in frontal and coronal axes were measured without significant deviation from standard values.

Main extensor mechanism complications are shown in table III. The most frequent complications were instability of the extensor mechanism and patellar fractures. However, most of the fractures were related to a traumatic event as patients in this series were old people, so this complication cannot be only linked to surgical aggression. Patellar tendon rupture was mostly related to knees with previous surgery as valgus osteotomy.

Instability of the extensor mechanism (patellar dislocation or subluxation)	**1.79% (15 cases)**
Patellar fracture	1.43% (12 cases)
Patellar tendon rupture	0.47% (4 cases)
Patella loosening	0.95% (8 cases)
Clunk syndrome	0.71 (6 cases)

Table 3. Extensor mechanism complications

4. Discussion

For many years dealing with the patella in total knee arthroplasties has been a controversial topic. Most of the non-resurfacers surgeons justify their choice based in the frequent complications related to surgery around the patella. It is true that surgical gestures used during patellar resurfacing can affect the patello-femoral tracking, weak patellar bone or alter vascularisation around the patella. Besides it has been remarked by many authors that some knee replacements failures are related to disorders in the mechanics of the patellofemoral joint.

Soft-tissue imbalance is shown as the responsible of patellar instability, the most frequent extensor mechanism complication with an incidence as high as 29% in some series after TKAs [6]. Muscle atrophy, weakness, more proximal attachment of the VMO after closure of the arthrotomy and predominance of the VL are considered the main causes of patellofemoral dysfunction [6]. However, forces from the different bellies of the quadriceps can modify patellofemoral function [7].

Aside from anatomical aspects of the quadriceps that are non surgical-dependant, some technical aspects on the patellar side should be observed during this step of the surgery. It is of main importance to restore patellar thickness to prevent from high mechanical pressures and increase de risk of patellar fracture [8]. It is recommended to maintain between 13 and 15 mm of patellar bone remained to adapt the all-polyethylene insert which has 8-10 mm thickness. Surgical technique is of crucial importance in patellar alignment. An increase combined thickness of the implant and patellar bone leads to higher forces on patellar side and close follow-up of these patients should be done. Postoperative lateral tilt increased when thickness after patella resurfacing was augment in 1 mm from the preoperative patella [9]. This lateral tilt is usually treated by lateral release that improves patellar alignment, but lateral release is related to complications as patellar fracture, vascular problems and postoperative pain [10].

Patellar fracture is not an exclusive complication of resurfaced patella and can be sustained in non-resurfaced cases but in rates as low as 0.05%. They are usually related to rheumatoid arthritis or advanced degenerative osteoarthritis [11]. Only in cases of a thin patella or sclerotic bone we advise not to resurface the patella.

Another important fact in this patellar reconstruction is the direction of the osteotomy. Changes in resection angle influence patellar tracking and favour lateral tilt that could require a subsequent lateral release. The goal is to get a flat bone cut with a symmetrical resection. This step could be done freehand, but we employ the cutting guide provides by the manufacturer to improve our results. Once the cut has been done, medial placement of the polyethylene offers better patellar tracking than if it is placed laterally. It is advisable to assess patellar tracking with the "no-thumb" rule placing the knee through full ROM. If the patella tracks laterally, lateral release should be taken into account trying to preserve superior lateral genicular vessels in order to avoid osteonecrosis, patellar fracture or post-operative pain [8, 10].

The fixation of the implant could be done with single or three pegs system depending on surgeon's preference. Today loosening of the patella is a rare complication. As we have said our knee models have only available "onlay" patellar prosthesis, though some authors recommend "inlay" inserts which make them more confident, but no significative differences are observed between the two models [12]. It is said that "inlay" implants allow increase the interface bone-cement, preserve more bone stock and are easy to use [13], but survivorship and clinical and radiological results are similar to the "onlay" designs [14]. In our series we have employed all-polyethylene patella without important complications and good functional outcomes.

Patellar instability, which may happen after TKA with or without patellar resurfacing, is a major cause of functional restraint that requires revision surgery. The incidence of symptomatic instability leading to revision is around 0.8%, lower than instability of the extensor mechanism in our series, but we want to remark that most of our cases were classified as subluxations (8 cases out of 15), not frank dislocations so revision rate was similar. Conservative methods as quadriceps exercises, braces or avoiding activities that aggravate instability were applied in subluxations and with time scarring of the retinacular tissues lead to resolutions of the symptoms. However in cases of frank dislocation revision surgery was mandatory. In these cases careful analysis of prosthesis sources of instability were cautious checked to avoid failed surgery. If problem was related to soft tissues, realignment of the extensor mechanism should be considered (lateral release plus proximal or distal realignment) [15].

We must remember that other issues as design and placement of the implants may predispose to extensor mechanism complications. Design of the femoral sulcus generated years ago high incidence of patellofemoral complications and led to debate if patella should be resurface and how to do this replacement [16]. Modern knee prostheses have got more anatomic designs, but even now there is no consensus about the size, shape and position of the femoral trochlea in relation to femorotibial compartment [17]. Furthermore it is important to restore sulcus position (0.7 mm lateral to the midline of the distal femoral cut) during surgery as best as possible [18].

As well as properties of the femoral and patellar designs, surgical details of the technique are also valuables. Restoration of the mechanical axis is of great importance in knee surgery, as it is selecting the appropriate size of the femur to avoid overstuffing of the anterior compartment [19] and placing the femoral implant lateralized. Femorotibial alignment influences patellar tracking in native knees as does after knee replacement. Navigation systems that allow surgeons to be more precise in coronal and sagittal planes alignment avoid problems in patellofemoral joints [10].

In our opinion getting the proper rotation for the femoral and tibial components is the main goal to avoid complications of the extensor mechanism [19, 20]. There are four ways for determining the rotational alignment of the femur, however we have only used in this series the trans-epicondylar axis and 3° of external rotation based on the posterior condyles. Rotational alignment of the tibia is as important as femoral placement, so neutral or external rotation of the tibial component in relation to the tibia decreases the Q angle and helps patellar tracking [20, 21]. Usually more attention is paid to rotational position of the femoral component than to the tibial baseplate and the goal to get proper coverage and good cortical support for the tibial implant could led to a wrong rotational tibial alignment. External rotation of the tibial component moves the tibial tubercle internally so less patellofemoral complications are detected in this situation [22]. Precise rotational tibial alignment can be obtained from a line perpendicular to the epicondylar axis of the femur [22].

Significance of implant position is crucial in order to avoid extensor mechanism problems, so navigation or personal guides system should offer some advantages at the time of prostheses placement. However many authors believe that proper accuracy can be obtain with traditional guides. X-ray allow to evaluate alignment of the components in the coronal and sagittal plane as well as patellar tracking in the axial view, but rotational position of the implants can't be assess by simple radiographies. In these cases we must employ CT to get a more precise image of the situation of the components that can justify extensor mechanism complications.

It is important to remark the importance of being careful with this resurfacing step as we are with the other ones. It's surprising as some surgeons are extremely cautious with bone cuts, implant alignment and gaps balancing, but not so watchful with patellar resurfacing. After patella evertion they made a non-controlled cut and leave the PE component on it, without taking into account cut direction, bone width or thickness and medialization of the PE implant.

Preoperative patellar tracking can be a measurement of great value in order to analyze patellar position after TKA. Lateral displacement of 3 mm is predictive of patellar maltracking when the knee is placed in full ROM after surgery. This is an evidence of the issue that patellar tracking is related to soft-tissue tension [23]. Lateral shift of the patella implies a contracture of the lateral tissues and this event can be detected in standard preoperative radiographic images. This can be help to identify patients at a higher likehood of experiencing maltracking after TKA [23]. Of course a valgus knee deformity is related to problems with patellar tracking, but a more careful analysis of the preoperative X-ray may help us in patellar replacement decision.

Resurfacing the patella by all-polyethylene implant can be questioned as this surgical gesture obviously affects patellar tracking, but on the other hand non-resurfacing the patella suppose a different pattern of contact at the patellofemoral joint. To assess intraoperatively patellar tracking a surgical navigation system with the aid of a computer have been designed but until now it is not routinely used. However, the system could be a valuable support to analyze one of the main reasons of failure in TKAs [5].

Until recent days it couldn't have been established a correlation between anterior knee pain and weight [24]. However there is some evidence of a relationship between knee pain and patella tilt. [25]. So "inlay" implants have been criticized for leaving a portion of the lateral facet uncovered by the implant that could be considered a source of pain as it articulates with the femoral component. This liaison may be linked to increase anterior knee pain or worse Knee Society Score. Though we have checked few problems with "onlay" insert in our series, some authors prefer the inset technique of patella resurfacing which for them is simple and safe [1]. We have no experience with the inset patella design proposed by Freeman in 1989 and improved over the years. It looks as this design would have less patellar tracking problems, would need less lateral releases and show less signs of instability in the axial X-rays. On the other hand the technique is more demanding and sacrifices more bone, but allow us to be more precise in restoring patellar thickness [1].

Many extensor mechanism complications can be evaluated through simple X-ray (patellofemoral instability, patellar fracture, loosening of the patellar insert, complete patellar o quadricipital tendon rupture...). US images and IRM help us in diagnosis of partial ruptures of the extensor mechanism, synovial effusions... and TC is of great aid in analyzing rotational position of the components. But what can we do in front of a painful total knee arthroplasty without positive results in conventional diagnostic techniques. The easiest decision is to resurface the patella in case it wasn't but if it was? Careful analysis of the different diagnostic tools is essential (X-ray, evaluation of patellar tracking, CT imaging to check components rotation...). Recently SPECT/CT imaging looks very helpful in establishing the diagnosis of painful knees after TKA, mainly when we are in front of patellofemoral problems without components malposition or loosening. A significantly higher tracer uptake in the patella is shown with this SPECT/CT technique in patients with painful knee due to patellofemoral problems [26].

Patella resurfacing is related to good clinical results but is also linked to some extensor mechanism complications and a possible need for revision surgery in the future [25]. On the other hand, non-resurfacing could avoid complications of the extensor mechanism but a high rate of anterior knee pain is perceived. This situation drives the surgeon to a predictable reoperation as patients increase their retrieval of pain relief. For this reason we consider the decision to resurface the patella as a subjective question [25]. Current literature on patellar resurfacing after TKA has not shown a clear advantage of patellar resurfacing if we analyzed clinical scores, though for many authors patellar replacement looks a better strategy in order to avoid reoperation and anterior knee pain. As the average reoperation rate for non-resurfaced cases was 7.2% compared to 2.8% for the resurfaced, resurfacing the patella would prevent one revision surgery for every 23 patella resurfaced. Knowing the cost of a revision surgery and taking into account that less than 50% of patients would benefit from a secondary resurfacing, primary replacement of the patella offers economic and clinical advantages [25].

The Swedish Knee Arthroplasty Registry shows statistically significant patient satisfaction in cases of patella resurfacing in 98% of about 27000 knees follow-up at 14 years. The Registry also shows that there is 1.27 risk ratio for unresurfaced patella to be revised. The Australian National Joint Registry reveals the same risk ratio (1.25). We must be careful with these numbers about unresurfaced patella being revised because our first option in front of a patient with anterior knee pain an unresurfaced patella is to resurface it. However, more than 50% of patients are dissatisfied with revision for only patella component [27, 28]. What looks evident from the different meta-analysis is that anterior knee pain is greater after non-resurfacing the patella, as well as patient dissatisfaction and increase revision rate. It looks positive resurfacing the patella at primary surgery based on functional results [27]. Some authors do not agree with this assertion and after an observational study from the Norwegian Arthroplasty Register they conclude that patella resurfacing has no clinical effect on function or anterior knee pain, which is debatable [29]. The Norwegian Register finds a lower risk of revision when the patella is resurfaced after a TKA although differences in rates of revision surgery are not significant. But improvement in new prosthesis designs that have substituted the older ones has been related to an increase in the survivorship of the knee prosthesis in Norway [30].

In a prospective cohort study that compares resurfaced vs. non-resurfaced patella in 65 patients that received bilateral total knee replacement, significant better scores were achieved on the resurfaced side at final follow-up. Anterior knee pain was a complaint in 4 patients on the non-resurfaced side and revision surgery was required in these patients. On the other hand no revision was performed in the resurfaced side. The author concluded that better patellofemoral functional outcomes, less anterior knee pain and lower rates of revision surgery could be obtained after patella resurfacing [31].

Nowadays, it looks as two great groups of surgeons are completely established and divided by a huge lake: the North American resurfacers and the European non-resurfacers, however it is not possible to reach a conclusion about which alternative is better. But we can add another group whose select when to resurface the patella. Which are their criteria? How can they determine which patients would need or not patellar resurfacing? The quality of the cartilage and joint congruence can be parameters that aid in the determination of selective patellar resurfacing [32, 33]. When could we advise not to resurface the patella? Park et al remark that non-resurfaced patella is possible if the patient is a young one, the patella is small and its cartilage is almost normal, the patient has no preoperative anterior pain and bone quality is good [34]. If some surgeon decides not to resurface the patella it looks advisable to remove osteophytes of the patella and carry a marginal electrocauterization. Selective resurfacing of patellar bone with specific criteria and the used a patella-friendly implant can be associated with satisfactory outcomes [34].

Reasons for resurfacing the patella are avoiding anterior knee pain, so reoperation rate can be reduced, improve results in some patients with RA and improve functional outcomes as going up stairs [35].

http://dx.doi.org/10.5772/53382

The great majority of evidences and experiences are in favour of patellar resurfacing, so we also recommend substituting the patella [36]. This surgical detail only add a short time (less than 8 minutes) to the surgery and warrant less complains of anterior knee pain [35].

However patellar resurfacing no longer should be considered a mandatory step in TKAs. We must consider femoral and patellar design before resurfacing patella as several authors have reported nice results with patella non-resurfacing [37]. The importance of the femoral design (patella-friendly component) is of maximum significance as coupling patella design provides better anterior knee pain results and improved knee functions. Routine patellar replacement in TKA cannot be defended when a coupling femoral component is available [37]. However, proper femoral component design is necessary in order to compare patellar resurfacing and non-resurfacing.

As we can see many features influence patellofemoral function after TKAs but surgical technique is one the primary factors affecting patellar alignment [10], so we can conclude that surgical technique and accurate placement of the implants are of crucial importance in patella resurfacing and a careful procedure improves outcomes.

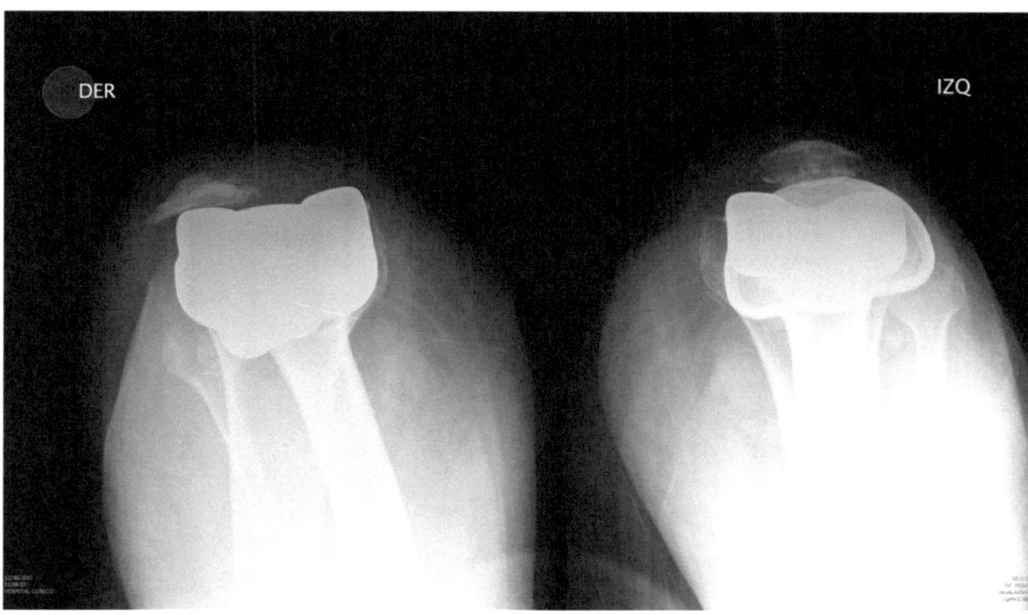

Figure 1. Advanced-age patient suffered subluxation of the extensor mechanism due to a patella infera, after total knee replacement. It was well tolerated; orthopedics measures were employed (a brace and avoiding activities that aggravate instability)

The determination whether to resurface the patella or not is still nowadays controversial [25]. Some trials have concluded there are no advantages in routine patellar resurfacing [38, 39] meanwhile other reports [40] and some meta-analyses [2-4] show less anterior knee pain, better functional outcomes and lower rates of revision after patella resurfacing.

We believe the ultimate result of the patella treatment in total knee replacement is multifactorial and depend on patient factors (illness, previous pain, age, weight, BMI...), surgical technique (features shown before), implant design (trochlear groove, tibial implant, patella size and thickness) and above all a proper placement of the components.

However pain is the main reason why the patients seek for a TKA. They accept undergo this procedure to alleviate pain and to restore as best function as possible. Literature reports better functional results and less pain after patellar resurfacing. It seems not fair to avoid patellar resurfacing for financial criterion or because longer surgical times. If extensor mechanical problems are not as frequent as our series shows and look like these complications could be an acceptable risk, why not to resurface the patella?

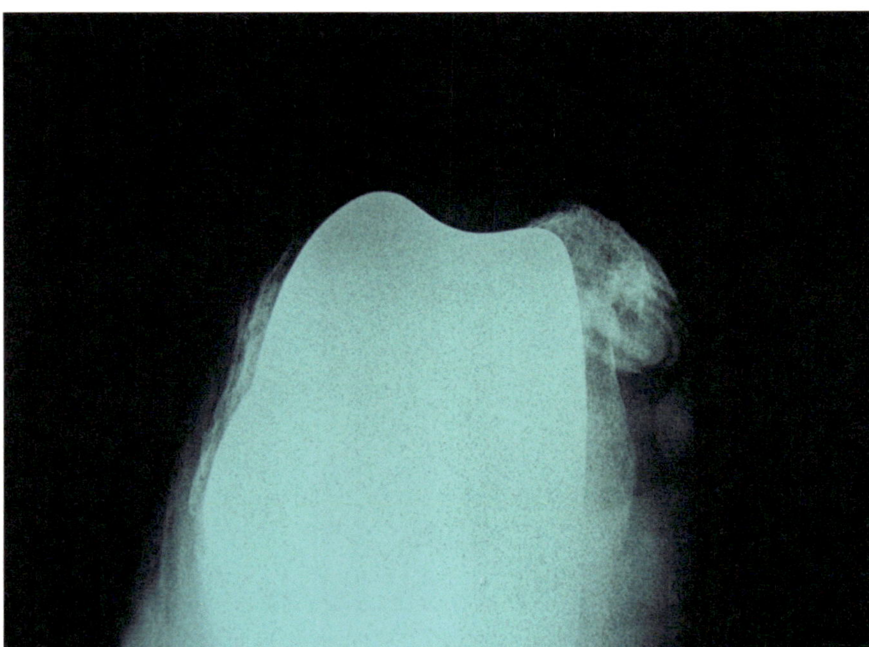

Figure 2. Frank dislocation of the patella who required revision surgery. Internal rotational alignment of the femoral component made us to revise it, getting good functional outcome after surgery.

http://dx.doi.org/10.5772/53382

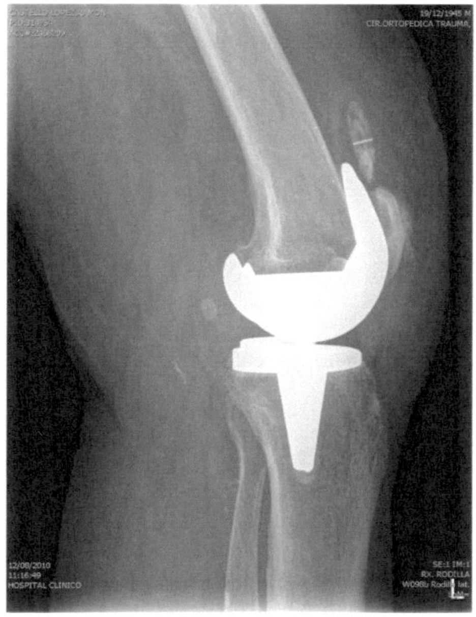

Figure 3. Loosening of the patellar insert that required removing of the polyethylene. As quality of remaining bone wasn't good, no other all-polyethylene implant was placed

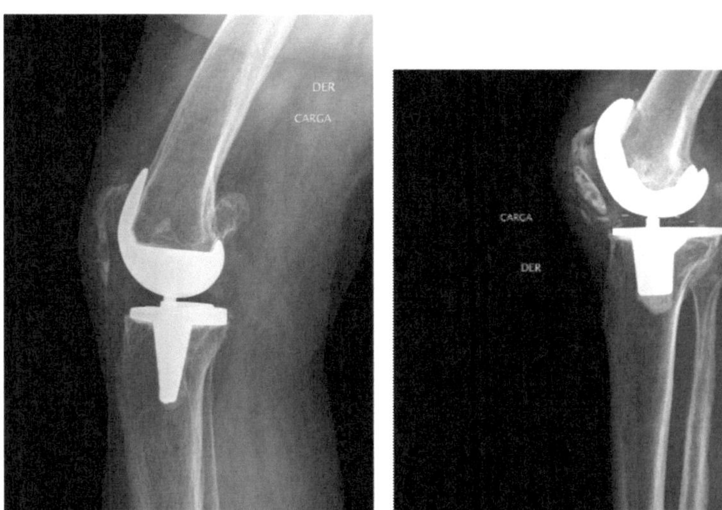

Figure 4. Two examples of fracture of the patella with loosening of the patella. The patients referred a previous trauma in both cases and revision surgery with extensor mechanism reconstruction was done.

Author details

Antonio Silvestre[1,2], Raúl Lopez[1], Fernando Almeida[1], Pablo Renovell[1], Francisco Argüelles[1] and Oscar Vaamonde[1]

1 Clinic Hospital of Valencia, Spain

2 Orthopedic Department, School of Medicine, University of Valencia, Spain

References

[1] Hurson C, Kashir A, Flavin R, Kelly I. Routine patellar resurfacing using an inset patellar technique. International Orthopaedics, 2010; 34: 955-58

[2] Parvizi J, Rapuri VR, Saleh KJ, Kuskowski MA, Sharkey PF, Mont MA. Failure to resurface the patella during total knee arthroplasty may result in more knee pain and secondary surgery. Clin Orthop, 2005; 438:191–96

[3] Pakos EE, Ntzani EE, Trikalinos TA. Patellar resurfacing in total knee arthroplasty. A meta-analysis. J Bone Joint Surg Am, 2005; 87 (7):1438–45

[4] Nizard R S, Biau D, Porcher R, Ravaud P, Bizot P, Hannouche D, Sedel L. A meta-analysis of patellar replacement in total knee arthroplasty. Clin Orthop 2005; 432: 196-203.

[5] Belvedere C, Catani F, Ensini A, Moctezuma de la Barrera JL, Leardini A. Paellar Trucking Turing total knee arthroplasty: an in Vitro feasibility stydu. Knee Surg Sports Traumatol Arthrosc 2007; 15: 985-93

[6] Walligora AC. Johanson NA, Hirsch BE. Clinical Anatomy of the quadriceps femoris and extensor apparatus of the knee. Clin Orthop. 2009 (467: 3297-306

[7] Amis AA. Current concepts on anatomy and biomechanics of patellar stability. Sports Med Arthrosc. 2007; 15:48–56

[8] Levai JP. Technical aspects: The patellar side. Knee Surg Sports Traumatol Arthrosc. 2011; 9 (suppl 1): S19-S20

[9] Youm YS, Cho WS, Woo JH, Kim BK. The effect of patellar thickness changes on patellar tilt in total knee arthroplasty. Knee Surg Sports Traumatol Arthrosc. 2010; 18: 923-7

[10] Fukagawa S, Matsuda S, Mizu-uchi H, Miura H, Okazaki K, Iwamoto Y. Cjanges in patellar alignment alter total knee arthroplasty. Knee Surg Sports Traumtol Arthrosc. 2011; 19: 99-104

[11] Seijas R, Orduña JM, Castro MC, Granados N, baliarda J, Alcantara E. Journal of Orthopeadic Surgery 2009; 17(2): 251-4

[12] Freeman MA, Samuelson K-M, Elias S-G, Mariorenzi LJ, Gokcay EI, Tuke M. The patellofemoral joint in total knee prostheses. Design considerations. J Arthroplasty, 1989; 4 [Suppl]:69–74

[13] Rosentein AD, Postak PD, Greenwald AS. Fixation strength comparision of onlay and inset patellar implants. Knee. 2007; 14 (3): 194-7

[14] Erak S, Rajgopal V, Mac Donald SJ, McCalden RW, Burne RB. Ten-year results o fan inset biconvex patella prosthesis in primary knee artrhoplasty. Clin Orthop, 2009; 467: 1781-92

[15] Motsis EK, Paschos N, Pakos EE, Georgoulis AD. Review article: Patellar instability alter total knee arthroplasty. Journal of Orthopaedic Surgesry. 2009; 17 (3):351-7

[16] Kulkarni SK, Freeman MAR, Poal-Manresa JC, Asencio JI, Rodriguez JJ. The patellofemoral Joint in total knee arthroplasty: is the designo f the trochlea the critical factor?. Knee Surg Sports Traumatol Arthrosc. 2001; 9 (Supp 1): S8-S12

[17] Iranpour F, Merican AM, Dandachii W, Amis AA, Cobb JP. The geometry of the trochlear groove. Clin Orthop. 2010; 468: 782-788

[18] Lingaraj K, Bartlett J. The femoral sulcus in total knee artrhoplasty. Knee Surg Sports Traumatol Arthrosc. 2009; 17: 499-502

[19] Gosh KM, Merican AM, Iranpour F, Deehan DJ, Amis AA. The effect of overstuffing the patellofemoral Joint on the extensor retinaculum of the knee. Knee Surg Sports Traumtol Arthrosc, 2009; 17: 1211-16

[20] Anglin C, Brimacombe JM, Hodgson AJ, Masri BA, Greidanus NV, Tonetti J, Wilson DR. Determinants of patellar tracking in total knee arthroplasty. Clin Biomech (Bristol, Avon). 2008; 23:900–910

[21] Luring C, Perlick L, Bathis H, Tingart M, Grifka J The effect of femoral component rotation on patellar tracking in total knee arthroplasty. Orthopedics, 2007; 30:965–967

[22] Rossi R, Bruzzone M, Bonasia DE, Marmottu A, Castoldi F. Evaluation of tibial rotacional alignment in total knee arthroplasty: a cadáver study. Knee Surg Sports Traumatol Arthrosc, 2010; 18: 889-93

[23] Chia SL, Merican AM, Devadasan B, Strachan RK, Amis AA. Radiographic features predicitive of patellar maltracking during total knee arthroplasty. Knee Surg Sports Traumtol Arthrosc 2009; 17: 1217-24

[24] Wood DJ, Smith AJ, Collopy D, White B, Brankov B, Bulsara MK. Patellar resurfacing in total knee arthroplasty: a prospective randomized trial. J Bone Jt Surg Am. 2002; 21 (2): 129-37

[25] Helmy N, Anglin C, Greidanus N, Masri B. To resurface or not resurface the patella in total knee arthroplasty. Clin Orthop, 2008; 466: 2775-83

[26] Hirschmann MT, Konala P, Iranour F, Kerner A, Rasch H, Friederich NF. Clinical value of SPECT/CT for evaluation of patients with painful knees after total knee ar-

throplasty – a new dimension of diagnostics? BMC Musculoskeletal disorders, 2011; 12: 36-46

[27] Clements WJ, Miller S, Whitehouse SL, Graves SE, Ryan P, Crawford RW. Early outcomes of patella resurfacing in total knee arthroplasty. A report from the Australian Orthopaedic Association National Joint Replacement Registry. Acta Orthopaedica 2010; 81 (1): 108-13

[28] Parvizi J, Mortazavi SM, Devulapalli C, Hozack WJ, Sharkey PF, Tithman RH. Secondary resurfacing of the patella after primary total knee arthroplasty does the anterior pain resolve? J Arthroplasty 2012; 27 (1): 21-6

[29] Lygre SHL, Espehaug B, Havelin LI, Vollset SE, Furnes O. Does patella resurfacing really matter? Pain and function in 972 patients alter primary total knee arthroplasty. An observational study from the Norwegian Arthroplasty Register. Acta Orttho-paedica 2010; 81(1): 99-107

[30] Lygre SHL, Espehaug B, Havelin LI, Vollset SE, Furnes O. Failure of total knee arthroplasty with or withpout patella resurfacing. A study from the Norwegian Arthroplasty Register with 0-15 of follow-up. Acta Orthopaedica 2011; 82 (2): 282-92

[31] Patel K, Raut V. Patella in total knee arthroplasty: to resurface or not to – a cohorte study of staged bilateral total knee arthroplasty. International Orthopaedics, 2011; 35: 349-53

[32] Atik OS. Is Soutine patellar resurfacing in total knee arthroplasty necessary?. Eklem Hastalikian ve Cerrahisi, 2010; 21: 61

[33] Sanchez-Marquez JM, Rodriguez-Merchan EC. Implantación del componente rotuliano en la artroplastia total de rodilla: situación actual. Rev esp cir ortop traumatol 2010; 54 (3): 186-92

[34] Se-Jin P, Young-Bok J, Hwa –Jae J, Hun-Kyu S, Ho-Joong J, Jong.Jum L, Ji-Woong Y, Kim E. Long-term results of primary total knee arthroplasty with and without patellar resurfacing. Acta Med Okayama 2010; 64 (5): 331-38

[35] Ghasemzadeh F, Mateescu C. Resurfacing patella in 140 TKA patients. Letter to the editor. IRCMJ, 2010; 12 (1): 76-8

[36] Li S, Chen Y, Su W, Zhao J, He S, Luo X. Systematic review of patellar resurfacing in total knee artrhoplasty. International Orthopaedics, 2011; 35: 305-16

[37] Whitesides LA. Patella resurfacing no longer considered routine in TKA. Orhtopaedics 2006; 29 (9): 833-5

[38] Campbell DG, Duncan WW, Ashworth M, Mintz A, Stirling J, Wakefield L, Stevenson TM. Patellar resurfacing in total knee replacement: a ten-year randomized prospective trial. J Bone Jt Surg Br. 2006; 88 /6): 734-9

[39] Maculé F, castillo F, Llopis-Miró R, Nogales J, Budeus Gonzalez-Solis JM, Lozano LM, Segur JM, Suso S. Sustitución patelar en artroplastia total de rodilla. Estudio prospectivo multicéntrico: resultados preliminares. Avances Traum, 2008; 38 (1): 30-4

[40] Waters TS, Bentley G. Patellar resurfacing in total knee arthroplasty. A prospective randomized study. J Bone Jt Surg Am. 2003 85 (2); 212-7

Chapter 21

Glenoid Loosening in Total Shoulder Arthroplasty

Nahum Rosenberg, Maruan Haddad and
Doron Norman

Additional information is available at the end of the chapter

http://dx.doi.org/10.5772/53438

1. Introduction

Inflammatory or degenerative processes in glenohumeral joint lead to pain and restriction of movements of the shoulder. Prosthetic replacement of the glenohumeral joint has gained in popularity because of its efficacy in relieving pain. The pioneering successful prostheses for total shoulder arthroplasty (TSA) have been based on an unconstrained design, i.e. a metal spherical head component fixed to a metal intramedullary stem articulating with a high-density polyethylene socket. These components are stabilized in the adjacent bone using polymethylmethacrylate (PMMA) bone cement [1]. The most important cause for failure of the cemented prostheses is related to the glenoid component, with a 0.01-6% rate of loosening [2, 3, 4].

The long term survivorship data of the prosthesis developed by C. Neer for the cemented total shoulder arthroplasty (TSA) show 87% fifteen year survivorship rate for Neer I & II cemented shoulder prostheses [5]. This implant has become the gold standard, against which all the successive prosthetic designs are compared.

Further developments of TSA implants have been aimed at enhancing longevity by addressing the following most critical issues: (1) Improving the incorporation of the glenoid component using a more "biological" type of fixation in order to reduce the rate of mechanical loosening; (2) Designing a better glenoid component to achieve the lowest possible rate of wear. But still the main cause of TSA failure has remained the aseptic loosening of the glenoid component [6].

2. Aseptic loosening

Aseptic loosening of endoprostheses occurs as a result of immune rejection response to an implanted foreign material. This response is enhanced when particles of polyethylene (from the glenoid insert), metal (from the glenoid metal backplate and/or from humeral component) or from fixating PMMA are released due to a mechanically abnormal gliding of the prosthesis. These particles, below 10μ in size, usually in 0.5-1.0μ range [7], induce local and systemic recruitment of macrophages and osteoclasts [8], with subsequential generation of reactive pseudomembrane and local lysis of the prosthesis-bone interface [9] (Figure 1). The lysis of the fixation interface of the prosthesis causes its eventual loosening. Since in the TSA prosthesis the glenoid component is exposed to the higher stresses and usually constructed, at least partly, from polyethylene, it's loaded surface is prone to wear and its surrounding is exposed to the wear particles' seeding. For this reason the immune rejection response is concentrated mainly around the glenoid component.

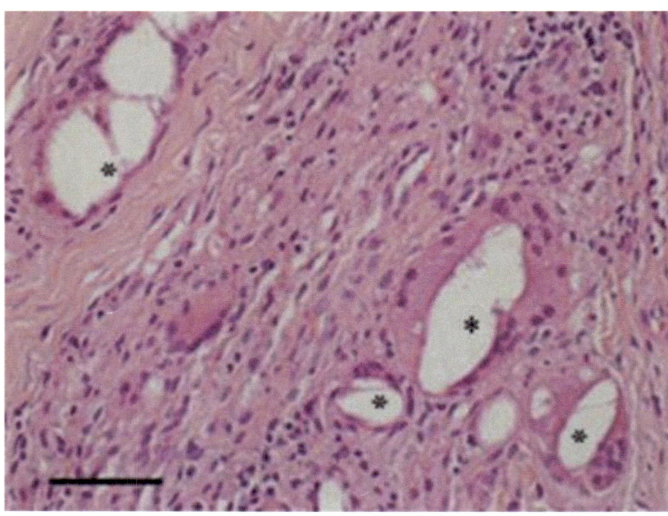

Figure 1. Micrograph (scale 200μ, HE staining) of pseodocapsule retrieved from the surface of a failed prosthesis. Characteristic foreign body reaction [10] is evident around areas of debris (*).

3. Mechanical considerations

The main cause of the wear of the glenoid component is its high loading by the eccentric forces. The excessive eccentric forces are generated when the transverse axis of the implanted glenoid is situated in a position which is incompatible with normal anatomical version of glenoid, e. g. between 2^0 of anteversion and 13^0 of retroversion [11]. This might happen when the prosthesis is implanted in an arthritic joint with advanced erosion of the posterior glenoid. Therefore care should be taken to reshape the glenoid towards an anteverted surface, in the physiological range, prior to implantation of the glenoid component [12].

In the longitudinal axis the excessive eccentric forces are generated when the superior stabilization of the humeral head is insufficient, therefore in patients with massive tears of the rotator cuff muscles an implantation of the glenoid component is contraindicated.

The full conformity between the TSA prosthesis components may also lead to an enhanced stress on the globoid rim due to the loss of the humeral head translation, which is possible in the normal shoulder joint, and as a consequence there is a higher risk for prosthetic loosening. [13,14]. The exact degree of optimal mismatch of the glenoid and the humeral head radii is not known. Furthermore the suboptimal mismatch of the glenoid and humeral component curvature can lead to a considerable rate of polyethylene wear due to an uneven force distribution between the components and a point loading and a point wear of the polyethylene [14].

4. Material considerations

There are several unique issues in TSA that should be addressed in the prosthesis design. First is a limited space and a limited bone stock for the glenoid component implantation. Two main difficulties arise due to this limitation:

1. The fixation area of the glenoid component is limited, either for cemented or cementless fixation. In order to increase fixation interface the glenoid components bear keels (central or in offset position), pegs (straight or tapered) and/or curved backsurface of the insert. It is not clear what type of fixation design is optimal for the cemented fixation [11]. There is some clinical evidence that a central tapered peg on a metal back-plate, covered by hydroxyapatite for enhanced ossiointegration, and initially fixed by two screws, might reduce loosening rate of glenoid component in cementless press fit fixation [15] (Figure 2).

2. The polyethylene gliding surface is essential in most designs of the glenoid component. The polyethylene surface should be at least 3 mm thick, preferably 4-6 mm thick, in order to diminish its wear following interaction with metal head of the humeral component [16]. This requirement prevents the versatile use of the cementless designs of a glenoid component, because they require the use of a metal back-plate under the polyethylene insert, with essential limitation of the later thickness in order to prevent the joint overstuffing. For this reason there is a high preference for use of all polyethylene made glenoid components for cemented implantation. This type of design allows the use of more thick polyethylene component, with lower wear rate. But the cemented fixation of this type of glenoid component might produce thermal mediated, adjacent to the implant, bone necrosis while PMMA polymerization and therefore eventually an enhanced loosening. Currently there is no clear information which of the fixation methods of the glenoid component is clinically advantageous.

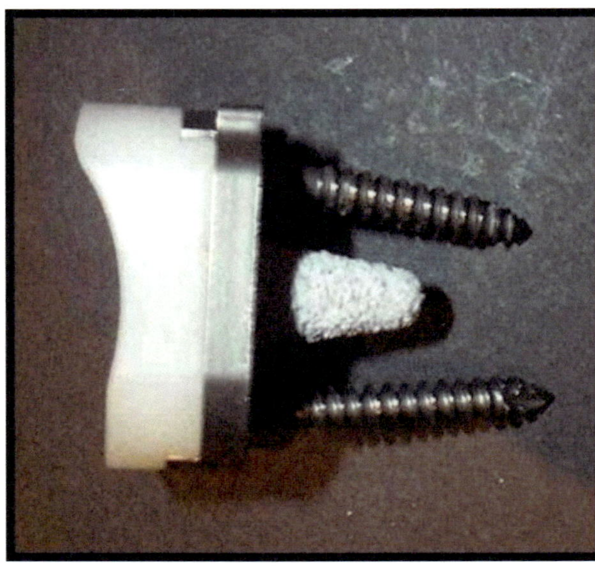

Figure 2. An example of glenoid component for cementless implantation: a polyethylene insert mounted on a metal back-plate with tapered peg covered by hydroxyapatite. The initial press fit fixation is enhanced by two screws. This design showed improved survivorship rates.

5. Clinical signs of the glenoid component loosening

The clinical signs of the TSA prosthesis failure include an increased level of pain during follow-up, that appeared to be related to the implant, with restriction of external rotation to under 20° and abduction to under 60° and/or newly developed radiolucency at the glenoid component interface with the underlying bone, more than 2mm in width [17]. The recognition of coexistence of both physical and radiographic signs is essential, since the isolated finding of periprosthetic radiolucency, without pain or significant restriction of movements of the shoulder, might not be of a high clinical importance (Figure 3). This consideration

http://dx.doi.org/10.5772/53438

should be undertaken carefully in order to avoid unnecessary revision surgery. In all the cases of suspected TSA prosthesis loosening a standard workup for possible periprosthetic infection should be done in order to avoid a devastating misdiagnosis [18] (the discussion of this topic is out of the scope of the present chapter).

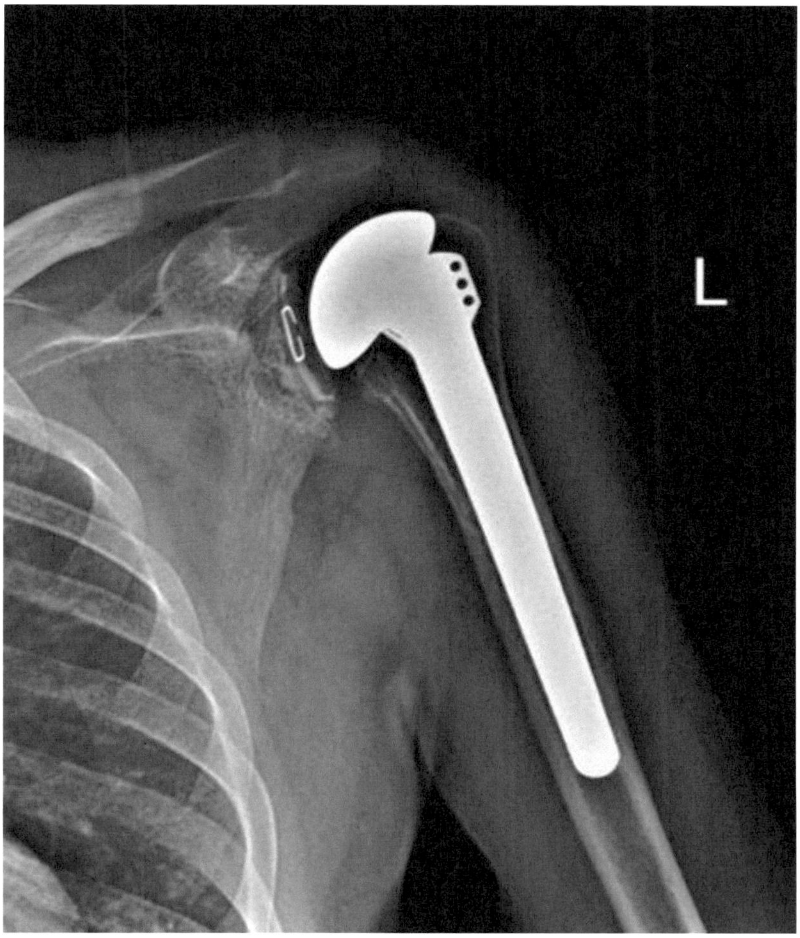

Figure 3. A shoulder radiograph (anterior-posterior view) of 60 years old male patient, three years after cemented TSA. Lucency is evident in the direct proximity to the glenoid component, but the patient is pain free and has good range of movements of the operated shoulder, without any laboratory evidence of infection and is satisfied from the function of the operated shoulder.

6. Survivorship data of TSA prostheses with special emphasis on glenoid loosening

In order to get a meaningful evaluation of the implanted prostheses longevity a powerful statistical tool of survivorship analysis is used [19]. Because the relative complicity in this method implementation, especially in defining the criteria for the "failure" of the implanted prostheses, only few reports on survivorship data of TSA exist, mainly with the parameter of a revision surgery as the indication of the failed prosthesis.

From the few reported survivorship data a short-term glenoid failure, requiring implant removal, reaches the rate of around 6% for cemented designs and 3% for cementless designs. Overall the glenoid component failure is the cause of between 20% - 60% of all failed TSAs, cemented or cementless (Table 1). Survivorship of TSA is the highest in patients with rheumatoid arthritis and the lowest in patients implanted following trauma and fracture. The reason is probably a lower demand for shoulder activity in the former group and expectations for nearly normal function in the latter group of patients [20, 21, 22, 23].

Reference	Type of prosthesis	No. of Patients	Survivorship	End point criteria	Glenoid failure rate	Overall failure rate
Tarchia et al [21]	Neer I & II cemented	113 [31=OA, 36=RA 12=2ary OA]	10years= 93% 15years= 87%	Revision – severe pain, abd<90°, ext rot<20°	7/113	14/113
Brenner et al [23]	Neer II & Gristina cemented	51 [37=OA 14=RA]	11years= 75%	Severe pain, radiographic evidence of component loosening	3/51	6/51
Cofield [22]	Cofield cementless	180 [110=OA 28=RA 30=2ary OA 12=revisions]	Not calculated	Revision	5/180	12/180
Pfahler et al [20]	Aequalis cemented	705 [418=OA 107=RA 180=2ary OA]	Not calculated	Revision	9/705	43/705

OA = osteoarthritis, RA = rheumatoid arthritis

Table 1. Long term survivorship data on cemented and the outcome of a large series of a cementless total shoulder replacement prostheses.

7. Treatment of loose glenoid

Surgical revision of failed glenoid should address several crucial factors. One of the main factors for consideration is the preservation of an adequate bone stock following the component removal. This is essential if replantation is considered, otherwise the component resection will be the definite procedure. Interestingly several authors reported that a resection of the failed glenoid component without subsequential replantation of a new component might cause a considerably favorable clinical outcome [24].

The second crucial factor is the preservation of adequate version of the remained glenoid in order to avoid future eccentric loads on the replanted glenoid component.

These two factors can be achieved by bone grafting, autologous or by allograft, with additional controlled reaming of the remained glenoid surface. The surgeon's arsenal of glenoid components for replantation includes parts for either cemented or cementless fixation, and biological soft tissue allografts for biological resurfacing. Several reports support the use of soft tissue allograft material, e.g. Achilles tendon, meniscus etc., for glenoid resurfacing in revision surgery [25]. Finally the replantation of the glenoid component might be immediate, during the revision surgery, or late, following initial bone grafting of cavitations and/ or bone deficiencies in the treated glenoid. Since this type of surgery has no standard guidelines because of the different patterns of the bone loss of the treated glenoids, a precise surgical protocol does not exist for this purpose and a lot of the decision making depends on the surgeon's experience and methodical preferences.

In order to avoid an extensive tissue damage during the glenoid revision surgery an arthroscopic approach has been suggested and reported in a small number of published reports. This method was popularized by O'Driscoll SW et al [26]. The authors used an arthroscopic approach through the standard anterior and posterior portals, with addition of another extended portal for the glenoid component remnants' retrieval. This method is suitable only for all-polyethylene components, because they should be cut in situ to at least 3 parts (by diagonal cuts using an inserted through the portal osteotom) in order to retrieve pieces in sizes which are compatible with the retrieval portal diameter. This method allows also a subsequential bone grafting of the exposed glenoid undersurface by using metal impactors which are inserted through the created portals [27]. This is a technically demanding technique, especially due to the optical interference, e.g. "mirror effect", that is caused by the metal humeral component head and due to the difficulty to control bleeding from the exposed glenoid surface. But because of the appealing tissue preservation this method might gain more widespread use in the future.

8. Prospective on the future improvement of the glenoid component design

Two main issues should be considered when seeking the improvement of the TSA survivorship. First of all the currently used TSA methods have already reached a high, above 90%, middle and long term survivorship rate, leaving a small, but important margin for improvement [21]. Secondary it is clear that this margin for improvement is related to the glenoid component design, since most of the failed TSAs are due to glenoid component failure. There is an example supporting this claim, when following a change of the design of the glenoid component a 10% increase in a short term survivorship of cementless TSA prosthesis has been achieved [15].

Clearly the main changes in the glenoid component design should address the rate of wear of this component and the efficiency of the component fixation. Therefore it is logical that the prospective for improvement of these issues will be related to finding the articulating surfaces generating less wear particles, even when subjected to excessive eccentric loading. Probably improving the biological osseous integration into the glenoid component will solve the complications of the current fixation either by the PMME or by the mechanical press fit fixation techniques. Some indications of the efficiency of biological fixation of the glenoid component have been already revealed in the devices coated by osteoconductive material, such as hydroxyapatite.

Author details

Nahum Rosenberg[1*], Maruan Haddad[2] and Doron Norman[2]

*Address all correspondence to: nahumrosenberg@Hotmail.Com

1 Rambam – Health Care Campus, Laboratory of Musculoskeletal Research, Department of Orthopaedic Surgery, Haifa, Israel

2 Rambam – Health Care Campus, Department of Orthopaedic Surgery. Haifa, Israel

References

[1] Neer CS: Replacement Arthroplasty for Glenohumeral Arthritis. J Bone Joint Surg Am 1974; 56-A113

[2] Brems J: The Glenoid Component in Total Shoulder Arthroplasty. J Shoulder Elbow Surg 1993; 2 47-54

[3] Crites BM, Berend ME, Ritter MA. Technical Considerations of Cemented Acetabular Components: a 30-year Evaluation. Clin Orthop 2000; 382 114-119

[4] Pfahler M, Jena F, Neyton L, Sirveaux F, Mole D, Cedex N: Hemiarthroplasty Versus Total Shoulder Prosthesis: Results of Cemented Glenoid Components. J Shoulder Elbow Surg 2006; 15 154-163.

[5] Tarchia ME, Cofield RH, Settergren CR . Total Shoulder Arthroplasty with the Neer Prosthesis: Long-Term Results. J Shoulder Elbow Surg 1997, 6:495-505.

[6] Hasan SS, Leith JM, Campbell B, Kapil R, Smith KL, Matsen FA. Characteristics of Unsatisfactory Shoulder Arthroplasties. J Shoulder Elbow Surg 2002; 11 431-41.

[7] Hallab NJ, Jacobs JJ. Biologic Effects of Implant Debris. Bul NYU Hosp Joint Dis 2009;67(2) 182-188

[8] Ren PG, Irani A, Huang Z, Ma T, Biswal S, Goodman SB. Continuous Infusion of UNMWPE Particles Induces Increased Bone Macrophages and Osteolysis. Clin Orthop Relat Res 2011; 469 113-122

[9] Purdue PE, Koulouvaris P, Nestor BJ, Sculco TP. The Central Role of Wear Debris In Periprosthetic Osteolysis. HSSJ 2006; 2 102-113

[10] Pandey R, Drakoulakis E, Athanasou NA. An Assessment of The Histological Criteria Used to Diagnose Infection in Hip Revision Artroplasty Tissue. J Clin Pathol 1999; 52 118-123

[11] Strauss EJ, Roche C, Flurin PH, Wright T, Zuckerman JD. The Glenoid In Shoulder Arthroplasty. J Shoulder Elbow Surg 2009; 18 819-833

[12] Farron A, Terrier A, Buchler P. Risks Of Loosening of a Prosthetic Glenoid Implanted In Retroversion. J Shoulder Elbow Surg 2006; 15 521-526

[13] Harryman DT, Sidles JA, Harris SL, Lippitt SB, Matsen FA. The Effect of Articular Conformity and the Size of the Humeral Head Component on Laxity and Motion after Glenohumeral Arthroplasty. J Bone Joint Surg Am 1995; 77-A 555-563

[14] Walch G, Edwards TB, Boulahia A, Boileau P, Mole D, Adeleine P. The Influence of Glenohumeral Prosthetic Mismatch on Glenoid Radiolucent Lines. Results of a multicenter study. J Bone Joint Surg Am 2002; 84-A 2186-2191.

[15] Rosenberg N, Neumann L Modi A, Mersich IJ, Wallace AW. Improvements In Survival of the Uncemented Nottingham Total Shoulder Prosthesis: A Prospective Comparative Study. BMC Musculoskeletal Disorders 2007; 8 76 - 87

[16] Brems J: The Glenoid Component In Total Shoulder Arthroplasty. J Shoulder Elbow Surg 1993; 2 47-54.

[17] Wallace AL, Walsh WR, Sonnabend DH: Dissociation of The Glenoid Component In Cementless Total Shoulder Arthroplasty. J Shoulder Elbow Surg 1999; 8 81-84

[18] Zimmerli W., Trampuz A., Ochsner PE. Prosthetic-joint Infections. N Engl J Med 2004; 351(16) 1645-1654

[19] Rosenberg N, Soudry M. Survivorship Analysis of Orthopaedc Procedures – Practical Approach. Arthroscopy 2011; 27(suppl 4) 16-24

[20] Pfahler M, Jena F, Neyton L, Sirveaux F, Mole D, Cedex N. Hemiarthroplasty Versus Total Shoulder Prosthesis: Results of Cemented Glenoid Components. J Shoulder Elbow Surg 2006; 15 154-163

[21] Tarchia ME, Cofield RH, Settergren CR . Total Shoulder Arthroplasty with the Neer Prosthesis: Long-Term Results. J Shoulder Elbow Surg 1997; 6 495-505

[22] Cofield RH: Uncemented Total Shoulder Arthroplasty. Clin Orthop 1994; 307 86-93

[23] Brenner BC, Ferlic DC, Clayton ML, Dennis DA. Survivorship of Unconstrained Total Shoulder Arthroplasty. J Bone Joint Surg Am 1989; 71-A 1289-1296

[24] Raphael BS, Dines JS, Warren RF , Figgie M, Craig EV. Symptomatic Glenoid Loosening Complicating Total Shoulder Arthroplasty. HSSJ 2010; 6 52 -56

[25] Namdari S, Gel DP, Wrner JJ. Managing Glenoid Bone Loss In Revision Total Shoulder Arthroplasty: A Review. UPOJ 2010; 20 44-49

[26] O'Driscoll SW, Petrie RS, Torchia ME. Arthroscopic Removal of the Glenoid Component for Failed Total Shoulder Arthroplasty. A Report of Five Cases. J Bone Joint Surg Am 2005; 87-A 858-863

[27] Namdari S, Glaser D. Arthroscopically Assisted Conversion of Total Shoulder Arthroplasty to Hemiarthroplasty with Glenoid Bone Grafting. Orthopedics 2011;34(11) 862-865

Section 6

Periprosthetic Infection

Chapter 22

Peri-Prosthetic Joint Infection: Prevention, Diagnosis and Management

Adrian J. Cassar Gheiti and Kevin J. Mulhall

Additional information is available at the end of the chapter

http://dx.doi.org/10.5772/53247

1. Introduction

Total Joint Arthroplasty (TJA) is a safe and effective procedure that improves the quality of life and restores function in most patients suffering from joint arthritis. Post-operative peri-prosthetic joint infections (PJI) are an uncommon and difficult complication of joint replacement surgery.

PJI affects 1-3% total joint replacements and is the most common indication for revision in total knee arthroplasty (TKA) and third most common indication for revision total hip arthroplasty (THA)[1-4]. PJI can be difficult to diagnose and can present at any time from the primary procedure[5, 6]. PJI is painful, disabling, costly and often requires multiple procedures[7], prolonged periods of rehabilitation, antibiotic treatment and poor functional outcome. It places a considerable burden on hospital and surgeon resources with an estimated annual cost of infected revisions in US hospitals increasing from $320 million in 2001 to $566 million in 2009, with a projected cost exceeding $1.62 billion by 2020[8]. Consistent efforts at prevention are mandatory, and treatment of infection requires appropriate assessment of its chronicity and causative factors, the status of the wound and the overall health of the patient.

We will first provide an overview on peri-prosthetic joint infection and the possible risk factors involved. Finally, we will provide an overview of the current evidence available in preventing, diagnosis and managing peri-prosthetic joint infection.

2. Pathophysiology

Peri-prosthetic joint infections are a result of an intricate interaction between the host, the pathogen and the implant[9-11]. There is a multitude of host factors, ranging from medical comorbidities to social economic status, which increase the risk of PJI[9, 10, 12-15].

2.1. Host and environmental factors

Predisposing factors for PJI can be sub classified into preoperative, intraoperative and post-operative factors (Table 1). Preoperative predisposing factors include medical conditions such as diabetes, inflammatory arthropathies, preoperative anemia, congestive heart disease and chronic pulmonary disease to mention few[9, 10, 12, 14]. Intraoperative predisposing factors include simultaneous bilateral joint arthroplasty, longer operative time, knee arthroplasty, increased operating room traffic and contamination by the surgical team during preparation and draping[12, 16-19].

Post-operative predisposing factors to PJI include immunosuppressive medications, allogenic blood transfusion, post-operative atrial fibrillation, myocardial infarction, urinary tract infection and longer hospital stay[9, 10, 12].

Peri-prosthetic joint infections are typically caused by microorganisms that grow in biofilms[36]. Within biofilms, microorganisms in a polymetric matrix and develop into organized complex communities resembling a multicellular organism[37]. In a biofilm, microbes are protected from antimicrobial agents and host immune responses. This may be related to the reduced growth rate of biofilm microorganisms, which enter a stationary phase of growth[38]. Different microbes have different interactions with the host and the prosthetic. Some have specific adhesion molecules which help them adhere to the implant until a biofilm is formed, which is mediated in part by intracellular adhesion molecules[39]. Initially, adherent microorganisms and early biofilms are relatively unstable and still susceptible to host defense and antimicrobial agents. In contrast, mature biofilms are more stable and resist to elimination[40]. Furthermore, implants are devoid of microcirculation, which is crucial for the immune system and antibiotics to interact with microbes. Implants also tend to activate neutrophils which release peptides that deactivate granulocytes, impairing the removal of microbes[41]. This effect on granulocytes reduces the minimal amount of microbes that are required to cause an infection[41]. Inoculation of implants, not only occurs during the time of surgery, but can occur in the presence of a bacteremia from any source in the human body during the entire lifetime of the implant[42].

2.2. Microbial profile in PJI

A multitude of organisms mostly bacteria and fungi are reported to cause PJI (Table.2). The most reported organisms responsible for PJI are Gram positive *cocci*, most commonly *Staphylococcus Aureus* and *Staphylococcus Epidermidis* as reported by various authors[12, 20, 22, 31, 43-45]. On certain occasions, Gram negative bacteria and Fungi can also be responsible for periprosthetic joint infections[46, 47]. In a recent study published by Buller et al., Methicillin Resistant *Staph. Aureus* (MRSA) and Methicillin Resistant *Staph. Epidermidis* (MRSE) account for about 15.5% of all PJIs[20] and according to other studies up to 19% of PJIs can be poly microbial[12, 22, 48]. These microorganisms can all be part of normal skin flora; hence, direct inoculation at the time of the operation as well as airborne contamination are the most likely causes of these infections.

Predisposing Factors	**Studies**
Preoperative	
Male sex	Buller et al.[20], Jämsen et al.[21]
Socioeconomic status	Pulido et al.[12], Berbari et al.[22]
ASA > 2	Pulido et al.[12], Buller et al.[20], Bozic et al.[9], Saleh et al.[23],
Diabetes and elevated blood sugars	Buller et al.[20], Bozic et al.[9], Jämsen et al.[24], Berbari et al[22]., Saleh et al.[23]
Inflammatory Arthropathy	Pulido et al.[12], Bozic et al.[9], Wilson et al.[10], Jämsen et al.[21] , Berbari et al.[22]
Immunosuppressant medication	Wilson et al.[10], Berbari et al.[22], Saleh et al.[23]
Preoperative Anaemia	Pulido et al.[12], Greenky et al.[14], Bozic et al.[9]
Poor Nutrition	Berbari et al.[22]
Higher BMI	Pulido et al.[12], Bozic et al.[9]
Other infected Joint Arthroplasty	Buller et al.[20], Jafari et al.[15], Berbari et al.[22]
History of malignancy/metastasis	Bozic et al.[9], Berbari et al.[22]
Skin ulcers/PVD	Bozic et al.[9], Wilson et al.[10], Berbari et al.[22], Poss et al.[25]
Intraoperative	
Knee arthroplasty	Pulido et al.[12], Buller et al.[20]
Simultaneous bilateral	Pulido et al.[12]
Longer operative time	Pulido et al.[12], Muilwijk et al.[26], Ong et al.[27], Berbari et al.[22], Saleh et al.[23]
No prophylactic antibiotic	Fogelberg et al.[28], Pavel et al.[29], Meehan et al.[30], Al-Maiyah et al.[31]
Cement with no antibiotics	Hanssen AD.[32], Jämsen et al.[21]
Skin Preparation and Draping	Johnson et al.[33], Katthagen et al.[16]
Contamination by operating room personnel	Ayers et al.[34], Rao et al.[35]
Operating Room Traffic	Panahi et al.[18]
Postoperative	
Renal impairment	Pulido et al.[12], Saleh et al.[23], Bozic et al.[9]
Allogenic blood transfusion	Pulido et al.[12], Berbari et al.[22], Saleh et al.[23]
Myocardial Infarction	Pulido et al.[12]
Atrial fibrillation	Pulido et al.[12], Berbari et al.[22]
Urinary tract infection	Pulido et al.[12], Wilson et al.[10], Poss et al.[25]
Haematoma	Pulido et al.[12], Jämsen et al.[21], Berbari et al.[22], Saleh et al.[23]
Continuous wound discharge	Pulido et al.[12], Jämsen et al.[21], Berbari et al.[22]
Prolonged Hospital stay	Pulido et al,[12]. Berbari et al.[22]

Table 1. Predisposing factors to PJI

Organism	**Study (number of cases)**							
	Buller et al [342]	Mahmud et al [250]	Romano et al [71]	Pulido et al [63]	Berbari et al [462]	Phillips et al [75]	Al-Maiyah et al [106]	Salvati et al [2330]
Staphylococcus								
MRSA	13.5%	3.2%	31%	19%	22%	4%	6.6%	27.3%
MSSA	19.6%	16%	21.1%	19%		25%		
MRSE	2%	21.2%	22.5%	11%	19%	36%	68.9%	27.8%
MSSE	19.9%							
α-Hemolytic Streptococcus	3.8%	2.8%	5.6%	12.7%	9%	7%		0.7%
β-Hemolytic Streptococcus	6.1%							7.2%
γ-Hemolytic Streptococcus	4.1%							5.6%
Enterococcus	2.9%		5.6%	1.6%	1.2%	9%		4.5%
VRE	0.6%							
Streptococcus milleri	0.6%							
Peptostreptococcus	2.4%		2.8%				12.3%	
Gram-positive rods								
Corynebacterium	0.3%		1.4%	1.6%	0.6%			3.2%
Enterobacter	4.1%	1.6%						1%
Propionibacterium	2.9%	0.8%	2.8%			1%		1.7%
Gram negative								
Escherichia coli	3.2%	1.2%		3.2%		4%	0.9%	5.5%
Haemophilus	0.3%							
Citrobacter koseri	0.3%							0.1%
Klebsiella	1.2%			3.2%		3%		1.3%
Proteus mirabilis	2.0%			1.6%				3.1%
Pseudomonas	3.2%	0.8%	5.6%	1.6%		4%	1.9%	5.6%
Salmonella	0.9%					1%		0.3%
Serratia marcescens	0.3%	1.2%	1.4%	1.6%				0.3%
Bacteroides fragilis	0.3%	0.4%						0.5%
Yeasts								
Candida	0.3%				0.2%			0.3%
Diphteroids						1%	9.4%	0.9%
Polymicrobial		0.02%		6.3%	19%			
Culture negative	8.8%	27.2%		9.5%	12%			
No Results		22.4%						

MRSA: Methicillin Resistant *Staph. aureus*, MSSA: Methicillin Sensitive *Staph. aureus,* MRSE: Methicillin Resistant *Staph. epidermis.* MSSE: Methicillin Sensitive *Staph. epidermis.*

Table 2. Percentage of microbes in PJI [12, 20, 22, 31, 43-45, 48]

While, the patient's endogenous flora is largely held accountable for surgical site infections, the surgical team personnel and operating room environment may also contribute to disperse organisms[49] and increase the bacterial count[18, 50]. Members of the surgical team who have direct contact with sterile field have been linked to outbreaks of unusual organism such as *Serratia Marcescens*[51]. Even though anesthesiologists, are not directly involved in the operative field, they perform a variety of procedures related to the operation and have been associated with outbreaks of bloodstream and surgical site infections linked to the re-use of propofol vials and other deviations from acceptable protocols[52].

2.3. Classification of PJI

The classification of PJI is based on, either the type of pathogenesis or the time of clinical manifestation. When PJI are classified according to the pathogenesis, inoculation of the surgical site occurs either exogenously or haematogenously[11]. Exogenous infection, are infections that occur during surgery or in the early post-operative period, usually in the presence of large hematomas. Haematogenous infections are acquired through the bloodstream at any time after surgery. As discussed in section 2.1, it has been reported that implants impair the immune defenses and decrease the minimal abscess-forming dose of *Staph. aureus* at least 10 000 fold both in an animal and human model[53, 54]. Patients with prosthetic joints have a reported risk of 30 - 40% for haematogenous device–associated infection during *Staph. aureus* sepsis[13, 42]. Even though patients, are mostly susceptible to PJI early after implantation, haematogenous infection can occur at any time after surgery.

More commonly, PJI is classified according to the time of clinical manifestation after total joint replacement. This classification is divided into 4 stages or groups[11, 55, 56]:

- Stage I or Early post-operative infection, which present acutely within the first 4 to 8 weeks after the operation
- Stage II or Delayed onset PJI and occurs between the 3rd month up to 24 months after surgery
- Stage III or Late onset PJI usually occur after 2 years from the procedure, the presentation is usually sudden in an otherwise well-functioning joint.
- Stage IV or Silent infection when a positive culture is found at time of revision without any previous evidence of infection.

Early (Stage I), delayed (Stage II) and silent (Stage IV) infections are commonly exogenous, while stage I infections are probably caused by virulent microorganisms such as *Staph. aureus* and *Escherichia coli*, Stage II and Stage IV are typically caused by low virulent bacteria such as coagulase negative staphylococci and *Propionbacterium acnes[56, 57]*. Stage III or Late onset PJI occur acutely in a well-functioning joint and are caused by haematogenous spread. The most common primary focus of infection is from skin and soft tissue infections, but seeding from urinary, respiratory, gastrointestinal tract and dental infections are also reported[58]. In a recent report by Sendi et al., 57.5% of cases with haematogenous PJI had no source identified either because of primary bacteremia, or because the primary infection has already healed by the time signs and symptoms of PJI present[13].

2.4. Definition of PJI

The Musculoskeletal Infection Society (MSIS) have recently analyzed the available evidenced and proposed a set of criteria to define peri-prosthetic joint infection.

Based on these criteria[59], a definite PJI exists when:

i. there is a sinus tract communicating with the prosthesis; or

ii. a pathogen is isolated by culture from 2 or more separate tissue or fluid samples obtained from the affected prosthetic joint; or

iii. when 4 of the following 6 criteria exist;

- **a.** elevated serum erythrocyte sedimentation rate and serum C-reactive protein (CRP) concentration,
- **b.** elevated synovial white blood cell count,
- **c.** elevated synovial polymorphonuclear percentage(PMN%),
- **d.** presence of purulence in the affected joint
- **e.** isolation of a microorganism in one culture of periprosthetic tissue or fluid, or
- **f.** greater than 5 neutrophils per high-power field in 5 high-power fields observed from histologic analysis of periprosthetic tissue at ×400magnification.

PJI may be present if less than 4 of these criteria re not met and that in certain infections with low virulent organisms such as *Propionibacetium acnes,* several of these criteria may not be routinely met despite the presence of PJI.

3. Prevention of PJI

Both the host and environmental factors described previously (Table. 1) can affect the risk for developing PJI. An effective strategy in preventing PJI is to improve both host and environmental factors during the pre, intra and post-operative period (Table. 3).

There are a number of host factors that increase the risk of PJI including conditions such as diabetes, inflammatory arthropathy, preoperative anaemia, poor nutrition and obesity to mention a few(Table. 1). Patients who present for elective orthopaedics procedures are in suboptimal health. Furthermore, the impact of various risk factors appears to be accumulative, such that each factor has an individual affect to increase the risk of infection and has a synergistic potential on the risk conferred by other factors[60, 61]. Thus, identifying such risk factors and addressing them in the preoperative setting is critical in reducing PJI and other postoperative complication.

http://dx.doi.org/10.5772/53247

Time			Strategy
Preoperative	Early	Host optimization	Improve Diabetic control
			Treat possible site of infections
			Improve possible Medical Comorbidities
			Obesity + Improve Nutritional Status
			Pre – operative anaemia
			Smoke Cessation
			MRSA screening
	Day of Surgery	Surgical Site Optimization	Surgical Site Shaving
			Skin decolonisation (CHG wipes/showers)
Intraoperative	Surgical factors		Prophylactic antibiotics
			Skin Preparation
			Draping
			Bleeding Control
			Antibiotic impregnated cement
			Skin Closure
			Wound Dressing
	Surgical team		Decolonization: Surgical scrubbing/rubbing
			Impermeable Gowns/PPS
			Double Gloving
	OR environment		Operating Room Traffic
			Laminar Airflow
Post-operative	Immediate		Antibiotics for 24 hours
			Wound management
			Blood Transfusion only where indicated
			Management of medical complications
	Late		Antibiotic prophylaxis before invasive procedures

CHG: Chlorhexadine Gluconate, OR: Operating Room, PPS: Personal Protection System, MRSA: Methicillin Resistant Staph. aureus Adopted from Matar et al. Preventing infection in total joint arthroplasty. J Bone Joint Surg Am. 2010;92 Suppl 2:36-46. Epub 2010/12/09.

Table 3. Preoperative, Intraoperative and Post-operative Strategies in preventing PJI

3.1. Pre-operative period

3.1.1. Health optimization

Pre-operative optimization of health is of crucial importance to ensure a satisfactory outcome following total joint arthroplasty. ASA scores >2, diabetes and rheumatoid arthritis among several factors have been associated with increased rates of perioperative complications and PJI after total joint arthroplasty[9, 12, 20, 21, 24]. Lei et al. and Malinzak et al. have both reported that diabetes and the total number of comorbidities were associated with a higher risk of infection and that medical conditions have a synergistic effect on the risk of developing a PJI[60, 62].

Prior to total joint arthroplasty, all patients should be assessed and managed in a multidisciplinary pre-assessment clinic to optimize their general health. These have been shown to significantly reduce both the post-operative mortality and costs per admission in orthopaedic surgery[63]. Pre Assessment Clinics (PAC), focus on optimizing the host health in the preoperative period such as improving nutritional status, optimizing diabetic control, cardiac and respiratory comorbidities and screening for possible source of infection and MRSA decolonization. In our institution, all patients are assessed in the pre assessment clinic by a consultant anesthesiologist, specialist nurse, nutritionist and physiotherapist, and if necessary further consultation with other medical specialists such as cardiologist, rheumatologist or neurologists is available to optimize the patients' health preoperatively. The anesthetic consultant also follows the patient during hospitalization and during the post-operative period whenever possible.

3.1.2. Bacterial decolonization

The Centre for Disease Control (CDC) guidelines for prevention of surgical site infection (SSIs) has strongly recommended that patients require to shower or bathe with an antiseptic agent on at least the night before the operative day in order to reduce bacterial load[64]. While whole body bathing with antiseptic has been shown to reduce bacterial load of the skin as well as reducing the risk of infections[35, 65-67], it presents challenges in achieving entire body coverage and in maintaining sufficiently high concentrations of solution on the skin for effective antisepsis[68]. Further more patient compliance with these protocols is an issue[69]. Recent studies have addressed the effectiveness of preoperative protocols with chlorhexidine gluconate (CHG) applied twice daily by patients at home before their joint replacement[33, 70] and one study reported reduction in SSI infection from 3.19% to 1.59% after the introduction of 2% CHG in place of povidone iodine antiseptic[71]. Based on the results of these studies, home skin preparation seems to be a simple and cost effective technique in reducing PJI but patient compliance is an issue and further randomized control trials are required to fully understand the effect on preventing PJI.

http://dx.doi.org/10.5772/53247

3.1.3. Prophylactic antibiotics

The benefits of prophylactic antibiotics have been widely reported in orthopaedic literature [28-30, 72]. In 1970, Foldberg et al. compared a group treated prophylactically with penicillin given preoperatively, intraoperatively and up to 5 days post operatively, with a control group not treated with antibiotics; both groups underwent a mixture of mold arthroplasties and spinal fusions[28]. The prevalence of infections was 1.7% in the treated group while 8.9% in the control group[28]. Furthermore during the period of the study these authors have noticed an increase in the prevalence of MRSA in all major orthopaedic wound infections, which demonstrates a delicate balance between the use and overuse of antibiotics in the prevention and treatment of infections.

The most common organisms responsible for PJI have been already discussed in section 2.2, and prophylactic antibiotics are targeted to cover this spectrum of organisms. Cefazolin and cefuroxamine are the antibiotics of choice because of their good tissue penetration and excellent activity against Staphylococci and Streptococci. The American Association of Orthopaedic Surgeons (AAOS) published guidelines regarding prophylactic choice, dosing and optimal postoperative duration[61]. The AAOS recommendations for the use of intravenous antibiotic prophylaxis are as follows:

- **Recommendation 1:** The antibiotic used for prophylaxis should be selected carefully, consistent with current recommendations in the literature, taking into account the issue of resistance and *patient allergies*. Currently, cefazolin and cefuroxamine are the preferred antibiotics for patients undergoing orthopaedic procedures. Clindamycin and vancomycin may be used in patients with known β-lactam allergy. Vancomycin may be used in patients with known colonization with MRSA or in facilities with recent MRSA outbreaks. In multiple studies, exposure to vancomycin is reported as a risk in the development of vancomycin resistant enterococcus (VRE) colonization and infection. Vancomycin should be reserved fir the treatment of serious infection with β-lactam resistant organisms or for treatment of infection in patients with life threatening allergy to β-lactam antimicrobials.

- **Recommendation 2:** Timing and dosage of antibiotics administration should optimize the *efficiency of the therapy*. Prophylactic antibiotics should be administered within 1 hour before skin incision. Owing to an extended infusion time, vancomycin should be started within 2 hours before incision. If a proximal tourniquet is used, the antibiotic must be completely infused before the inflation of the tourniquet. Dose amount should be proportional to the patients' weight; for patients who weigh more than 80Kg, Cefazolin dose should be doubled. Additional intraoperative doses of antibiotics are advised is [1] the duration of the procedure exceeds one to two tines the antibiotic's half-life or [2] there is significant blood loss during the procedure. The general guidelines for frequency of intraoperative antibiotic administration are as follows: cefazolin every 2-5 hours, cefuroxamine every 2-4 hours, clindamycin every 2-6 hours and vancomycin every 6-12 hours.

- **Recommendation 3:** Duration of prophylactic antibiotic administration should not exceed *the 24 hour postoperative period*. Prophylactic antibiotics should be discontinued within 24 hours of the end of surgery. The medical literature does not support the continuation of antibiotics until all drains or catheters are removed and provides no evidence of benefit when they are continued past the 24 hours.

3.2. Intra-operative period

3.2.1. Pre-operative hair removal

Pre-operative hair removal is of common practice, and a meta-analysis by the Cochrane group showed that the relative risk of surgical site infection following hair removal with a razor was significantly higher than that following hair removal with clippers, but there was no difference reported in the rate of post-operative infections between procedures preceded by hair removal and those performed without hair removal[73]. It is recommended that whenever hair is removed clippers rather than a razor should be used at the time of surgery[73].

3.2.2. Pre-operative skin preparation

3.2.2.1. Patients

Three main types of skin antiseptic agents are used; mainly chlorohexidine gluconate (CHG), alcohol based solutions and povidone-iodine. Chlorohexidine is favored due to its long lasting and cumulative activity against gram-positive and gram negative organisms found on human flora. Povidone iodine it is also effective in reducing skin flora but in becomes ineffective on contact with blood and duration of activity is shorter the CHG. Alcohol is an excellent antimicrobial but its effectiveness is limited by the lack of any residual activity after drying and the risk of flammability. A Cochrane meta-analysis carried out in 2004 showed no difference in efficiency among skin antiseptics used in clean surgery[74]. Recent studies strongly suggest that CHG combined with alcohol is superior to povidone-iodine combined with alcohol in antisepsis for patients[75-77]. Ostrander et al. reported reduced bacterial count on feet prepared with Chloraprep (2% CHG and 70% isopropyl alcohol; Medi-Flex, Overland Park, Kansas) than on those prepared with Duraprep (0.7% iodin and 74% isopropyl alcohol; 3M Healthcare, St. Paul, Minnesota) or Techni-Care[3.0% chloroxylenol; Care-Tech Laboratories, St. Louis, Missouri) but there was no difference in infection rates among the 3 groups[77].

3.2.2.2. Surgeon

Antiseptic agents for surgeons can be classified into hand scrubs agents and hand rub agents. Hand scrubs are typically solutions of CHG or povidone-iodine while hand rubs are typically alcohol based solutions. Most data indicates that povidone–iodine and CHG have equal efficacy in decreasing bacterial colony forming units from the skin of surgeons; furthermore no difference was found between hand rubs and hand scrub solutions[78, 79]. Some studies report better cost effectiveness of alcoholic hand rub by saving on water consumption and better physician compliance [78].

3.2.3. Draping

There is strong evidence in the literature for the use of plastic surgical adhesive tapes and nonpermeable paper drapes for surgical site draping [16, 80-83]. Nonpermeable drapes are used to prevent bacterial penetration during surgery, which was found to increase when traditional cloth drapes got wet[80]. Iobhan iodophor-impregnated drapes (3M Health Care) have been shown a reduction in wound contamination without any decrease in wound infection rate after total joint arthroplasty[84]. In their review of 4 000 patients in seven different trials, the Cochrane Wounds Group, found no evidence that adhesive drapes (plain or impregnated with antimicrobials) reduce surgical site infection rates[85].

3.2.4. Double gloving

Sterile surgical gloves aim to protect the patient from contamination from residual bacteria from members of the surgical team after hand scrubbing and protect the surgical team from the patient's body fluids[86]. Double gloving has been recommended because it has been shown that it reduces perforations in the innermost glove especially in orthopaedic procedures where sharp surfaces are easily formed[86-88]. Beldame et al. have reported that, 80% of glove perforations occur during surgical incision and changing the outer glove after surgical incision and before implantation of the prosthesis can reduce the risk of contamination and perforation and resulted in a sterile state in 80% of cases[89].

3.2.5. Laminar flow, operating room traffic and personal protection system

Operating theatres are designed to reduce bacterial exposure to patients during surgery. Vertical laminar airflow (LAF) provides directional airflow through a higher efficiency particulate air (HEPA) filters and positive air pressure within the surgical field. Multiple studies have reported reduced PJI rates with LAF[17, 90-92]. Brandt et al. reported no benefit from using LAF, and it was even associated with increased risk of surgical site infection after total hip arthroplasty. A recent systematic review on SSI following hip and knee arthroplasty included 8 studies over the past 10 years and showed no improvement on PJI rates and recommends against the installation of LAF systems in new operating theatres[93].

The opening of the operating room door disrupts the laminar airflow, allowing pathogens to enter the space surrounding the site of the operation with increased risk of PJI[17, 94, 95]. Panahi et al. have reported a mean rate of 0.69 door opening per minute for primary and 0.84 openings per minute for revision total joint arthroplasty. Only 8% of the traffic was determined to be due to scrubbing in and out, demonstrating a high rate of unjustifiable traffic, the authors further advise to implement strategies in reducing operating room traffic in an attempt to decrease one etiology of PJI[18].

The human exhaust system or personal protection system (PPS) was initially introduced by Sir J Charnley in the 1960s and designed to decrease airborne bacteria and intraoperative contamination in total joint arthroplasty[96]. No uniform opinion exists with regard to the use of PPS and the incidence of PJI[97-101]. One of the main issues with PPS is that, they are bulky and tend to get contaminated. In a recent study, Kearns et al. have reported that 53 out of 102 PPS tested were contaminated with staphylococcus and one with MRSA, which means that the PPS does not remain externally sterile in half of the cases[19]. These authors recommend refraining from touching the PPS during surgery and the need to change gloves if hand contact with the PPS occurs[19].

3.2.6. Operative time

Long operative times have been found to increase the risk for PJI after total joint arthroplasty[27, 102, 103]. From a cohort of 9245 patients undergoing total joint arthroplasty, Pulido et al reported longer operative time as a predisposing factor for PJI, a finding which is also supported Kurtz et al. and Peersman et al[104, 105]. Furthermore, surgeons volume seems to be inversely proportional to the rate of infection, were the higher the surgeon volume the lower the rate of infection, but this was only found to be statistically significant after total knee arthroplasty[26].

3.2.7. Addition of antibiotics to cement

In recent years antibiotic impregnated cement has become a standard for use in cemented primary arthroplasty. According to recent studies, the rate of PJI was lower when a combination of intravenous antibiotic prophylaxis and antibiotic impregnated cement was used for primary cemented arthroplasty[21, 106]. Antibiotic impregnated cement seems to be of particular use in the revision setting[107-109]. Nevertheless there is strong evidence to support the efficiency of combined regime of prophylactic antibiotic and cement impregnated antibiotic when compared to prophylactic antibiotic only in patients with other risk factors for PJI[32, 110, 111].

3.2.8. Wound closure and surgical dressing

Various methods of skin closure are used in arthroplasty surgery, ranging from skin staples, subcuticular closure with absorbable suture and recently the use of knotless barbed sutures. A recent meta-analysis by Smith et al. reported that closure with skin staples had a significant risk of wound infection when compared to traditional suturing, but out of the six studies reviewed only one study had acceptable methodology[112]. Newman et al has reviewed 181 patients after total knee arthroplasty and reported significant fewer complications after closure with skin staples when compared with absorbable subcuticular sutures[113]. A prospective randomized control trial comparing staples to subcuticular absorbable suture and tissue adhesives after TKA, showed highest superficial infection rate for subcuticular suture (26%) and the lowest for skin staples (5%), although none of them required any treatment with antibiotics[114]. Furthermore, staple based wound closure was fastest and the least expensive after TKA but had the longest hospital stay when compared to the other methods[114]. Recently there has been increased interest in knotless barbed sutures for wound closure after total joint arthroplasty[115-117]. Most studies reported faster closure times for the barbed sutures when compared to traditional methods[116, 117]. Patell et al. have reported a significant increase risk of major wound complications especially after TKA, when barbed sutures (4.3%) were used compared to staples 1.1% and standard absorbable subcuticular closure (4.2%)[115]. However, debate still exists on which is the optimal method of closure.

Surgical technique with careful tissue handling and wound closure is important in wound healing, as well as the type of dressing that is applied postoperatively[118, 119]. Wound dressing assist with healing by acting as a physical barrier to bacteria, splinting the wound to protect it from subsequent injury, helping with haemostasis, reducing dead space and minimizing pain. The use of occlusive dressings is well known to improve re-epithelisation and subsequent collagen synthesis when compared to wound exposed to air[120, 121]. In a recent Cochrane review, Dumville et al. reported no evidence to suggest that one dressing is better than any other in preventing surgical site infection and advised that the choice of dressing should be based on costs and the need for management of specific symptoms[122]. After total joint arthroplasty, a hydrofiber/hydrocolloid dressing using the jubilee method has been shown to reduce the rate of blister formation but no significant reduction in surgical site infection[118]. Burke et al. have carried out a prospective randomized study comparing the jubilee dressing method with standard adhesive dressing after total joint arthroplasty and reported a significant reduction in blister formation, leakage and dressing changes in the group treated with the jubilee method but no significant reduction in SSI. The authors of this study recommend the use of the hydrofiber/hydrocolloid dressing combination after total joint arthroplasty due to the associated lower complication rate[123].

3.3. Post-operative period

Most medical complications in the post-operative period have been to increased rates of PJI, mainly elevated blood creatinine levels, allogenic blood transfusion, myocardial infarction, atrial fibrillation and urinary tract infections[9, 10, 12, 21, 22, 25]. Adequate hydration is critical in post-operative period and allogenic blood transfusion is indicated in the presence of symptomatic anaemia, a haemoglobin level <8g/dL, or when it is medically indicated[124]. Control and monitoring of blood sugar levels is important in diabetic patients and should follow the same principles used in the preoperative period. Persistent wound drainage has been has been found as a contributing factor in the development of PJI[12, 21, 22], however there is little or no supportive evidence for the continues use of antibiotics[61] or antimicrobial impregnated dressings[122]. Furthermore, post-operative complication can result in delayed rehabilitation after a total joint arthroplasty with resultant delay in discharge from hospital, which has been reported by various studies as a risk factor for the development of PJI[12, 22].

4. Diagnosing PJI

Currently there is no diagnostic modality, which is 100% reliable in diagnosis PJI. An assessment using a combination of clinical findings and investigations is necessary.

4.1. Clinical

A careful history and physical examination are crucial in making a diagnosis of PJI. Although the diagnosis of early postoperative or acute haematogenous infection is not difficult, late infections can be challenging to distinguish from other causes of pain in a patient with previous total joint arthroplasty. Clinically, early or acute infections are characterized by pain, fever, wound drainage or erythema. While the only feature of chronic infection, can be pain unrelieved by a seemingly well-functioning arthroplasty. Loosening during the first year post implantation or a consistently painful arthroplasty should be considered infected until proven otherwise.

4.2. Diagnostic investigations

4.2.1. Serology

Erythrocyte Sedimentation Rate (ESR) and C-Reactive Protein (CRP) are baseline screening tests for any patient planned for revision arthroplasty regardless of the cause of failure[5]. Diagnostic value of ESR and CRP has been widely reported, and their combined use is a very good 'rule out' test [125, 126]. When both ESR and CRP are negative, periprosthetic infection is unlikely, however when both tests are positive PJI must be considered, and this warrants further investigations [5]. Ghanem et al. have reported that values higher than an ESR of 30 mm/h and CRP 10 mg/l combined to gather had 97.6% sensitivity for a positive diagnosis of PJI[127].

A full blood count including a white blood cell (WBC) count is part of the routine workout for patients with suspected PJI, however recent evidence suggests that serum WBC and differential carries a very low sensitivity (55% and 52% respectively) and specificity (66% and 75% respectively)[128]. Accordingly, routine serum WBC count and differential have no role in the diagnosis of PJI..

4.2.2. Joint aspiration

Joint aspiration is recommended as part of the work up in diagnosing PJI in patients with combined elevation of ESR and CRP levels in the hip and elevation of ESR and/or CRP levels in the knee joint[5]. Joint aspiration is usually carried out under sterile conditions, and synovial fluid should be for culture and sensitivity, WBC count and neutrophil percentage. Some patients with abnormal ESR and CRP may require more than one aspiration. A WBC count higher than 1700 cell/μl or a neutrophil percentage greater than 65% is highly suggestive of chronic PJI, however these values are not applicable when diagnosis acute PJI[129, 130]

4.2.3. Imaging studies

Imaging studies such as plain radiographs, computed tomography (CT) or magnetic resonance imaging (MRI) scans are useful in sub classifying patient into high and low probability of PJI. Radiolucent lines, focal osteolysis, periosteal bone formation or early loosening may all suggest PJI[131], however differentiating between PJI and aseptic loosening may not be possible using imaging modalities on their own. Nuclear scintigraphy detects inflammation in peri-prosthetic tissue, and although technetium-99m bone scintigraphy has very high sensitivity, it lacks specificity for infection[132]. A technetium bone scan can remain positive more than a year after implantation because of increased periprosthetic bone remodelling.

http://dx.doi.org/10.5772/53247

Love et al. reported increased sensitivity (96%), specificity (87%) and accuracy (91%) when a leukocyte/marrow scintigraphy was used to identify PJI. The test was significantly more accurate than bone (50%), bone/gallium (66%) and leuckocyte/bone (70%) scintigraphy in diagnosing PJI[133]. It seems that a Leukocyte/marrow scintigraphy will remain the procedure of choice in diagnosing PJI until agents capable of differentiating infection from aseptic inflammation are developed[133].

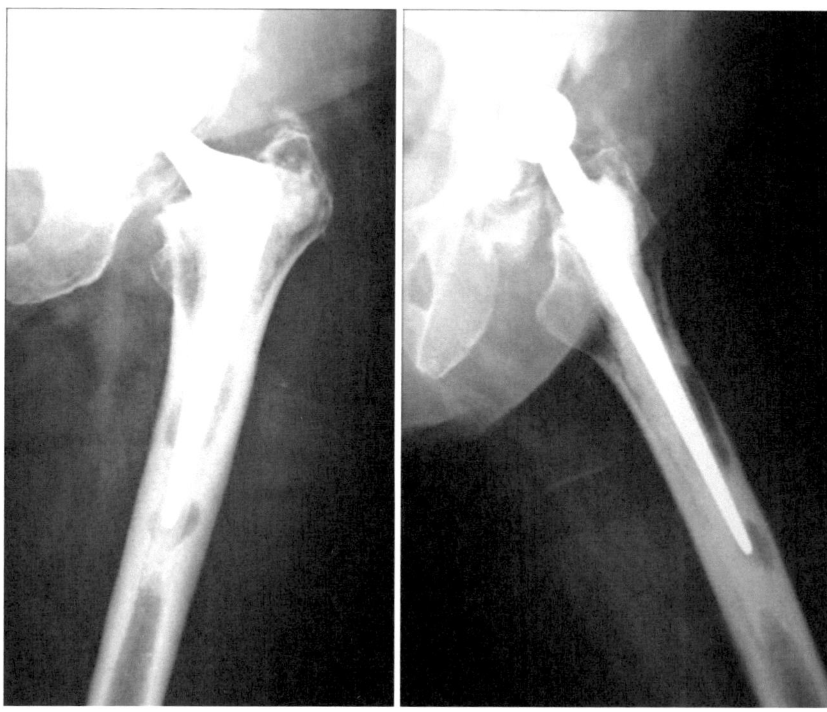

Figure 1. Plain AnteroPosterior and Lateral Radiographs showing focal areas of osteolysis, suspicious of PJI.

4.2.4. *Intraoperative techniques*

Various techniques can be used intraoperatively during revision arthroplasty to diagnose infection. These techniques include synovial fluid biomarkers, cultures and frozen sections.

4.2.4.1. *Cultures and Gram stain*

Cultures of periprosthetic tissues provide the most reliable means of detecting that pathogen and are often used as a reference standard in diagnosing PJI. Multiple samples should be taken at the time of the procedure from various regions, at least 3 samples for culture are recommended[134-136]. Cultures may be negative because prior antibiotic exposure, low number of organisms, an inappropriate culture medium, fastidious organisms or prolonged transport time to the laboratory[11]. Grams stains have high specificity (97%) but extreme low sensitivity (less than 26%)[137, 138]. The AAOS guidelines recommend against the routine use of intraoperative gram stain for the diagnosis of PJI[5].

4.2.4.2. Frozen sections

A meta-analysis by Della Valle et al reported that frozen sections are very good in ruling in but have low value in ruling out and infection[5]. These studies have more than 80% sensitivity and more than 90% specificity, but they also have high interobserver variability. The degree of inflammatory cells infiltrations varies among specimens from the same patient, sometimes even within individual tissue samples[11].

4.2.4.3. Synovial fluid biomarkers

Synovial fluid can used to analyse for various biomarkers such as leukocyte esterase, synovial CRP and white blood cell count, interleukin 6 (IL-6) and interleukin 8 (IL-8). Leukocyte esterase is an enzyme secreted by activated neutrophils that migrate at the site of infections. This enzyme is usually found on colorimetric dipsticks to diagnose urinary tract infections. Potential advantages of this diagnostic tool include wide availability, low cost and potential of an accurate diagnosis within minutes. Parvizi et al. have initially reported preliminary data on using leukocyte esterase as a diagnostic tool. These authors reported 80.6% sensitivity and 100% specificity in diagnosing PJI, with 100% positive predictive value and 93.3% negative predictive value[139]. Wetters et al also reported similar results when they used leukocyte esterase for diagnosis PJI[140]. In both studies, the leukocyte esterase strip was unreadable in on third off cases due to synovial blood or debris. Even though, these results are promising, both of these studies have their limitations in the methodology used, and further on, none of studies identifies whether the leukocyte esterase strip is able to differentiate between inflammation and infection.

Measurement of synovial CRP has been shown to be a sensitive (85%) and specific (95%) marker in diagnosis PJI[141, 142]. Recent studies report IL-6 levels to be more accurate in diagnosis PJI than ESR, CRP level, or synovial fluid WBC count and can be useful in diagnosis of PJI in patients with confounding systemic variables. Jacovides et al. have also reported higher specificity and sensitivity for both IL-6 (100% and 87.1%) and IL-8 (97.7% and 90.3%) when compared to synovial CRP (97.7% and 87.1%)[143]. Based on these studies synovial fluid biomarkers could provide an additional valuable resource for the diagnosis of PJI, but further studies are required.

4.3. AAOS guidelines

The American Academy of Orthopaedic Surgeons (AAOS), based on the current clinical evidence, has proposed clinical guidelines in the diagnosis of peri-prosthetic joint infection[144]. On the bases of the clinical features, the patients are classified into those who have a high or low probability of PJI (Table 4). The guidelines consist of 15 recommendations, with the majority being supported strongly in the literature. The guidelines advocate an algorithmic approach to the diagnosis of PJI, beginning with baseline investigations such the Erythrocyte Sedimentation Rate (ESR) and the C Reactive Protein (CRP) that carry high sensitivity and specificity when combined together[125, 126].

Higher Probability of Infection	One or more symptoms, AND at least one or more:
	• risk factor* OR
	• physical exam finding; OR
	• early implant loosening/osteolysis (as detected by x-ray)
Lower Probability of Infection	Pain or joint stiffness only and none of the following:
	• risk factors;* OR
	• physical exam findings; OR
	• early implant loosening/osteolysis (as detected by x-ray)

*risk factor supported by evidence or expert opinion. Adopted from the AAOS clinical practice guidelines for the diagnosis of periprosthetic infections[144]

Table 4. Stratification of patients into High or low probability of infection[144]

Further investigations, such as joint aspiration, are recommended in a stepwise manner depending on the ESR and CRP levels. The AAOS clinical guidelines and algorithms for the diagnosis peri-prosthetic infections, are available free to download from http://www.aaos.org/research/guidelines/guide.asp.

5. Management of PJI

The management of total joint arthroplasty consists of one or more of the following techniques:

i. Antibiotic therapy

ii. Debridement and Irrigation of the joint with component retention or linear exchange

iii. Single Stage Revision Arthroplasty (SSRA)

iv. Two Stage Revision Arthroplasty (TSRA)

v. Arthrodesis

vi. Amputation

Management decisions are made on severity, chronicity of the infection, virulence of the infecting organism, status of surrounding soft tissue and physiological status of the patient.

5.1. Unexpected positive intraoperative cultures

Unexpected positive intraoperative cultures are found in cases where pre-operative assessment fails to show infection, these cases usually undergo revision for aseptic loosening. Tsukayama eta al. reported up to 11% of cases were infection was diagnosed with positive intraoperative cultures and were all treated with 6 weeks of antibiotics without additional operation. Antibiotic therapy failed in 3 of these cases, and the patients required further surgical treatment with 2 patient showing evidence of recurrent infection at 2 year follow up[56]. In another study, 15 patients with positive intraoperative cultures were not treated with antibiotics, recurrence of infection was reported in 6 patients[145]. Based on these studies, patients with unexpected positive cultures should be treated with antibiotics for 6 weeks while monitoring their ESR and CRP values to assess response to treatment under the supervision of a specialist microbiologist[146].

5.2. Antibiotic suppression

When patients have poor state of health, have a high risk of complications after surgery and the infective organism is of low virulence and susceptible to antibiotic therapy, suppression by antibiotic alone may be the best option. Rao et al. investigated the rates of eradication of antibiotic resistant organisms with suppression therapy and noted eradication in 86% at mean follow up of five years, with five recurrent infections all within the first 3 years[147]. Antibiotic suppression is also indicated in patient with persistent PJI following surgical intervention if they decline or cannot tolerate further surgery[6, 11, 148, 149]. The literature on antibiotic suppressive therapy without any surgical intervention is poor; despite this, patients who cannot tolerate surgery have no other option than suppressive therapy.

5.3. Debridement and Irrigation with component retention or linear exchange

Operative debridement and irrigation with component retention should be reserved of acute infections (Stage II and occasionally stage III). Early infections may range in severity from superficial cellulitis to deep infections. Superficial infections associated with wound dehiscence or purulent drainage and infections with wound necrosis or infected haematomas often require surgical debridement. Reported eradication rate has been between 24% to 71 % following open debridement and irrigation[56, 150, 151]. Even though, some case reports show excellent results from irrigation and debridement[152], a recent multicentre retrospective study showed that irrigation and debridement with component retention is not affected by organism type and that this technique had a failure rate as high as 70%, with the authors questioning the actual role of irrigation and debridement in the treatment of PJI[151]. Prostheses retention is also contraindicated in those with multiple joint arthroplasty or when the duration of symptoms is more than 1 month[7, 15].

5.4. Single stage revision arthroplasty

Single stage revision with removal of components, debridement, irrigation and reimplantation of new components provides removal of infected prosthesis while limiting the number of surgeries, recovery time and costs. Callaghan et al. reports 8.3% rate of recurrence after single stage revision arthroplasty with a minimum follow up of 10 years[153]. The local therapy, is achieved by adding antibiotics to the cement used for fixation of the implant, this is followed by a minimum of 6 weeks antibiotic therapy. Two studies comparing one-stage to two stage revision arthroplasty favoured the two stage technique[154, 155]. Failure rates in SSRA ranged from 10.1% to 12.4%, compared to 3.5% to 5.6% in TSRA. A recent meta-analysis comparing SSRA to TSRA reported the presence of nearly three additional reinfections per 100 revisions when performing a one stage compared to a two stage procedure[156]. However, not enough evidence is available to demonstrate that one technique is superior to the other[156].

5.5. Two stage revision arthroplasty

Two stage revision arthroplasty (TSRA) is currently the gold standard technique for the treatment of infected joint arthroplasty[107, 157-159]. TSRA involves initial removal of the infected components and all foreign material including cement, cement restrictors and cables or wires whenever possible with meticulous debridement and irrigation. All necrotic tissue is excised, and sinus tracts are debrided. After irrigation the joint should be inspected for any remaining debris. A cement spacer loaded with antibiotics is used, this is either pre-manufactured or constructed at the time of surgery[160, 161]. Various techniques described in the construction of a cement loaded spacer, the technique used depends on the joint involved and the level of bone loss encountered during the first stage[109, 161-164]. These custom spacers allow antibiotic elution locally to eradicate the infective organism and maintain soft tissue balance to accommodate the definitive implant during the second stage. A minimum course of six weeks of antibiotics is usually required, and resolution of infection is confirmed through serial ESR and CRP and repeated aspiration of the joint. A further aspiration of the joint before the second stage is recommended in one study, which reported recurrence rate of 3% among those who underwent aspiration compared with 14% in those who did not[165].

The advantages of TSRA[166] include:

i. meticulous debridement of soft tissue, necrotic bone and cement during the first stage and during the second stage before reimplantation

ii. identification of offending organism, sensitivities are determined and appropriate antibiotic therapy is given for a prolonged period before reimplantation

iii. evaluation of distant foci of infection and eradication of sites responsible for haematogenous spread

iv. informed decision can be made as to whether the degree of disability from resection arthroplasty or arthrodesis would justify the risks involved in the implantation of a new prosthesis

The disadvantages[166] include:

i. prolonged period of disability and hospital stay

ii. increased costs

iii. delayed rehabilitation

iv. technically difficult second procedure due to loss soft tissue balance, loss of bone stock shortening and scarring

TSRA has been associated with lower rates of recurrent infections in most studies[6, 167, 168]. The duration of antibiotics between the two stages has not been determined, but a minimum of 6 weeks is usually standard and is guided by serial ESR and CRP levels. Management of bone stock deficiency at the time of revision is a problem. Impaction bone grafting with cemented prosthesis has been used for reconstruction during the second stage with good results. English et al. reported eradication in 49 out of 53 cases treated with impaction bone grafting during the second stage with a minimum follow up of 2 years[169] and a recurrence rate up to 7.5%[169, 170]. Use of antibiotic loaded cement for fixation of the implant during the second stage has been shown to reduce rates of reinfection. Garvin et al. reported eradication in 95% of patients at 5 year interval when gentamicin loaded cement was utilised during the second stage[171]. Highest success rates for TSRA were found for patients treated with antibiotics-eluting spacer or beads between the first and second stage, followed by a second reconstruction with an antibiotic loaded cemented reconstruction[55, 167, 172].

Data on uncemented implants has generally been less positive, with early studies reporting rates of infection as high as 18% and additional cases of loosening[43, 173]. Studies that are more recent have reported reinfection rates between 6% and 11%[174]. The decision regarding cemented or uncemented reimplantation is guided by the available bone stock, physiological age and expected longevity of the patient. To minimize loss of bone stock during the first stage, the Exeter group adopted a cement in cement revision technique for hip arthroplasty, where an excision arthroplasty with antibiotic impregnated cement beads is carried out during the first stage. In this technique if the cement mantle from the previous arthroplasty is well fixed, is left alone. During the second stage, the cement beads are removed, and the existing cement mantle is reamed to remove any membrane or microfilm and to create space for the new antibiotic augmented cement and the new implant. Sixteen patients with at least three years follow up underwent this procedure with one patient requiring revision due to recurrent infection[175].

5.6. Arthrodesis and amputation

Salvage procedures are reserved for patients whose medical condition such as immunocompromised patients or in patients where successful reconstruction is impossible. Successful reconstruction is limited those patients with insufficient bone stock, inadequate muscle function and poor soft tissue coverage. Eradication of infection after salvage procedures is reported between 86% to 96% although they are usually associated with poor functional outcomes[176-178]. Above knee amputation provides good return to function with a fitted pros-

http://dx.doi.org/10.5772/53247

thesis, especially in patients who cannot tolerate multiple procedures. Arthrodesis allows the patient to retain the extremity at the cost of reducing ambulation especially in patients with a fused knee.

6. Conclusion

Infection of a total Joint arthroplasty is considered a major complication in orthopaedic surgery with significant morbidity and places a considerable burden on hospitals and surgeons. Prevention is better than treatment and improving the patients' health prior to surgery is important in reducing the risk of infection. Furthermore, prompt diagnosis, permits early treatment that is important in acute infections. In the absence of a perfect test, the evidence based algorithmic approach brought forward by the AAOS guidelines should enable diagnosis of infection to be made with a high degree of confidence. There is clearly a role for surgical intervention, and so far a two-stage revision arthroplasty demonstrates the lowest rates of recurrent infection and as such is regarded as the 'gold standard'.

Author details

Adrian J. Cassar Gheiti and Kevin J. Mulhall

Orthopaedic Research and Innovation Foundation, Republic of Ireland

References

[1] Bozic KJ, Kurtz SM, Lau E, Ong K, Chiu V, Vail TP, et al. The epidemiology of revision total knee arthroplasty in the United States. Clin Orthop Relat Res. 2010;468[1]: 45-51. Epub 2009/06/26.

[2] Bozic KJ, Kurtz SM, Lau E, Ong K, Vail TP, Berry DJ. The epidemiology of revision total hip arthroplasty in the United States. J Bone Joint Surg Am. 2009;91[1]:128-33. Epub 2009/01/06.

[3] Clohisy JC, Calvert G, Tull F, McDonald D, Maloney WJ. Reasons for revision hip surgery: a retrospective review. Clin Orthop Relat Res. 2004[429]:188-92. Epub 2004/12/04.

[4] Vessely MB, Whaley AL, Harmsen WS, Schleck CD, Berry DJ. The Chitranjan Ranawat Award: Long-term survivorship and failure modes of 1000 cemented condylar total knee arthroplasties. Clin Orthop Relat Res. 2006;452:28-34. Epub 2006/08/29.

[5] Della Valle C, Parvizi J, Bauer TW, Dicesare PE, Evans RP, Segreti J, et al. Diagnosis of periprosthetic joint infections of the hip and knee. J Am Acad Orthop Surg. 2010;18[12]:760-70. Epub 2010/12/02.

[6] Parvizi J, Adeli B, Zmistowski B, Restrepo C, Greenwald AS. Management of Periprosthetic Joint Infection: The Current Knowledge: AAOS Exhibit Selection. J Bone Joint Surg Am. 2012;94[14]:e1041-9. Epub 2012/07/20.

[7] Parvizi J, Zmistowski B, Adeli B. Periprosthetic joint infection: treatment options. Orthopedics. 2010;33[9]:659. Epub 2010/09/16.

[8] Kurtz SM, Lau E, Watson H, Schmier JK, Parvizi J. Economic Burden of Periprosthetic Joint Infection in the United States. J Arthroplasty. 2012. Epub 2012/05/05.

[9] Bozic KJ, Lau E, Kurtz S, Ong K, Rubash H, Vail TP, et al. Patient-related risk factors for periprosthetic joint infection and postoperative mortality following total hip arthroplasty in Medicare patients. J Bone Joint Surg Am. 2012;94[9]:794-800. Epub 2012/05/04.

[10] Wilson MG, Kelley K, Thornhill TS. Infection as a complication of total knee-replacement arthroplasty. Risk factors and treatment in sixty-seven cases. J Bone Joint Surg Am. 1990;72[6]:878-83. Epub 1990/07/01.

[11] Zimmerli W, Trampuz A, Ochsner PE. Prosthetic-joint infections. N Engl J Med. 2004;351[16]:1645-54. Epub 2004/10/16.

[12] Pulido L, Ghanem E, Joshi A, Purtill JJ, Parvizi J. Periprosthetic joint infection: the incidence, timing, and predisposing factors. Clin Orthop Relat Res. 2008;466[7]:1710-5. Epub 2008/04/19.

[13] Sendi P, Banderet F, Graber P, Zimmerli W. Clinical comparison between exogenous and haematogenous periprosthetic joint infections caused by Staphylococcus aureus. Clin Microbiol Infect. 2011;17[7]:1098-100. Epub 2011/05/21.

[14] Greenky M, Gandhi K, Pulido L, Restrepo C, Parvizi J. Preoperative Anemia in Total Joint Arthroplasty: Is It Associated with Periprosthetic Joint Infection? Clin Orthop Relat Res. 2012. Epub 2012/07/10.

[15] Jafari SM, Casper DS, Restrepo C, Zmistowski B, Parvizi J, Sharkey PF. Periprosthetic joint infection: are patients with multiple prosthetic joints at risk? J Arthroplasty. 2012;27[6]:877-80. Epub 2012/03/06.

[16] Katthagen BD, Zamani P, Jung W. [Effect of surgical draping on bacterial contamination in the surgical field]. Z Orthop Ihre Grenzgeb. 1992;130[3]:230-5. Epub 1992/05/01. Einfluss der Inzisionsfolie auf das Keimverhalten im Operationsgebiet.

[17] Evans RP. Current concepts for clean air and total joint arthroplasty: laminar airflow and ultraviolet radiation: a systematic review. Clin Orthop Relat Res. 2011;469[4]:945-53. Epub 2010/12/17.

[18] Panahi P, Stroh M, Casper DS, Parvizi J, Austin MS. Operating Room Traffic is a Major Concern During Total Joint Arthroplasty. Clin Orthop Relat Res. 2012. Epub 2012/02/04.

[19] Kearns KA, Witmer D, Makda J, Parvizi J, Jungkind D. Sterility of the personal protection system in total joint arthroplasty. Clin Orthop Relat Res. 2011;469[11]:3065-9. Epub 2011/06/15.

[20] Buller LT, Sabry FY, Easton RW, Klika AK, Barsoum WK. The preoperative prediction of success following irrigation and debridement with polyethylene exchange for hip and knee prosthetic joint infections. J Arthroplasty. 2012;27[6]:857-64 e1-4. Epub 2012/03/10.

[21] Jamsen E, Huhtala H, Puolakka T, Moilanen T. Risk factors for infection after knee arthroplasty. A register-based analysis of 43,149 cases. J Bone Joint Surg Am. 2009;91[1]:38-47. Epub 2009/01/06.

[22] Berbari EF, Hanssen AD, Duffy MC, Steckelberg JM, Ilstrup DM, Harmsen WS, et al. Risk factors for prosthetic joint infection: case-control study. Clin Infect Dis. 1998;27[5]:1247-54. Epub 1998/11/25.

[23] Saleh K, Olson M, Resig S, Bershadsky B, Kuskowski M, Gioe T, et al. Predictors of wound infection in hip and knee joint replacement: results from a 20 year surveillance program. J Orthop Res. 2002;20[3]:506-15. Epub 2002/06/01.

[24] Jamsen E, Nevalainen P, Eskelinen A, Huotari K, Kalliovalkama J, Moilanen T. Obesity, diabetes, and preoperative hyperglycemia as predictors of periprosthetic joint infection: a single-center analysis of 7181 primary hip and knee replacements for osteoarthritis. J Bone Joint Surg Am. 2012;94[14]:e1011-9. Epub 2012/07/20.

[25] Poss R, Thornhill TS, Ewald FC, Thomas WH, Batte NJ, Sledge CB. Factors influencing the incidence and outcome of infection following total joint arthroplasty. Clin Orthop Relat Res. 1984[182]:117-26. Epub 1984/01/01.

[26] Muilwijk J, van den Hof S, Wille JC. Associations between surgical site infection risk and hospital operation volume and surgeon operation volume among hospitals in the Dutch nosocomial infection surveillance network. Infect Control Hosp Epidemiol. 2007;28[5]:557-63. Epub 2007/04/28.

[27] Ong KL, Lau E, Manley M, Kurtz SM. Effect of procedure duration on total hip arthroplasty and total knee arthroplasty survivorship in the United States Medicare population. J Arthroplasty. 2008;23[6 Suppl 1]:127-32. Epub 2008/06/17.

[28] Fogelberg EV, Zitzmann EK, Stinchfield FE. Prophylactic penicillin in orthopaedic surgery. J Bone Joint Surg Am. 1970;52[1]:95-8. Epub 1970/01/01.

[29] Pavel A, Smith RL, Ballard A, Larsen IJ. Prophylactic antibiotics in clean orthopaedic surgery. J Bone Joint Surg Am. 1974;56[4]:777-82. Epub 1974/06/01.

[30] Meehan J, Jamali AA, Nguyen H. Prophylactic antibiotics in hip and knee arthroplasty. J Bone Joint Surg Am. 2009;91[10]:2480-90. Epub 2009/10/03.

[31] Al-Maiyah M, Hill D, Bajwa A, Slater S, Patil P, Port A, et al. Bacterial contaminants and antibiotic prophylaxis in total hip arthroplasty. J Bone Joint Surg Br. 2005;87[9]: 1256-8. Epub 2005/09/01.

[32] Hanssen AD. Prophylactic use of antibiotic bone cement: an emerging standard--in opposition. J Arthroplasty. 2004;19[4 Suppl 1]:73-7. Epub 2004/06/11.

[33] Johnson AJ, Daley JA, Zywiel MG, Delanois RE, Mont MA. Preoperative chlorhexidine preparation and the incidence of surgical site infections after hip arthroplasty. J Arthroplasty. 2010;25[6 Suppl):98-102. Epub 2010/06/24.

[34] Ayers DC DD, Johanson NA, Pellegrini.VD Jr. Instructional Course Lectures, The American Academy of Orthopaedic Surgeons - Common Complications of Total Knee Arthroplasty. J Bone Joint Surg Am. 1997;79[2]:278-311.

[35] Rao N, Cannella B, Crossett LS, Yates AJ, Jr., McGough R, 3rd. A preoperative decolonization protocol for staphylococcus aureus prevents orthopaedic infections. Clin Orthop Relat Res. 2008;466[6]:1343-8. Epub 2008/04/12.

[36] Gristina AG. Biomaterial-centered infection: microbial adhesion versus tissue integration. Science. 1987;237[4822]:1588-95. Epub 1987/09/25.

[37] Costerton JW, Stewart PS, Greenberg EP. Bacterial biofilms: a common cause of persistent infections. Science. 1999;284[5418]:1318-22. Epub 1999/05/21.

[38] Anderl JN, Zahller J, Roe F, Stewart PS. Role of nutrient limitation and stationary-phase existence in Klebsiella pneumoniae biofilm resistance to ampicillin and ciprofloxacin. Antimicrob Agents Chemother. 2003;47[4]:1251-6. Epub 2003/03/26.

[39] Darouiche RO. Device-associated infections: a macroproblem that starts with microadherence. Clin Infect Dis. 2001;33[9]:1567-72. Epub 2001/09/29.

[40] Hoiby N, Ciofu O, Johansen HK, Song ZJ, Moser C, Jensen PO, et al. The clinical impact of bacterial biofilms. International journal of oral science. 2011;3[2]:55-65. Epub 2011/04/13.

[41] Zimmerli W, Lew PD, Waldvogel FA. Pathogenesis of foreign body infection. Evidence for a local granulocyte defect. J Clin Invest. 1984;73[4]:1191-200. Epub 1984/04/01.

[42] Murdoch DR, Roberts SA, Fowler Jr VG, Jr., Shah MA, Taylor SL, Morris AJ, et al. Infection of orthopedic prostheses after Staphylococcus aureus bacteremia. Clin Infect Dis. 2001;32[4]:647-9. Epub 2001/02/22.

[43] Salvati EA, Gonzalez Della Valle A, Masri BA, Duncan CP. The infected total hip arthroplasty. Instr Course Lect. 2003;52:223-45. Epub 2003/04/15.

[44] Phillips JE, Crane TP, Noy M, Elliott TS, Grimer RJ. The incidence of deep prosthetic infections in a specialist orthopaedic hospital: a 15-year prospective survey. J Bone Joint Surg Br. 2006;88[7]:943-8. Epub 2006/06/27.

[45] Romano CL, Romano D, Logoluso N, Meani E. Septic versus aseptic hip revision: how different? J Orthop Traumatol. 2010;11[3]:167-74. Epub 2010/09/03.

[46] Zmistowski B, Fedorka CJ, Sheehan E, Deirmengian G, Austin MS, Parvizi J. Prosthetic joint infection caused by gram-negative organisms. J Arthroplasty. 2011;26[6 Suppl):104-8. Epub 2011/06/07.

[47] Anagnostakos K, Kelm J, Schmitt E, Jung J. Fungal periprosthetic hip and knee joint infections clinical experience with a 2-stage treatment protocol. J Arthroplasty. 2012;27[2]:293-8. Epub 2011/07/15.

[48] Mahmud T, Lyons MC, Naudie DD, Macdonald SJ, McCalden RW. Assessing the Gold Standard: A Review of 253 Two-Stage Revisions for Infected TKA. Clin Orthop Relat Res. 2012. Epub 2012/04/28.

[49] Hare R, Thomas CG. The transmission of Staphylococcus aureus. Br Med J. 1956;2[4997]:840-4. Epub 1956/10/13.

[50] Ritter MA. Operating room environment. Clin Orthop Relat Res. 1999[369]:103-9. Epub 1999/12/28.

[51] Passaro DJ, Waring L, Armstrong R, Bolding F, Bouvier B, Rosenberg J, et al. Postoperative Serratia marcescens wound infections traced to an out-of-hospital source. J Infect Dis. 1997;175[4]:992-5. Epub 1997/04/01.

[52] Veber B, Gachot B, Bedos JP, Wolff M. Severe sepsis after intravenous injection of contaminated propofol. Anesthesiology. 1994;80[3]:712-3. Epub 1994/03/01.

[53] Elek SD, Conen PE. The virulence of Staphylococcus pyogenes for man; a study of the problems of wound infection. Br J Exp Pathol. 1957;38[6]:573-86. Epub 1957/12/01.

[54] Zimmerli W, Waldvogel FA, Vaudaux P, Nydegger UE. Pathogenesis of foreign body infection: description and characteristics of an animal model. J Infect Dis. 1982;146[4]: 487-97. Epub 1982/10/01.

[55] Fitzgerald RH, Jr., Nolan DR, Ilstrup DM, Van Scoy RE, Washington JA, 2nd, Coventry MB. Deep wound sepsis following total hip arthroplasty. J Bone Joint Surg Am. 1977;59[7]:847-55. Epub 1977/10/01.

[56] Tsukayama DT, Estrada R, Gustilo RB. Infection after total hip arthroplasty. A study of the treatment of one hundred and six infections. J Bone Joint Surg Am. 1996;78[4]: 512-23. Epub 1996/04/01.

[57] Zimmerli W, Moser C. Pathogenesis and treatment concepts of orthopaedic biofilm infections. FEMS Immunol Med Microbiol. 2012;65[2]:158-68. Epub 2012/02/09.

[58] Maderazo EG, Judson S, Pasternak H. Late infections of total joint prostheses. A review and recommendations for prevention. Clin Orthop Relat Res. 1988[229]:131-42. Epub 1988/04/01.

[59] Workgroup Convened by the Musculoskeletal Infection S. New definition for periprosthetic joint infection. J Arthroplasty. 2011;26[8]:1136-8. Epub 2011/11/15.

[60] Malinzak RA, Ritter MA, Berend ME, Meding JB, Olberding EM, Davis KE. Morbidly obese, diabetic, younger, and unilateral joint arthroplasty patients have elevated total joint arthroplasty infection rates. J Arthroplasty. 2009;24[6 Suppl):84-8. Epub 2009/07/17.

[61] Fletcher N, Sofianos D, Berkes MB, Obremskey WT. Prevention of perioperative infection. J Bone Joint Surg Am. 2007;89[7]:1605-18. Epub 2007/07/04.

[62] Lai K, Bohm ER, Burnell C, Hedden DR. Presence of medical comorbidities in patients with infected primary hip or knee arthroplasties. J Arthroplasty. 2007;22[5]: 651-6. Epub 2007/08/11.

[63] Kamal T, Conway RM, Littlejohn I, Ricketts D. The role of a multidisciplinary preassessment clinic in reducing mortality after complex orthopaedic surgery. Ann R Coll Surg Engl. 2011;93[2]:149-51. Epub 2011/11/02.

[64] Control CfD. Guidline For Prevention of Surgical Site Infection. 1999; Available from: http://www.cdc.gov/HAI/ssi/ssi.html.

[65] Bleasdale SC, Trick WE, Gonzalez IM, Lyles RD, Hayden MK, Weinstein RA. Effectiveness of chlorhexidine bathing to reduce catheter-associated bloodstream infections in medical intensive care unit patients. Arch Intern Med. 2007;167[19]:2073-9. Epub 2007/10/24.

[66] Climo MW, Sepkowitz KA, Zuccotti G, Fraser VJ, Warren DK, Perl TM, et al. The effect of daily bathing with chlorhexidine on the acquisition of methicillin-resistant Staphylococcus aureus, vancomycin-resistant Enterococcus, and healthcare-associated bloodstream infections: results of a quasi-experimental multicenter trial. Crit Care Med. 2009;37[6]:1858-65. Epub 2009/04/23.

[67] Rao N, Cannella BA, Crossett LS, Yates AJ, Jr., McGough RL, 3rd, Hamilton CW. Preoperative screening/decolonization for Staphylococcus aureus to prevent orthopedic surgical site infection: prospective cohort study with 2-year follow-up. J Arthroplasty. 2011;26[8]:1501-7. Epub 2011/04/22.

[68] Edmiston CE, Jr., Seabrook GR, Johnson CP, Paulson DS, Beausoleil CM. Comparative of a new and innovative 2% chlorhexidine gluconate-impregnated cloth with 4% chlorhexidine gluconate as topical antiseptic for preparation of the skin prior to surgery. Am J Infect Control. 2007;35[2]:89-96. Epub 2007/03/01.

[69] Ramos N, Skeete F, Haas JP, Hutzler L, Slover J, Phillips M, et al. Surgical site infection prevention initiative - patient attitude and compliance. Bull NYU Hosp Jt Dis. 2011;69[4]:312-5. Epub 2011/12/27.

[70] Zywiel MG, Daley JA, Delanois RE, Naziri Q, Johnson AJ, Mont MA. Advance preoperative chlorhexidine reduces the incidence of surgical site infections in knee arthroplasty. Int Orthop. 2011;35[7]:1001-6. Epub 2010/06/22.

[71] Eiselt D. Presurgical skin preparation with a novel 2% chlorhexidine gluconate cloth reduces rates of surgical site infection in orthopaedic surgical patients. Orthop Nurs. 2009;28[3]:141-5. Epub 2009/06/06.

[72] Mauerhan DR, Nelson CL, Smith DL, Fitzgerald RH, Jr., Slama TG, Petty RW, et al. Prophylaxis against infection in total joint arthroplasty. One day of cefuroxime compared with three days of cefazolin. J Bone Joint Surg Am. 1994;76[1]:39-45. Epub 1994/01/01.

[73] Tanner J, Norrie P, Melen K. Preoperative hair removal to reduce surgical site infection. Cochrane Database Syst Rev. 2011[11]:CD004122. Epub 2011/11/11.

[74] Edwards PS, Lipp A, Holmes A. Preoperative skin antiseptics for preventing surgical wound infections after clean surgery. Cochrane Database Syst Rev. 2004[3]:CD003949. Epub 2004/07/22.

[75] Ostrander RV, Brage ME, Botte MJ. Bacterial skin contamination after surgical preparation in foot and ankle surgery. Clin Orthop Relat Res. 2003[406]:246-52. Epub 2003/02/13.

[76] Keblish DJ, Zurakowski D, Wilson MG, Chiodo CP. Preoperative skin preparation of the foot and ankle: bristles and alcohol are better. J Bone Joint Surg Am. 2005;87[5]:986-92. Epub 2005/05/04.

[77] Ostrander RV, Botte MJ, Brage ME. Efficacy of surgical preparation solutions in foot and ankle surgery. J Bone Joint Surg Am. 2005;87[5]:980-5. Epub 2005/05/04.

[78] Tanner J, Swarbrook S, Stuart J. Surgical hand antisepsis to reduce surgical site infection. Cochrane Database Syst Rev. 2008[1]:CD004288. Epub 2008/02/07.

[79] Larson EL, Butz AM, Gullette DL, Laughon BA. Alcohol for surgical scrubbing? Infect Control Hosp Epidemiol. 1990;11[3]:139-43. Epub 1990/03/01.

[80] French ML, Eitzen HE, Ritter MA. The plastic surgical adhesive drape: an evaluation of its efficacy as a microbial barrier. Ann Surg. 1976;184[1]:46-50. Epub 1976/07/01.

[81] Johnston DH, Fairclough JA, Brown EM, Morris R. Rate of bacterial recolonization of the skin after preparation: four methods compared. Br J Surg. 1987;74[1]:64. Epub 1987/01/01.

[82] Blom AW, Gozzard C, Heal J, Bowker K, Estela CM. Bacterial strike-through of reusable surgical drapes: the effect of different wetting agents. J Hosp Infect. 2002;52[1]:52-5. Epub 2002/10/10.

[83] Blom A, Estela C, Bowker K, MacGowan A, Hardy JR. The passage of bacteria through surgical drapes. Ann R Coll Surg Engl. 2000;82[6]:405-7. Epub 2000/12/05.

[84] Ritter MA, Campbell ED. Retrospective evaluation of an iodophor-incorporated antimicrobial plastic adhesive wound drape. Clin Orthop Relat Res. 1988[228]:307-8. Epub 1988/03/01.

[85] Webster J, Alghamdi AA. Use of plastic adhesive drapes during surgery for preventing surgical site infection. Cochrane Database Syst Rev. 2007[4]:CD006353. Epub 2007/10/19.

[86] Guo YP, Wong PM, Li Y, Or PP. Is double-gloving really protective? A comparison between the glove perforation rate among perioperative nurses with single and double gloves during surgery. Am J Surg. 2012;204[2]:210-5. Epub 2012/02/22.

[87] Tanner J, Parkinson H. Double gloving to reduce surgical cross-infection. Cochrane Database Syst Rev. 2006[3]:CD003087. Epub 2006/07/21.

[88] Ersozlu S, Sahin O, Ozgur AF, Akkaya T, Tuncay C. Glove punctures in major and minor orthopaedic surgery with double gloving. Acta Orthop Belg. 2007;73[6]:760-4. Epub 2008/02/12.

[89] Beldame J, Lagrave B, Lievain L, Lefebvre B, Frebourg N, Dujardin F. Surgical glove bacterial contamination and perforation during total hip arthroplasty implantation: when gloves should be changed. Orthop Traumatol Surg Res. 2012;98[4]:432-40. Epub 2012/05/15.

[90] Lidwell OM, Elson RA, Lowbury EJ, Whyte W, Blowers R, Stanley SJ, et al. Ultraclean air and antibiotics for prevention of postoperative infection. A multicenter study of 8,052 joint replacement operations. Acta Orthop Scand. 1987;58[1]:4-13. Epub 1987/02/01.

[91] Dharan S, Pittet D. Environmental controls in operating theatres. J Hosp Infect. 2002;51[2]:79-84. Epub 2002/07/02.

[92] Ayliffe GA. Role of the environment of the operating suite in surgical wound infection. Rev Infect Dis. 1991;13 Suppl 10:S800-4. Epub 1991/09/01.

[93] Gastmeier P, Breier AC, Brandt C. Influence of laminar airflow on prosthetic joint infections: a systematic review. J Hosp Infect. 2012;81[2]:73-8. Epub 2012/05/15.

[94] Lynch RJ, Englesbe MJ, Sturm L, Bitar A, Budhiraj K, Kolla S, et al. Measurement of foot traffic in the operating room: implications for infection control. Am J Med Qual. 2009;24[1]:45-52. Epub 2009/01/14.

[95] Parikh SN, Grice SS, Schnell BM, Salisbury SR. Operating room traffic: is there any role of monitoring it? J Pediatr Orthop. 2010;30[6]:617-23. Epub 2010/08/25.

[96] Charnley J, Eftekhar N. Penetration of gown material by organisms from the surgeon's body. Lancet. 1969;1[7587]:172-3. Epub 1969/01/25.

[97] Der Tavitian J, Ong SM, Taub NA, Taylor GJ. Body-exhaust suit versus occlusive clothing. A randomised, prospective trial using air and wound bacterial counts. J Bone Joint Surg Br. 2003;85[4]:490-4. Epub 2003/06/10.

[98] Howard JL, Hanssen AD. Principles of a clean operating room environment. J Arthroplasty. 2007;22[7 Suppl 3]:6-11. Epub 2007/11/21.

[99] Pasquarella C, Pitzurra O, Herren T, Poletti L, Savino A. Lack of influence of body exhaust gowns on aerobic bacterial surface counts in a mixed-ventilation operating theatre. A study of 62 hip arthroplasties. J Hosp Infect. 2003;54[1]:2-9. Epub 2003/05/28.

[100] Sanzen L, Carlsson AS, Walder M. Air contamination during total hip arthroplasty in an ultraclean air enclosure using different types of staff clothing. J Arthroplasty. 1990;5[2]:127-30. Epub 1990/06/01.

[101] Shaw JA, Bordner MA, Hamory BH. Efficacy of the Steri-Shield filtered exhaust helmet in limiting bacterial counts in the operating room during total joint arthroplasty. J Arthroplasty. 1996;11[4]:469-73. Epub 1996/06/01.

[102] Urquhart DM, Hanna FS, Brennan SL, Wluka AE, Leder K, Cameron PA, et al. Incidence and risk factors for deep surgical site infection after primary total hip arthroplasty: a systematic review. J Arthroplasty. 2010;25[8]:1216-22 e1-3. Epub 2009/11/03.

[103] Ong KL, Kurtz SM, Lau E, Bozic KJ, Berry DJ, Parvizi J. Prosthetic joint infection risk after total hip arthroplasty in the Medicare population. J Arthroplasty. 2009;24[6 Suppl):105-9. Epub 2009/06/06.

[104] Peersman G, Laskin R, Davis J, Peterson M. Infection in total knee replacement: a retrospective review of 6489 total knee replacements. Clin Orthop Relat Res. 2001[392]: 15-23. Epub 2001/11/22.

[105] Kurtz SM, Ong KL, Lau E, Bozic KJ, Berry D, Parvizi J. Prosthetic joint infection risk after TKA in the Medicare population. Clin Orthop Relat Res. 2010;468[1]:52-6. Epub 2009/08/12.

[106] Engesaeter LB, Lie SA, Espehaug B, Furnes O, Vollset SE, Havelin LI. Antibiotic prophylaxis in total hip arthroplasty: effects of antibiotic prophylaxis systemically and in bone cement on the revision rate of 22,170 primary hip replacements followed 0-14 years in the Norwegian Arthroplasty Register. Acta Orthop Scand. 2003;74[6]:644-51. Epub 2004/02/07.

[107] Romano CL, Romano D, Logoluso N, Meani E. Long-stem versus short-stem preformed antibiotic-loaded cement spacers for two-stage revision of infected total hip arthroplasty. Hip Int. 2010;20[1]:26-33. Epub 2010/03/18.

[108] Dairaku K, Takagi M, Kawaji H, Sasaki K, Ishii M, Ogino T. Antibiotics-impregnated cement spacers in the first step of two-stage revision for infected totally replaced hip joints: report of ten trial cases. J Orthop Sci. 2009;14[6]:704-10. Epub 2009/12/10.

[109] Cassar Gheiti AJ, Baker JF, Brown TE, Mulhall KJ. Management of Total Femoral Bone Loss Using a Hybrid Cement Spacer Surgical Technique. J Arthroplasty. 2012. Epub 2012/07/04.

[110] Chiu FY, Lin CF, Chen CM, Lo WH, Chaung TY. Cefuroxime-impregnated cement at primary total knee arthroplasty in diabetes mellitus. A prospective, randomised study. J Bone Joint Surg Br. 2001;83[5]:691-5. Epub 2001/07/31.

[111] Hanssen AD, Spangehl MJ. Practical applications of antibiotic-loaded bone cement for treatment of infected joint replacements. Clin Orthop Relat Res. 2004[427]:79-85. Epub 2004/11/24.

[112] Smith TO, Sexton D, Mann C, Donell S. Sutures versus staples for skin closure in orthopaedic surgery: meta-analysis. BMJ. 2010;340:c1199. Epub 2010/03/18.

[113] Newman JT, Morgan SJ, Resende GV, Williams AE, Hammerberg EM, Dayton MR. Modality of wound closure after total knee replacement: are staples as safe as sutures? A retrospective study of 181 patients. Patient Saf Surg. 2011;5[1]:26. Epub 2011/10/21.

[114] Eggers MD, Fang L, Lionberger DR. A comparison of wound closure techniques for total knee arthroplasty. J Arthroplasty. 2011;26[8]:1251-8 e1-4. Epub 2011/05/03.

[115] Patel RM, Cayo M, Patel A, Albarillo M, Puri L. Wound complications in joint arthroplasty: comparing traditional and modern methods of skin closure. Orthopedics. 2012;35[5]:e641-6. Epub 2012/05/17.

[116] Stephens S, Politi J, Taylor BC. Evaluation of Primary Total Knee Arthroplasty Incision Closure with the Use of Continuous Bidirectional Barbed Suture. Surg Technol Int. 2011;XXI:199-203. Epub 2012/04/17.

[117] Eickmann T, Quane E. Total knee arthroplasty closure with barbed sutures. J Knee Surg. 2010;23[3]:163-7. Epub 2011/02/19.

[118] Clarke JV, Deakin AH, Dillon JM, Emmerson S, Kinninmonth AW. A prospective clinical audit of a new dressing design for lower limb arthroplasty wounds. J Wound Care. 2009;18[1]:5-8, 10-1. Epub 2009/01/10.

[119] Cosker T, Elsayed S, Gupta S, Mendonca AD, Tayton KJ. Choice of dressing has a major impact on blistering and healing outcomes in orthopaedic patients. J Wound Care. 2005;14[1]:27-9. Epub 2005/01/20.

[120] Cho CY, Lo JS. Dressing the part. Dermatol Clin. 1998;16[1]:25-47. Epub 1998/02/14.

[121] Mertz PM, Marshall DA, Eaglstein WH. Occlusive wound dressings to prevent bacterial invasion and wound infection. J Am Acad Dermatol. 1985;12[4]:662-8. Epub 1985/04/01.

[122] Dumville JC, Walter CJ, Sharp CA, Page T. Dressings for the prevention of surgical site infection. Cochrane Database Syst Rev. 2011[7]:CD003091. Epub 2011/07/08.

[123] Burke NG, Green C, McHugh G, McGolderick N, Kilcoyne C, Kenny P. A prospective randomised study comparing the jubilee dressing method to a standard adhesive dressing for total hip and knee replacements. J Tissue Viability. 2012;21[3]:84-7. Epub 2012/06/05.

[124] Matar WY, Jafari SM, Restrepo C, Austin M, Purtill JJ, Parvizi J. Preventing infection in total joint arthroplasty. J Bone Joint Surg Am. 2010;92 Suppl 2:36-46. Epub 2010/12/09.

[125] Greidanus NV, Masri BA, Garbuz DS, Wilson SD, McAlinden MG, Xu M, et al. Use of erythrocyte sedimentation rate and C-reactive protein level to diagnose infection before revision total knee arthroplasty. A prospective evaluation. J Bone Joint Surg Am. 2007;89[7]:1409-16. Epub 2007/07/04.

[126] Schinsky MF, Della Valle CJ, Sporer SM, Paprosky WG. Perioperative testing for joint infection in patients undergoing revision total hip arthroplasty. J Bone Joint Surg Am. 2008;90[9]:1869-75. Epub 2008/09/03.

[127] Ghanem E, Antoci V, Jr., Pulido L, Joshi A, Hozack W, Parvizi J. The use of receiver operating characteristics analysis in determining erythrocyte sedimentation rate and C-reactive protein levels in diagnosing periprosthetic infection prior to revision total hip arthroplasty. Int J Infect Dis. 2009;13[6]:e444-9. Epub 2009/05/29.

[128] Toossi N, Adeli B, Rasouli MR, Huang R, Parvizi J. Serum White Blood Cell Count and Differential Do Not Have a Role in the Diagnosis of Periprosthetic Joint Infection. J Arthroplasty. 2012. Epub 2012/05/23.

[129] Trampuz A, Hanssen AD, Osmon DR, Mandrekar J, Steckelberg JM, Patel R. Synovial fluid leukocyte count and differential for the diagnosis of prosthetic knee infection. Am J Med. 2004;117[8]:556-62. Epub 2004/10/07.

[130] Ghanem E, Parvizi J, Burnett RS, Sharkey PF, Keshavarzi N, Aggarwal A, et al. Cell count and differential of aspirated fluid in the diagnosis of infection at the site of total knee arthroplasty. J Bone Joint Surg Am. 2008;90[8]:1637-43. Epub 2008/08/05.

[131] Tigges S, Stiles RG, Roberson JR. Appearance of septic hip prostheses on plain radiographs. AJR Am J Roentgenol. 1994;163[2]:377-80. Epub 1994/08/01.

[132] Smith SL, Wastie ML, Forster I. Radionuclide bone scintigraphy in the detection of significant complications after total knee joint replacement. Clin Radiol. 2001;56[3]: 221-4. Epub 2001/03/15.

[133] Love C, Marwin SE, Palestro CJ. Nuclear medicine and the infected joint replacement. Semin Nucl Med. 2009;39[1]:66-78. Epub 2008/11/29.

[134] Pandey R, Berendt AR, Athanasou NA. Histological and microbiological findings in non-infected and infected revision arthroplasty tissues. The OSIRIS Collaborative Study Group. Oxford Skeletal Infection Research and Intervention Service. Arch Orthop Trauma Surg. 2000;120[10]:570-4. Epub 2000/12/08.

[135] Atkins BL, Athanasou N, Deeks JJ, Crook DW, Simpson H, Peto TE, et al. Prospective evaluation of criteria for microbiological diagnosis of prosthetic-joint infection at revision arthroplasty. The OSIRIS Collaborative Study Group. J Clin Microbiol. 1998;36[10]:2932-9. Epub 1998/09/17.

[136] Spangehl MJ, Masri BA, O'Connell JX, Duncan CP. Prospective analysis of preoperative and intraoperative investigations for the diagnosis of infection at the sites of two hundred and two revision total hip arthroplasties. J Bone Joint Surg Am. 1999;81[5]: 672-83. Epub 1999/06/09.

[137] Johnson AJ, Zywiel MG, Stroh DA, Marker DR, Mont MA. Should gram stains have a role in diagnosing hip arthroplasty infections? Clin Orthop Relat Res. 2010;468[9]: 2387-91. Epub 2010/01/06.

[138] Oethinger M, Warner DK, Schindler SA, Kobayashi H, Bauer TW. Diagnosing periprosthetic infection: false-positive intraoperative Gram stains. Clin Orthop Relat Res. 2011;469[4]:954-60. Epub 2010/10/01.

[139] Parvizi J, Jacovides C, Antoci V, Ghanem E. Diagnosis of periprosthetic joint infection: the utility of a simple yet unappreciated enzyme. J Bone Joint Surg Am. 2011;93[24]:2242-8. Epub 2012/01/20.

[140] Wetters NG, Berend KR, Lombardi AV, Morris MJ, Tucker TL, Della Valle CJ. Leukocyte Esterase Reagent Strips for the Rapid Diagnosis of Periprosthetic Joint Infection. J Arthroplasty. 2012. Epub 2012/05/23.

[141] Parvizi J, Jacovides C, Adeli B, Jung KA, Hozack WJ. Mark B. Coventry Award: synovial C-reactive protein: a prospective evaluation of a molecular marker for periprosthetic knee joint infection. Clin Orthop Relat Res. 2012;470[1]:54-60. Epub 2011/07/26.

[142] Parvizi J, McKenzie JC, Cashman JP. Diagnosis of Periprosthetic Joint Infection Using Synovial C-Reactive Protein. J Arthroplasty. 2012. Epub 2012/05/09.

[143] Jacovides CL, Parvizi J, Adeli B, Jung KA. Molecular markers for diagnosis of periprosthetic joint infection. J Arthroplasty. 2011;26[6 Suppl):99-103 e1. Epub 2011/05/17.

[144] Della Valle C, Parvizi J., Bauer T.W., DiCesare, P.E., Evans, R.P., Segreti, J., Spangehl, M. Diagnosis of Periprosthetic Joint Infections of the Hip and Knee. 2010; Available from: http://www.aaos.org/research/guidelines/PJIguideline.asp.

[145] Dupont JA. Significance of operative cultures in total hip arthroplasty. Clin Orthop Relat Res. 1986[211]:122-7. Epub 1986/10/01.

[146] Toms AD, Davidson D, Masri BA, Duncan CP. The management of peri-prosthetic infection in total joint arthroplasty. J Bone Joint Surg Br. 2006;88[2]:149-55. Epub 2006/01/26.

[147] Rao N, Crossett LS, Sinha RK, Le Frock JL. Long-term suppression of infection in total joint arthroplasty. Clin Orthop Relat Res. 2003[414]:55-60. Epub 2003/09/11.

[148] Segreti J, Nelson JA, Trenholme GM. Prolonged suppressive antibiotic therapy for infected orthopedic prostheses. Clin Infect Dis. 1998;27[4]:711-3. Epub 1998/11/03.

[149] Goulet JA, Pellicci PM, Brause BD, Salvati EM. Prolonged suppression of infection in total hip arthroplasty. J Arthroplasty. 1988;3[2]:109-16. Epub 1988/01/01.

[150] Crockarell JR, Hanssen AD, Osmon DR, Morrey BF. Treatment of infection with debridement and retention of the components following hip arthroplasty. J Bone Joint Surg Am. 1998;80[9]:1306-13. Epub 1998/10/06.

[151] Odum SM, Fehring TK, Lombardi AV, Zmistowski BM, Brown NM, Luna JT, et al. Irrigation and debridement for periprosthetic infections: does the organism matter? J Arthroplasty. 2011;26[6 Suppl):114-8. Epub 2011/05/31.

[152] Baker JF, Vioreanu MH, Harty JA. Clostridium perfringens infection complicating periprosthetic fracture fixation about the hip: successful treatment with early aggressive debridement. Hip Int. 2012;22[1]:122-5. Epub 2012/02/22.

[153] Callaghan JJ, Katz RP, Johnston RC. One-stage revision surgery of the infected hip. A minimum 10-year followup study. Clin Orthop Relat Res. 1999[369]:139-43. Epub 1999/12/28.

[154] Elson RA. Exchange arthroplasty for infection. Perspectives from the United Kingdom. Orthop Clin North Am. 1993;24[4]:761-7. Epub 1993/10/01.

[155] Garvin KL, Fitzgerald RH, Jr., Salvati EA, Brause BD, Nercessian OA, Wallrichs SL, et al. Reconstruction of the infected total hip and knee arthroplasty with gentamicin-impregnated Palacos bone cement. Instr Course Lect. 1993;42:293-302. Epub 1993/01/01.

[156] Lange J, Troelsen A, Thomsen RW, Soballe K. Chronic infections in hip arthroplasties: comparing risk of reinfection following one-stage and two-stage revision: a systematic review and meta-analysis. Clin Epidemiol. 2012;4:57-73. Epub 2012/04/14.

[157] Younger AS, Duncan CP, Masri BA, McGraw RW. The outcome of two-stage arthroplasty using a custom-made interval spacer to treat the infected hip. J Arthroplasty. 1997;12[6]:615-23. Epub 1997/11/05.

[158] Garvin KL, Backstein D, Pellegrini VD, Jr., Kim RH, Lewallen DG. Dealing with complications. J Bone Joint Surg Am. 2009;91 Suppl 5:18-21. Epub 2009/08/08.

[159] Pignatti G, Nitta S, Rani N, Dallari D, Sabbioni G, Stagni C, et al. Two stage hip revision in periprosthetic infection: results of 41 cases. Open Orthop J. 2010;4:193-200. Epub 2010/08/20.

[160] Wan Z, Momaya A, Karim A, Incavo SJ, Mathis KB. Preformed Articulating Knee Spacers in 2-Stage Total Knee Revision Arthroplasty: Minimum 2-Year Follow-Up. J Arthroplasty. 2012. Epub 2012/03/20.

[161] Duncan CP, Beauchamp C. A temporary antibiotic-loaded joint replacement system for management of complex infections involving the hip. Orthop Clin North Am. 1993;24[4]:751-9. Epub 1993/10/01.

[162] Richards C, Bell CJ, Viswanathan S, English H, Crawford RW. Use of a cement-loaded Kuntscher nail in first-stage revision hip arthroplasty for massive femoral bone

loss secondary to infection: a report of four cases. J Orthop Surg (Hong Kong). 2010;18[1]:107-9. Epub 2010/04/30.

[163] Yoo J, Lee S, Han C, Chang J. The modified static spacers using antibiotic-impregnated cement rod in two-stage revision for infected total knee arthroplasty. Clin Orthop Surg. 2011;3[3]:245-8. Epub 2011/09/13.

[164] Morgan M TA, Hubble M.J.W. Diagnosis and Management of Infection. In: Ling RSM, Princess Elizabeth Orthopaedic Hospital. Exeter Hip U, editors. The Exeter hip : 40 years of innovation in total hip arthroplasty. Exeter: Exeter Hip Publishing; 2010. p. 369 p.

[165] Mont MA, Waldman BJ, Hungerford DS. Evaluation of preoperative cultures before second-stage reimplantation of a total knee prosthesis complicated by infection. A comparison-group study. J Bone Joint Surg Am. 2000;82-A[11]:1552-7. Epub 2000/11/30.

[166] Canale ST, Beaty JH. Part III - Arthroplasty. Campbell's operative orthopaedics. 11th ed. St. Louis, Mo. ; London: Mosby Elsevier; 2008.

[167] Hanssen AD, Rand JA. Evaluation and treatment of infection at the site of a total hip or knee arthroplasty. Instr Course Lect. 1999;48:111-22. Epub 1999/03/31.

[168] Choi HR, Malchau H, Bedair H. Are Prosthetic Spacers Safe to Use in 2-Stage Treatment for Infected Total Knee Arthroplasty? J Arthroplasty. 2012. Epub 2012/04/17.

[169] English H, Timperley AJ, Dunlop D, Gie G. Impaction grafting of the femur in two-stage revision for infected total hip replacement. J Bone Joint Surg Br. 2002;84[5]: 700-5. Epub 2002/08/22.

[170] Alexeeff M, Mahomed N, Morsi E, Garbuz D, Gross A. Structural allograft in two-stage revisions for failed septic hip arthroplasty. J Bone Joint Surg Br. 1996;78[2]: 213-6. Epub 1996/03/01.

[171] Garvin KL, Evans BG, Salvati EA, Brause BD. Palacos gentamicin for the treatment of deep periprosthetic hip infections. Clin Orthop Relat Res. 1994[298]:97-105. Epub 1994/01/01.

[172] Hanssen AD, Spangehl MJ. Treatment of the infected hip replacement. Clin Orthop Relat Res. 2004[420]:63-71. Epub 2004/04/02.

[173] Nestor BJ, Hanssen AD, Ferrer-Gonzalez R, Fitzgerald RH, Jr. The use of porous prostheses in delayed reconstruction of total hip replacements that have failed because of infection. J Bone Joint Surg Am. 1994;76[3]:349-59. Epub 1994/03/01.

[174] Mitchell PA, Masri BA, Garbuz DS, Greidanus NV, Duncan CP. Cementless revision for infection following total hip arthroplasty. Instr Course Lect. 2003;52:323-30. Epub 2003/04/15.

[175] Hubble MJW, Whittaker, J.P., Blake, S.M., Briant-Evans, T. Cement In Cement revision. In: Ling RSM, Princess Elizabeth Orthopaedic Hospital. Exeter Hip U, editors.

The Exeter hip : 40 years of innovation in total hip arthroplasty. Exeter: Exeter Hip Publishing; 2010. p. 369 p.

[176] Bourne RB, Hunter GA, Rorabeck CH, Macnab JJ. A six-year follow-up of infected total hip replacements managed by Girdlestone's arthroplasty. J Bone Joint Surg Br. 1984;66[3]:340-3. Epub 1984/05/01.

[177] Castellanos J, Flores X, Llusa M, Chiriboga C, Navarro A. The Girdlestone pseudarthrosis in the treatment of infected hip replacements. Int Orthop. 1998;22[3]:178-81. Epub 1998/09/05.

[178] Conway JD, Mont MA, Bezwada HP. Arthrodesis of the knee. J Bone Joint Surg Am. 2004;86-A[4]:835-48. Epub 2004/04/08.

Chapter 23

Management of Prosthetic Infection According to Organism

Trisha Peel, Kirsty Buising, Michelle Dowsey and Peter Choong

Additional information is available at the end of the chapter

http://dx.doi.org/10.5772/53244

1. Introduction

Since the advent of prosthetic joint replacement surgery, patients with arthritis have had significant improvement in pain-relief, mobility and quality of life. Approximately 90,000 Australians undergo joint replacement surgery each year [1]. With an ageing population, this number will increase (figure 1). Similar data from USA predicts that by 2030 the number of procedures per year will increase to 4.05 million [2]. Despite the overall success of this surgery, infection of the prosthesis remains a devastating complication [3]. Of concern, the incidence of prosthetic joint infection is increasing, in proportion to the number of procedures being performed [4]. Significant patient morbidity is associated with prosthetic joint infections, including the need for further operative procedures, long-term antibiotic therapy with associated toxicity, and prolonged hospitalisation [3]. In addition, the cost to the health system is substantial. The cost of treating infection is 3-5 times the cost of primary arthroplasty [5, 6]. In Australia, the annual additional expenditure incurred as a result of this devastating complication is estimated at AUD $90 million per year [6]. In the United States, the annual cost of treatment of prosthetic joint infection is projected to exceed US$1.6 billion dollars by 2020[7].

The incidence of prosthetic joint infection is estimated at 1-3% of all prosthetic joint replacements [3]. In prosthetic hip replacement, the rate of infection is estimated at 0.88% and in knee replacement at 0.92%[4]. The incidence of prosthetic joint infections is higher for upper limb arthroplasty; in shoulders the incidence of infection is 1.8-4% and in elbow replacements the incidence of infection is 3-7.5% of patients [8-10].

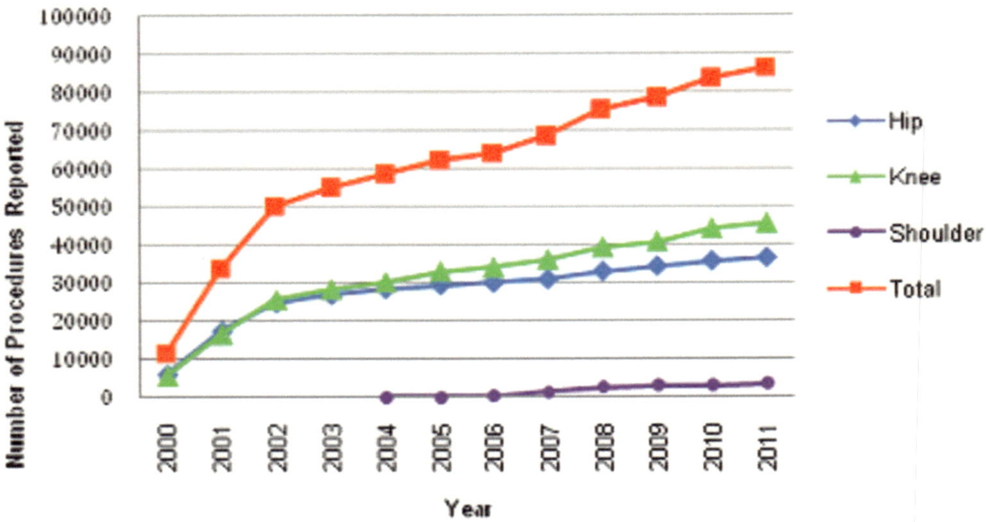

Figure 1. Prosthetic Joint Replacement Surgery in Australia *(adapted from AOA National Joint Replacement Registry[1])*

A number of pre-operative factors have been implicated in the development of prosthetic joint infection, including revision arthroplasty, diabetes mellitus and rheumatoid arthritis [11-16]. The risk factors for prosthetic joint infection differ according to the joint replaced. Obesity plays a greater role in the evolution of prosthetic joint infection in lower limb arthroplasty [17-19]. The presence of post-operative wound complications, including high drain tube losses, wound discharge and superficial surgical site infection have been implicated as risk factors for development of prosthetic joint infection in hip and knee arthroplasty[11, 20]. In addition the presence of a drain tube appears to be protective for prosthetic knee infections [17, 18]. Underlying inflammatory arthritis and concomitant steroid use increases the risk of infections in all arthroplasty surgery but the association is particularly marked in the upper limb [16, 17]. In addition male gender has been identified as a risk factor in shoulder arthroplasty infection, potentially through the interaction with *Propionibacterium acnes* (see below)[12].

2. Pathogenesis

There are two main mechanisms of acquisition of prosthetic joint infection; (i) direct inoculation of the prosthesis at the time of surgery or with manipulation of the joint and (ii) seeding from the blood stream at a later time[3]. The pathogenesis of prosthetic joint infections differs to that of many other bacterial infections through the property of microorganisms to form biofilms[3]. Microorganisms can exist in two phenotypic forms: the planktonic form which is encountered in the majority of acute bacterial infections such as bacterial septicaemia or pneumonia, and the sessile form associated with medical device infections such as prosthetic joint infections[21]. In medical device associated infections, the planktonic bacteria seed the device and undergo a phenotypic change transforming into the sessile bacteria. The biofilm is comprised of the sessile bacteria and the extracellular matrix they secrete[21]. This matrix protects the microorganisms from antibiotics and the host immune response and is thought to be the underlying reason for persistence of infections[21].

3. Microbiology

Staphylococcus aureus and coagulase negative Staphylococcus species are the most common aetiological agents of prosthetic joint infections. The incidence of methicillin resistant strains such as methicillin resistant *Staphylococcus aureus* (MRSA) differ globally; the rate of MRSA prosthetic joint infections across Europe and the Americans MRSA ranges from 8% to 30%[22-24]. In Australia, 26% of prosthetic joint infections are due to MRSA. In addition, methicillin resistant coagulase negative Staphylococci account for a further 22% of isolates [25, 26].

Gram negative bacilli such as *Escherichia coli* and *Pseudomonas aeruginosa* are the next most common isolates[3, 26]. Other microorganisms such as enterococci, streptococci, corynebacterium, fungal species and mycobacterial species are reported less commonly [3, 27]. Of note, the microbiology of prosthetic joint infection differs between upper limb and lower limb arthroplasty: *Propionibacterium acnes* is one of the most common microorganisms encountered in shoulder prosthetic joint infection, occurring in up to 40% of shoulder arthroplasty infections [16, 28, 29]. This association may be due to the increased occurrence of *Propionibacterium acnes* around the head and neck, in particular in the sebaceous glands and hair bulbs [12].

From a review of 6,282 prosthetic hip and knee replacements performed at St Vincent's Hospital Melbourne (SVHM) between 2000 and 2012, there were 138 definite infections (table 1). Prosthetic joint infection was defined by the typical diagnostic criteria which include those discussed further in table 2. Microorganisms were defined as the causative pathogen/s if isolated on two or more intra-operative specimens.

The microbiology of hip and knee prosthetic joint infection was similar, except for an increased number of culture negative infections in prosthetic knee joints and increased isolation of *Enterococcus faecalis* from prosthetic hip infections. From SVHM data there was an increased rate of incisional surgical site infections in knee arthroplasties that later developed prosthetic joint infections compared to hip arthroplasty (28% versus 12%)[17, 30]. Therefore it is postulated that the increased number of culture negative infections in the knee replacement patients may reflect increased antibiotic exposure for superficial wound complications or for unrecognised prosthetic joint infection.

	Number (%) of Prosthetic Knee Infections (n=66)	Number (%) of Prosthetic Hip Infections (n=72)	Number (%) of All Prosthetic Joint Infections (n=138)
Gram positive organisms	48 (73%)	60 (83%)	108 (78%)
Staphylococcus aureus	25 (38%)	35 (49%)	60 (43%)
Methicillin sensitive	16 (24%)	17 (24%)	33 (24%)
Methicillin resistant	9 (14%)	18 (25%)	27 (20%)
CNS	14 (21%)	13 (18%)	26 (19%)
Methicillin sensitive	1 (2%)	0	1 (1%)
Methicillin resistant	13 (20%)	13 (18%)	26 (19%)
Streptococcus species	4 (6%)	2 (3%)	6 (4%)
Enterococcus faecalis	4 (6%)	10 (14%)	14 (10%)
Other gram positive organisms*	3 (5%)	1 (1%)	4 (3%)
Gram negative organisms	9 (14%)	14 (19%)	23 (17%)
Escherichia coli	1 (2%)	3 (4%)	4 (3%)
Morganella morganii	4 (6%)	0	4 (3%)
Klebsiella pneumoniae	0	1 (1%)	1 (1%)
Serratia marcescens	2 (3%)	0	2 (1%)
Pseudomonas aeruginosa	0	1 (1%)	1 (1%)
Citrobacter koseri	0	1 (1%)	1 (1%)
Enterobacter cloacae	0	3 (4%)	3 (2%)
Proteus mirabilis	2 (3%)	4 (6%)	6 (4%)
Bacteroides fragilis	0	1 (1%)	1 (1%)
Culture negative	17 (26%)	11 (15%)	28 (20%)

CNS = Coagulase negative Staphylococcus species

* Other gram positive isolates included 1 Peptostreptococcus species, 1 Bacillus cereus and 2 Corynebacterium species

Table 1. Microbiology of 138 prosthetic hip and knee joint infections seen at SVHM between 2000 and 2012

4. Clinical classification and presentation

Prosthetic joint infections are classified as (i) early (developing in the first three months after implantation), (ii) delayed (occurring 3 to 24 months after surgery) and (iii) late (greater than 24 months) or (iv) haematagenous [3]. Haematogenous seeding of the prosthesis typically occur late (after 24 months) but can occur at any time point following implantation [3, 31].

http://dx.doi.org/10.5772/53244

The clinical manifestation differs according to time of presentation. In early prosthetic joint infection, patients typically present with surgical wound complications such as purulent discharge, erythema and swelling of the affected joint (Figure 2) [3, 32]. In delayed and late infections, pain is the predominant feature with patients reporting a history of slowly increasing pain involving the prosthetic joint [32]. Haematogenous infections in contrast, typically are associated with a history of a joint that was free of any problems for several months to years before an acute onset of fever, erythema around the surgical wound and pain in the affected joint[33].

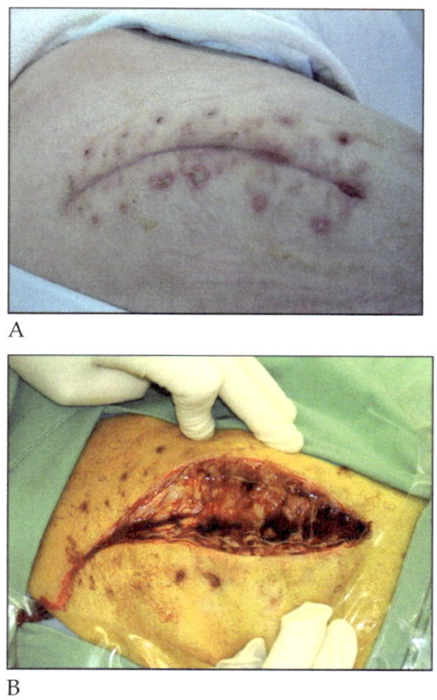

Figure 2. Early Prosthetic Hip Joint Infection (A) at presentation with infection showing wound erythema, swelling and purulent discharge and (B) intra-operative appearance showing purulence surrounding the prosthetic joint.

The presentation of shoulder arthroplasty infection due to *Propionibacterium* acnes is generally delayed or late[12]. The classic features of infection are frequently absent with pain and stiffness of the joint the predominant symptoms [12, 34]. Bruising along the surgical wound has been described as a pathognomonic sign of *Propionibacterium acnes* shoulder arthroplasty infection [34].

5. Diagnosis of prosthetic joint infections

The diagnosis of infections is challenging due to the absence of an internationally accepted gold standard for defining arthroplasty infection. Current definitions rely on a number of parameters including clinical, microbiological and histopathological features (Table 2) [3, 35-39].

Prompt recognition and diagnosis of prosthetic joint infection is imperative to minimize patient suffering and to improve patient outcomes [40]. Isolation of the causative microorganism is the most important diagnostic test as it allows confirmation of diagnosis and assessment of antimicrobial susceptibilities. Infection of the prosthesis is suggested by the isolation of the same microorganism from 2 or more intra-operative specimens [3, 35, 36] To increase the likelihood of diagnosis, ≥5 peri-prosthetic tissue specimens should be obtained intra-operatively with each specimen placed in separate sterile containers [35, 36]. This is of particular importance for skin commensals such as *Propionibacterium acnes* and coagulase negative Staphylococcus species to aid in distinguishing true infection from specimen contamination.

The diagnosis of prosthetic joint infection should be considered in patients with any of the following [3, 36-39]:
Presence of peri-prosthetic purulence observed intra-operatively; OR
Isolation of indistinguishable micro-organism/s on ≥2 intra-operative specimens (tissue or joint aspirate cultures); OR
Presence of a sinus tract in communication with the prosthetic joint; OR
Histopathological features of acute infections with ≥5 neutrophils per-high power field (x 500 magnifications) in 5 different microscopic fields.

Table 2. Diagnosis of Prosthetic Joint Infection

Prior exposure to antibiotic therapy increases the risk of culture negative prosthetic joint infection [30, 37, 41]. Therefore antibiotic therapy should not be commenced until after obtaining multiple intra-operative specimens, except in the case of the septic patient in whom commencement of antibiotic therapy should not be delayed. In patients with delayed and late infections, who have received antibiotic therapy prior to obtainment of intra-operative cultures, definitive surgery may be delayed for 2-4 weeks after cessation of antibiotics to increase the intra-operative yield[30, 37, 41].

Sonication of the explanted prosthesis disrupts the biofilm and may increase the diagnostic yield of microbiological culture. Sonication is particularly useful in patients who have received antibiotics in 14 days preceding surgery [37]. Prolongation of microbiological cultures from 3 to 14 days also increases the diagnostic yield, particularly of more fastidious organisms such as *Propionibacterium acnes* [42].

6. Management of prosthetic joint infection

The goal of treatment of prosthetic joint infection is to eradicate the biofilm dwelling microorganisms, whilst maintaining function of the joint and patient quality of life[3].

The surgical strategies to manage prosthetic joint infection include: (i) one-stage or two-stage exchange procedures, (ii) debridement and retention of the prosthesis in conjunction with biofilm active antibiotics, (iii) removal of the prosthesis +/- arthrodesis, (iv) amputation of the affected limb and (v) chronic suppression without surgical debridement of the infected joint. Removal of the prosthesis and amputation are associated with significant impairment of mobility. Chronic suppression is association with a high rate of recurrence of infection. Therefore these strategies are reserved for patients with significant co-morbidities or in patients with recalcitrant infection [3, 33]. Exchange procedures and debridement and retention are the two strategies that best meet the goals of treatment [3, 33].

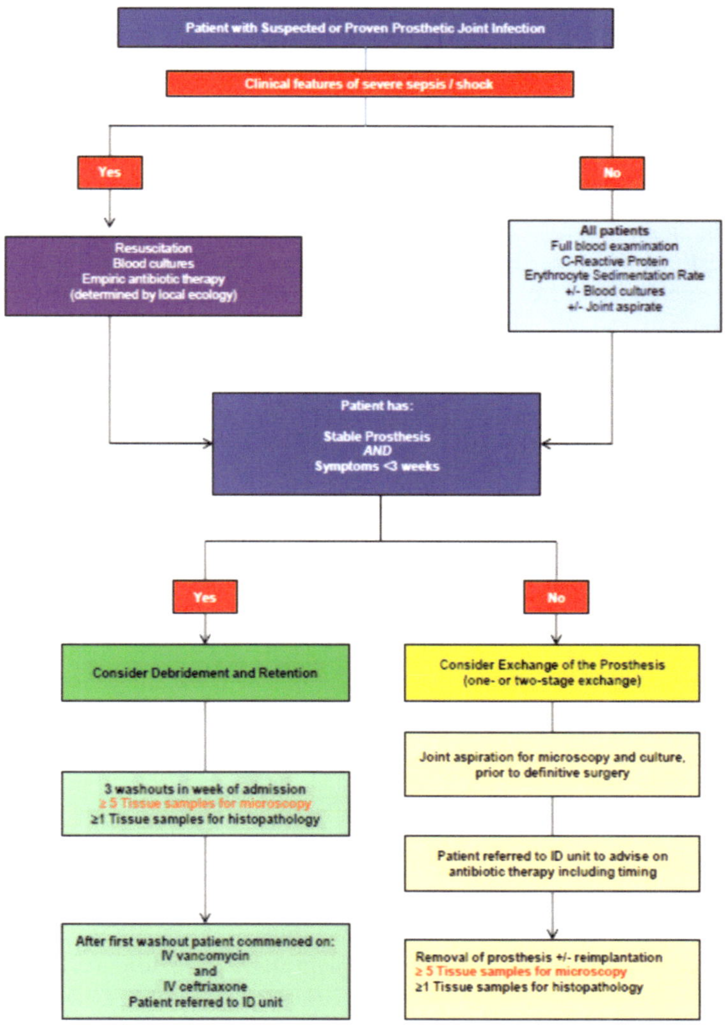

Figure 3. SVHM Protocol Algorithm for Management of Prosthetic Joint Infection

Given the heterogeneous nature of prosthetic joint infections there are no large randomized control trials to guide recommendations. Surgical strategies differ significantly worldwide; exchange procedures are the favoured treatment modality in Northern America, whereas debridement and retention is more commonly performed in Australia and parts of Europe [3, 26, 33]. A number of treatment algorithms exist to guide management decisions and these are based on factors such as duration of symptoms, the stability of implant, patient co-morbidities and the type of infecting microorganism[3, 33]. Compared to the exchange procedures, patients managed with debridement and retention of the implant undergo fewer and less extensive surgical procedures and have shorter duration of hospitalisation and immobilisation [3, 33, 43]. Therefore early and haematogenous infections can be managed by debridement and retention. However, if the implant is loose, if the duration of symptoms prior to presentation exceed 21 days or if the isolated pathogen is resistant to biofilm-active antibiotics, the likelihood of treatment success for debridement and retention is markedly reduced[3, 33]. Therefore if the patient has any of the above features, expert opinion recommends patients undergo prosthesis exchange (either as a one-stage or two-stage procedure). Delayed or late prosthetic joint infections should be managed by one- or two-stage exchange; debridement and retention of the prosthesis in this setting is associated with a high failure rate[3, 33].

At SVHM, a management protocol was established through collaboration between the Orthopaedic and Infectious Diseases Departments. The abbreviated algorithm is shown in Figure 3. The antibiotic regimens for different pathogens are detailed in Table 3. At SVHM patients managed by debridement and retention of the prosthesis undergo 3 debridements of the infected joint. The liner is changed, where feasible, but other mobile parts are not routinely changed. This differs from other protocols for debridement and retention, in which patients undergo a single debridement with exchange of all mobile parts and liners [33]. Regardless of technique, the aim of the debridement/s is to reduce the microbial burden prior to instigation of antibiotic therapy with activity against the biofilm-dwelling microorganisms.

7. Staphylococcus aureus and coagulase negative Staphylococcus species

Rifampicin has excellent activity against Staphylococcal biofilms and is the mainstay of treatment in these infections, particularly with debridement and retention [3, 33, 44-46]. Older treatment algorithms recommended against debridement and retention for MRSA however, emerging evidence suggests that this is a suitable strategy in carefully selected patients [33, 46, 47].

Staphylococcus becomes rapidly resistant to rifampicin if this antibiotic is used alone, therefore rifampicin must always be administered with a second agent (companion drug) [48]. Fluoroquinolones, such as ciprofloxacin, are frequently used as companion drugs however fluoroquinolone resistance is increasing thus limiting the utility of this combination[25]. Alternate companion drugs for rifampicin include fusidic acid, trimethoprim-sulfamethoxazole, minocycline, daptomycin and linezolid [33, 47-52]. There are no clinical studies comparing the efficacy of different drugs used in combination with rifampicin. In Australia including SVHM, fusidic acid is commonly prescribed as a companion drug for rifampicin [47] [26].

Rifampicin based regimens are recommended even for methicillin sensitive isolates. Given the high oral bioavailability of rifampicin, a move to oral therapy is suggested as soon as the patient can reliably take oral diet after completion of surgical debridements. For those few patients who are bacteraemic, however, more prolonged intravenous therapy may be required along with appropriate investigation to exclude other foci of infection, such as endocarditis.

In patients with MRSA infections managed with two-stage exchange; the insertion of a spacer should be avoided as there is an increased rate of treatment failure [3, 33, 53]. In addition, an association between the presence of a spacer and the development of rifampicin resistance in MRSA strains has been reported [53].

8. Streptococcus

Streptococcus are the causative agent in 8% of prosthetic joint infections[26]. In general the treatment outcomes are excellent for all surgical strategies for Streptococcal arthroplasty infection [54-58]. However, the outcomes with group B streptococcal infections are mixed with some studies reporting poorer outcomes with these isolates [58-60]. In general intravenous benzylpenicillin or ceftriaxone can be used (often for 2 weeks) before a shift to high dose oral amoxicillin. In some circumstances, with typable streptococci where susceptibility to rifampicin is expected, rifampicin can be added to the amoxicillin as part of the oral regimen although the evidence for this practice is still not clear.

9. Enterococcus

Enterococcus is an uncommon cause of prosthetic joint infection however, the incidence of these infections is increasing[61]. At our institution, *Enterococcus faecalis* was isolated in 10% of all infections. It is a common isolate in polymicrobial infections of the prosthetic hip joint. There are little published data to guide treatment of enterococcal prosthetic joint infection. Some experts recommend treatment strategies extrapolated from other enterococcal infections, in particular enterococcal endocarditis [61]. Beta-lactam antibiotics, such as penicillin are bacteriostatic against enterococci, therefore combination therapy with aminoglycosides such as gentamicin, is recommended for management of enterococcal endocarditis[62]. However data from retrospective studies suggest there is no additional benefit with combination therapy with aminoglycosides in enterococcal prosthetic joint infections and, of great concern, there was significant nephrotoxicity and ototoxicity associated with aminoglycoside therapy[61]. Euba et al examined the role of ampicillin-ceftriaxone combination therapy, however, only 3 patients with enterococcal prosthetic joint infection were included in this study and 2 of those patients had late infections[63]. Therefore the role of this combination therapy remains unclear and further studies are required. Recent in-vitro models have suggested rifampicin in combination either with ciprofloxacin or linezolid are the most efficacious antibiotic combinations against biofilm dwelling Enterococcus faecalis, although there are no reports at present of the use of these combinations in patients[64].

Enterococcus faecium is infrequently involved in prosthetic joint infections; however, it presents significant treatment challenges, owing to increased resistance when compared to *Enterococcus* faecalis. In particular, *Enterococcus faecium* is increasingly resistant to benzylpenicillin and amoxicillin[62]. There is little clinical data outlining management approaches for *Enterococcus faecium,* however, exchange procedures are likely to be the optimal strategy in these infections. Other resistant enterococcal prosthetic joint infection including vancomycin resistant enterococcus (VRE), also are very uncommon. In a statewide review of 163 prosthetic joint infections, VRE was isolated once (0.6%). Two-stage exchange of the prosthesis is recommended for VRE arthroplasty infections in conjunction with agents such as daptomycin, linezolid or pristinamycin. In all enterococcal infections, including VRE, the use of spacers in two-stage exchange procedures is not recommended due to the increased risk of treatment failure [3, 33].

10. Gram negative bacilli

For gram-negative bacilli infections, ciprofloxacin has been shown to be effective in guinea pig tissue cage models[65]. There is conflicting data on the clinical outcomes of gram-negative bacilli infections, particularly with debridement and retention. The reported success rate for debridement and retention ranges from 27%-94% with a similar range reported for exchange procedures [66-70]. The likelihood of success may relate to the quality of the debridement and meticulous care should be taken to ensure removal of all dead and devitalised tissue and removal of all cement in the exchange procedures [69]. In addition, gram-negative bacteria, particularly *Pseudomonas aeruginosa,* have a propensity to develop resistance to fluoroquinolones in-vivo[62]. In light of this, many experts recommend a 2-4 week course of beta-lactam antibiotic prior to commencement of ciprofloxacin to reduce the bacterial load and thus reduce the likelihood of generation of in-vivo resistance [33].

11. Propionibacterium

As with all other infections, the duration of symptoms dictates the most appropriate surgical strategy for *Propionibacterium acnes* prosthetic joint infection. In *Propionibacterium* arthroplasty infection, the majority of cases are delayed or late presentations, with a long duration of symptoms[12]. Therefore prosthesis exchange is the surgical modality of choice.

Evidence of the ability of *Propionibacterium acnes* to form biofilms is emerging. A number of in-vitro models have been developed to assess the activity of antibiotics against biofilm-associated *Propionibacterium.* As with staphylococcal biofilm models, the activity of rifampicin is preserved with *Propionibacterium* biofilms[71]. The emergence of rifampicin resistance with monotherapy has not been demonstrated[71]. In one study combination therapy with daptomycin and rifampicin was the most effective treatment regimen[71]. Other studies have demonstrated penicillin alone or combination therapy with rifampicin and linezolid are also effective against *Propionibacterium* biofilms[72].

http://dx.doi.org/10.5772/53244

The antibiotic regimens reported to treat patients with *Propionibacterium acnes* prosthetic joint infection are diverse and include: penicillin, amoxicillin, ceftriaxone, clindamycin and rifampicin-fluoroquinolone or rifampicin-clindamycin combination therapy [73, 74]. In general, we recommend IV benzylpenicillin followed by high dose oral amoxicillin combined with rifampicin.

12. Fungi

Fungal prosthetic joint infections are rare. The majority of fungal prosthetic joint infections are due to Candida species however, other fungal species have been reported including Aspergillus species, *Cryptococcus neoformans*, Zygomycetes, *Histoplasma capsulatum, Rhodotorula minuta* [75-78] (figure 4).

The results for debridement and retention and exchange procedures for management of fungal prosthetic joint are poor. In treatment guidelines from the Infectious Diseases Society of America, resection arthroplasty is recommended for prosthetic joint infection due to candidal species[79]. In addition, the use of a spacer following resection of the prosthesis is associated with a high rate of failure and should be avoided [75, 80]. If reimplantation is considered following prosthesis resection, a prolonged period (3-6 months) prior to reinsertion is recommended [81]. Finally, in candidal prosthetic joint infections, there is emerging evidence that the activity of caspofungin is better preserved in the presence of biofilm, compared to fluconazole [80, 82]. For other non candidal fungi, individualized expert advice should be sought to guide antimicrobial choice.

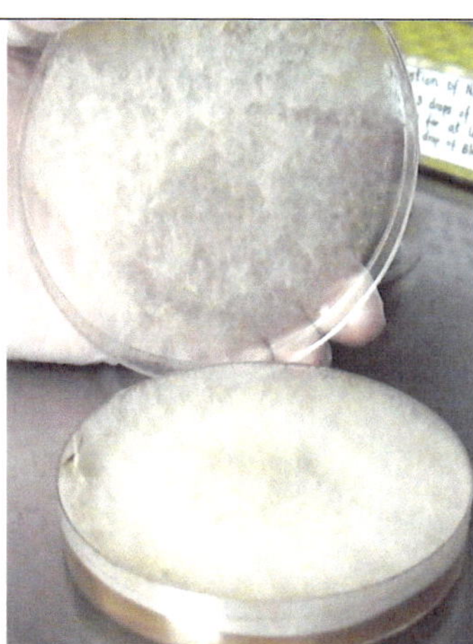

These microbiological cultures were obtained from a patient with disseminated Rhizopus infection including prosthetic hip joint involvement. The patient had significant comorbidities and was managed with debridement and retention of the prosthesis and long-term posaconazole therapy[76].

Figure 4. Rhizopus species cultured from an infected prosthetic hip joint. Photo courtesy of Dr Harsha Sheorey, Microbiology Department, St Vincent's Hospital Melbourne.

13. Culture negative

One of the greatest challenges in management is the 'culture negative' prosthetic joint infection. In published case series, the reported rate of culture-negative prosthetic joint infection ranges from 5-41% [3, 27, 83]. A number of factors contribute to the failure of microbiological cultures to isolate a pathogen including poor culture technique (including obtaining fewer than 5 intra-operative specimens), fastidious organisms that are difficult to culture and prior antibiotic exposure that impedes bacterial growth. Of these mechanisms, prior antibiotic exposure is the most common reason for failing to isolate a causative pathogen. In some studies, 44% of patients with culture negative prosthetic joint infection were receiving antibiotic therapy at the time of obtainment of microbiological specimens[30]. Indeed, the receipt of antibiotics in the 3 months prior to presentation with prosthetic joint infection, lead to a 5-fold increased chance of culture-negative prosthetic joint infection [41].

The choice of antibiotic treatment in culture negative prosthetic joint infection should be guided by local ecology. In addition, if patients had prior exposure to antibiotic therapy, the spectrum of these antibiotics may also influence subsequent antibiotic selection. The results for culture negative prosthetic joint infection are generally similar to culture positive prosthetic joint infection [41].

14. Conclusion

With an ageing population and the increasing popularity of arthroplasty, prosthetic joint infection will continue to present a diagnostic and management challenge to clinicians. Treatment approaches for arthroplasty infection are still under debate, in particular, optimal treatment strategy for different microorganisms. Increasing understanding of the role of biofilm in the pathogenesis of prosthetic joint infections and investigation of the activity of different antimicrobial agents against biofilm associated microorganisms will provide important information to guide therapy. In addition, multicentre studies and collaborative research groups are key to providing more detailed treatment particularly for less commonly encountered pathogens.

Author details

Trisha Peel, Kirsty Buising, Michelle Dowsey and Peter Choong

University of Melbourne, St. Vincent's Hospital Melbourne, Australia

References

[1] Australian Orthopaedic Association. National Bone and Joint Registry Annual Report 2011. Adelaide 2011.

[2] Kurtz S, Ong K, Lau E, Mowat F, Halpern M. Projections of primary and revision hip and knee arthroplasty in the United States from 2005 to 2030. Journal of Bone and Joint Surgery 2007;89-A(4):780-5.

[3] Zimmerli W, Trampuz A, Ochsner PE. Prosthetic-joint infections. New England Journal of Medicine. 2004;351(16):1645-54.

[4] Kurtz SM, Lau E, Schmier J, Ong KL, Zhao K, Parvizi J. Infection burden for hip and knee arthroplasty in the United States. Journal of Arthroplasty. 2008;23(7):984-91.

[5] Bozic KJ, Ries MD. The impact of infection after total hip arthroplasty on hospital and surgeon resource utilization. Journal of Bone and Joint Surgery. 2005;87-A(8): 1746-51.

[6] Peel TN, Dowsey MM, Buising KL, Liew D, Choong PF. Cost analysis of debridement and retention for management of prosthetic joint infection. Clinical Microbiology and Infection. 2011;in press.

[7] Kurtz SM, Lau E, Watson H, Schmier JK, Parvizi J. Economic burden of periprosthetic joint infection in the United States. Journal of Arthroplasty. 2012;in press.

[8] Coste JS, Reig S, Trojani C, Berg M, Walch G, Boileau P. The management of infection in arthroplasty of the shoulder. Journal of Bone and Joint Surgery 2004;86-Br(1):65-9.

[9] Vergidis P, Greenwood-Quaintance KE, Sanchez-Sotelo J, Morrey BF, Steinmann SP, Karau MJ, et al. Implant sonication for the diagnosis of prosthetic elbow infection. Journal of Shoulder and Elbow Surgery. 2011;20(8):1275-81.

[10] Achermann Y, Vogt M, Spormann C, Kolling C, Remschmidt C, Wust J, et al. Characteristics and outcome of 27 elbow periprosthetic joint infections: results from a 14-year cohort study of 358 elbow prostheses. Clinical Microbiology and Infection. 2011;17(3):432-8.

[11] Berbari EF, Hanssen AD, Duffy MC, Steckelberg JM, Ilstrup DM, Harmsen WS, et al. Risk factors for prosthetic joint infection: case-control study. Clinical Infectious Diseases. 1998;27(5):1247-54.

[12] Kanafani ZA, Sexton DJ, Pien BC, Varkey J, Basmania C, Kaye KS. Postoperative joint infections due to Propionibacterium species: a case-control study. Clinical Infectious Diseases. 2009;49(7):1083-5.

[13] Poss R, Thornhill TS, Ewald FC, Thomas WH, Batte NJ, Sledge CB. Factors influencing the incidence and outcome of infection following total joint arthroplasty. Clinical Orthopaedics and Related Research. 1984;182:117-.

[14] Bengtson S, Knutson K. The infected knee arthroplasty. Acta Orthopaedica Scandinavica. 1991;62(4):301-11.

[15] Yang K, Yeo SJ, Lee BP, Lo NN. Total knee arthroplasty in diabetic patients: a study of 109 consecutive cases. Journal of Arthroplasty. 2001;16(1):102-6.

[16] Topolski MS, Chin PYK, Sperling JW, Cofield RH. Revision shoulder arthroplasty with positive intraoperative cultures: the value of preoperative studies and intraoperative histology. Journal of Shoulder and Elbow Surgery. 2002;15(4):402-6.

[17] Peel TN, Dowsey MM, Daffy JR, Stanley PA, Choong PF, Buising KL. Risk factors for prosthetic hip and knee infections according to arthroplasty site. Journal of Hospital Infection. 2011;79(2):129-33.

[18] Dowsey MM, Choong PFM. Obese diabetic patients are at substantial risk for deep infection after primary TKA. Clinical Orthopaedics and Related Research. 2009;467(6):1577-81.

[19] Dowsey MM, Choong PF. Obesity is a major risk factor for prosthetic infection after primary hip arthroplasty. Clinical Orthopaedics and Related Research. 2008;466(1): 153-8.

[20] Surin VV, Sundholm K, Backman L. Infection after total hip replacement. With special reference to a discharge from the wound. Journal of Bone and Joint Surgery 1983;65-Br(4):412-8.

[21] Costerton JW. Bacterial biofilms: a common cause of persistent infections. Science. 1999;284(5418):1318-22.

[22] Parvizi J, Ghanem E, Azzam K, Davis E, Jaberi F, Hozack W. Periprosthetic infection: are current treatment strategies adequate? Acta Orthopedica Belgium. 2008;74(6): 793-800.

[23] Pulido L, Ghanem E, Joshi A, Purtill JJ, Parvizi J, Pulido L, et al. Periprosthetic joint infection: the incidence, timing, and predisposing factors. Clinical Orthopaedics and Related Research. 2008;466(7):1710-5.

[24] Moran E, Masters S, Berendt aR, McLardy-Smith P, Byren I, Atkins BL. Guiding empirical antibiotic therapy in orthopaedics: The microbiology of prosthetic joint infection managed by debridement, irrigation and prosthesis retention. Journal of Infection. 2007;55(1):1-7.

[25] Nimmo GR, Pearson JC, Collignon PJ, Christiansen KJ, Coombs GW, Bell JM, et al. Prevalence of MRSA among Staphylococcus aureus isolated from hospital inpatients, 2005: report from the Australian Group for Antimicrobial Resistance. Communicable Diseases Intelligence. 2007;31(3):288-96.

[26] Peel TN, Cheng AC, Buising KL, Choong PF. The microbiological aetiology, epidemiology and clinical profile of prosthetic joint infections: are current antibiotic prophy-

laxis guidelines effective? Antimicrobial Agents and Chemotherapy. 2012;56(5): 2386-91.

[27] Steckelberg JM, Osmon DR. Prosthetic Joint Infections. In: Waldvogel FA, Bisno AL, editors. Infections Associated with Indwelling Medical Devices. 3rd ed. Washington DC: ASM Press; 2000. p. 173-209.

[28] Weber P, Utzschneider S, Sadoghi P, Andress HJ, Jansson V, Muller PE. Management of the infected shoulder prosthesis: a retrospective analysis and review of the literature. International Orthopaedics. 2011;35(3):365-73.

[29] Piper KE, Jacobson MJ, Cofield RH, Sperling JW, Sanchez-Sotelo J, Osmon DR, et al. Microbiologic diagnosis of prosthetic shoulder infection by use of implant sonication. Journal of Clinical Microbiology. 2009;47(6):1878-84.

[30] Berbari EF, Marculescu C, Sia I, Lahr BD, Hanssen AD, Steckelberg JM, et al. Culture-negative prosthetic joint infection. Clinical Infectious Diseases. 2007;45(9):1113-9.

[31] Murdoch DR, Roberts SA, Fowler VG, Shah MA, Taylor SL, Morris AJ, et al. Infection of orthopedic prostheses after Staphylococcus aureus bacteremia. Clinical Infectious Diseases. 2001;32(4):647-9.

[32] Inman RD, Gallegos KV, Brause BD, Redecha PB, Christian CL. Clinical and microbial features of prosthetic joint infection. American Journal of Medicine. 1984;77(1): 47-53.

[33] Trampuz A, Zimmerli W. Diagnosis and treatment of implant-associated septic arthritis and osteomyelitis. Current Infectious Disease Reports. 2008;10(5):394-403.

[34] Kanafani ZA. Invasive Propionibacterium infections. In: UpToDate, Basow, DS (Ed), UpToDate, Waltham, MA; 2012.

[35] Atkins BL, Athanasou N, Deeks JJ, Crook DWM, Simpson H, Peto TEA, et al. Prospective evaluation of criteria for microbiological diagnosis of prosthetic-joint infection at revision arthroplasty. Journal of Clinical Microbiology 1998;36(10):2932-9.

[36] Parvizi J, Zmistowski B, Berbari E, Bauer T, Springer B, Della Valle C, et al. New definition for periprosthetic joint infection: from the workgroup of the musculoskeletal infection society. Clinical Orthopaedics and Related Research. 2011;469(11):2992-4.

[37] Trampuz A, Piper KE, Jacobson MJ, Hanssen AD, Unni KK, Osmon DR, et al. Sonication of removed hip and knee prostheses for diagnosis of infection. New England Journal of Medicine. 2007;357(7):654-63.

[38] Mirra JM, Amstutz HC, Matos M, Gold R. The pathology of the joint tissues and its clinical relevance in prosthesis failure. Clinical Orthopaedics and Related Research. 1976;117:221-40.

[39] Peel TN, Buising KL, Choong PF. Diagnosis and management of prosthetic joint infection. Current Opinion in Infectious Diseases. 2012;in press.

[40] Marculescu CE, Berbari EF, Hanssen AD, Steckelberg JM, Harmsen SW, Mandrekar JN, et al. Outcome of prosthetic joint infections treated with debridement and retention of components. Clinical Infectious Diseases. 2006;42(4):471-8.

[41] Malekzadeh D, Osmon DR, Lahr BD, Hanssen AD, Berbari EF. Prior use of antimicrobial therapy is a risk factor for culture-negative prosthetic joint infection. Clinical Orthopaedics and Related Research. 2010;468(8):2039-45.

[42] Schafer P, Fink B, Sandow D, Margull A, Berger I, Frommelt L. Prolonged bacterial culture to identify late periprosthetic joint infection: a promising strategy. Clinical Infectious Diseases. 2008;47(11):1403-9.

[43] Brandt CM, Sistrunk WW, Duffy MC, Hanssen aD, Steckelberg JM, Ilstrup DM, et al. Staphylococcus aureus prosthetic joint infection treated with debridement and prosthesis retention. Clinical Infectious Diseases. 1997;24(5):914-9.

[44] Zimmerli W, Frei R, Widmer AF, Rajacic Z. Microbiological tests to predict treatment outcome in experimental device-related infections due to Staphylococcus aureus. Journal of Antimicrobial Chemotherapy. 1994;33:959-67.

[45] Zimmerli W, Widmer AF, Blatter M, Frei R, Ochsner PE. Role of rifampin for treatment of orthopedic implant-related staphylococcal infections: a randomized controlled trial. Journal of the American Medical Association. 1998;279(19):1537-41.

[46] Senneville E, Joulie D, Legout L, Valette M, Dezeque H, Beltrand E, et al. Outcome and predictors of treatment failure in total hip/knee prosthetic joint infections due to Staphylococcus aureus. Clinical Infectious Diseases. 2011;53(4):334-40.

[47] Aboltins CA, Page MA, Buising KL, Jenney AWJ, Daffy JR, Choong PFM. Treatment of staphylococcal prosthetic joint infections with debridement, prosthesis retention and oral rifampicin and fusidic acid. Clinical Microbiology and Infection. 2007;13(6): 586-91.

[48] Forrest GN, Tamura K. Rifampin combination therapy for nonmycobacterial infections. Clinical Microbiology Reviews. 2010;23(1):14-34.

[49] Segreti J, Nelson JA, Trenholme GM. Prolonged suppressive antibiotic therapy for infected orthopedic prostheses. Clinical Infectious Diseases. 1998;27(4):711-3.

[50] Soriano a, Gomez J, Gomez L, Azanza JR, Perez R, Romero F, et al. Efficacy and tolerability of prolonged linezolid therapy in the treatment of orthopedic implant infections. European Journal of Clinical Microbiology and Infectious Diseases. 2007;26(5): 353-6.

[51] Rao N, Regalla DM. Uncertain efficacy of daptomycin for prosthetic joint infections. Clinical Orthopaedics and Related Research. 2006;451:34-7.

[52] John A-K, Baldoni D, Haschke M, Rentsch K, Schaerli P, Zimmerli W, et al. Efficacy of daptomycin in implant-associated infection due to methicillin-resistant Staphylo-

coccus aureus: importance of combination with rifampin. Antimicrobial Agents and Chemotherapy. 2009;53(7):2719-24.

[53] Achermann Y, Clauss M, Derksen L, Raffeiner P, Zellweger C, Eigenmann K, et al. Risk factors for rifampin resistance of staphylococci causing periprosthetic joint infections S 7.4. 29th Annual Meeting of the European Bone and Joint Infection Society; September 2 – 4 Heidelberg, Germany2010.

[54] Deirmengian C, Greenbaum J, Stern J, Braffman M, Lotke PA, Booth RE, Jr., et al. Open debridement of acute gram-positive infections after total knee arthroplasty. Clinical Orthopaedics and Related Research 2003;416(11):129-34.

[55] Meehan AM, Osmon DR, Duffy MC, Hanssen AD, Keating MR. Outcome of penicillin-susceptible streptococcal prosthetic joint infection treated with debridement and retention of the prosthesis. Clinical Infectious Diseases. 2003;36(7):845-9.

[56] Everts RJ, Chambers ST, Murdoch DR, Rothwell AG, McKie J. Successful antimicrobial therapy and implant retention for streptococcal infection of prosthetic joints. ANZ Journal of Surgery 2004;74(4):210-4.

[57] Gaunt PN, Seal DV. Group G streptococcal infection of joints and joint prostheses. Journal of Infection. 1986;13(2):115-23.

[58] Sendi P, Christensson B, Uckay I, Trampuz A, Achermann Y, Boggian K, et al. Group B streptococcus in prosthetic hip and knee joint-associated infections. Journal of Hospital Infection. 2011;79(1):64-9.

[59] Zeller V, Lavigne M, Leclerc P, Lhotellier L, Graff W, Ziza JM, et al. Group B streptococcal prosthetic joint infections: a retrospective study of 30 cases. Presse Medicale. 2009;38(11):1577-84.

[60] Zeller V, Lavigne M, Biau D, Leclerc P, Ziza JM, Mamoudy P, et al. Outcome of group B streptococcal prosthetic hip infections compared to that of other bacterial infections. Joint Bone Spine. 2009;76(5):491-6.

[61] El Helou OC, Berbari EF, Marculescu CE, El Atrouni WI, Razonable RR, Steckelberg JM, et al. Outcome of enterococcal prosthetic joint infection: is combination systemic therapy superior to monotherapy? Clinical Infectious Diseases 2008;47(7):903-9.

[62] Mandell GL, Bennett JE, Dolin R. Principles and Practice of Infectious Diseases. 7th ed. Philadelphia, PA, USA: Churchill Livingstone Elsevier; 2010.

[63] Euba G, Lora-Tamayo J, Murillo O, Pedrero S, Cabo J, Verdaguer R, et al. Pilot study of ampicillin-ceftriaxone combination for treatment of orthopedic infections due to Enterococcus faecalis. Antimicrobial Agents and Chemotherapy. 2009;53(10):4305-10.

[64] Holmberg A, Morgelin M, Rasmussen M. Effectiveness of ciprofloxacin or linezolid in combination with rifampicin against Enterococcus faecalis in biofilms. Journal of Antimicrobial Chemotherapy. 2012;67(2):433-9.

[65] Widmer AF, Wiestner A, Frei R, Zimmerli W. Killing of nongrowing and adherent Escherichia coli determines drug efficacy in device-related infections. Antimicrobial Agents and Chemotherapy. 1991;35(4):741-6.

[66] Hsieh P-H, Lee MS, Hsu K-Y, Chang Y-H, Shih H-N, Ueng SW. Gram-negative prosthetic joint infections: risk factors and outcome of treatment. Clinical Infectious Diseases. 2009;49(7):1036-43.

[67] Aboltins CA, Dowsey MM, Buising KL, Peel TN, Daffy JR, Choong PF, et al. Gram-negative prosthetic joint infection treated with debridement, prosthesis retention and antibiotic regimens including a fluoroquinolone. Clinical Microbiology and Infection. 2011;17(6):862-7.

[68] Legout L, Senneville E, Stern R, Yazdanpanah Y, Savage C, Roussel-Delvalez M, et al. Treatment of bone and joint infections caused by gram-negative bacilli with a cefepime-fluoroquinolone combination. Clinical Microbiology and Infection. 2006;12(10): 1030-3.

[69] McDonald DJ, Fitzgerald RH, Ilstrup DM. Two-stage reconstruction of a total hip arthroplasty because of infection. Journal of Bone and Joint Surgery. 1989;71(6):828-34.

[70] Salvati EA, Chekofsky KM, Brause BD, Wilson PD. Reimplantation in infection. Clinical Orthopaedics and Related Research. 1982;170:62-75.

[71] Tafin UF, Corvec S, Betrisey B, Zimmerli W, Trampuz A. Role of rifampin against Propionibacterium acnes biofilm in vitro and in an experimental foreign-body infection model. Antimicrobial Agents and Chemotherapy 2012;56(4):1885-91.

[72] Bayston R, Nuradeen B, Ashraf W, Freeman BJ. Antibiotics for the eradication of Propionibacterium acnes biofilms in surgical infection. Journal of Antimicrobial Chemotherapy 2007;60(6):1298-301.

[73] Lutz MF, Berthelot P, Fresard A, Cazorla C, Carricajo A, Vautrin AC, et al. Arthroplastic and osteosynthetic infections due to Propionibacterium acnes: a retrospective study of 52 cases, 1995-2002. European Journal of Clinical Microbiology and Infectious Diseases 2005;24(11):739-44.

[74] Zeller V, Ghorbani A, Strady C, Leonard P, Mamoudy P, Desplaces N. Propionibacterium acnes: an agent of prosthetic joint infection and colonization. Journal of Infection. 2007;55(2):119-24.

[75] Azzam K, Parvizi J, Jungkind D, Hanssen A, Fehring T, Springer B, et al. Microbiological, clinical, and surgical features of fungal prosthetic joint infections: a multi-institutional experience. Journal of Bone and Joint Surgery. 2009;91-A Suppl 6:142-9.

[76] Peel T, Daffy J, Thursky K, Stanley P, Buising K. Posaconazole as first line treatment for disseminated zygomycosis. Mycoses. 2008;51(6):542-5.

[77] Johannsson B, Callaghan JJ. Prosthetic hip infection due to Cryptococcus neoformans: case report. Diagnostic Microbiology and Infectious Disease. 2009;64(1):76-9.

[78] Marculescu CE, Berbari EF, Cockerill FR, 3rd, Osmon DR. Fungi, mycobacteria, zoonotic and other organisms in prosthetic joint infection. Clinical Orthopaedics and Related Research. 2006;451(10):64-72.

[79] Rex JH, Walsh TJ, Sobel JD, Filler SG, Pappas PG, Dismukes WE, et al. Practice guidelines for the treatment of candidiasis. Infectious Diseases Society of America. Clinical Infectious Diseases. 2000;30(4):662-78.

[80] Garcia-Oltra E, Garcia-Ramiro S, Martinez JC, Tibau R, Bori G, Bosch J, et al. Prosthetic joint infection by Candida spp. Rev Esp Quimioter. 2011;24(1):37-41.

[81] Phelan DM, Osmon DR, Keating MR, Hanssen AD. Delayed reimplantation arthroplasty for candidal prosthetic joint infection: a report of 4 cases and review of the literature. Clinical Infectious Diseases. 2002;34(7):930-8.

[82] Uppuluri P, Srinivasan A, Ramasubramanian A, Lopez-Ribot JL. Effects of fluconazole, amphotericin B, and caspofungin on Candida albicans biofilms under conditions of flow and on biofilm dispersion. Antimicrobial Agents and Chemotherapy. 2011;55(7):3591-3.

[83] Bejon P, Berendt A, Atkins BL, Green N, Parry H, Masters S, et al. Two-stage revision for prosthetic joint infection: predictors of outcome and the role of reimplantation microbiology. Journal of Antimicrobial Chemotherapy. 2010;65(3):569-75.

Chapter 24

Periprosthetic Infection Following Total Knee Arthroplasty

Michael Soudry, Arnan Greental, Gabriel Nierenberg, Mazen Falah and Nahum Rosenberg

Additional information is available at the end of the chapter

http://dx.doi.org/10.5772/53250

1. Introduction

One of the most devastating complications of prosthetic knee arthroplasty is a periprosthetic infection. This complication occurs in 1-2% of knee arthroplasties [1,2] and can exceed 4% in immunocompromized individuals [3] and 7% after revision surgery [4]. Prosthetic infection leads to loosening of the implant, [5,6]. In this circumstances revision surgery is required. Because of the diversity of the clinical presentation, i.e. early, intermediate or late infection [1], different surgical methods to treat infected knee prostheses were developed [5,6]. Several treatment methods became well accepted but others are still controversial. In the present review we intend to describe mainly the diagnostic tools for detection of infection and commonly used treatment methods in failed total knee arthroplasty due to infection, with special emphasis on the surgical techniques. Additionally we will describe some trends for the future improvement of the treatment modalities.

2. Pathology and microbiology

The main infecting pathogens, around 50%, of knee prostheses, are the different strains of *Staphylococci*, e.g. coagulase negative *Staphylococci* cause around 27% of knee prostheses infections and *Staphylococcus aureus* is responsible for 23% of infections, according to pooled data from nine different studies [7]. Most of the clinically significant infections are caused by biofilm producing microorganisms. The role of biofilms in pathogenesis of periprosthetic infection is the masking of the pathogens from bodily immune response and antibiotic access. Biofilm is a biological structure containing bacteria in a planktonic form imbedded in extracellular matrix made of different polysaccharide molecules, proteins and extracellular DNA (Figure 1). Biofilm generation goes through four consecutive steps: adherence of the pathogens to the surface of prosthesis, accumulation of the biofilm components, maturation of the biofilm and finally its detachment and spread of the microorganisms [8]. The ability of the microorganism to produce masking biofilm defines its virulence in prosthetic infection. Commensal bacteria, such as coagulase negative *Staphylococci* are more frequent in immediate and early prosthetic infections, when spread from the surgical wound edges and in late low grade infections. In late infections by hematogeous spread the *Staphylococcus aureus* is the most important causative factor [9].

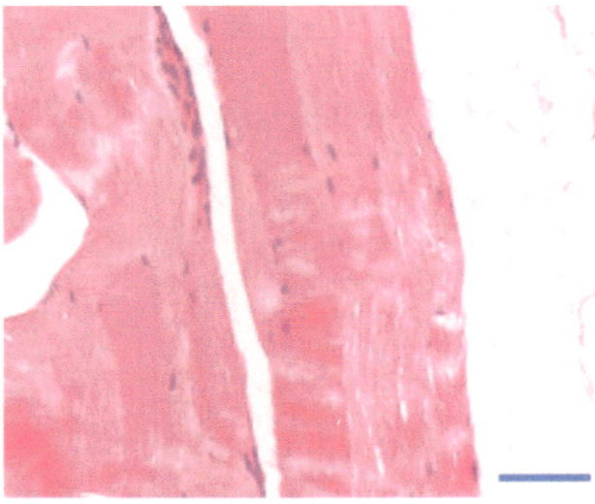

Figure 1. Microscopic image (H&E staining, scale 100µ) of biofilm found at the edge of retrieved tibial component of infected knee prosthesis. Amorphous fibrin-like substance, mostly acellular, is evident

3. Timing of occurence

Infections associated with prosthetic joints are classified according to time at detection as: early (develop less than 3 months after surgery), delayed [3 to 24 months after surgery) or late (more than 24 months after surgery) [10]. Clinical manifestations are in relation with timing [11]. In early cases clinical manifestations are joint pain, effusion, erythema and warmth of the joint. In delayed cases there are subtle signs such as implant loosening, persistent joint pain. Infection is generally provoked by less virulent microorganism. Late are acquired during hematogenous seeding. In a study of infection with THA during a 16 years period, 29 % of cases were early infections, 41 % delayed and 30% late infections [12].

4. Diagnosis

Accurate and early diagnosis is the first step in effectively managing patients with prosthetic joint infection. Clinical history, physical examination, laboratory data and imaging studies are all taken into consideration. In addition to cultures, the most commonly used laboratory tests include serum inflammatory markers and synovial fluid cytology.

http://dx.doi.org/10.5772/53250

Plain films: The appearance of rapidly progressive radiolucent lines surrounding an implant may be present during an infection. The resorption of subchondral bone and patchy osteoporosis are strong elements of suspicion (Figure 2).

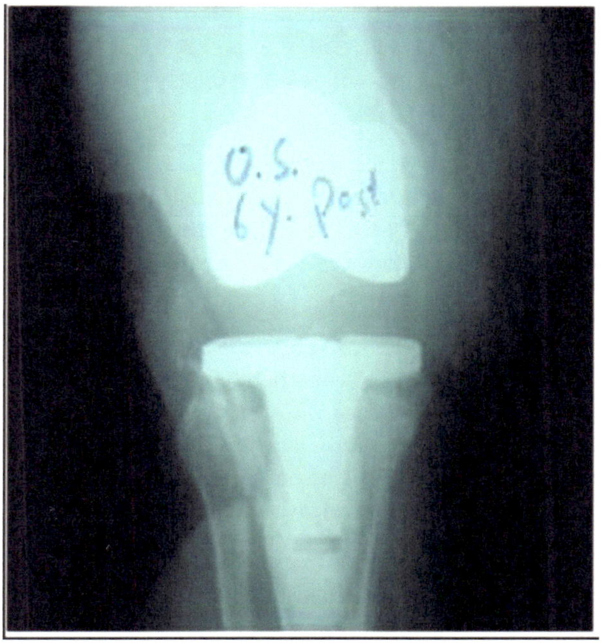

Figure 2. Radiograph of right knee (anterior-posterior view) showing radiolucency under the tibial component indicating periprosthetic infection.

Bone scan: bone scan can help confirm a diagnosis. However its high cost and its inability to provide acceptable levels of sensitivity and specificity have restricted its use. Although bone scintigraphy with technetium 99 m – labeled methylene diphosphonate has a high sensitivity, it lacks specificity for infection [13]. A technetium bone scan remains positive more than one year after implantation because of increased periprosthetic bone remodeling. Bone scan alone without labeling of the white cell has been found to have no role in diagnosing prosthetic joint infection. However, the use of indium 111 labeled leucocyte is time consuming and requires specialized labelling facility [14].

Laboratory tests: There is no evidence supporting the role of WBC and/or white cell blood differential in diagnosis of presence or absence of infection. ESR and CRP are valuable markers for both diagnosing and monitoring periprosthetic infection. After surgery the C Reactive protein level is elevated and return to normal within weeks. Serial postoperative measurements are more informative than single values [15].

Elevated serum interleukin-6 level correlated positively with the presence of periprosthetic infection in patients undergoing a reoperation at the site of a total hip or knee arthroplasty.

In a prospective, case-control study of 58 patients undergoing revision surgery of total hip and knee arthroplasties, serum Interleukin-6 values >10 pg/mL was reported to have a sensitivity of 100%, specificity of 95%, positive predictive value of 89%, negative predictive value of 100% and accuracy of 97% [16].

Knee aspirate cell count and differential: Synovial fluid cell count and differential is a very useful diagnostic test. Antibiotics should be suspended, if possible, for 10 to 14 days before carrying out the aspiration. Traumatic aspirations will result in falsely elevated leukocyte counts.

Polymerase chain reaction (PCR): This method is used to detect and amplify the presence of bacterial DNA. It is thought to be a quick method since it is not affected by whether the patient takes antibiotics or not. However, a high percentage of false negative test results has been detected [17]. Therefore currently this technique can be used as a complementary diagnostic tool to the methods described above.

Sonication: Organisms associated with prosthetic-joint infection are found attached to the prosthesis, where they often form biofilms. This suggests that obtaining a sample from the implant might improve the diagnosis of prosthetic joint infection by unmasking adherent bacteria from explanted prosthesis by sonication. It was found that culture of samples obtained by sonication of prostheses were more sensitive than conventional periprosthetic-tissue culture for the microbiologic diagnosis of prosthetic joint infection, especially in patients who had received antimicrobial therapy within 14 days before surgery [18].

Intraoperative Frozen Section: The analysis of frozen histological sections is a valuable tool for diagnosing infection. It most often used to assist decision-making in cases with equivocal serum inflammatory makers and aspirate cytology. The cutoff value of >5 neutrophils per high power field at a magnification of 400 is most commonly used for the diagnosis of infection. The sensitivity is more than 80 percent and a specificity of of more than 80 percent [19].

Intraoperative Gram Stain: This modality is unreliable (sensitivity = 27%) and should not be used routinely. The AAOS guideline recommends against the use of intraoperative gram stain to rule out periprosthetic infection [20].

5. Management of total knee arthroplasty infection

There are several options when it comes to managing an infected TKA. But before we select any of these, we must take into consideration a series of factors. These factors include the amount of time elapsed from infection, host-related factors, condition of the soft tissues, condition of the implant, virulence of microorganism present and its degree of sensitivity and, last but not least, the patient's expectations and functional needs.

Planning for any one option requires having detailed clinical records, cultures, x-rays and information of previously received treatment. It is important to identify high-risk patients, i.e. those receiving immunosuppressive treatment or suffering from malnutrition or systemic disease, trying to improve their general condition as much as possible before surgery.

Physical examination should provide information about the patient's neurovascular situation, articular mobility, the condition of their extensor mechanism and their soft tissues as well as about any previous incisions or the need of skin coverage by a plastic surgeon. Preoperative planning is important. The final goal of treatment is to eradicate infection, ease the pain and preserve the limb's function.

5.1. Antibiotic suppressive therapy

Efficiency of infection eradication with antibiotic therapy only is limited mainly due to the presence of foreign bodies, as implant and acrylic cement, and bacterial biofilm, therefore its use should be restricted to specific circumstances [21,22].

Indications for this type of treatment are as follows: 1) High operative risk due to medical co-morbidities; 2) Presence of low-virulence micro-organisms susceptible oral antibiotics that can be tolerated by the patient; 3) Mechanically stable prosthesis.

Antibiotic treatment should follow 3 basic principles: 1) Use of antibiotics of proven intracellular efficacy such as rifampicin, and new anti-staphylococcal agents. 2) Antibiotics should be combined, using a minimum of two to enhance the possibility of therapeutic success. 3) Long-standing administration, i.e. treatment should last a minimum of 6 months.

The use of new antibiotics could improve results for resistant bacteria. The oxazolidinone linezolid is a new wide-spectrum antibiotic with very attractive pharmacokinetic and activity profiles. It is an antibiotic that acts against methicillin-resistant staphylococci and vancomycin-resistant enterococci.

5.2. Surgical treatment

In early infection debridement and irrigation, without removing the implant, are usually chosen for surgical treatment.

The approach is through the previous surgical wound. Following division the subcutaneous tissue the knee is aspirated again.

Beforehand, the surgeon should carefully evaluate the knee radiographs for any sign of loosening, slight change in the components position, heterotrophic bone formation. All these may indicate chronic situation. Following the surgical exposure the stability of the implant should be evaluated. If reactive tissue found to sprout at the edge of the implant, it also might indicate on chronicity of the infection.[23, 24, 25]

Extensive debridement should be performed followed with vigorous irrigation. The debrided tissue is sent for cultures and pathology while the implant preserved. When no reactive tissue left, last survey should include the gutters, the patellar tracking and the back fold of the knee.

Closure of the knee might need multi layers sutures, using non absorbable materials over heavy drain, which could be left in place for several days to the discharge to stop. Most surgeons allow regular rehabilitation and long term IV antibiotics. Some surgeons leave antibiotic beads and perform recurrent debridement prior to knee rehabilitation [23]

5.3. Delayed or late infections

With delayed or late infection the orthopedic surgeon might face various clinical uncertainties with regard of decision making. The following are the most common clinical situations that are usually encountered:

Suppurating knee with positive cultures

Clinically infected knee with positive laboratory data but negative cultures

Clinically suspected infected knee without support of laboratory data

Clinically not infected knee with positive cultures

5.3.1. Suppurating knee with positive cultures

Identification of the infective germ prior to surgery allows preparation of appropriate antibiotics use within the operation. In some centers single stage revision preferred in cases of low virulence germ, effective antibiotics available both for embedding in the cement and the parenteral line.

Most surgeons favor a two-stage revision instead of a one-stage procedure [26, 27]

5.3.1.1. The two stage procedure

The two-stage procedure is indicated particularly to treat overt infections with an active discharge and virulent organism on culture such as *Staphylococus aureus* and mainly in methicillin-resistant staphylococcus (MRSA). Removal of the implant is done in first stage and implantation of the new prosthesis is performed later and delayed for a variable period of time until all parameters of inflammation disappear (Figure 3).

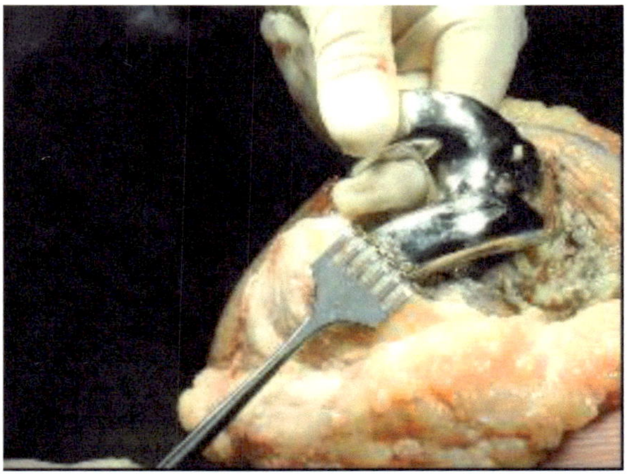

Figure 3. Intraoperative image of the grossly infected knee prosthesis before retrieval

The use of tourniquet without Esmarch bandage is advisable. Careful marking of the scars allows excision of the scars with old suture material. The arthrotomy should follow the original cut with extended lengths if necessary. Careful dissection is utilized in order to protect the vulnerable subcutaneous flaps. If open sinuses exist they should be debrided through the track. Pus and soft tissue are sent to culture with long incubation [28]. Extensive meticulous debridement is performed to the level of natural tissue, removing all synovial necrotic and non viable tissue. [27,29]. All prosthetic components and acrylic cement are removed.

After the implants are exposed from all soft tissue, the anterior surface of the femoral component is gently released as with Gigli saw, the distal part of it is detached by thin osteotome and gentle mallet percussions saving the bone stock, without leaning on the soft infected bone. Following removal of the femoral component the undersurface of the tibial tray is released with a saw and osteotomes which are inserted medially and laterally. Then hammering of the tray away from the tibia is performed. Meticulous removal of **all** pieces of cement **is a must** and,although can be technically demanding, should be accomplished. Thorough debridement is performed again with excision and removal of all remnants of infected tissue. Then the dressing is changed and the knee is draped again. Irrigation should follow with 3 to 4 liters of saline. Five minutes of betadine soaking of the wound should be followed by insertion of antibiotic-impregnated spacers.

A cement spacer impregnated with eluting antimicrobial drugs, according the sensitivity of the infective microorganism, is then interposed between distal femur and proximal tibia. This keeps the limb at its correct length and allows partial joint mobility Non-articulating, or articulated, spacers, can be used according to preference. Few spacer types are used: antibiotic cemented beads, antibiotic cement block, articulating spacer etc [30, 31, 32] (Figure 4).

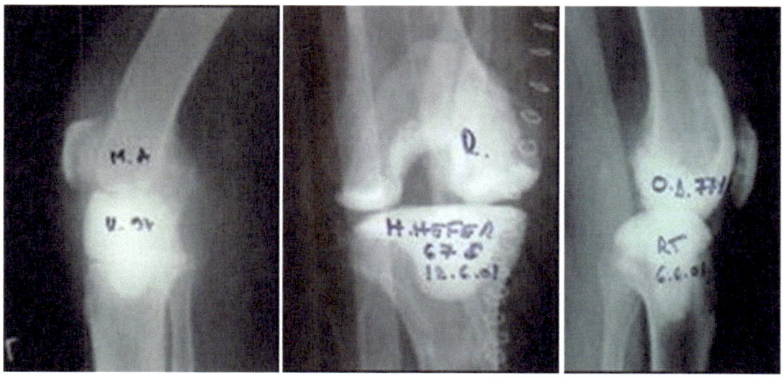

Figure 4. Knee radiographs showing different types of cement spacers

The non articulated spacer is a fixed one, with inherited stability that allows post op full weight bearing but no knee movement. Sometimes an intramedullary nail (abut 30-36 cm long) used to bridge the knee with cement for the enhanced stability. Care should be taken to prevent thermal injuries by the inserted cement at its' extension under the patella.

A divided or articulated spacer contains two parts: one piece should be attached to the proximal tibia and the other to the distal femur. The articulating cement spacer allows the patient to bend his knee, to exercise for range of movement, thus preventing joint contractures and keeping the extensor mechanism integrity.

Adequate hemostasis should follow tourniquet release, irrigation and closure of the wound over a large bore drain.

Antibiotics are administered intravenously according to microbial sensitivity for an average of six weeks. The interval can vary between the two stages, e.g. between six weeks to three months, when the clinical condition is settled. During this period, the clinical recovery is carefully evaluated by the laboratory tests for infection control (ESR and CRP). If there is no clear evidence of clinical improvement, re-arthrotomy and debridement should be considered.

The second stage requires re-arthrotomy through the old scar, tissue is sent for cultures, for pathologic examination, including high power field microscopic examination. The cement spacer is removed; the surgeon should patiently repeat the meticulous debridement. Intense irrigation and change of knee dressing followed by bone preparation and revision implant cementing are performed. A constrained rotating knee prosthesis is generally the most suitable implant particularly in cases of bone loss.

5.3.1.2. The one stage procedure

The use of a single-stage revision is advocated by some in certain patients with known causative organism, when no discharging sinuses are present, the patient is not immunocompromized, and there is no radiological evidence of component loosening or osteitis.

This type of revision is considered when pathogen germ has been definitely identified with appropriate sensitive antibiotic. The cement should contain suitable antibiotics according the sensitivity of the infective pathogen, if it is known; antimicrobial treatment is given 2-3 weeks before prosthesis exchange.

Technically one stage revision procedure includes removal of all foreign material, implant components and cement, thorough the same steps of meticulous debridement, as stated above, and re-implantation of a new prosthesis at the same surgical session.

5.3.2. Clinically infected knee with positive laboratory data but negative cultures

Clinical infection with negative cultures is not rare. A patient may present painful and swollen knee, with synovitis and intraarticular fluid, elevated ESR and CRP, with positive leukocyte bone scan, while aspirated fluid reveal negative cultures. In such a case the aspiration should be repeated, and microbiological studies for rare microorganisms, including PCR should be performed.

The clinical suspicion mandates the type of surgery: The surgical process should be identical to 1st stage revision with extensive debridement and removal of the implant. Multiple bone and soft tissue cultures and pathology should be obtained intraoperatively. Sonication of the prosthesis might be indicated. The cement spacer should contain antibiotics relevant against the common bacteria. Post operative intravenous antibiotics should be administered for six weeks. The 2nd stage is similar to those performed for the positive culture group.

The one-stage type of revision can also be considered in presence of low grade clinical expression, such as long relentless pain, local heat, tenderness and slow rehabilitation milestones, negative preoperative aspiration cultures and intraoperative gram stains, as well as frozen section demonstrating less than 5 polymorphonuclears per high power field. Aged patients with positive cultures for low virulence strains, such as *Staphylococcus epidermidis* and *Streptococcus type* A, are sometimes allocated for revision in a single stage.

5.3.3. Clinically suspected infected knee without support of laboratory data

This group of patients is presented with swollen painful knee, sometimes with synovitis and loosening. Usually not long from the primary surgery, with no sign of polyethylene wear, normal laboratory tests as CRP or ESR, normal blood leukocytes count and negative leukocytes bone scan. Knee aspiration could reveal not clear fluid but with negative culture. In such circumstances repeated aspiration performed and the workup should be extended for material allergy such as nickel and chrome. If the clinical suspicion for infection is significant the surgeon might take steps as for fully infected case, performing two or single stage revision. The decision making in these circumstances lacks a high level of evidence support.

5.3.4. Clinically not infected knee with positive cultures

Bone and soft tissue cultures are part of all knee revision as well as routine sonication of the retrieved implants. Sometimes a positive culture might be discovered in routine, not infected, with normal blood tests, negative leukocyte bone scan and without gross intraoperative signs of infected knee prosthesis. The finding should be carefully evaluated for contamination. If high suspicion for masked infection exists, six weeks of parenteral antibiotic should be administered.

6. Outcome of treatment with surgical revision

As a rule, revision Total Knee Arthroplasty offers inferior results and higher complication rates compared to primary arthroplasty [33].

According to the published data the successful functional results following the treatment of late infection of a total knee arthroplasty by a two-stage re-implantation of a new prosthesis should be expected in about 90% of patients [34, 35, 36, 37].

In spite of its high personal and financial burden the two-stage re-implantation is recognized as the most reliable method for eradicating infection [38]. Although one-stage revision is appealing and less technically demanding, the risk of re-infection is a deterring factor.

Two-stage revision procedures may encounter bone loss, obscure landmarks, structural weakness and soft tissue deficiency, which may result in continued pain, decreased mobility and rarely fractures. Nevertheless, the success rate of this method was found to be in the range of 82-93%, whereas the success rate of the one-stage procedure was of 71-81% [34]. Therefore two-stage re-implantation technique represents the procedure of choice for definitive eradication of infection and preservation of knee function.

According to the published data on one-stage revisions (Table 1) in the large series of patients, with mid-term follow up, around 80% success rate in eradication of infection should be expected.

Author	Year	No. of patients	Follow-up duration	Success rate*
Foerster et al[39]	1991	104	5-15 years	80%
Lu et al[49]	1997	8	20.1 months	100%
Siegel et al[50]	2000	31	2-15 years	71% (22/31)
Buechel et al[27]	2004	22	10.2 years	90.9%
Soudry et al[42]	2009	20	8 years	80% (16/20)

* Rates of infection eradication

Table 1. Results of one-stage knee revision arthroplasty

As early as 1983, Windsor and Insall reported a success rate of 97.4% in two-stage revision surgery in 38 patients, with four years of follow-up, but other reports had slightly lower success rates, around 90% (Table 2).

Author	Year	No. of patients	Average follow-up	Success rate*
Windsor & Insall [40]	1983	384	4 years	97.4%
Hannsen et al [51]	1994	36	52 months	89%
Goldman et al [52]	1996	64	7.5 years	97%
Gacon et al [53]	1997	29	3.5 years	82.7%
Hirakawa et al [53]	1998	55	61.9 months	87.2%
Siebel et al [55]	2002	10	13.5 months	100%
Pietsch et al [56]	2003	24	14.8 months	95.8%
Haleem et al [37]	2004	96	7.2 years	91%
Soudry et al [42]	2009	21	8 years	100%

* Rates of infection eradication

Table 2. Results of two-stage knee revision arthroplasty

http://dx.doi.org/10.5772/53250

In our series of 43 patients with infected TKA, with characteristic 50% rate of infection with Staphylococcal strains [7], twenty patients underwent a one-stage procedure and 21 patients underwent a two-stage procedure. Our overall data indicate 83% postoperative satisfaction with 87% good and excellent results after revision [41,42]. After an average follow-up of 8 years, subjective satisfaction was reported by 80% of patients without any evidence of re-infection in the whole group of these patients. However in one-stage group a recurrent infection was noted in 20% of cases. We use a constrained design of revision prosthesis in order to overcome the expected soft tissue insufficiency in the revised knee (Figure 5).

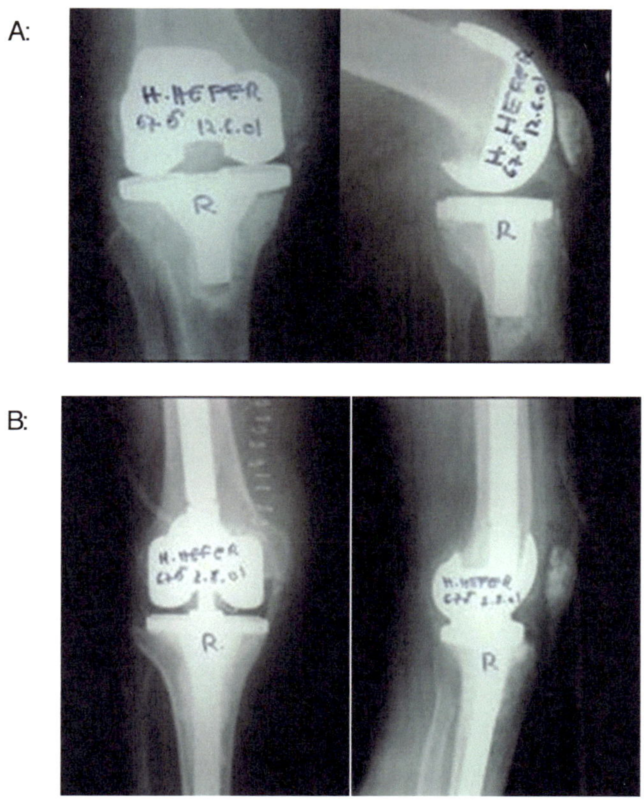

Figure 5. A : Knee radiographs (Anterior-Posterior and Lateral views). Radiolucency is evident around the tibial component indicating septic loosening. B: Knee radiographs (Anterior-Posterior and Lateral views) following revision with a constrained type prosthesis (CCK).

7. Salvage surgical procedures

In failed treatment of revision TKA or in case of a multioperated knee and a debilitated patient another surgical procedure might be required for limb salvage.

7.1. Knee arthrodesis

Knee arthrodesis should be considered as a therapeutic option when other described above techniques have failed, especially in young patients with high functional demands or in patients with extensive deformities, advanced alterations of the extensor mechanism, deficient soft tissues, immunosuppression or infections by highly virulent bacteria. Arthrodesis provides a stable and pain-free limb. However, there is no flexion and the function of the knee is sacrificed, causing an advanced functional impairment. This is generally an irreversible situation. The procedure can be performed with intramedullary nail, metallic plate or external fixation [43, 44] (Figure 6). We have a good clinical experience using the Ilizarov external fixator for this purpose. We used this method in twelve consecutive patients following failed revision TKA surgery performed as treatment for infected initial knee prosthesis. Solid fusion was achieved in all patients within an average healing time of 27.6 weeks. Average shortening of the affected lib was 3.7 cm. We concluded that the Ilizarov fixator for knee arthrodesis after failed TKR produced favorable results and should be considered for the use by surgeons who are familiar with this technique [44]. The success is dependent on the proficiency of the surgeons in Ilizarov method and patient cooperation.

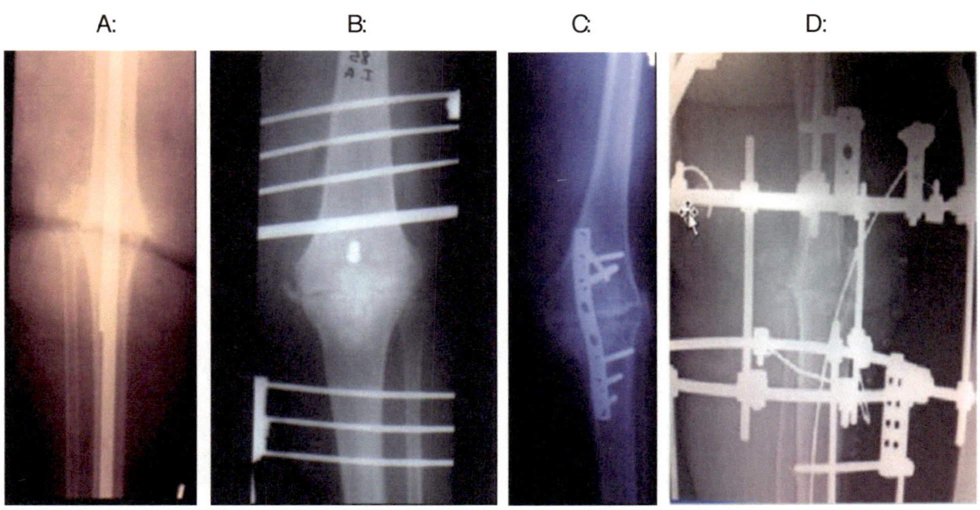

Figure 6. Radiographs of fused knees, following failed revision of TKA, by: A: Intramedullary nail, B: Tubular external fixator. C: Internal fixation by plate and screws, D: Ilizarov external fixator.

7.2. Resection arthroplasty

By this salvage method a permanent removal of the implant and cement with local debridement, without re-implantation, are performed. The purpose of this technique is to create a false joint that may allow a certain range of motion. The leg is immobilized for a period between 3 and 6 months in order to allow the soft tissues retraction with creation of free area for movement with a certain degree of stability. Candidates for this type of treatment are patients with low functional demands [45].

7.3. Limb amputation

This technique should be considered the last resort when dealing with salvage of a prosthetic infection. Its indications are as follows: an uncontrolled infection that threatens the patient's life, large bone loss and severe soft tissue defects [46]. Functional results tend to be extremely poor and patients often end up in a wheelchair. However a successful above knee amputation may provide the best function for patients who otherwise would have a functionless knee joint. In the past limb amputation was required most frequently in infected TKA with cemented stem hinges.

8. Future: Prosthetic design "tuned" to prevention of periprosthetic infection

The best solution is to prevent infection rather than treat it. Nowadays the trend is to design an implant that is less susceptible to infection by using surfaces that will be resistant to bacterial adhesion and generation of biofilm. These designs will be appropriate to prevent infection originating via hematogeous spread. Another approach is to use local slowly released antibacterial agents, such as antibiotics or chemical free radicals, that will keep an efficient periprosthetic high concentration antimicrobial milieu in order to prevent biofilm bacterial masking [47]. This is a very important factor since the effective concentration of antibiotics for penetration of biofilm masking should be 1000 times higher than can be achieved following they usual oral or parenteral administration.

Most of the efforts for generation of anti-biofilm surfaces of the prostheses are still in development stage and still have not gain wide clinical use. Currently three main directions are utilized for this purpose. The most common method is to use titanium surfaces that release bactericidal superoxide radicals [48]. This method is especially appealing since TiO_2 is has no significant cytotoxic effect on mammalian cells. We observed that human osteoblast-like cells in culture remain viable after exposure to high concentration of TiO_2 0.1 mm granules in culture media (10% v:v). Another metal that has bactericidal properties is silver. There are a lot of efforts in designing prosthetic surfaces containing silver [48]. We found that it has a bactericidal effect on different *Staphylococci* strains, but *Pseudomonas aeruginosa* remained resistant to its high concentration (10% v:v). The main problem with the use of silver for prosthetic coating is its toxicity to the host cells. We observed a profound cytotoxic effect in cultures of human osteoblast-like cells exposed to 0.1 mm granules of silver in culture media in bactericidal concentration. For this reason the surfaces coated by TiO_2 have a better bactericidal potential for clinical use.

There is also a possibility to use immobilized antibiotic coverage for prosthetic surfaces. This method is still has not reached a proved clinical use [48].

Currently the widespread method of prosthetic fixation with methyl methacrylate bone cement, containing broad spectrum antibiotics, is the only proven way to create an antimicrobial periprosthetic surrounding. The uncontrolled release of the antibiotics and potential reduced fixation characteristics of the cement containing antibiotics are the main disadvantage of this method, but it is no clinical evidence that might support these concerns.

9. Conclusion

Despite considerable advances in surgical techniques and preoperative care, a 0.5-2% prevalence of infection in total knee arthroplasty (TKA) still poses a great challenge in the treatment of this devastating and costly complication. Current solutions to treat periprosthetic infection remain imperfect. Treatment strategy varies from conservative lifelong antibiotic suppression therapy in the very high risk patient, arthroscopic or surgical debridement, revision in one or two-stage, arthrodesis or resection arthroplasty as a salvage procedure, and amputation in life-threatening conditions. The decision on the best method of treatment should be personalized to the patient's general health, the severity of the infection and the complexity of the surgery. Currently most of the surgeons have adopted the two-stage protocol, where prosthetic removal, debridement and culture-specific I.V. therapy prior to re-implantation are regarded as standards of care. Although one-stage revision procedure is practiced by some, there is no clear evidence to define when this procedure can be safely applied, because there is no sufficient reliable data on a clinical reliability of this approach. The quest to perform one-stage revision should be continued, as two-stage operations classify the patient in a multiple operations category, with all the resulting potential complications, such as arthrodesis and amputation. Nevertheless, the threat of re-infection after the one-stage procedure surpasses the potential benefits. Judicious selection of patients is the key for successful mode of treatment. Currently the two-stage exchange arthroplasty, with all its inherent problems and drawbacks, allows only a partial success in treatment of TKA infection. New modalities or avenues for treatment of prosthetic infection are desirable.

Author details

Michael Soudry[1*], Arnan Greental[2], Gabriel Nierenberg[2], Mazen Falah[2] and Nahum Rosenberg[2]

*Address all correspondence to: michael.soudry@gmail.com

1 Department of Orthopaedic Surgery, Hillel Yaffe Medical Center, Hadera, Israel

2 Rambam Health Care Campus, Dept of Orthopaedic Surgery. Haifa, Israel

References

[1] Zimmerli W., Trampuz A., Ochsner PE. Prosthetic-joint infections. N Engl J Med 2004;351(16):1645-54.

[2] Kurtz SM., Ong KL., Lau E., Bozic KJ., Berry D., Parvizi J. Prosthetic joint infection risk after TKA in the Medicare population. Clin Orthop Relate Res 2010: 468(1):52-56.

[3] Bengtson S., Knutson K. The infected knee arthroplasty. A 6-year follow-up of 357 cases. Acta Orthop Scand 1991; 62(4): 301-11.

[4] Hansen AD., Rand JA. Evaluation and treatment of the infection at the site of a total hip and knee arthroplasry. Instr Course Lect 1999;48:111-122.

[5] Ellenrieder et al. Two-stage revision of implant-associated infections after total hip and knee arthroplasty. GMS Krankenhaushygiene Interdisziplinar 2011;6(1):1-8.

[6] Chiang ER et al. Comparison of articulating and static spacers regarding infection with resistant organisms in total knee arthroplasty .Acta Orthopaedica 2011; 82(4): 460-64.

[7] Peel TN., Buising KL., Choong PFM. Prosthetic joint infection: challenges of diagnosis and treatment. ANZ J Surg ;81: 32-39.

[8] Fey PD., Olson ME. Current concepts in biofilm formation of Staphylococcus epidermidis. Future Microbiol 2010 5(6): 917-933.

[9] Sendi P., Zimmerli W. Challenges in periprosthetic knee-joint infection. Int J Artif Organs 2011; 34(9):947-956.

[10] Schafroth M., Zimmerli W., Brunazzi M., Ochsner PE. Infections. In: Ochsner PE ed. Total hip replacement . Berlin: Springer Verlag; 2003. p65-90.

[11] Zimmerli W., Trampuz A., Ochsner PE. Prosthetic-joint infections. N Engl J Med 2004;351(16):1645-54.

[12] Giuleri SG., Graber P., Ochsner PE., Zimmerli W. Management of infection associated with THA according to a treatment algorithm. Infection; 2004; 32(4):222-8.

[13] Smith SL., Wastle ML., Forster I. Radiolonuclide bone scintigraphy in the detection of significant complications after total knee joint replacement. Clin Radiol; 2001: 56: 221-4.

[14] Hain SF., O'Doherty MJ., Smith MA. Functional imaging and the orthopedic surgeon. J. Bone Joint Surg Br. 2002; 84:315-21.

[15] Shih LY., Wu JJ., Yang DJ. Erythrocyte sedimentation rate and CRP values with THA. Clinic Orthop 1987:225:238-46.

[16] Di Cesare PE., Chang E., Preston CF., Liu CJ. Serum Interleukin-6 as a Marker of Periprosthetic Infection Following Total Hip and Knee Arthroplasty. J Bone Joint Surg Am 2005; 87(9):1921-1927.

[17] Marian BD., Martin DS., Levine MJ., Booth RE., Tuan RS. Polymerase Chain. Reaction Detection of Bacterial Infection in Total Knee Arthroplasty. Clinical Orthop 1996; 331: 11-22.

[18] Trampuz A., Piper K., Jacobson M. et al. Sonication of removed hip and knee prostheses for diagnosis of infection. N Engl J Med 2007;357:654-63.

[19] Tampuz A., Hansen AD., Osmon DR., Mandrekar J., Steckekberg JM., Patel R. Advances in the laboratory diagnosis of prosthetic joint infection. Rev Med Microbiol 2003; 14:1-14.

[20] Parvizi J., Della Valle CJ. In: AAOS Clinical Practice Guideline. Diagnosis and Treatment of periprosthetic joint infections of the hip and knee. J. Am Acad Orthop Surg 2010;18:771-772.

[21] Grogan TJ., Dorey F., Rollins J. et al. Deep sepsis following TKA. JBJS A, 1986: 68:226-234.

[22] Johnson DP., Bannister GC. The outcome of infected arthoplasty of the knee. JBJS B 1986:68;289-291.

[23] Do CSO., Beauchamp CP., Clarke HD., Spangehl MJ. A Two-stage Retention Debridement Protocol for Acute Periprosthetic joint infection. Clin Orthop Relat Res. 2010: Aug;468(8):2029-38.

[24] Parvizi J., Ghanem E., Sharkey P. Prosthetic Joint Infections. Clin Orthop Relat Res 2007; 461:44-47.

[25] Coventry MB., Beckenbaugh RD., Nolan DR., Ilstrup DM. 2,012 total hip arthroplasties. A study of postoperative course and early complications. J Bone Joint Surg Am. 1974;56(2):273-84.

[26] Parkinson RW., Kay PR., Rawal A. A case for one-stage revision in infected totalknee arthroplasty. Knee 2011; 18:1–4.

[27] Buechel FF. The Infected Total Knee Arthroplasty. Just When You Thought It Was Over. The Journal of Arthroplasty 2004; Suppl 4: 19.

[28] Fink B., Gebhard A., Fuerst M., Berger I., Schafer P. High Diagnostic Value of Synovial Biopsy in Periprosthetic Joint Infection of the Hip. Clin Orthop Relat Res. in press.

[29] Nickinson RS.J, Board TN., Gambhir AK., Porter ML., Kay PR. Two stage revision knee arthroplasty for infection with massive bone loss. A technique to achieve spacer stability. Knee 2012;19: 24–27.

[30] Kohl S., Evangelopoulos DS., Kohlhof H., Krueger A., Hartel M., Roeder C., Eggli S. An intraoperatively moulded PMMA prostheses-like spacer for two-stage revision of infected total knee arthroplasty. Knee 2011;18: 464–469.

[31] Choi HR., Malchau H., Bedair H. Are Prosthetic Spacers Safe to Use in 2-Stage Treatment for Infected Total Knee Arthroplasty? J of Arthroplasty 2012; in press.

[32] Macmull S., Bartlett W., Miles GW., Blunn J., Pollock RC., Carrington RWJ., Skinner JA., Cannon SR., Briggs TWR. Custom-made hinged spacers in revision knee surgery for patients with infection, bone loss and instability. Knee 2010;17: 403–406.

[33] Joseph TN., Chen AL., Di Cesare PE. Use of antibiotic-impregnated cement in total joint arthroplasty. J Am Acad Orthop Surg 2003;11:38-47.

[34] Hanssen AD., Rand JA. Evaluation and treatment of infection at the site of a total hip or knee arthroplasty. J Bone Joint Surg 1998; 80:910-922.

[35] Hoad-Reddick DA., Evans CR., Norman .P, Stockly I. Is there a role for extended antibiotic therapy in a two-stage revision of the infected knee arthroplasty?. J Bone Joint Surg Br 2005; 87-B:171-174.

[36] Freeman MA., Sudlow RA., Casewell MW., Radcliff SS. The management of infected total knee replacements. J Bone Joint Surg Br 1985; 67:764-768.

[37] Haleem AA., Berry DJ., Hanssen AD. Mid-term to long-term follow-up of two-stage reimplantation for infected total knee arthroplasty. Clin Orthop. 2004: 428:35-39.

[38] Wilde AH., Ruth JT. Two-stage reimplantation in infected total knee arhroplasty. Clin Orthop 1988; 236:23-35.

[39] Von Foerster G., Klüber D., Käbler U. Mid- to long-term results after treatment of 118 cases of periprosthetic infections after knee joint replacement using one-stage exchange surgery]. Orthopade. 1991 Jun;20(3):244-52.

[40] Windsor R., Insall J. Management of the infected total knee arthroplasty. In: Insall-Scott, eds. Surgery of the Knee. 1st ed. Churchill Livingstone, New York, 1983. 959-974.

[41] Soudry M., Greental A., Niereberg G., Falah M. One and two-stage revision in infected TKA. JBJS B. 2005: Vol 87-B. Supp III: 389.

[42] Soudry M., Nierenberg G., Msika C., Jontschew DA., Falah M. One vs two-stage revision of infected knee arthroplasty. Portugese Journal of Orthopaedics. 2009: Vol 17 (4): 1-11.

[43] Klinger HM., Spahn G., Schultz W., Baums MH. Arthrodesis of the knee after failed infected total knee arthroplasty. Knee Surg Sports Traumatol Arthrosc.2006; 14(5): 447-53.

[44] David R., Shtarker H., Horesh Z., Tsur A., Soudry M. Knee Arthrodesis with the Ilizarov after failed knee arthroplasty. Orthopedics, 2001 Jan: 24(1):33-6.

[45] Falahee MH., Matthews LS., Kaufer H. Resection Arthroplasty as a salvage procedure for a knee with infection after TKA. JBJS A 1987: 69: 1013-1021.

[46] Pring DJ., Marks, Angel JC. Mobility after amputation for failed knee replacement. JBJS B 1988: 70: 770-771).

[47] Vasilev K., Cook .J, Griesser HJ. Antibacterial surfaces for biomedical devices. Expert Rev Med Devices 2009; 6(5): 553-567.

[48] Visai L., De Nardo L., Punta C., Melone L., Cigada A., Imbriani M., Arciala CR. Titanium oxide antibacterial surfaces in biomedical devices. Int J Artif Organs 2011; 34(9):929-946.

[49] Lu H., Kou B., Lin J. One-stage reimplantation for the salvage of total knee arthroplasty complicated by infection. Zhonghua Wai Ke Za Zhi. 1997 Aug;35(8):456-8.

[50] Siegel A., Frommelt L., Runde W. Therapy of bacterial knee joint infection by radical synovectomy and implantation of a cemented stabilized knee joint endoprosthesis. Chirurg. 2000 Nov;71(11):1385-91.

[51] Hanssen AD., Rand JA., Osmon DR. Treatment of the infected total knee arthroplasty with insertion of another prosthesis. The effect of antibiotic-impregnated bone cement. Clin Orthop Relat Res. 1994 Dec;(309):44-55.

[52] Goldman RT., Scuderi GR., Insall JN. 2-stage reimplantation for infected total knee replacement. Clin Orthop Relat Res. 1996 Oct;(331):118-24.

[53] Gacon G., Laurencon M., Van de Velde D., Giudicelli DP. Two stages reimplantation for infection after knee arthroplasty. Apropos of a series of 29 cases. Rev Chir Orthop Reparatrice Appar Mot. 1997;83(4):313-23.

[54] Hirakawa K., Stulberg BN., Wilde AH., Bauer TW., Secic M. Results of two-stage reimplantation for infected total knee arthroplasty. J Arthroplasty. 1998 Jan;13(1):22-8.

[55] Siebel T., Kelm J., Porsch M., Regitz T., Neumann WH. Two-stage exchange of infected knee arthroplasty with a prosthesis-like interim cement spacer. Acta Orthop Belg. 2002 Apr;68(2):150-6.

[56] Pietsch M., Wenisch C., Traussnig S., Trnoska R., Hofmann S. Temporary articulating spacer with antibiotic-impregnated cement for an infected knee endoprosthesis. Orthopade. 2003 Jun;32(6):490-7.

Chapter 25

Articulating Spacers in Infection of Total Knee Arthroplasty — State of the Art

Manuel Villanueva-Martínez, Antonio Ríos-Luna, Francisco Chana-Rodriguez, Jose A. De Pedro and Antonio Pérez-Caballer

Additional information is available at the end of the chapter

http://dx.doi.org/10.5772/53243

1. Introduction

Infection is one of the most devastating complications of total knee arthroplasty. It is also the leading cause of early revision after knee arthroplasty, ahead of instability and aseptic loosening [1].

Treatment of an infected total knee arthroplasty requires 3 to 6 times more hospital resources than a primary arthroplasty and 2 times more than an aseptic revision [2]. The goal of treatment is to eradicate infection and maintain joint function.

Two-stage exchange remains the treatment of choice in cases of late infection, with good or excellent results in 80% to 100% of cases; nevertheless, it is aggressive, costly, and long. It is also considered the treatment of choice in cases of fungal infection, infection by virulent organisms, inflammatory diseases, immunosuppression, and reinfection after reimplantation.

Compared with direct replacement, 2-stage revision of infected arthroplasty has several disadvantages: longer hospital stay, higher cost, longer surgical time, tissue retraction, instability, and functional limitation between procedures. From a technical standpoint, surgical reimplantation may be hampered by retraction of soft tissue and loss of tissue planes.

Most authors agree that almost all of these problems can be minimized using antibiotic-loaded articulating cement spacers, although 2-stage exchange can be used to eradicate infection both with and without cement spacers.

The most consistent results have been published with 2-stage exchange, regardless of variations in the type of spacer, causal microorganism, or duration of infection. In a systematic review of the literature between 1980 and 2005, Jämsen et al. [3] found 31 original articles describing the results of 154 direct exchanges and 926 2-stage exchanges. Eradication rates were 73%-100% for 1-stage exchange and 82%-100% for 2-stage exchange. Final range of motion and reinfection rates were lower in the series that used antibiotic-loaded articulating spacers. No correlation was observed with the type of spacer or functional outcome between direct revision and 2-stage exchange.

2. Spacer types: Nonarticulating and articulating

The 2-stage exchange protocol was designed by Insall in 1983. Since the first report in 1990, long-term results have shown two-stage exchange to be the treatment of choice for infection after total knee arthroplasty [4]. The outcome of the original procedure was poor to fair in 20% of cases, mainly owing to functional disability and retraction of soft tissue. Atrophy, stiffness, bone loss, and increased extensile exposure were observed at reimplantation.

The use of antibiotic-loaded articulating spacers helped to reduce these complications and improve the possibilities of eradicating infection [5-9]. The choice of spacer depends on many factors, including degree of bone loss, state of the soft tissue, choice of antibiotics, and financial and technical restraints. A benefit that is common to both articulating and nonarticulating antibiotic-loaded spacers is the fact that greater intra-articular levels of antibiotic can be delivered than with parenteral antibiotics [10-11].

The approach aims to be above breakpoint sensitivity (ie, the level of antibiotic that sets the boundary between bacterial susceptibility and the development of resistance) and to eradicate infection.

Nonarticulating spacers enable local administration of a high concentration of antibiotic, improve patient autonomy, facilitate outpatient treatment, and maintain the joint space for future procedures.

Borden and Gearen [5], Booth and Lotke [7], and Cohen et al. [12] reported data for antibiotic-loaded beads and cement spacers, which are molded to adapt to the defect created by removal of the infected prosthesis. Although in some cases these authors made the spacer in 2 semi-blocks, thus forming a partial joint, neither the design of the blocks nor the rehabilitation protocol included controlled mobility. Calton et al. [9] modified this approach, although disadvantages were still observed (eg, bone loss when the spacer sank into the tibia).

Other disadvantages of this system are the minimal range of motion of the joint, which can lead to shortening of the quadriceps, capsule, and ligaments, thus increasing the need for extensile approaches with longer surgical time during reimplantation.

Antibiotic-loaded articulating cement spacers can improve function between operations and facilitate the second stage.

Although this approach remains open to debate, most authors agree that articulating spacers provides better functional results and enable more efficacious eradication of infection than nonarticulating spacers [3], [13-15].

The shape and features of articulating spacers vary considerably, from fully manual spacers made in preformed molds to modular spacers, which include plastic and metal surfaces. Spacers differ in price, complexity, and degree of constraint. The advantages of articulating spacers are as follows: retraction of soft tissue and extensor mechanisms is prevented, high doses of antibiotics can be added in the time between operations, bone mass is preserved better than with nonarticulating spacers[9], [16], the need for expanded approaches at reimplantation is reduced, and the success rate is increased. These approaches also enable greater controlled mobility of the joint and application of a partial support brace, thus facilitating acceptable function between procedures.

3. Historical development of articulating spacers

Use of antibiotic-loaded articulating spacers was first reported by Wilde and Ruth [6] in 1988. This was the first attempt to reduce complications due to functional disability between operations, as observed in the initial work by Windsor and Insall [4].

Preformed articulating systems (PROSTALAC®) first appeared in 1992. Their main advantage was excellent tolerability and function between procedures, thanks to high joint congruence and reduced friction [17]. Their disadvantages include high cost, presence of metal and plastic surfaces that could facilitate bacterial growth, and size limitations. Preformed articulating systems are not widely used because of their price and the theoretical risk that the presence of metal and plastic components facilitates persistence of infection, although this has not been confirmed in clinical practice. Therefore, other factors (eg, aggressiveness of the microorganism, addition of high proportions of cement, and antibiotic treatment) may be more important than the type of spacer used.

Hand-made cement articulating spacers, however, maintain almost all the advantages of preformed spacers, although they also have a series of drawbacks.

Between these extremes, many authors have developed modifications to minimize the disadvantages of hand-made spacers and PROSTALAC® spacers, by adapting them to their technical and economic possibilities. The real impact of the theoretical advantages of the different types of spacer is unknown.

The main forms are as follows:

1. Manual construction of a spacer with cement in the operating room by recreating the normal anatomy of the patient [18], [19] (Figure 1) or more congruent systems (ball and socket) [20] (Figure 2).

2. Construction of customized spacers in the operating room using prefabricated silicone or aluminum molds [21], [22], or using trial components to shape the spacer [23]. Cement

molds can be made during surgery using trial components, and the definitive spacer can be made using these cement molds [24], [25].

3. Prefabricated spacers made of cement only [26].
4. Cement components in combination with modular components made of plastic and metal (PROSTALAC®, DePuy, Warsaw, Indiana) [27], [28].
5. Resterilization of the prosthesis and insertion of a femoral component and a tibial polyethylene insert with cement or a new prosthesis as a spacer (prosthesis-spacer) with high antibiotic loads [29], [30].
6. Combinations of these approaches for moderate or massive defects [31], [32].

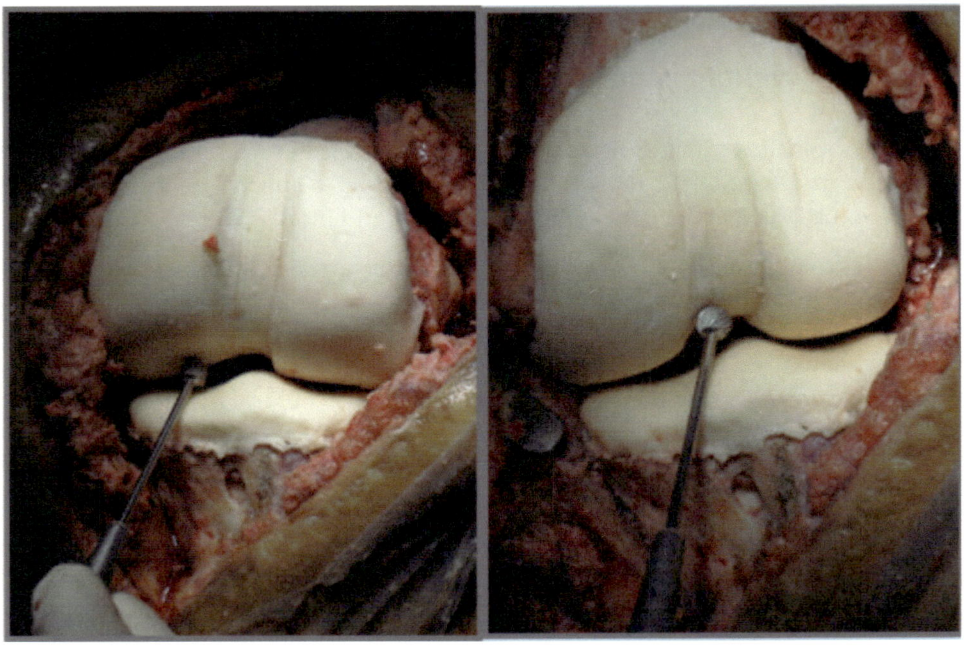

Figure 1. Remodeling prominent areas of a hand-made spacer with a high-speed burr.

Favorable results have been reported with each of these types of spacers. The more rudimentary a spacer is, the lower its congruence and the greater the sensation of popping, giving way, or instability. In contrast, it is cheaper, more widely available, and versatile. The specific advantage of spacers built manually with cement only is that the whole spacer is loaded with antibiotics, and these can be tailored to the causative organism. The spacer does not include plastic, metal, or resterilized parts and can be applied in any operating room with no need for specific instruments. The main disadvantage of cement spacers is the lack of optimal congruence, instability, and the difficulty in modeling, especially with high antibiotic loads (>10%-15%) (Figure3). In addition, cement-on-cement spacers can cause more inflammatory reactions as a result of particle generation; however, this has not been considered a real problem in published series [18], [21], [24].

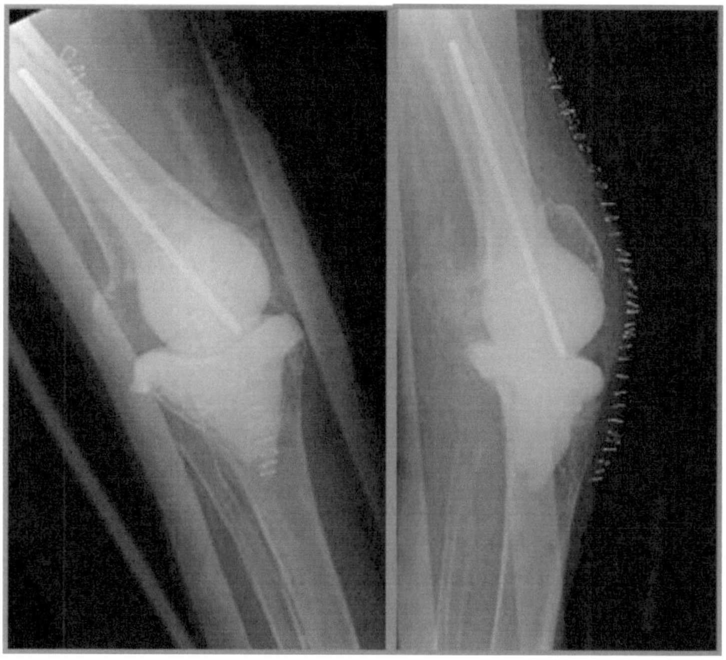

Figure 2. Ball and socket spacer.

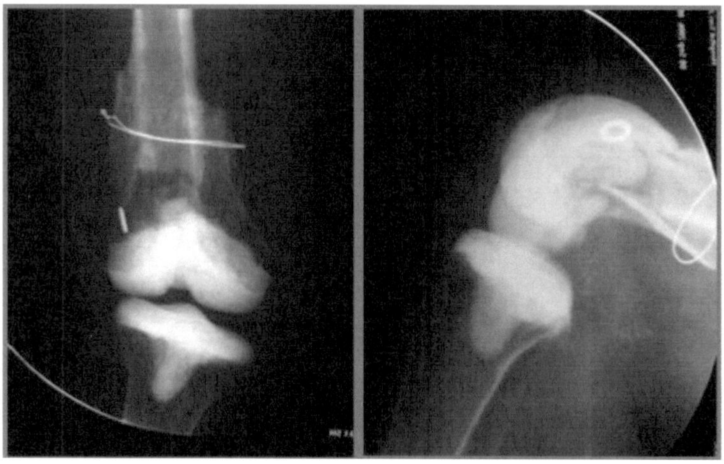

Figure 3. Hand-made spacer for a segmental defect. Excellent range of motion. Due to instability or giving way the patients usually walks with a brace.

Customized spacers constructed completely of cement using prefabricated silicone or aluminum molds are not difficult to shape with greater antibiotic loads.

By contrast, preformed spacers including metal or plastic elements or resterilized prostheses have a limited antibiotic load, which is not tailored to the patient. These spacers involve the insertion of foreign material into a septic environment. In these cases, only the cement fixing the metal components, the prosthesis, or the preformed spacer takes the maximum load of tailored antibiotics.

Also important is the degree of constriction of the spacer. All spacers made intraoperatively with a mold design lack a tibial post and femoral bar; at most, they have a tibial post that gives them some medial-lateral stability. The bar, or lever, which provides anteroposterior stability, is exclusive to PROSTALAC® systems or prosthesis-spacers.

4. Characteristics of antibiotic-loaded spacers

Elution of antibiotics from bone cement depends on several factors: the type of antibiotic, the concentration and combination of antibiotics, the porosity and type of the cement, and the surface of the spacer [33], [34].

4.1. Cement type: Commercially available vs. custom antibiotic-loaded cement

Most commercially available antibiotic-loaded cements, have a low dose of antibiotic, which can act as prophylaxis in patients at risk (ie, double prophylaxis in combination with parenteral antibiotics), or during reimplantation in a 2-stage revision of an infected total knee arthroplasty, but not for the treatment of infection when it is diagnosed[35].

Therefore, surgeons should add antibiotics to the cement to achieve the appropriate doses needed for the treatment of periprosthetic joint infection and to tailor the drug to the causative microorganism.

In comparison with commercial presentations, manually mixed cement releases less antibiotic [33], [34].

Manual mixing of cement and antibiotics increases the porosity of the cement. In theory, this approach weakens the cement, but increases the elution surface, since the antibiotic is released from the surface of the spacer and from cracks in the surface. On the other hand, distribution is not homogeneous (unlike commercially available preloaded cements), thus decreasing the rate of elution from a given surface [36], [37]. One study showed that increasing the surface area of bone cement by 40% yielded a 20% increase in the elution rate of vancomycin [38].

The addition of dextran increases porosity and elution rates. Kuechle et al. [39] noted that when dextran was added at 25%, the release of antibiotics during the first 48 hours was about 4 times greater, and the duration of elution reached 10 days instead of only 6, compared with the routine preparation. The same effect was observed with the addition of lactose and xylitol (or other sugars), which increase the release of daptomycin, vancomycin, and gentamicin [33].

Vacuum mixing decreases the porosity of the cement and thus potentially decreases the elution rate. However, this is not true for all cements, because other factors, such as hydrophilicity or viscosity, may be more important than the area of elution.

In a recent study, Meyer et al. [34] compared the elution of 6 commercially available vacuum-mixed and manually mixed antibiotic-loaded cements. All showed detectable antimicrobial activity during the 5 days of the trial, with peak activity on the first day and levels above breakpoint sensitivity. Levels decreased rapidly thereafter. Cumulative antimicrobial activity during the trial was similar with the manually mixed Cemex Genta and the vacuum-mixed Cobalt G-HV and Palacos RG and higher than that of VersaBond AB, Simplex P with Tobramycin, and SmartSet GMV. The cumulative antimicrobial activity of manually mixed Cemex Genta over 5 days was significantly higher than that of Cobalt G-HV and Palacos RG, which in turn significantly higher cumulative antimicrobial activity than VersaBond AB, Simplex P with Tobramycin, and SmartSet GMV. Vacuum mixing increased the cumulative antimicrobial activity of Cobalt G-HV, Palacos RG, and Simplex P with Tobramycin and decreased the activity of Cemex Genta, SmartSet GMV, and VersaBond AB. The antimicrobial activity was similar for Cobalt G-HV and Palacos RG and significantly higher than that of the other cements. Furthermore, vacuum mixing also increased the number of days of elution above the breakpoint sensitivity necessary to eliminate 99% of methicillin-susceptible *Staphylococcus aureus* (MSSA) and methicillin-resistant *S. aureus* (MRSA) and 85% of coagulase-negative staphylococci (CNS) recorded between 2009 and 2010. For Palacos RG, the number of days of elution increased from 2 days for manually mixed cements to 5 days for vacuum-mixed cements. For Cobalt G-HV, this value increased from 2 to 3 days; for Simplex P with Tobramycin it increased from 1 to 2 days. By contrast, vacuum mixing reduced the number of days' elution above this limit for Cemex Genta from 3 days to 1 day. The authors concluded that vacuum mixing had adverse effects on elution with low-viscosity cement (Cemex Genta), positive effects on elution with high-viscosity cements (Cobalt G-HV and Palacos RG), and unpredictable effects on elution with medium-viscosity cements (Simplex P with Tobramycin, SmartSet GMV, and VersaBond AB). Only manually mixed Cemex Genta and vacuum-mixed Palacos RG eluted antibiotics above breakpoint sensitivity on the third day; the remainder did so only on the first day. Although Cobalt G-HV and Palacos RG have a lower gentamicin load, they have greater antimicrobial activity and elution rates than other cements with a higher antibiotic load.

Other studies confirm differences between cements. Stevens et al. [40] studied the *in vitro* elution of antibiotics from Simplex and Palacos cements and noted that Palacos was a more effective vehicle for local administration [41], [42].

4.2. Choice of antibiotic

Antibiotic-loaded cement spacers release high concentrations of drug and enable higher intra-articular concentrations to be reached than parenteral antibiotics alone, with little effect on serum or urine concentrations and therefore with minimal risk of systemic damage [29], [43], [44]. It is essential to achieve local bactericidal concentrations that make it possible to eradicate infection or prevent colonization of the new implant during the reimplantation phase (the "race for the surface").

The antibiotic used must have 2 fundamental properties:

- Thermostability: Polymerization of the cement is an exothermic reaction. The cement increases in temperature within 10-13 minutes, and this change may alter the properties of the antibiotic.
- Water solubility: The antibiotic is disseminated in the tissues surrounding the infected joint. By maintaining the spacer in the joint for no less than 8 weeks, the antibiotic is released at a constant rate. However, the bactericidal effect is concentrated in the early days. Subsequently, spacers fulfill mainly a mechanical function.

The most frequently used antibiotics are tobramycin, gentamicin, vancomycin, and cephalosporins. Antibiotics can be combined to achieve broad-spectrum coverage, depending on the nature of the causative microorganism. Aminoglycoside in powder is recommended, as it does not weaken the cement; however, it is difficult to obtain in some countries. The surgeon's options are therefore limited when combining antibiotics.

Periprosthetic infections are caused mainly by gram-positive microorganisms (*S. aureus* and CNS). When the pathogen and its antibiotic sensitivity profile are clearly identified, a single antibiotic should be administered. When the pathogen is unknown, treatment is more difficult, and a combination of antibiotics can improve the chances of eradicating infection. Vancomycin covers MRSA, gentamicin covers Enterobacteriaceae and *Pseudomonas aeruginosa*, and cefotaxime destroys microorganisms resistant to gentamicin.

In addition to increasing the range of coverage, some combinations of antibiotics have a synergistic effect. Penner et al. [41] observed that the combination of vancomycin and tobramycin acted synergistically, although they discouraged the use of vancomycin in monotherapy. However, other authors have reported excellent results for CNS and MRSA with cement loaded with only 5-7.5% vancomycin (Simplex P, Howmedica, Rutherford, New Jersey, USA: 2-3 g of vancomycin per bag), both in static and in articulating spacers [45].

Synergy between aminoglycosides and vancomycin and, occasionally, a cephalosporin can make it possible to cover a broad spectrum of microorganisms. These antibiotics are usually available in powder form; however, antibiotic-loaded cements are not commercially available. Heraeus are working on a commercial presentation of gentamicin with vancomycin for commercial use in Europe in 2012.

The only commercial presentation with a synergistic effect is Copal, which combines clindamycin and gentamicin. Copal enables increased release of antibiotic and greater ability to inhibit the formation of biofilm than gentamicin alone. Ensing et al. [46] showed that the elution rate of Copal (clindamycin + gentamicin) is much greater than that of other cements, which are also considered excellent [47]. At 7 days, the elution rate was 65% for clindamycin and 41% for gentamicin; for Palacos RG the value for release was 4% for preloaded gentamicin. This increased release of antibiotic resulted in greater and more prolonged inhibition of bacterial growth on agar plates. Gentamicin-susceptible *S. aureus* strains were "small colony variants" that were resistant to gentamicin in Palacos RG and less so to the gentamicin in Copal. Elution of gentamicin in Palacos RG ceased after 72 hours, in contrast with Copal, which maintained bacterial inhibition during the study period. In addition, unlike Copal, Palacos RG was unable to inhibit bacterial growth of gentamicin-resistant CNS. The addition of clindamycin to gentamicin-loaded cement had an additive effect on the inhibition of biofilm. Conversely, although both cements fulfill ISO norms, the mechanical properties of Palacos RG are superior.

The study by Ensing et al. [46] has several practical implications. Synergy can enable the release of greater amounts of antibiotic, thus making inhibition of bacterial growth more effective and increasing the chances of winning the "race for the surface". By achieving high rates of antibiotic elution, even resistant bacteria can be eradicated when the dose rises sufficiently. Finally, given its worse biomechanical properties, Copal seems ideal for articulating spacers, which are withdrawn after a few weeks, but not as appropriate as Palacos RG for definitive reimplantation once the infection has been cured.

Effective elution from cement has also been observed with quinolones, daptomycin, and linezolid, although these agents are difficult to obtain in powder form or are too expensive [48]. Anguita-Alonso et al. [48] compared quinolones, cefazolin, and linezolid and found linezolid to be the most stable antibiotic after polymerization of PMMA. It achieved high peak concentrations at 7.5% and 15%. All detectable concentrations of linezolid were always above the cutoff sensitivity of *Staphylococcus* spp. (≤4 μg/mL).

Daptomycin has also demonstrated the ability to elute in local bactericidal concentrations for *S. aureus* and CNS, with a release profile similar to that of vancomycin [39], [49], [50].

4.3. Fungal infections

In the case of fungal infections, the recommended antibiotic is amphotericin B or fluconazole (Figure 4). 5-Flucytosine is not stable and is therefore not valid for use in cement. Amphotericin can cause nephrotoxicity, hepatotoxicity, chills, nausea, and blood disorders, thus necessitating lower doses and more prolonged treatment. Fortunately, the incidence of fungal infection is low. Most infections are by *Candida* species, of which *C. albicans* accounts for 60%, *C. parapsilosis* 20%, and *C. tropicalis* 20%. More uncommon species include *Coccidioides immitis, Sporothrix schenckii*, and *Blastomyces dermatitidis*.

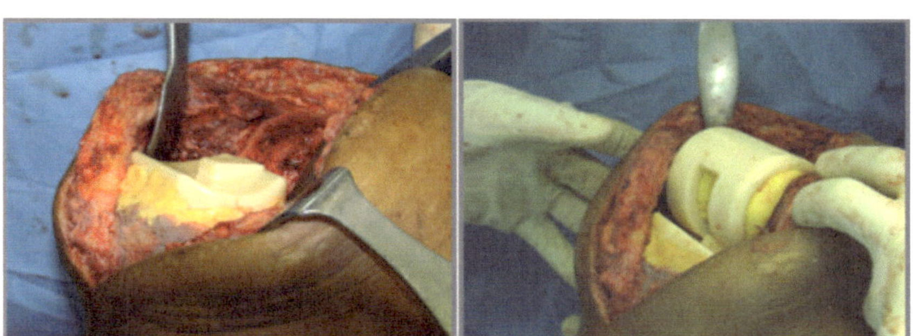

Figure 4. Preformed cement spacer with amphotericin B and fluconazole in a prosthesis with fungal infection.

Immunosuppression, prolonged hospitalization, prolonged intravenous therapy, drug dependence, and inflammatory diseases are risk factors for the development of fungal infections; however, in most published cases the patients did not present these risk factors. A reasonable postulate is that infection is caused by intraoperative inoculation rather than by hematogenous spread. The symptoms are those of a subacute infection, namely, mild to moderate pain or discomfort, effusion, and, occasionally, progressive osteolysis [51]. Published series are very short [52]-[54]. Phelan et al. [55] performed a 2-stage revision procedure with systemic administration of antifungal agents to treat 4 *Candida* infections of total joint arthroplasties. They also identified 6 other cases in the literature that had been treated with the same regimen. In addition to resection arthroplasty, 8 patients received amphotericin B alone or in combination with other antifungal agents, and 1 patient was treated with fluconazole in monotherapy. Eight patients had no recurrence of infection at a mean of 50.7 months after reimplantation.

4.4. Dose of antibiotic

Lewis [33] studied the properties of antibiotic-loaded cements. Elution typically occurs in 3 phases: an exponential phase (during the first 24 hours), a declining phase, and a final low constant elution phase. The exponential phase depends on the diffusion area of the surface of the spacer, although porosity and hydrophilicity of the cement also play a role. Porosity determines the amount of liquid that comes into contact with the surface of the cement, which in turn determines the elution rate of the antibiotic from the surface or from deeper cracks in the cement.

The addition of high doses of antibiotic to the cement is a key element of treatment when attempting to reach maximum intra-articular concentrations in the exponential phase, although some authors have observed persistent effective levels of antibiotics until 4 months after surgery [56].

The antibiotic should not exceed 20% of the total mass of cement. In addition, it should be in powder form, since liquid forms hinder polymerization. No standard ideal dosage of each drug to be mixed with bone cement has been established. Addition of 2 antibiotics to the cement is superior to the addition of 1. The most frequently used doses vary from 2.4 g of tobramycin with 1 g of vancomycin per 40 g of cement to 4 g of vancomycin with 4.6 g of tobramycin per 40 g of cement. These doses have been associated with success rates of above 90% [41], [56].

As the amount of antibiotic powder increases, the strength of the cement decreases. However, antibiotic load seems to be yet another factor within 2-stage exchange, and consistent results have been obtained using unloaded antibiotic spacers or spacers with only minimal loads. Fehring et al. [15] reported efficacious results with 1.2 g of tobramycin per 40 g of bone cement. Mean follow-up was 36 months for patients who received a nonarticulating spacer (88% eradication) and 27 months for patients treated with an articulating spacer (93% eradication).

4.5. Resistance: Mechanical properties of cement

The factors affecting the mechanical properties of the cement are type of cement, proportion and combination of antibiotics, administration in liquid or powder form, and mixing method (manual or vacuum). Cement mixed with cloxacillin, cefazolin, gentamicin, vancomycin, and tobramycin has been shown to maintain good resistance to tension and compression [57], [58].

However, adding liquid antibiotic interferes with early polymerization, leading to a significant deterioration in the properties of the cement, because of the effect of the water and not the properties of the antibiotic itself. For example, addition of liquid gentamicin instead of powder can decrease the resistance of the cement to compression by 49% and the tensile strength by 46%. Tobramycin powder, on the other hand, had not detrimental effects on the spacers [59], [60].

Manually adding antibiotic also weakens the cement. Vacuum-mixed antibiotic-impregnated cement improves its mechanical properties by reducing porosity by up to 20%. It has been estimated that manual mixing causes a 30-40% reduction in resistance and that vacuum mixing can reduce 10-fold the rate of fracture during cyclic loading with spacers [61], [62].

Commercial antibiotic-loaded cements retain their mechanical properties, although the dose may not be sufficient for the treatment of an infection or for the manufacture of spacers, except for some commercial forms, such as Copal.

Duncan [17] reported that manual mixing decreased resistance by 36% with respect to commercially available cement, while the resistance of the latter did not differ from that of nonloaded cement.

Lewis [33] compared several cements and their biomechanical properties after combination with different antibiotics. The composition of the cement was a major factor. The elution rate of vancomycin and tobramycin from Palacos RG is superior to that of Simplex, and the elution rate of Simplex is superior to that of CMW. The combination of antibiotics is also important. Vancomycin combined with tobramycin increases elution with Palacos (the same is true of gentamicin), but with Simplex P, elution of tobramycin decreases, not vice versa. Vacuum mixing also affects elution. CMW variants decrease elution of gentamicin when vacuum-mixed; however, with Palacos the opposite occurs, as confirmed by a recent study [34]. The concentration of vancomycin did not differ significantly depending on whether the cement was mixed manually or by vacuum. These authors also studied the effect of loading and impact cycles, which can lead to minor porosity and cracks in the spacer, thus increasing the elution rate. Among the cements studied, elution only increased with Palamed G, whose porosity is higher. For the remainder, no statistically significant differences were observed between load and lack of impact on the patient.

Also important is the way in which the mixture is made. Hanssen and Spangehl [63] proposed a method for adding high doses of antibiotics to bone cement powder. Polymethylmethacrylate monomer and cement powder must first be mixed to form the liquid cement, and the antibiotic is added afterwards. It is important to leave as many large crystals as possible intact in order to create a more porous mix that increases the elution rate of the antibiotics.

This approach is not applicable when using antibiotic-loaded cement prophylactically, as crystals weaken the cement. Moreover, manual mixing decreases the elution rate in some types of cement. Therefore, commercial forms are preferred.

The method of Frommelt and Kühn [64], namely, fractional addition of antibiotic (now generally recommended), involves the gradual addition of cement and antibiotic powder and mixture of the two until the expected load of antibiotic is complete. The mixture can then be made manually or by vacuum, depending on the type of cement and the availability of vacuum systems. Once mixed, the cement has to be applied in the doughy phase or late phase of polymerization to prevent excessive interdigitation with the bone, thus facilitating extraction during surgery and providing the surgeon with a certain degree of freedom to shape the articular surface of the spacer.

4.6. Safety

As with any treatment, the surgeon must be aware of the possible side effects of the antibiotics used in spacers. Despite the large number of infected arthroplasties treated annually and the widespread use of antibiotic-loaded cement, complications are rare.

Evans [54] used 4 g of vancomycin and 4.6 g of tobramycin in powder per batch of 40 g of polymethylmethacrylate cement in 44 patients with a total of 54 periprosthetic joint infections. Follow-up to a minimum of 2 years showed no renal, vestibular, or auditory effects. Springer et al. [43] studied the systemic safety of cement loaded with high doses of antibiotic over time and reported that an average dose of 10.5 g of vancomycin and 12.5 g of gentamicin was clinically safe, with no signs of acute renal failure or other systemic side effects. In contrast, Van Raaij et al. [65] reported a case of acute renal failure that affected an 83-year-old woman after treatment with 2 g of gentamicin in a 240-g cement block combined with 7 strings of gentamicin-loaded polymethylmethacrylate beads. Serum levels of gentamicin were high, leading to removal of the spacer and eventual recovery of renal function. Ceffa et al. [66] reported 2 cases of mucormycosis after treatment with antibiotic-loaded cement spacers.

The complications reported are rare events in which other factors (eg, blood volume or intravenous antibiotics) could play a role, since the normalization profile of serum antibiotic levels, when using antibiotic-loaded spacers, is exponential and reaches normal values in 24 hours.

5. Results

The use of a polymethylmethacrylate antibiotic-loaded spacer provides not only more effective treatment of periprosthetic infection, with eradication rates ranging from 90% to 100% in the literature, but also improved function, reduced pain, greater patient satisfaction, shorter hospital stay, and lower costs. Few studies analyze developments in the medium-to-long term. Although the results remain more or less stable, up to 30% of patients require revision for loosening, reinfection, or other causes in the medium term [67].

Several studies compare the results of 2-stage exchange with articulating spacers and 28 studies compare the results with a static spacer [3].

Park et al. [68] compared 20 prosthetic knee infections treated with monoblock spacers and 16 treated with articulating spacers. The reinfection rate was 6.3% for the articulating group and 15% for the fixed group. The range of motion with the spacer was 80º and 9º, respectively (final range, 108º and 92º). The clinical and functional score according to the HSS scale was significantly better with the articulating spacer, and the number of extensile exposures was lower. In the static spacer group, 75% of patients (65% of the femurs and 50% of the tibias) had bone loss. This complication was not observed for the articulating spacers.

Meek et al. [27] retrospectively analyzed the results of 2-stage exchange with a PROSTALAC articulating spacer in 47 patients with infected knee prosthesis and a mean follow-up of 41 months. The eradication rate was 96%. The Western Ontario and McMaster Universities Osteoarthritis scale and the Oxford-12 and Short Form-12 scales showed better scores for articulating spacers.

Calton et al. [9] compared the outcomes of patients treated with articulating spacers and patients treated with nonarticulating spacers. Among the 24 patients with a nonarticulating spacer, 60% had an average bone loss of 6.2 mm in the tibia and 12.8 mm in the femur, often with invagination and migration of the spacer and problems of soft tissue retraction. The authors recommended intramedullary extension of the spacer to prevent migration and obtain the appropriate thickness. They also recommended tightening the collateral ligaments to prevent contracture and a block that is sufficiently wide to rest on the cortical rim and prevent migration to cancellous bone. No differences were observed between the groups in eradication rates, time of surgery, or functional outcome.

Fehring et al. [15] studied 25 nonarticulating spacers and 30 articulating spacers and found that articulating spacers facilitated reimplantation and were not associated with bone loss.

Emerson et al. [13] reported that range of motion was greater with articulating knee spacers than with nonarticulating spacers; flexion of the knee averaged 107.8° and 93.7°, respectively, and no evidence of higher complication rates was found.

Therefore, a comprehensive review of the literature provides more arguments for articulating spacers than for static spacers. Articulating spacers seem to be the most widespread form of treatment. The method of making the spacer does not seem to affect eradication rates or functional outcome.

Durbhakula et al. [21] treated 4 patients with antibiotic-loaded articulating spacers made in vacuum-injected silicone molds designed to produce articulating femoral and tibial components. The final average range of motion was 104° and the HSS score was 82. The rate of eradication of infection was 92% after an average of 33 months. A system of this type does not require a metal-polyethylene articulation surface and reduces costs by applying reusable molds that cost about $300 each. The authors reported no problems of dislocation, retraction, bone loss, fracture, or fragmentation of the spacer.

Goldstein et al. [23] formed spacers intraoperatively using cement and test components on aluminum foil to prevent interdigitation. The femoral condyles were molded with the tibial trial implant, and the tibial implant was used to calculate the size and thickness of the cemented tibial component. The authors reported initial success in 5 patients.

MacAvoy and Ries [20] described an inexpensive mold-based method for manufacturing a spherical articulating spacer (ball and socket). They used this method in cases with severe bone deficiency and damage to the ligaments because of its high congruence. The average load was 3.6 g to 4 g of tobramycin + 1 g of vancomycin per bag of Palacos. For an average of 4 cements, this represents a dose of more than 14 g. In 12 patients with severe comorbidities, infection was eradicated in 9 of 13 knees with a mean follow-up of 28 months. All patients could walk with minimal assistance. The average range of motion of the knee with the spacer was 79°, which increased to 98° at the end of treatment. The authors rarely used hinge models, despite serious injury to the ligaments and bone loss.

Using cement spacer molds created intraoperatively with Palacos RG loaded with 0.5 g of gentamicin plus 3 g of vancomycin, Shen et al. [25] obtained 10 reimplantations in 17 cases followed for 30 months. In 5 cases, the spacer was the definitive treatment, in 1 case the joint merged, and 1 patient required amputation. The average range of motion with the spacer was 82° (97° after reimplantation).

Excellent results have been reported with the Hoffman prosthesis-spacer system. Anderson et al. [30] reported a range of motion of 2° to 115°; Huang et al. [69] reported 97.6°, which was smaller than in previous publications (104º to 115º). As for eradication with this type of spacer, reinfection rates are variable: 4% according to Anderson et al. [30] (25 knees), 0%-12% according to Hofmann et al. [29] (22 and 50 patients; Simplex cement with 4.8 g of vancomycin per bag), 9% according to Emerson et al. [13] (22 patients), and 2% according to Cuckler [70] (44 patients).

Ha [24] reported motion ranging from 2° to 104° with manually modeled cement spacers. The study included 12 cases treated with spacers made using the double mold (a cement negative is made with trial components and the definitive spacer is modeled on the negative) and using doses of 4.8 g of tobramycin and 4 g of vancomycin per cement bag. The antibiotic load accounted for 20% of the cement-antibiotic composite.

In addition to the type of spacer, range of motion is influenced by preoperative mobility, the state of the soft tissues, surgical technique, implant selection, early rehabilitation, and patient cooperation. Our group [18] found the range of motion to be 107° after reimplantation using manual spacers and 7.5% antibiotic load.

Soft tissue damage, severe bone loss or general health status, appear to be more important than the treatment method, and the results of 2-stage exchange, which are generally excellent, are much worse in patients with a less favorable health status.

Macmull et al. [71] published 19 cases with the SMILES spacer, which was based on an antibiotic-loaded hinge coated with antibiotic-loaded cement (Palacos RG, Heraeus Medical GmbH, Wehrheim, Germany). The spacer was used in the early stages of chronic infection associated with severe bone loss on revision arthroplasty in 11 cases (58%), tumor endoprostheses in 4 (21%), primary arthroplasty in 2 (11%), and infection on fracture or osteotomy in 2. The eradication rate at 38 months was 63% (12 cases), Four patients (21%) suffered reinfection and 2 were amputees. Jeys et al. [72] reported an eradication rate of 72% in primary infection of massive tumor prosthesis with a 2-stage protocol.

Reinfection after reimplantation has not been adequately studied in the literature, although the high percentage of rescue treatments indicates that reinfection has its own prognostic implications. Therefore, it could be classified as a separate type of infection and independently studied in the future.

Hanssen et al. [73] published a series of 24 reinfections after infected total knee prosthesis. The infection was eradicated in only 1 case. Another patient received suppressive therapy after a new reimplantation, and the rest underwent arthrodesis.

Hart and Jones [74] reported 6 cases of reinfection following 2-stage revision. The infection was eradicated in 2 cases (with another 2-stage revision), 2 patients had bone fusions, and 2 had suppressive treatments.

6. Conclusions

1. Two-stage exchange is considered the treatment of choice in the following circumstances: late infection, unidentified causal microorganisms, fungal infections, infections by virulent organisms, underlying inflammatory diseases, immunosuppression, and reinfection after reimplantation.

2. Articulating spacers can minimize complications between procedures, thus enhancing patient autonomy and mobility, preventing retraction of the soft tissues, and facilitating reimplantation.

3. In addition, articulating spacers seem to improve eradication rates and functional outcomes and reduce complications.

4. The way the spacer is constructed does not seem to affect eradication rates and functional outcome. The surgeon's choice of spacer will depend on technical and financial restraints. Despite their advantages and disadvantages, all types of spacer have demonstrated consistent and reproducible results.

5. Not all cements are equally suitable for the prevention and treatment of infection.

6. The antibiotic should be added as powder to avoid weakening the cement. Appropriate use of synergies increases the spectrum of coverage and elution rate of certain antibiotics.

7. Once fractionated addition is complete, vacuum mixing increases the elution of the antibiotic from the spacer when high-viscosity cements are used. Manual mixing is preferred when low-viscosity cements are used.

Author details

Manuel Villanueva-Martínez[1*], Antonio Ríos-Luna[2], Francisco Chana-Rodriguez[1], Jose A. De Pedro[3] and Antonio Pérez-Caballer[4]

*Address all correspondence to: mvillanuevam@yahoo.com

1 Hospital General Universitario Gregorio Marañón, Universidad Complutense de Madrid, Madrid, Spain

2 Orthoindal Center, El Ejido, Almería University, Almería, Spain

3 Hospital Universitario Salamanca, Salamanca University, Spain

4 Hospital Infanta Elena, Francisco de Vitoria University, Madrid, Spain

References

[1] Sharkey, P. F, Hozack, W. J, Rothman, R. H, Shastri, S, & Jacoby, S. M. Why Are Total Knee Arthroplasties Failing Today?. Clin Orthop (2002). , 404, 7-13.

[2] Iorio, R, Healy, W. L, & Richards, J. A. Comparison of the hospital cost of primary and revision total knee arthroplasty after cost containment. Orthopedics (1999). , 22, 195-199.

[3] Jämsen, E, Stogiannidis, I, Malmivaara, A, Pajamäki, J, Puolakka, T, & Konttinen, Y. T. Outcome of prosthesis exchange for infected knee arthroplasty: the effect of treatment approach. A systematic review of the literature. Acta Orthopaedica (2009). , 80, 67-77.

[4] Windsor, R. E, Insall, J. N, Urs, W. K, Miller, D. V, & Brause, B. D. Two-stage reimplantation for the salvage of total knee arthroplasty complicated by infection: further follow-up and refinement of indications. J Bone Joint Surg Am (1990). A.: 272-8., 72.

[5] Borden, L. S. Gearen PF: Infected total knee arthroplasty: A protocol for management. J Arthroplasty (1987). , 2, 27-36.

[6] Wilde, A. H, & Ruth, J. T. Two stage reimplantation in infected total knee arthroplasty. Clin Orthop (1988). , 23-35.

[7] Booth, R. E, & Lotke, P. A. The results of spacer block technique in revision of infected total knee arthroplasty. Clin Orthop (1989).

[8] Hoffman, A. A, Kane, K. R, Tkach, T. K, Plaster, R. L, & Camargo, M. P. Treatment of infected total knee replacement arthroplasty using an articulating spacer. Clin Orthop (1995). , 321, 44-54.

[9] Calton, T. F, Fehring, T. K, & Griffin, W. L. Bone loss associated with the use of spacer blocks in infected total knee arthroplasty. Clin Orthop (1997). , 345, 148-54.

[10] Jiranek, W. A, Arlen, D, Hanssen, A. D, & Greenwald, A. S. Antibiotic-loaded bone cement for infection prophylaxis in total joint replacement. J Bone Joint Surg Am. (2006). , 88, 2487-2500.

[11] Alt, V, Bechert, T, & Steinrücke, P. In vitro testing of antimicrobial activity of bone cement. Antimicrob Agents Chemother (2004). , 48, 4084-8.

[12] Cohen, J. C, Hozack, W. J, Cucker, J. M, & Booth, R. E. Two stage reimplantation of septic total knee arthroplasty: report of three cases using an antibiotic PMMA spacer block. J Arthroplasty (1988). , 3, 369-77.

[13] Emerson Jr RHMuncie M, Tarbox TR, Higgins LL. Comparison of a static with a mobile spacer in total knee infection. Clin Orthop (2002). , 404, 132-8.

[14] Cui, Q, Mihalko, W. M, Shields, J. S, Ries, M, & Saleh, K. J. Antibiotic-impregnated cement spacers for the treatment of infection associated with total hip or knee arthroplasty. J Bone Joint Surg Am (2007). , 89, 871-82.

[15] Fehring, T. K, Odum, S, Calton, T. F, & Mason, J. B. Articulating versus static spacers in revision total knee arthroplasty for sepsis. The Ranawat Award. Clin Orthop (2000). , 380, 9-16.

[16] Chiang, E. R, Su, Y. P, Chen, T. H, Chiu, F. Y, & Chen, W. M. Comparison of articulating and static spacers regarding infection with resistant organisms in total knee arthroplasty. Acta Orthopaedica (2011). , 82, 460-464.

[17] Duncan, C. P, Beauchamp, C. P, & Masri, B. The antibiotic loaded joint replacement system: A novel approach to the management of the infected knee replacement. J Bone Joint Surg Br (1992). suppl III): 296

[18] Villanueva-martínez, M, Ríos-luna, A, Pereiro, J, & Fahandez-saddi, H. Hand-made articulating spacers in two-stage revision for infected total knee arthroplasty: good outcome in 30 patients. Acta Orthop Scand (2008). , 79, 674-82.

[19] Mcpherson, E. J, Lewonowski, K, & Dorr, L. D. Techniques in arthroplasty. Use of an articulated PMMA spacer in the infected total knee arthroplasty. J Arthroplasty (1995). , 10, 87-89.

[20] MacAvoy MCRies MD. The ball and socket articulating spacer for infected total knee arthroplasty. J Arthroplasty (2005). , 20, 757-62.

[21] Durbhakula, S. M, Czajka, J, Fuchs, M. D, & Uhl, R. L. Antibiotic-loaded articulating cement spacer in the 2-stage exchange of infected total knee arthroplasty. J Arthroplasty (2004). , 19, 768-74.

[22] Hsu, Y. C, Cheng, H. C, & Ng, T. P. Antibiotic-loaded cement articulating spacer for 2-stage reimplantation in infected total knee arthroplasty: a simple and economic method. J Arthroplasty (2007). , 22, 1060-6.

[23] Goldstein, W. M, Kopplin, M, Wall, R, & Berland, K. Temporary articulating methyl-methacrylate antibiotic spacer (TAMMAS): a new method of intraoperative manufacturing of a custom articulating spacer. J Bone Joint Surg. (2001). S, 2, 92-97.

[24] Ha, C. W. A technique for intraoperative construction of antibiotic spacers. Clin Orthop (2006). , 445, 204-9.

[25] Shen, H, Zhang, X, Jiang, Y, Wang, Q, & Chen, Y. Qi Wang Q, Shao J. Intraoperatively-made cement-on-cement antibiotic-loaded articulating spacer for infected total knee arthroplasty. The Knee (2010). , 17(2010), 407-411.

[26] Pitto, R. P, Castelli, C. C, Ferrari, R, & Munro, J. Pre-formed articulating knee spacer in two-stage revision for the infected total knee arthroplasty. Int Orthop (2005). , 29, 305-8.

[27] Meek, R. M, Masri, B. A, Dunlop, D, Garbuz, D. S, Greidanus, N. V, Mcgraw, R, & Duncan, C. P. Patient satisfaction and functional status after treatment of infection at the site of a total knee arthroplasty with use of the PROSTALAC articulating spacer. J Bone Joint Surg Am (2003). , 85, 1888-92.

[28] Haddad, F. S, Masri, B. A, Campbell, D, Mcgraw, R. W, Beauchamp, C. P, & Duncan, C. P. The PROSTALAC functional spacer in two-stage revision for infected knee replacements: prosthesis of antibiotic-loaded acrylic cement. J Bone Joint Surg Br (2000). , 82, 807-12.

[29] Hofmann, A. A, Goldberg, T, Tanner, A, & Kurtin, S. M. Treatment of infected total knee arthroplasty using an articulating spacer: 2- to 12-year experience. Clin Orthop (2005). , 430, 125-31.

[30] Anderson, J. A, Sculco, P. K, Heitkemper, S, Mayman, D. J, Bostrom, M. P, & Sculco, T. P. An articulating spacer to treat and mobilize patients with infected total knee arthroplasty. J Arthroplasty (2009). , 24, 631-5.

[31] Incavo, S. J, Russell, R. D, Mathis, K. B, & Adams, H. Initial Results of Managing Severe Bone Loss in Infected Total Joint Arthroplasty Using Customized Articulating Spacers. J Arthroplasty. (2009). , 24, 607-13.

[32] Macmull, S, Bartlett, M. J, Blunn, G. W, Pollock, R. C, Carrington, R. W, Skinner, J. A, Cannon, S. R, & Briggs, T. W. Custom-made hinged spacers in revision knee surgery for patients with infection, bone loss and instability. The Knee (2010). , 17, 403-406.

[33] Lewis, G. Review Properties of Antibiotic-Loaded Acrylic Bone Cements for Use in Cemented Arthroplasties: A State-of-the-Art Review. J Biomed Mater Res Part B: Appl Biomater (2009). B: , 558-574.

[34] Meyer, J, Piller, G, Spiegel, C. A, Hetzel, S, & Squire, M. Vacuum-Mixing Significantly Changes Antibiotic Elution Characteristics of Commercially Available Antibiotic-Impregnated Bone Cements. J Bone Joint Surg Am (2011). , 93, 2049-56.

[35] Dunne, N, Hill, J, Mcafee, P, Todd, K, Kirkpatrick, R, Tunney, M, & Patrick, S. In vitro study of the efficacy of acrylic bone cement loaded with supplementary amounts of gentamicin. Effect on mechanical properties, antibiotic release, and biofilm formation. Acta Orthopaedica (2007). , 78(6), 774-785.

[36] Nelson, C. L, Griffin, F. M, Harrison, B. H, & Cooper, R. E. In vitro elution characteristics of commercially and noncommercially prepared antibiotic PMMA beads. Clin Orthop Relat Res. (1992). , 284, 303-9.

[37] Kuehn, K. D, Ege, W, & Gopp, U. Acrylic bone cements: composition and properties. Orthop Clin North Am. (2005). , 36, 17-28.

[38] Greene, N, Holtom, P. D, Warren, C. A, Ressler, R. L, Shepherd, L, Mcpherson, E. J, & Patzakis, M. J. In vitro elution of tobramycin and vancomycin polymethylmethacrylate beads and spacers from Simplex and Palacos. Am J Orthop (1998). , 27, 201-205.

[39] Kuechle, D. K, Landon, G. C, Musher, D. M, & Noble, P. C. Elution of vancomycin, daptomycin, and amikacin from acrylic bone cement. Clin Orthop Relat Res (1991). , 264, 302-8.

[40] Stevens, C. M, Tetsworth, K. D, Calhoun, J. H, & Mader, J. T. An articulated antibiotic spacer used for infected total knee arthroplasty: a comparative in vitro elution study of Simplex and Palacos bone cements. Journal of Orthopaedic Researh (2005). , 23, 27-33.

[41] Penner, M. J, Masri, B. A, & Duncan, C. P. Elution characteristics of vancomycin and tobramycin combined in acrylic bone-cement. J Arthroplasty. (1996). , 11, 939-44.

[42] Greene, N, Holtom, P. D, Warren, C. A, Ressler, R. L, Shepherd, L, Mcpherson, E. J, & Patzakis, M. J. In vitro elution of tobramycin and vancomycin polymethylmethacrylate beads and spacers from Simplex and Palacos. Am J Orthop. (1998). , 27, 201-5.

[43] Springer, B. D, Lee, G. C, Osmon, D, Haidukewych, G. J, Hanssen, A. D, & Jacofsky, D. J. Systemic safety of high-dose antibiotic-loaded cement spacers after resection of an infected total knee arthroplasty. Clin Orthop Relat Res (2004). , 427, 47-51.

[44] Hanssen, A. D, & Spangehl, M. J. Practical applications of antibiotic-loaded bone cement for treatment of infected joint replacements. Clin Orthop Relat Res (2004). , 427, 79-85.

[45] Chiang, E. R, Su, Y. P, Chen, T. H, Chiu, F. Y, & Chen, W. M. Comparison of articulating and static spacers regarding infection with resistant organisms in total knee arthroplasty. Acta Orthopaedica (2011). , 82(4), 460-464.

[46] Ensing, G. T, Van Horn, J. R, Van Der Mei, H. C, Busscher, H. J, & Neut, D. Copal Bone Cement Is More Effective in Preventing Biofilm Formation than Palacos R-G. Clin Orthop Relat Res (2008). , 466, 1492-1498.

[47] Neut, D, De Groot, E. P, Kowalski, R. S, Van Horn, J. R, Van Der Mei, H. C, & Busscher, H. J. Gentamicin-loaded bone cement with clindamycin or fusidic acid added: biofilm formation and antibiotic release. J Biomed Mater Res (2005). , 165-170.

[48] Anguita-alonso, P, Rouse, M. S, Piper, K. E, Jacofsky, D. J, Osmon, D. R, & Patel, R. Comparative study of antimicrobial release kinetics from polymethylmethacrylate. Clin Orthop Relat Res (2006). , 445, 239-244.

[49] Webb, N. D, Mccanless, J. D, Courtney, H. S, Bumgardner, J. D, & Haggard, W. O. Daptomycin Eluted From Calcium Sulfate Appears Effective Against Staphylococcus. Clin Orthop Relat Res. (2008). , 466(6), 1383-1387.

[50] Hall, E. W, Rouse, M. S, Jacofsky, D. J, Osmon, D. R, Hanssen, A. D, Steckelberg, J. M, & Patel, R. Release of daptomycin from polymethylmethacrylate beads in a continuous flow chamber. Diagnostic Microbiology and Infectious Disease (2004). , 50, 261-265.

[51] Wyman, J, Mcgough, R, & Limbird, R. Fungal infection of a total knee prosthesis: Successful treatment using articulating cement spacers and staged reimplantation. Orthopedics (2002). , 25, 1391-4.

[52] Baumann, P. A, Cunningham, B, Patel, N. S, & Finn, H. A. Aspergillus fumigatus infection in a mega prosthetic total knee arthroplasty: salvage by staged reimplantation with 5-year follow-up. J Arthroplasty (2001). , 16, 498-503.

[53] Langer, P, Kassim, R. A, Macari, G. S, & Saleh, K. J. Aspergillus infection after total knee arthroplasty. Am J Orthop (2003). , 32, 402-4.

[54] Evans, R. P. Successful treatment of TH and TK infection with articulating antibiotic components. A modified treatment method. Clin Orthop Relat Research. (2004). , 427, 37-46.

[55] Phelan, D. M, Osmon, D. R, Keating, M. R, & Hanssen, A. D. Delayed reimplantation arthroplasty for candidal prosthetic joint infection: a report of 4 cases and review of the literature. Clin Infect Dis (2002). , 34, 930-8.

[56] Masri, B. A, Duncan, C. P, & Beauchamp, C. P. Long-term elution of antibiotics from bone-cement: an in vivo study using the prosthesis of antibiotic-loaded acrylic cement (PROSTALAC) system. J Arthroplasty (1998). , 13, 331-8.

[57] Armstrong, M. S, Spencer, R. F, Cunningham, J. L, Gheduzzi, S, Miles, A. W, & Learmonth, I. D. Mechanical characteristics of antibiotic-laden bone cement. Acta Orthop Scand (2002). , 73, 688-90.

[58] Klekamp, J, Dawson, J. M, Haas, D. W, Deboer, D, & Christie, M. The use of vancomycin and tobramycin in acrylic bone cement: biomechanical effects and elution kinetics for use in joint arthroplasty. J Arthroplasty (1999). , 14, 339-46.

[59] Seldes, R. M, Winiarsky, R, Jordan, L. C, Baldini, T, Brause, B, Zodda, F, & Sculco, T. P. Liquid gentamicin in bone cement: a laboratory study of a potentially more cost-effective cement spacer. J Bone Joint Surg Am (2005). , 87, 268-72.

[60] Deluise, M, & Scott, C. P. Addition of hand-blended generic tobramycin in bone cement: effect on mechanical strength. Orthopedics (2004). , 27, 1289-91.

[61] Kuehn, K. D, Ege, W, & Gopp, U. Acrylic bone cements: mechanical and physical properties. Orthop Clin North Am (2005). , 36, 29-39.

[62] Kuehn, K. D, Ege, W, & Gopp, U. Acrylic bone cements: composition and properties. Orthop Clin North Am (2005). , 36, 17-28.

[63] Hanssen, A. D, & Spangehl, M. J. Treatment of the infected hip replacement. Clin Orthop Relat Res (2004). , 420, 63-71.

[64] Frommelt, L, & Kühn, K. D. Antibiotic-loaded cement. In: Breusch SJ, Malchau M. The well-cemented total hip arthroplasty. Heidelberg: Springer, (2005). , 86-92.

[65] Van Raaij, T. M, Visser, L. E, Vulto, A. G, & Verhaar, J. A. Acute renal failure after local gentamicin treatment in an infected total knee arthroplasty. J Arthroplasty (2002). , 17, 948-50.

[66] Ceffa, R, Andreoni, S, Borre, S, Ghisellini, F, Fornara, P, Brugo, G, & Ritter, M. A. Mucoraceae infections of antibiotic-loaded cement spacers in the treatment of bacterial infections caused by knee arthroplasty. J Arthroplasty (2002). , 17, 235-8.

[67] Haleem, A. A, Berry, D. J, & Hanssen, A. D. Mid-Term to Long-Term Followup of Two-stage Reimplantation for Infected Total Knee Arthroplasty. Clin Orthop Relat Research (2004). , 428, 35-39.

[68] Park, S. J, Song, E. K, Seon, J. K, Yoon, T. R, & Park, Y. H. Comparison of static and mobile antibiotic-impregnated cement spacers for the treatment of infected total knee arthroplasty. International Orthopaedics (SICOT) (2010). , 34, 1181-1186.

[69] Huang, H, Su, J, & Chen, S. The results of articulating spacer technique for infected total knee arthroplasty. J Arthroplasty (2006). , 21, 1163-8.

[70] Cuckler, J. M. The infected total knee. Management options. J Arthroplasty (2005). S , 2, 33-6.

[71] Macmull, S, Bartlett, W, Miles, W, Blunn, J, Pollock, G. W, Carrington, R. C, Skinner, R. W, Cannon, J. A, Briggs, S. R, & Custom-made, T. W. hinged spacers in revision knee surgery for patients with infection, bone loss and instability. The Knee (2010). , 17, 403-406.

[72] Jeys, J L. M, Grimer, S. R, & Tillman, R. M. Periprosthetic infection in patients treated for an orthopaedic oncological condition. Bone Jt Surg Am (2005). , 87, 842-9.

[73] Hanssen, A. D, Trousdale, R. T, & Osmon, D. R. Patient outcome with reinfection following reimplantation for the infected total knee arthroplasty. Clin Orth Relat Res (1995). , 321, 55-67.

[74] Hart, W. J, & Jones, R. S. Two-stage revision of infected total knee replacements using articular cement spacers and short-term antibiotic therapy. J Bone J Surg Br (2006). , 88, 1011-5.

Chapter 26

The Role of Knee Arthrodesis After TKA Infection

Pablo Renovell, Antonio Silvestre and
Oscar Vaamonde

Additional information is available at the end of the chapter

http://dx.doi.org/10.5772/53690

1. Introduction

Infection after total knee arthroplasty (TKA) is a devastating complication posing substantial clinical and financial burden, which incidence is increasing in line with the rise of the number of TKAs performed worldwide. The incidence of this complication rates from 1% in primary TKAs to 5.8% after TKAs revision in long series [1]. The lowest reinfection rate after a prior reimplantation for septic TKA has been reported near 30% [2].

The goals in the treatment of chronic infected TKA are control of the disease and restoring knee function. Alternative techniques in the management of reinfected knee prosthesis are another two-stage prosthesis reimplantation, arthrodesis, resection arthroplasty, and supra-condylar amputation [3]. Although two-stage surgery is generally believed as the most successful decision, chronic infection forces surgeons to look for other alternatives.

Recurring infection at the site of a total knee arthroplasty should be treated by knee arthrodesis unless control of the disease and good functional recover could be possible [4]. Arthrodesis of the knee can provide a stable painless joint for an independent lifestyle that would not be possible after a failed total knee replacement. Whereas reimplantation of a TKA shows better limb function, arthrodesis achieves better pain relief, not finding significant differences in knee scores between the two procedures (Oxford knee score) [5, 6]. Knee arthrodesis can be achieved with a cemented or uncemented intramedullary nail, inserted from great trochanter or through the knee, with two plates applied in two planes or using an external fixator to produce a joint fusion [4]. Intramedullary nails provide greater stability, avoid pin-track infection, allow faster weight bearing and generally are better accepted by the patients than external fixators [7]. Illizarov method is more desirable when soft tissues conditions are poor or after failing of intramedullary nail [8, 9].

There are few and short series of cemented modular nail for knee arthrodesis after TKA infection in literature [10, 11]. The purpose of this study is to report the role of knee arthrodesis after chronic infection of knee prostheses and show our results with the use of a modular cemented nail inserted through the knee.

2. Material and methods

We review retrospectively twenty-one patients who have undergone knee arthrodesis with a cemented modular nail for chronic infection of knee prosthesis, from January 2003 until January 2011 in our Department. Three senior surgeons performed all procedures.

Endo-Model® Knee Fusion Nail (Newsplint, UK/Waldemar Link®, GmbH & Co. KG, Hamburg, Germany) was used in all cases. Twelve of those cases received previous surgery in our Hospital (a reference institution for knee reconstruction) but the other nine cases came from others Hospitals. The decision to undertake knee fusion was arranged after analyzing the different options with the patient.

The first surgical stage was exhaustive debridement and placement of a double antibiotic-loaded (clindamycin and gentamicin) bone cement as a static spacer (Rofabacin® Revision, Biomet®). Systemic antibiotics according to the culture results were given to the patients for at least six weeks. When the patient was recovered from the first-stage surgery, no signs of infection were observed and values of inflammatory markers (PCR and ESR) were decreased, the cemented modular nail was inserted through the knee after reaming tibial and femoral canals. Tibial and femur implants are cemented with antibiotic loaded cement. Nineteen cases were performed according to this two-stage procedure, but two cases were done in just one-stage.

Hospital records and serial radiographies of all patients were reviewed to evaluate patient status and outcomes. We have excluded a patient lost on follow-up.

Number of previous surgeries per patient, comorbidities and microorganisms responsible for the infection were recorded.

In order to assess functional outcome, the Oxford Knee Score (OKS) [12] was checked before removal of the implants and at final follow-up. Successful outcome was defined as not or slight pain on the operated limb and able to walk with or without aids at the time of the last follow-up.

3. Results

Twenty-one patients were treated with cemented modular nail for knee arthrodesis from 2003 to 2011 for chronic infection of the prostheses (Figure 1.). One patient was lost during follow-up and was excluded from this series. Mean follow-up of patients was 3.2 years (range, six months to eight years).

http://dx.doi.org/10.5772/53690

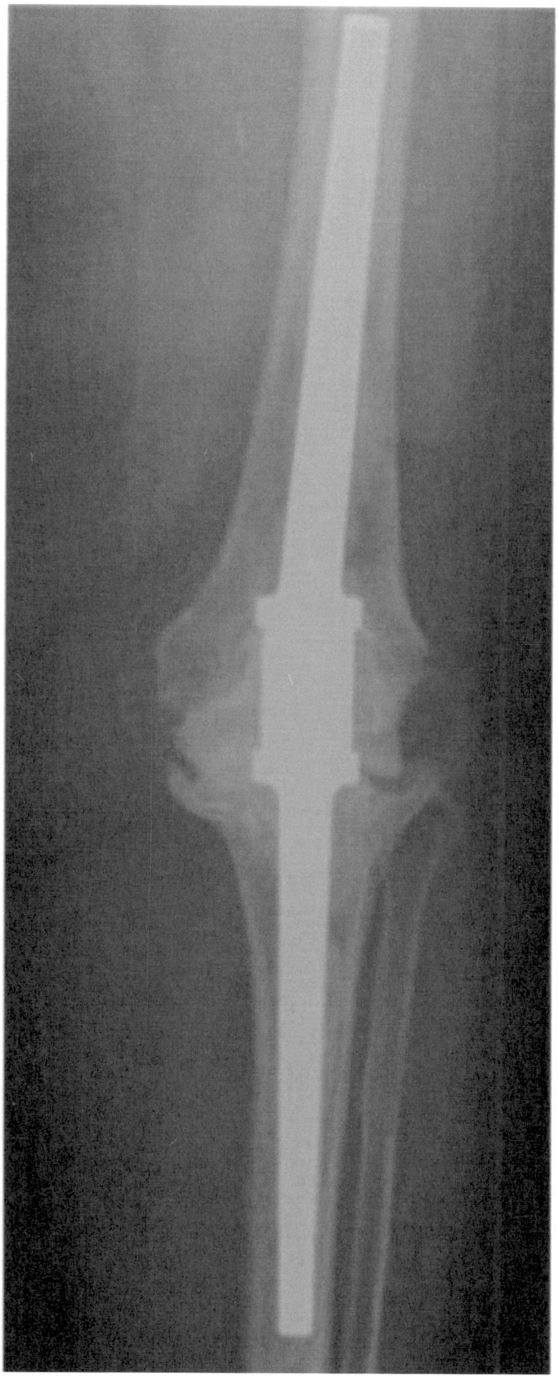

Figure 1. Cemented modular nail for knee arthrodesis.

Twenty patients were fully recorded. The series includes eleven women and nine men with a mean age of seventy-six years (range 68-86 years) at the time of arthrodesis. Time since primary knee arthroplasty until knee arthrodesis, ranged from eight months to nine years (mean 4.4 years). The number of procedures carried out before definitive arthrodesis ranged from 2 to 7 (mean 3.3 surgeries).

Most frequent comorbidities were hypertension (65%), obesity [BMI>30kg/m^2] (45%) and Diabetes Mellitus (40%). Demographics of the patients are shown in Table 1.

Number of patients fully recorded	20
Age	76.8±10.2
Sex (M/F)	11/9
Side (R/L)	12/8
Body mass index (Kg/m^2)	29.8±1.4
Comorbidities	
HTA	13 (65%)
Obesity	9 (45%)
DM	8 (40%)
Mean nº of knee prior surgeries	3.3(2-7)
Preoperative OKS	17.1 (9-32)

Table 1. Demographics of the study population

Intraoperative cultures were positive on 19 cases (95%). In eight of the cases (40%) only one bacteria could be checked, but on the other hand two or more microorganisms yielded on cultures in eleven cases (55%). The predominant microorganisms were *staphylococcus epidermidis* in 11 cases (55%) and *staphylococcus aureus* in 7 cases (35%), 10 of which (8 *s. epidermidis* and 2 *s. aureus*) were *methicillin-resistant staphylococcus (MRS),* so we can conclude that 50% of fused knees were positive to MRS. Other microorganism included in this series was *Escherichia coli* in 4 cases (20%).

Fifteen patients (75%) healed without problems and they did not need more surgeries, four (20%) showed inadequate control of infection so required new performances (one case one-stage debridement, two arthrodesis with external fixators and one case supracondylar amputation), and two cases (10%) suffered a tibial shaft fracture below the tip of the nail. One of the fractures was resolved changing the nail for a longer one (Figure 2), and the other was treated with immobilization. Two of the four cases (50%) with persistence of of infection were operated in one-stage surgery.

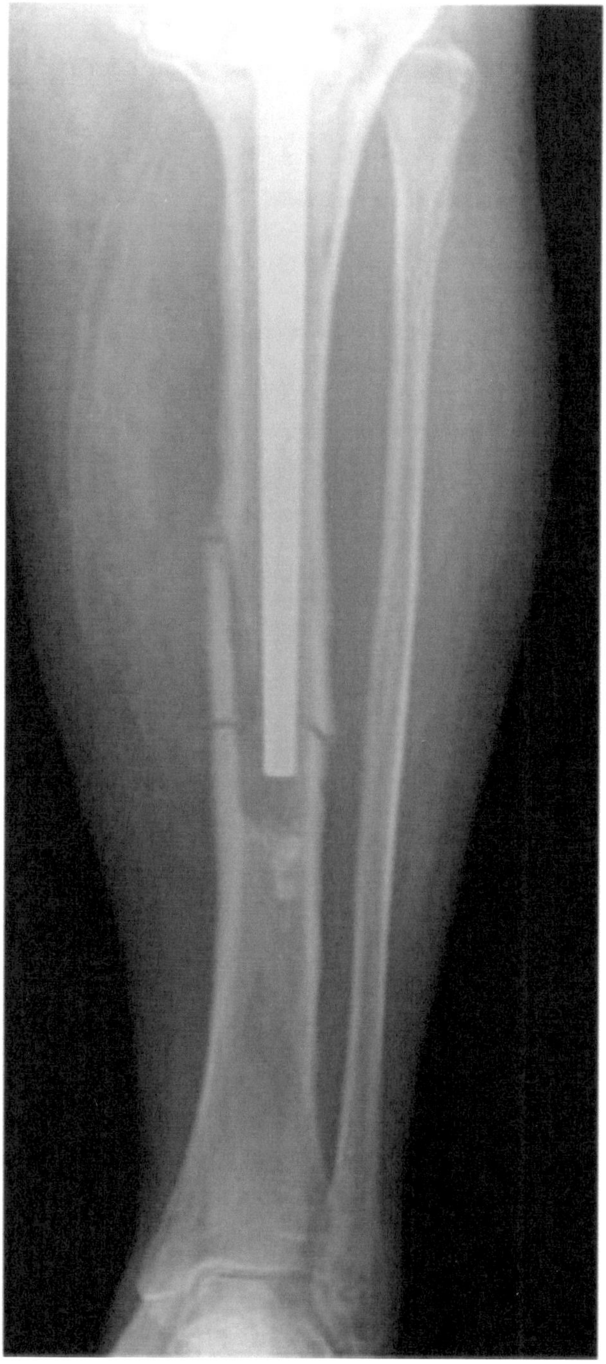

Figure 2. Tibia fracture and bone loosening below the nail.

The mean Oxford knee score improved from 17.1 points (range, 9 to 32 points) before removal of the prosthesis, to 27.4 points (range, 6 to 41 points) postoperatively. Successful outcome was 95% at the time of the last follow-up. Results of the series are shown in Table 2.

Number of cases infected by MRS	10 (50%)
Patients healed without problems	15 (75%)
Causes of reoperations	
Persistent infection	4 (20%)
Fracture on tibia below the nail (and bone loosening)	1 (5%)
Reoperations	
Arthrodesis with external fixator	2
One-stage debridement	1
Supracondylar amputation	1
Change for a longer nail	1
Postoperative OKS	27.4 (6-41)

Table 2. Results of knee arthrodesis with cemented modular nail

4. Discussion

The reason to turn a TKA into arthrodesis due to a chronic infection is not clear nowadays, and the decision-making process is sometimes difficult. When a second infection happens, the number of surgeries performed in the knee reaches until 9.3 of average [1], so this detail must be always present on surgeon's mind when re-infection occurs. Infection of primary TKA has been related with hyperglycaemia, prolonged operative time, obesity, rheumatoid arthritis and others [1], however in TKA reinfection, the main factors related to this condition are previous infection with tough microorganisms, poor soft tissue coverage and number of previous surgeries [2].

Although surgeon might consider joint fusion as a poor result, comparing to other choices, knee with a fusion is more efficient and functional [13]. Supracondylar amputation as a consequence of a failed total knee revision arthroplasty is a salvage procedure in front of a severe infection, uncontrolled pain or massive bone loss. This radical surgery should not be related knee prosthesis complications but to peripheral vascular disease or recurrence of a malignant tumor [14]. Functional outcome after supracondylar amputation carried out ought to an infected total knee replacement is poor. Patients with a supracondylar amputation after chronic infection of prosthesis show low functional status. Only 50% of these patients are able to walk after the surgery [15]. The awful OKS of our amputated patients (6 points), confirms this fact.

The alternative of resection arthroplasty in case of recalcitrant TKA infection is only an option when the patient previously was not able to walk, due to a medical infirmity or other limb pathology. Results on pain and functional scores are always lower than two-stage reimplatation or arthrodesis [16].

Clinical outcomes of revision TKA after aseptic loosening are better than knee prosthesis revision after chronic infection [17]. Wang et al [5] asserted, comparing clinical outcomes of the different alternatives in the treatment of infected TKA, that Oxford Knee Score after revision TKA is similar to knee arthrodesis. He reported just about mild-to-moderate knee pain on almost 50% of the reimplanted TKAs. Knee arthrodesis shows better pain relief but worse function than revision TKA, whereas reimplanted TKA reveals better function and worse pain relief than knee fusion. Anyway, knee arthrodesis allows the patient an independent lifestyle with few complications [18]. And it is important to keep in mind that re-infection rate after TKA revision is 68.6%, lessen to 52.6% in case of resistant microorganisms [2]. The rate can be reduced to only 18% when these microorganisms are identified and properly treated [19]. Maheshwari et al [2] reported that supracondylar amputation was performed on 14.2% of his cases, whereas only on 5.7% of his patients arthrodesis was the final operation. Our results show that infection was controlled in 75% of our patients with a knee arthrodesis done with a cemented modular nail and no more re-operations were needed. In our series, just one case of amputation was performed (5%). We agree with others authors [13, 20] that after a second TKA infection due to high virulence microorganisms or after multiple attempts of failed revision arthroplasty, knee arthrodesis should be the therapeutic choice in most of the cases or at least in those cases with low functional demanding patients in order to avoid a possible supracondylar amputation.

The three most frequent surgical techniques used to achieved knee arthrodesis after failed TKA are internal plate fixation, intramedullary rod fixation and external fixation [4]. Subsequent conversion of a knee arthrodesis to a total knee arthroplasty is not advisable, as almost of the reimplanted arthroplasties fail [21, 22].

Internal plate fixation is rarely used to achieve knee fusion due to the requirement of a broad soft tissue exposure, long time weight-bearing and because of the incidence of pseudoarthrosis is high.

External fixation has been the method of choice to attained knee arthrodesis following chronic infected TKA [8, 9, 23-25]. Advantages of external fixation include the fact that produces proper bone compression, the surgical procedure can be performed in one operative stage, and no implants remain inside the body after the external fixator removal. These details presume less recurrent infection rate than other arthrodesis techniques. Problems related to this treatment are carrying the device for long periods of time, usually more than six months, the subsequent shortening of the limb, the pin site infection or the possibility of a fracture through the weakened bone [7]. Nowadays this alternative is used in chronic infected knees after arthrodesis with bad tolerance of the nail. [4]. Two of our patients (10% of cases) needed an external fixator (Illizarov method) to achieve a useful limb.

Intramedullary nail is actually the most widespread option to fuse the knee [4, 20, 26-29]. Rate of fusion near 100% has been well documented in literature, as well as the satisfactory results in case of persistent infection that rarely forces the surgeon to take out the nail [30]. Complications of intramedullary nail fixation include periprosthetic fracture, hardware-related pain, bone loosening and persistent infection. Arthrodesis performed with a nail should be done according to a two-staged protocol in order to reduce the incidence of reinfection. Two of our four cases (50%), which showed inadequate infection control, were treated in first instance through a one-stage surgery; this fact supports previous reports and remarks the requirement of two stage-surgery to get a free-infected arthrodesis [4,31,32].

The preference of achieving knee fusion with an external fixator or with the aid of an intramedullary rod should be based on surgeon's experience and on the review of the advantages and disadvantages of each techniques [7].

There are different models of knee nails used to achieve arthrodesis. In the beginning long Küntscher nail was introduced through the great trochanter after debridement of the infected joint [33, 34]. This double approach is rarely used nowadays, and is reserved to failures of previous arthrodesis, fractures of the tibia or femur or cases of bone loosening that requires extended fixation [35, 36]. One patient (5%) of our series needed this procedure.

Modular nail can be inserted through the knee and it is at the present time the most frequent surgical technique to achieve a knee fusion; it shows fusion rates of nearly 95% of cases [37-39]. Modular nails could be cemented or uncemented but there is no literature that compares results of these models. When an uncemented nail is used, maximum bone contact is extremely important in order to get knee arthrodesis and usually autologous bone graft is required. After using an uncemented device shortening of the limb is frequent, as occurs with external fixators. Fractures around the tip of the rod or the locked screws are possible [40], as well as loosening of the implant. Few reports and small number of cases with the use of cemented nails have been published, so hardly any conclusions about this procedure can be obtained [10, 11]. The technique of cementing the nail could avoid shortening of the limb, compensate bone loss and provide an artificial joint fusion without employing bone graft. Fractures around the nail are probably less frequent than in uncemented nails, but when cemented nails must be removed surgery is quite tougher and bone loss bone could be a problem for the revision surgeries. Neuerburg et al [11] have published a review with the same number of cases than us, with similar results and conclusions, advising of clinical and radiological follow-up to allow appropriate surgery in case of loosening.

5. Conclusion

Recurrent infection after a previously exchange arthroplasty for chronic infected TKA is a challenging problem. This devastating complication is associated to infection due to high virulence resistant microorganisms, poor soft tissue coverage and a high number of previous surgeries. When this complication occurs, surgeons must always have in mind the possibility of an above knee amputation as a final result if we insist on revising to a knee arthroplasty. In order to avoid this terrible result, knee arthrodesis, preferably in two-stages, could be an option to achieve a useful and stable painless limb. Among the different alternatives to obtain knee arthrodesis, we believe that the best procedure is inserting a cemented modular nail through the knee, which provides a strong fixation, has a low rate of reinfection and allows to restore the length of the limb though significant bone loss due to previous surgeries.

Author details

Pablo Renovell, Antonio Silvestre and Oscar Vaamonde

Orthopaedic Department. Hospital Clínico of Valencia, Spain

References

[1] Blom, A. W, Brown, J, Taylor, A. H, Pattison, G, Whitehouse, S, & Bannister, G. C. Infection after total knee arthroplasty. J Bone Joint Surg Br. (2004). Jul;, 86(5), 688-91.

[2] Maheshwari, A. V, Gioe, T. J, Kalore, N. V, & Cheng, E. Y. Reinfection after prior staged reimplantation for septic total knee arthroplasty: is salvage still possible? J Arthroplasty. (2010). Sep; 25(6 Suppl): , 92-7.

[3] Morrey, B. F, Westholm, F, Schoifet, S, Rand, J. A, & Bryan, R. S. Long-term results of various treatment options for infected total knee arthroplasty. Clin Orthop Relat Res. (1989). Nov;(248): 120-8.

[4] Conway, J. D, Mont, M. A, & Bezwada, H. P. Arthrodesis of the knee. J Bone Joint Surg Am. (2004). Apr;A(4):835-48., 86.

[5] Wang, C. J, Huang, T. W, Wang, J. W, & Chen, H. S. The often poor clinical outcome of infected total knee arthroplasty. J Arthroplasty. (2002). Aug; , 17(5), 608-14.

[6] Husted, H. Toftgaard Jensen T. Clinical outcome after treatment of infected primary total knee arthroplasty. Acta Orthop Belg. (2002). , 68, 500-7.

[7] Mabry, T. M, Jacofsky, D. J, Haidukewych, G. J, & Hanssen, A. Comparison of intramedullary nailing and external fixation knee arthrodesis for the infected knee replacement. Clin Orthop Relat Res. (2007). Nov; , 464, 11-5.

[8] Oostenbroek, H. J, & Van Roermund, P. M. Arthrodesis of the knee after an infected arthroplasty using the Ilizarov method. J Bone Joint Surg Br. (2001). Jan;, 83(1), 50-4.

[9] Manzotti, A, Pullen, C, Guerreschi, F, & Catagni, M. A. The Ilizarov method for failed knee arthrodesis following septic TKR. Knee. (2001). Jun;, 8(2), 135-8.

[10] Rao, M. C, Richards, O, Meyer, C, & Jones, R. S. Knee stabilisation following infected knee arthroplasty with bone loss and extensor mechanism impairment using a modular cemented nail. Knee. (2009). Dec; , 16(6), 489-93.

[11] Neuerburg, C, Bieger, R, Jung, S, Kappe, T, Reichel, H, & Decking, R. Bridging knee arthrodesis for limb salvage using an intramedullary cemented nail: a retrospective outcome analysis of a case series. Arch Orthop Trauma Surg. (2012). May 13.

[12] Dawson, J, Fitzpatrick, R, Murray, D, & Carr, A. Questionnarie on the perceptions of patients about total knee replacement. J Bone Joint Surg (Br) (1998). B: 63-9., 80.

[13] Klinger, H. M, Spahn, G, Schultz, W, & Baums, M. H. Arthrodesis of the knee after failed infected total knee arthroplasty. Knee Surg Sports Traumatol Arthrosc. (2006). May;, 14(5), 447-53.

[14] Sierra, R. J, Trousdale, R. T, & Pagnano, M. W. Above-the-knee amputation after a total knee replacement: prevalence, etiology, and functional outcome. J Bone Joint Surg Am. (2003). Jun; A(6):1000-4., 85.

[15] Fedorka, C. J, Chen, A. F, Mcgarry, W. M, & Parvizi, J. Klatt BA Functional ability after above-the-knee amputation for infected total knee arthroplasty. Clin Orthop Relat Res. (2011). Apr; , 469(4), 1024-32.

[16] Falahee, M. H, Matthews, L. S, & Kaufer, H. Resection arthroplasty as a salvage procedure for a knee with infection after a total arthroplasty. J Bone Joint Surg Am. (1987). , 69, 1013-21.

[17] Barrack, R. L, Engh, G, Rorabeck, C, et al. Patient satisfaction and outcome after septic versus aseptic revision total knee arthroplasty. J Arthroplasty 15:990, (2000).

[18] Benson, E. R, Resine, S. T, & Lewis, C. G. Functional outcome of arthrodesis for failed total knee arthroplasty. Orthopedics. (1998). , 21, 875-9.

[19] Kilgus, D. J, Howe, D. J, & Strang, A. Results of periprosthetic hip and knee infections caused by resistant bacteria. Clin Orthop Relat Res. (2002). Nov;(404):116-24.

[20] Wiedel, J. D. Salvage of infected total knee fusion: the last option. Clin Orthop Relat Res. (2002). Nov;(404):139-42.

[21] Naranja RJ JrLotke PA, Pagnano MW, Hanssen AD. Total knee arthroplasty in a previously ankylosed or arthrodesed knee. Clin Orthop. (1996). , 331, 234-7.

[22] Clemens, D, Lereim, P, & Holm, I. Reikerås O Conversion of knee fusion to total arthroplasty: complications in 8 patients. Acta Orthop. (2005). Jun;, 76(3), 370-4.

[23] Phillips, H. T, & Mears, D. C. Knee fusion with external skeletal fixation after an infected hinge prosthesis: a case report. Clin Orthop Relat Res. (1980). Sep;(151):147-52.

[24] Garberina, M. J, Fitch, R. D, Hoffmann, E. D, Hardaker, W. T, Vail, T. P, & Scully, S. P. Knee arthrodesis with circular external fixation. Clin Orthop Relat Res. (2001). Jan;(382): 168-78.

[25] Vanryn, J. S, & Verebelyi, D. M. One-stage débridement and knee fusion for infected total knee arthroplasty using the hybrid frame. J Arthroplasty. (2002). Jan;, 17(1), 129-34.

[26] Wilde, A. H, & Stearns, K. L. Intramedullary fixation for arthrodesis of the knee after infected total knee arthroplasty. Clin Orthop Relat Res. (1989). Nov;(248):87-92.

[27] Gore, D. R, & Gassner, K. Use of an intramedullary rod in knee arthrodesis following failed total knee arthroplasty. J Knee Surg. (2003). Jul;, 16(3), 165-7.

[28] MacDonald JHAgarwal S, Lorei MP, Johanson NA, Freiberg AA. Knee arthrodesis. J Am Acad Orthop Surg. (2006). Mar;, 14(3), 154-63.

[29] Talmo, C. T, Bono, J. V, Figgie, M. P, Sculco, T. P, Laskin, R. S, & Windsor, R. E. Intramedullary arthrodesis of the knee in the treatment of sepsis after TKR. HSS J. (2007). Feb;, 3(1), 83-8.

[30] Schoifet, S. D, & Morrey, B. Persistent infection after successful arthrodesis for infected total knee arthroplasty. A report of two cases. J Arthroplasty. (1990). Sep;, 5(3), 277-9.

[31] Knutson, K, Hovelius, L, Lindstrand, A, & Lidgren, L. Arthrodesis after failed knee arthroplasty. Clin Orthop. (1984).

[32] Elligsen, D. E. Rand, JA Intramedullary arthrodesis of the knee after failed total knee arthroplasty. J Bone Joint Surg (1994). A:870-877., 76.

[33] Mazet R JrUrist MR. Arthrodesis of the knee with intramedullary nail fixation. Clin Orthop. (1960). , 18, 43-53.

[34] Knutson, K, & Lidgren, L. Arthrodesis after infected knee arthroplasty using an intramedullary nail. Reports of four cases. Arch Orthop Trauma Surg. (1982). , 100(1), 49-53.

[35] Jorgensen, P. S, & Torholm, C. Arthrodesis after infected knee arthroplasty using long arthrodesis nail. A report of five cases. Am J Knee Surg. (1995). , 8, 110-3.

[36] Bargiotas, K, Wohlrab, D, Sewecke, J. J, Lavinge, G, Demeo, P. J, & Sotereanos, N. G. Arthrodesis of the knee with a long intramedullary nail following the failure of a total knee arthroplasty as the result of infection. Surgical technique. J Bone Joint Surg Am. (2007). Mar;89 Suppl 2 Pt., 1, 103-10.

[37] Waldman, B. J, Mont, M. A, Payman, K. R, Freiberg, A. A, Windsor, R. E, Sculco, T. P, & Hungerford, D. S. Infected total knee arthroplasty treated with arthrodesis using a modular nail. Clin Orthop. (1999). , 367, 230-7.

[38] Mcqueen, D. A, Cooke, F. W, & Hahn, D. L. Knee arthrodesis with the Wichita Fusion Nail: an outcome comparison. Clin Orthop Relat Res. (2006). May;, 446, 132-9.

[39] Iacono, F, & Bruni, D. Lo Presti M, Raspugli G, Bondi A, Sharma B, Marcacci M. Knee arthrodesis with a press-fit modular intramedullary nail without bone-on-bone fusion after an infected revision TKA. Knee. (2012). Oct;Epub 2012 Feb 15., 19(5), 555-9.

[40] Hinarejos, P, Ginés, A, Monllau, J. C, Puig, L, & Cáceres, E. Fractures above and below a modular nail for knee arthrodesis. A case report. Knee. (2005). Jun;, 12(3), 231-3.

Section 7

Alternatives to Arthroplasty

Chapter 27

Proximal Interphalangeal Joint Arthrodesis with Tendon Transfer of the Flexor Digitorum Brevis

Ricardo Becerro de Bengoa Vallejo,
Marta Elena Losa Iglesias and
Miguel Fuentes Rodriguez

Additional information is available at the end of the chapter

http://dx.doi.org/10.5772/52752

1. Introduction

Hammer toe is a deformity characterized by dorsiflexion of the metatarsophalangeal (MTP) joint, plantarflexion of the proximal interphalangeal (PIP) joint, and dorsiflexion of the distal interphalangeal (DIP) joint. Claw toe is a similar deformity characterized by dorsiflexion of the MTP and plantarflexion of the PIP and DIP joints. These terms are often used interchangeably because both deformities involve the MTP joint. [1]

The causes of dorsiflexion of the metatarso- and interphalangeal joint have been described by various authors. [3], [4], [5], [6] Sandeman [2] reported that when the proximal phalanx is in the dorsal position at the expense of MTP dorsiflexion, the axis of the intrinsic musculature shifts. This causes a loss of competence of the intrinsic musculature of the foot, and the proximal phalanx can no longer be maintained in a plantar position. In the presence of concurrent flexor digitorum longus (FDL) contraction, the intrinsic musculature loses its ability to plantarflex the MTP joint. In a closed kinetic chain, this causes pathologic dorsiflexion of the MTP joint and places the proximal phalanx in a dorsal position. The result is claw or hammer deformity of the involved digits. Surgical correction of claw and hammer toe deformities utilize the action of the FDL tendon transferred to transform the deforming forces into corrective forces.

Correction of this flexible digital deformity by means of tendinous transposition of the flexor musculature to the extensor region of the toes has been described. [7], [8], [9], [10], [11], [12], [13] In each instance two cutaneous incisions have been utilized, one dorsal and another plantar. Only Barbari and Brevig [9] have described FDL tendon transfer to the dorsum of the extensor digitorum longus (EDL) tendon through a single incision approach. In this approach the dorso-lateral incision over the MTP joint extends about 3 cm distally from the neck of the metatarsal bone when there is only a single involved digit. When the procedure is undertaken in multiple digits, a transverse incision at the level of the digit crease is performed and the FDL tendon is sutured end-to-side to the EDL tendon. The authors stated that care must be taken to avoid injuring the neurovascular axes which are retracted laterally. The authors also advocated, when indicated, performing plantar capsulotomies for the DIP and PIP joints as described by Pyper [12] and Taylor. [13] The additional incision, however, increases the risk for injuring the principal plantar vessels of the involved digits..

Thus far, it has been recommended that correction of claw and hammer toe deformities be performed by transferring the FDL tendon to the dorsum of the proximal phalanx. Transposition of the FDL tendon via the dorsal approach through a unique longitudinal dorsal cutaneous incision without performing plantar incisions for capsulotomies of the DIP and PIP joints has not been previously described. To determine the feasibility of transferring the FDL tendon as an approach to correct claw and hammer toe deformities with this approach, it is necessary to determine whether these fascicles are long enough to transpose to the plantar aspect of the EDL tendon in the dorsal area of the proximal phalanx, and directly to the dorsum of the proximal phalanx of the second and third toes. We hypothesized that the FDL tendon, when incised at the level of the PIP joint, has adequate anatomical length to be transferred to the dorsal aspect of the proximal phalanx via a single longitudinal dorsal cutaneous incision and it would not be necessary to perform plantar capsulotomies at the interphalangeal joints, thus decreasing the risk of injury to the principal plantar vessels of the digits.

2. Materials and methods

Sixty cadaveric foot specimens (Total N, 60; 30 right, 30 left) were used for study procedures, including fourteen fresh and forty-six embalmed specimens. Transfer of the FDL tendon to the dorsum of the proximal phalanx via dorsal approach was attempted in 120 toes (60 each second and third toes).

The surgical technique performed in this study was a modification of a previously described method to transfer the flexor digitorum brevis (FDB) tendon. [14] To perform the FDL transfer a central longitudinal incision was made on the dorsal aspect of the digit, preserving the medial and lateral vessels and nerves. The incision was along the dorsum of the proximal phalanx of the digit from the base to the PIP joint. Once the EDL tendon was exposed, it was tenomiced and released along with the transverse aponeurosis that shapes the digital extensor apparatus. Proximal phalanx arthroplasty and hood ligament and MTP joint release were then performed by means of a dorsal, medial, and lateral capsulotomy. Section of the collateral and suspensory ligaments was performed to reduce the fixed extension deformity of the MTP joint in the specimens with fixed claw or hammer toe deformities.

After arthroplasty of the proximal phalanx was completed the dorsal aspect of the distal tendon sheath of the FDL and FDB tendons was exposed (Fig. 1). The vincula from the plantar aspect of the proximal phalanx to the dorsal aspect of the FDL and FDB tendons were released to further expose the flexor tendon sheath (Fig. 2). The tendon sheath was then incised and split longitudinally to the base of the middle phalanx (Fig. 3A), and the medial and lateral hemitendons of the FDB were exposed dorsally to the FDL (Fig. 3B). Plantar exposure of the FDB tendon was performed by inserting a curved hemostat by means of a blunt technique to identify and isolate the medial and lateral fascicles (Fig. 4 A, B). If the hemitendons of the FDB were not split adequately to permit passage of the FDL tendon, the FDB was divided longitudinally and proximally using a #15 blade (Fig. 5). The lateral and medial FDB hemitendons were then retracted to expose the FDL tendon (Fig. 6). Using a curved hemostat the FDL was collected dorsally between the medial and lateral FDB hemitendons (Fig. 7). Using a mini-osteotome, the FDL tendon was released from the plantar aspect of the distal middle phalanx to maximize the available tendon length (Fig. 8). This technique maximizes the length of the free distal tendinous stump to facilitate transfer to the dorsal aspect of the proximal phalanx (Fig. 9). The free proximal end of the tendon was clamped for later transfer (Fig 10). Next, using a #15 blade, the long flexor was split longitudinally in two portions, lateral and medial, proximal to distal (Fig. 11). Both free proximal FDL tendons were exposed between the plantar aspect of the proximal phalanx and the dorsal aspect of the FDB tendons (Fig 12).

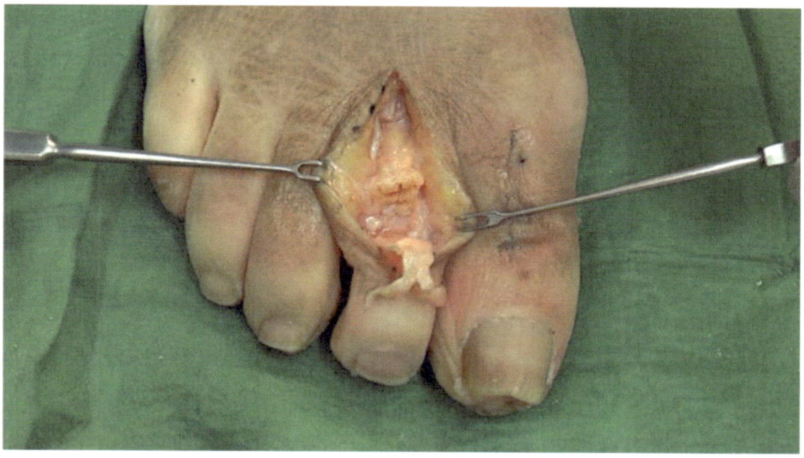

Figure 1. Dorsal aspect of the second digit after arthroplasty of the proximal phalanx and release of the metatarso-phalangeal joint. The base of the middle phalanx is exposed. The proximal phalanx with the head resected is shown, and plantarly is the digital segment of the distal tendon sheath of the flexor digitorum longus and brevis tendons.

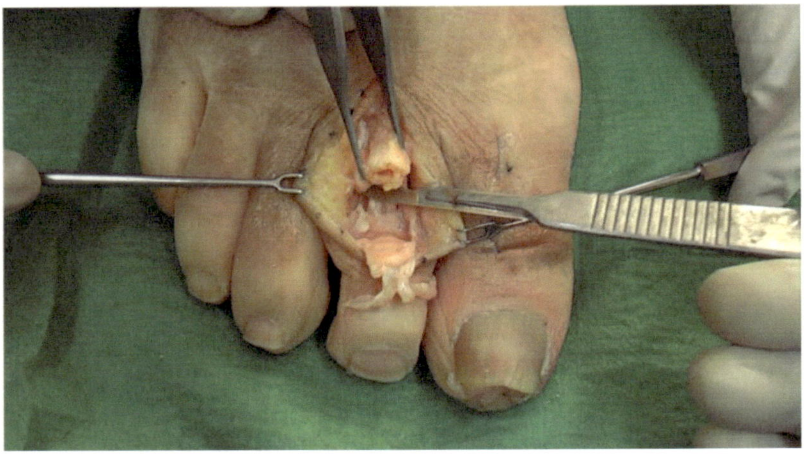

Figure 2. The plantar vincula are sectioned to release the flexor tendon sheath at the plantar aspect of the proximal phalanx of the second digit.

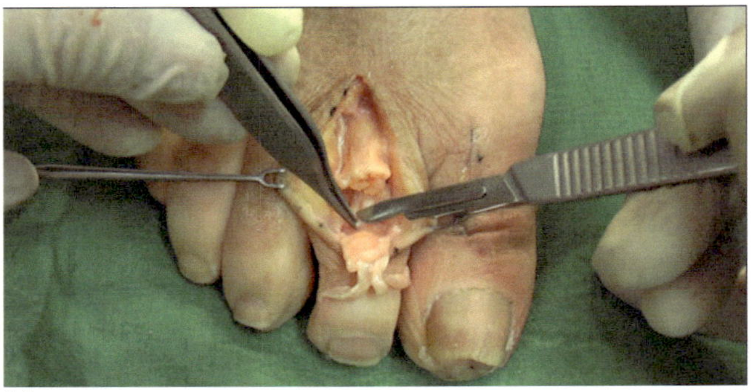

(a)

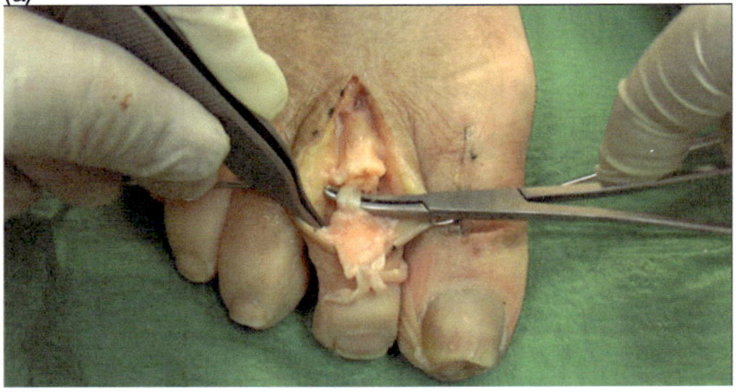

(b)

Figure 3. (a) The tendinous sheath is cut longitudinally, proximally and distally to the base of the middle phalanx. **(b)** The tendinous sheath is opened, and the flexor digitorum brevis hemitendons, lateral and medial, are exposed over the curved hemostat.

http://dx.doi.org/10.5772/52752

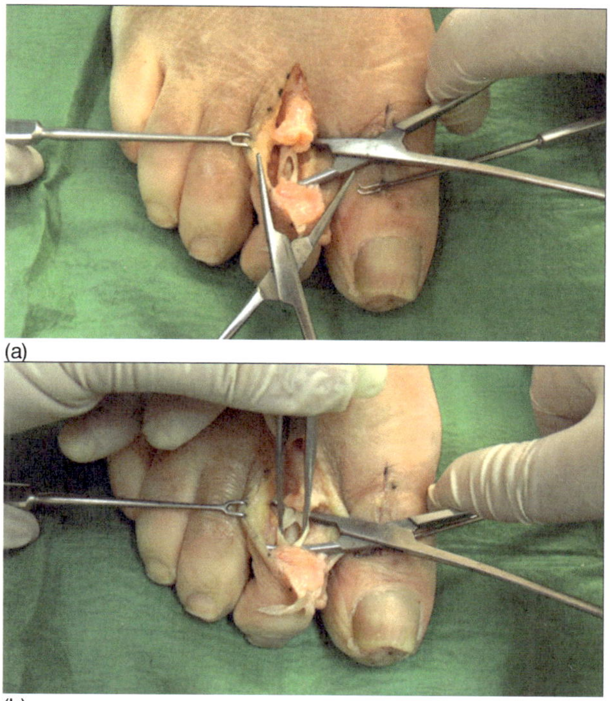

(a)

(b)

Figure 4. (a) The medial and lateral fascicles of the flexor digitorum brevis tendon are isolated using a curved hemostat. The flexor digitorum longus is localized plantarly. **(b)** Dorsal view of the hemitendons of flexor digitorum brevis with inadequate separation.

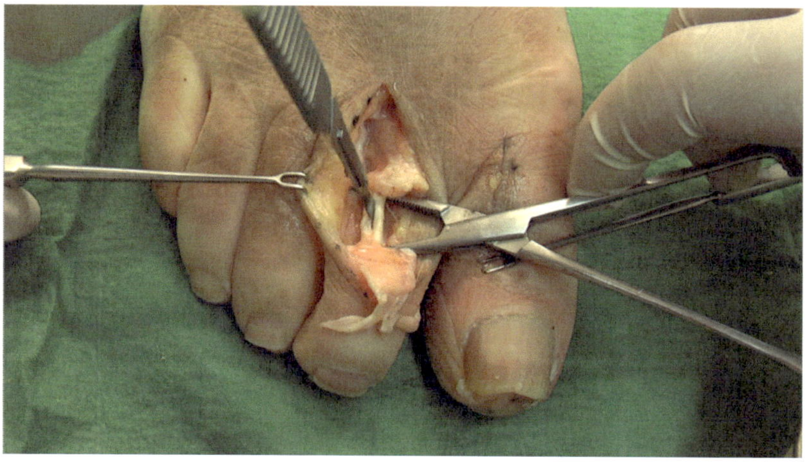

Figure 5. Flexor digitorum brevis is divided longitudinally and proximally using a blade #15 to permit passage of the flexor digitorum longus tendon.

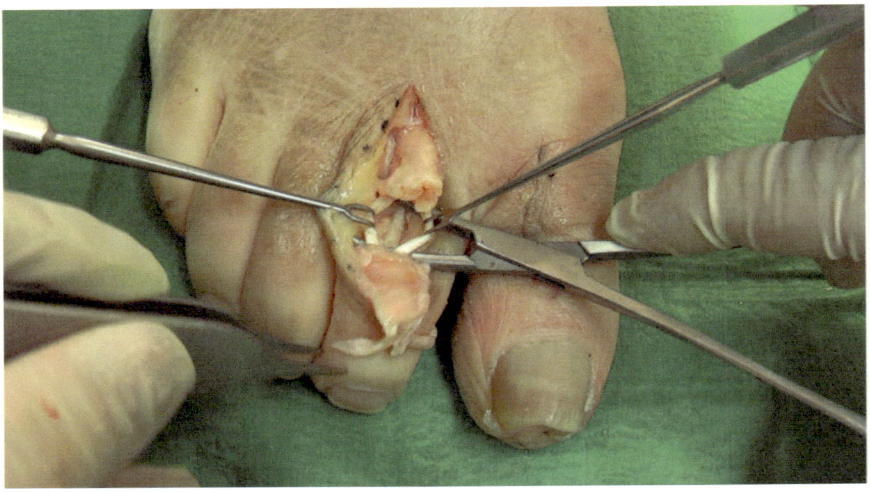

Figure 6. Medial and lateral hemitendon of the flexor digitorum brevis are retracted for plantar exposure of the flexor digitorum longus tendon.

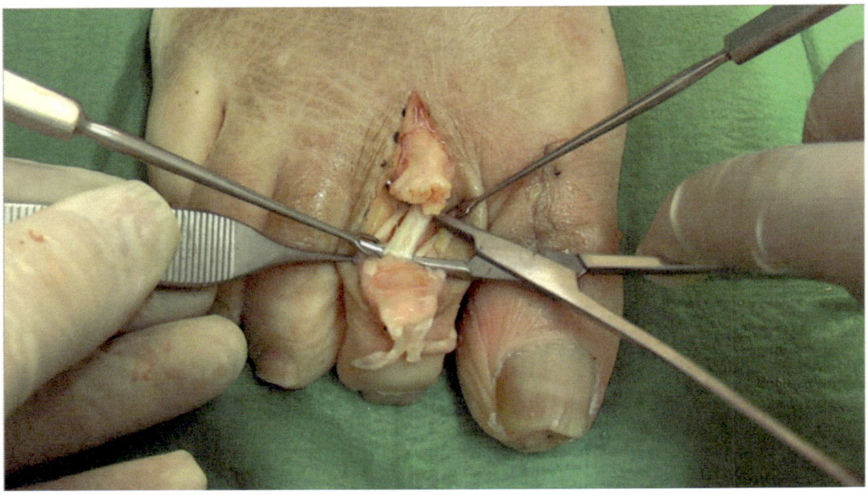

Figure 7. Using a curved hemostat and situating it plantar to the flexor digitorum longus is collocated dorsally between the medial and lateral hemitendons of flexor digitorum brevis.

http://dx.doi.org/10.5772/52752

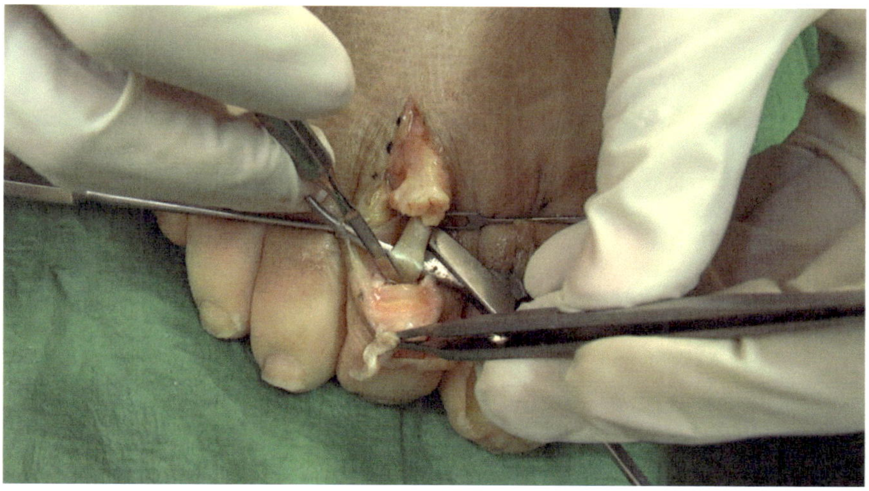

Figure 8. Using a mini-osteotome, the flexor digitorum longus tendon is released from the plantar aspect of the middle phalanx distally to obtain more tendon to facilitate the transfer.

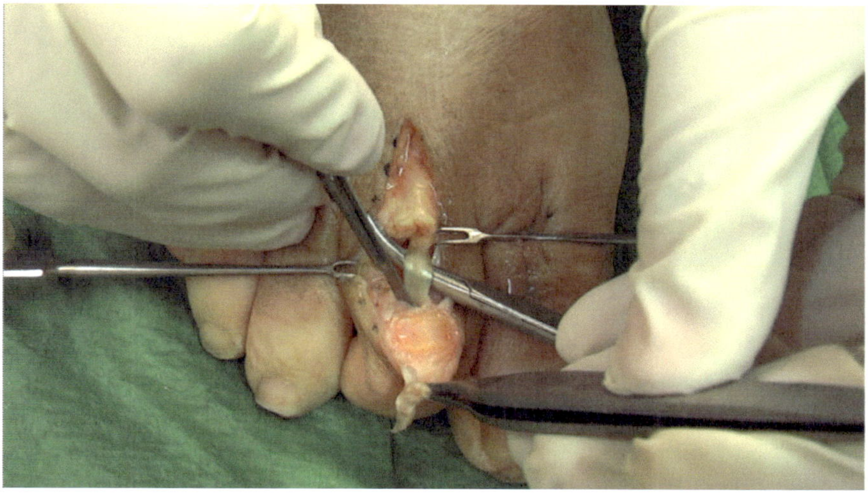

Figure 9. Flexor digitorum longus tendon is cut through its insertion point as distally as possible to the middle phalanx to maximize the length of the free distal tendinous stump.

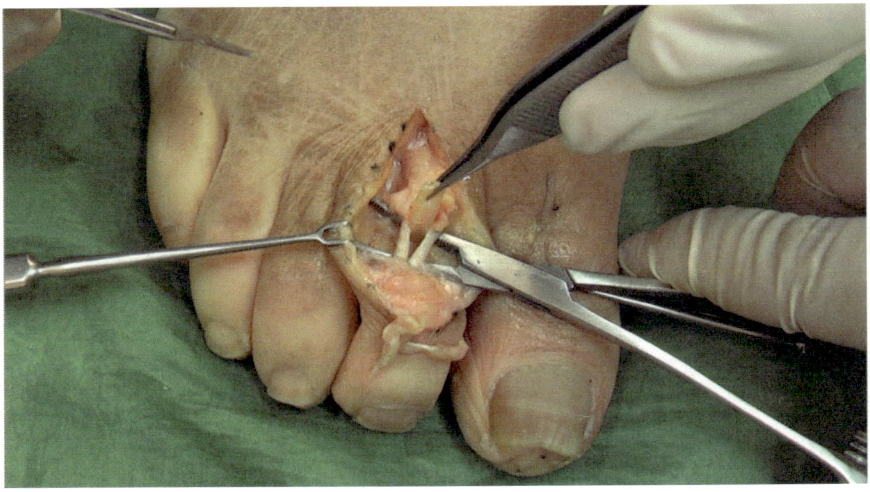

Figure 10. The stump of the proximal flexor digitorum longus tendon is clamped.

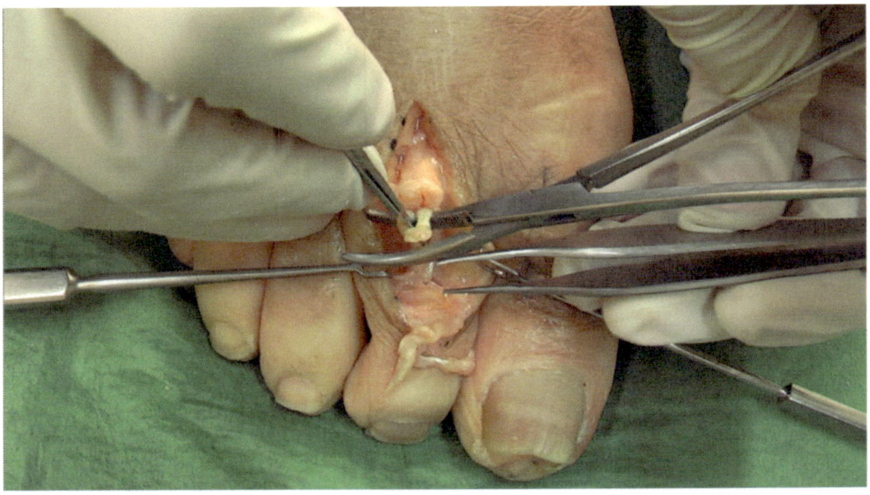

Figure 11. The long flexor is split longitudinally using a #15 blade.

http://dx.doi.org/10.5772/52752

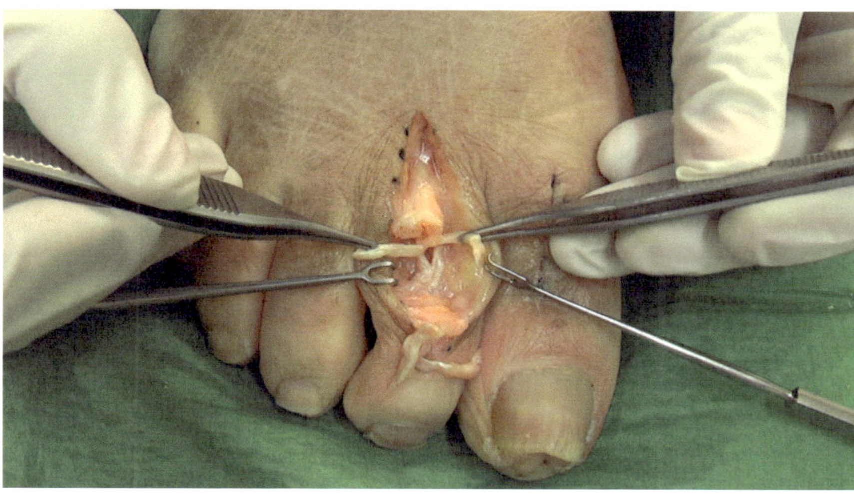

Figure 12. The flexor digitorum longus tendon has been split longitudinally in two portions, lateral and medial.

Once the medial and lateral fascicles of the FDL tendon had been clamped they were transferred to the dorsal aspect of the medial and lateral proximal phalanx, respectively. During this procedure the length of the split tendinous fascicles of the FDL tendon were evaluated to ascertain whether the length was sufficient to permit transposition over the dorsal proximal phalanx. If the length was not adequate, a major incision was made in the proximal flexor tendon sheath. The medial and lateral FDL tendon stumps were sutured to itself in the dorsum of the proximal phalanx (Fig. 13 A,B,C,D).

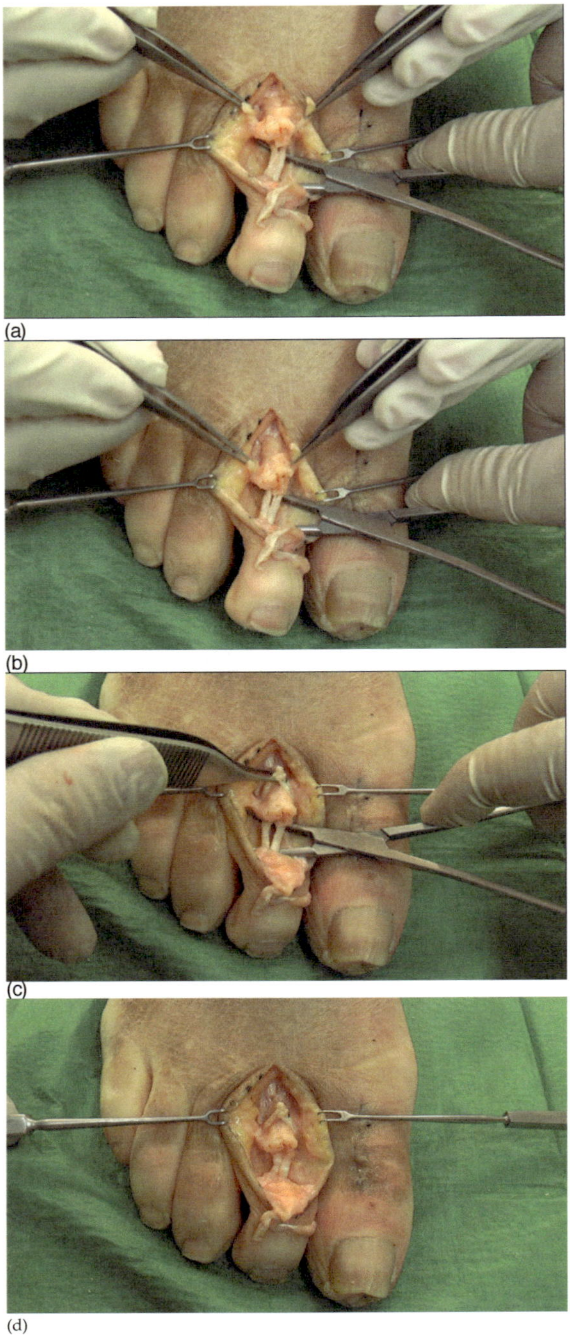

Figure 13. (a and b) The medial and lateral fascicles of the flexor digitorum longus tendon are transferred to the dorsal area of the proximal phalanx. The hemostat is showing the flexor digitorum brevis hemitendons. **(c)** Dorsal view of the medial and lateral stumps of the flexor digitorum longus tendon transferred to the medial and lateral aspects of

the proximal phalanx, respectively, and clamped with a pick up. The hemostat is showing the flexor digitorum brevis hemitendons intact. **(d)** Dorsal view of the flexor digitorum longus transferred to the dorsal aspect of the proximal phalanx

The toe was pinned using a double-pointed 0.54-mm Kirschner wire in a retrograde manner driven antegrade from the PIP joint, out the tip of the toe, and then retrograde into the proximal phalanx and the metatarsal head. The EDL stumps were sutured over the transferred FDL tendon (Fig. 14), and cutaneous suturing was performed in a usual manner.

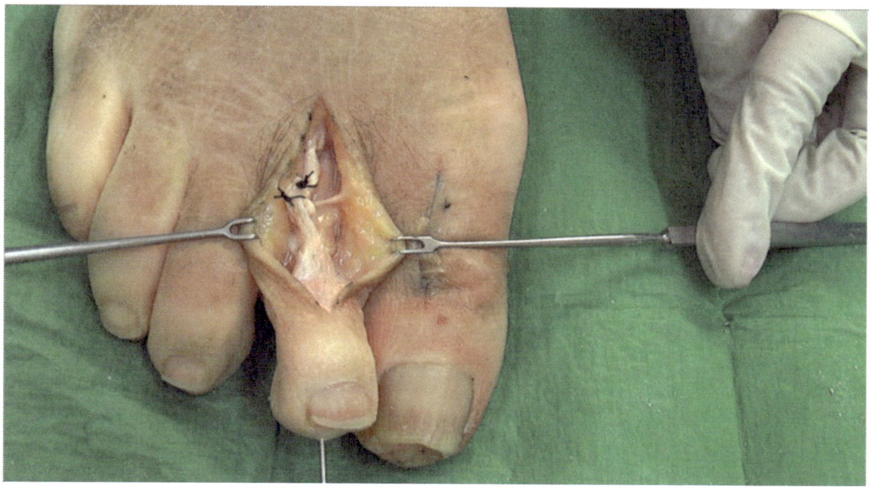

Figure 14. The extensor digitorum longus tendon stumps are sutured over the transferred flexor digitorum longus tendon.

3. Results

The FDL tendon transfer by the unique longitudinal dorsal approach attempted on 120 cadaveric toes (60 second toes and 30 third toes) was successful in 100% of the cases.

4. Discussion

The results of this study indicate that transfer of the FDL tendinous fascicles between the FDB hemitendons can be performed on second and third digits via a unique dorsal incision. Success of the procedure is predicated, in part, on an adequate longitudinal incision of the flexor tendon sheath that permits exposure and separation of the FDB hemitendons. We believe the indications for FDL tendon transfer between FDB hemitendons are the same as those for the FDL tendon transfer that other authors [28]- [36] are using for the correction of sagittal plane lesser MTP joint instability and loss of digital purchase. We do not, however, advocate this approach when the fifth digit is involved. In the current investigation, the FDB tendon was absent in 3 cases (7%), thus the dorsal approach was not possible. Any hammer toe or claw toe deformity that is accompanied by a semi-rigid or rigid MTP joint requires accompanying correction. This correction may be accomplished via PIP joint fusion or FDL tendon transfer, which moves the lever arm to the MTP joint and holds the proximal phalanx in a plantarflexed position.

Based on the results of this investigation, we believe the surgical technique for FDL tendon transfer should utilize a dorsal approach to minimize the risk of compromising the principal blood supply to the involved digits. Chen et al [37] evaluated the vasculature of 20 foot specimens focusing on the second, third, and fourth toes. Findings from the study suggest that plantar circulation is predominant in the second, third, and fourth toes, while dorsal circulation predominated in the first digit. Chen et al [37] further stated that the plantar digital arteries of the lesser toes provide the predominant arterial supply of the PIP joints through a system of transverse and longitudinal arches. Thus, when a claw or hammer toe deformity correction is performed via FDL tendon transfer through a two-incision plantar approach, a decision must be made regarding whether to continue or discontinue surgery when there is a risk of vascular compromise to the digit due to two incisions. Emphasizing the potential deleterious consequences of multiple incisions, Coughlin [18] recommended that it is far better to offer a 2-stage repair of the deformity than to incur a vascular insult with excessive surgery on a digit.

Surgical correction of hammer and claw toe deformity has been described extensively. Transposition of the flexor tendon to the extensor musculature through a dorso-lateral cut, with FDL tendon transfer to the dorso-lateral area of the proximal phalanx, was originally performed by Girdlestone in 1947 and developed by Taylor. [13] In his study, Taylor included 68 patients with claw or hammer toe deformity treated with this technique and associated procedures, such as dorsal capsulotomy of the MTP joint. Taylor also performed plantar capsulotomy of the interphalangeal joints and stabilization of the proximal phalanx using an external splint. Several modifications of the procedure have subsequently been reported. In 1970, Sgarlato [16] reported 53 cases of FDL tendon transfer through 3 skin incisions. Pyper [12] performed the technique described by Taylor [13] on 45 feet in 23 patients. To correct the digital deformity, he combined it with lengthening of the EDL tendon and dorsal capsulotomy of the MTP joint. Subsequently, Parrish [11] modified this technique by detaching the FDL tendon and dividing the proximal tendinous stump longitudinally and repositioning its medial and lateral aspects in the extensor area. He performed FDL and FDB tendon transfer on the first 5 patients in his series but not on the remaining 18 patients, stating that "the FDB tendon had a smaller calibre and its length was insufficient for the transposition." [11]

Marcinko et al [17] described the FDL tendon transfer using two incisions in the toe, one plantar and another dorsal. Barbari and Brevig [9] performed 39 FDL transpositions to the extensor area in 31 patients; 11 of the 39 procedures were performed in accordance with the technique of Taylor, [13] with the remaining 28 following the modified technique described by Parrish. [11] The approach was through a dorso-lateral incision over the MTP joint extending approximately 3 cm distally from the neck of the metatarsal bone. Dissection was then performed on each side of the proximal phalanx. The sheath of the flexor tendons was located, and the long flexor was then isolated, drawn out using a blunt hook, and divided near its distal insertion. It was then sutured end to end to the extensor tendon.

Coughlin [18], [19] performed an FDL tendon transfer by first making a transverse incision at the MTP joint, and then a second incision at the dorsal aspect of the digit. Kuwada [20] performed 81 procedures to transfer the FDL tendon via a dorsolateral incision along the digit beginning proximally at the MTP joint and extending distally to least the proximal PIP joint. Thompson and Deland [21] performed transfer of the FDL tendon in 13 digits following the indications of Coughlin [18] via the plantar and dorsal approach. Gazdag and Cracchiolo [22] in 11 feet performed an isolating tendon transfer of the FDL through the 2-cm longitudinal midline incision on the plantar side of the base of the proximal phalanx and performed another dorsal incision at the base of the proximal phalanx. Recently, Boyer and DeOrio [23] treated 70 toes with fixed or flexible hammer toes with a flexor-to-extensor tendon transfer making a longitudinal incision on the plantar aspect of the proximal phalanx and at the dorsal aspect of the toe.

The literature up to now reveals no attempts to discover why Parrish [11] found FDB tendon transfer to be a non-viable option. His findings, however, have been accepted by the scientific community without confirmation or challenge. Furthermore, many of the authors cited, except Barbari and Brevig, [9] performed the double plantar and dorsal incision approach as described by Girdlestone in 1947. [13]

In a cadaveric study we found [14] that it is possible to correct flexible claw and hammer toe deformity by transposing the FDB tendon to the extensor, or dorsal, area of the base of the proximal phalanx. This is a modification of the procedure used by Parrish [11] using a plantar and dorsal incision approach of the digit. We sought to transfer the FDB tendon to the dorsal aspect of the proximal phalanx via the dorsal approach through a unique incision, as described by Barbari and Brevig. [9]A search of the indexed literature found no previous reports of this procedure.

It is possible anatomical variations in the insertion of the FDB tendon may prohibit the popularity of this transfer approach. Three variations have been described: 1) absence of the tendon; 2) absence of the lateral and medial tendinous fascicles but presence of a single tendon running parallel to the FDL tendon; and 3) fusion of the FDB tendon to the FDL tendon. [24]-[27] LeDouble [24] and Nathan and Gloobe [25] found the FDB tendon to be absent in the fifth toe in 21.5% of cases. Testut [27] found the FDB tendon to be absent in the fourth and fifth toes in 3% of the dissections performed. In two separate studies [26], [27] Testut found that the FDB medial and lateral fascicles are not divided. Rather, the fascicles run parallel to the FDL tendon before inserting into a side of the intermediate phalanx of the fifth or fourth toe in 5% of patients. Although Testut [26], [27] did not specify individual percentages for variability in attachment for each of these digits, he established that the FDB tendon of the fifth toe is fused to the FDL tendon in 2% of cases. Thus, the anatomical variations found occur more frequently in the FDB tendon insertion of the fifth toe.

Anomalies or variations in the insertion of the FDB tendon in the third and second toes have not, however, been described. We reported [14] on transposition of the FDB tendon via the plantar approach in 180 digits of cadaveric feet, including 45 second digits, 45 third digits, 45 fourth digits, and 45 fifth digits. We found no cases of variation in the insertion of the FDB tendon in the second, third, or fourth digits, and the FDB tendon was present in all 45 cases. There was variability in FDB tendon presentation in the fifth digit, including FDB tendon absence in 3 of 45 digits (7%), which is a recognized anatomical variation. Thus, we performed the dorsal FDL tendon transfer via the dorsal approach between the FDB hemitendons in only the second and third digits.

Another potential factor prohibiting the tendon transfer approach described in this study may be inadequate space for FDL passage through the FDB hemitendons. After arthroplasty the tendon sheath is exposed and opened longitudinally, and the hemitendons of the FDB are identified just over the FDL tendon. Once the hemitendons are identified they are carefully separated (Fig. 4). If there is not adequate room for FDL passage, the FDB hemitendons must be incised longitudinally (Fig. 5). We believe this additional surgical step is the primary challenge associated with this technique, and may potentially explain why this technique has not previously been described.

Available FDL tendon length may also impact the surgical approach. Once the FDL tendon is detached distally from the distal phalange, it must be long enough to be transposed to the dorsal aspect of the proximal phalanx. When the MTP joint is rigidly dorsiflexed, it is necessary to perform a dorsal capsulotomy and MTP joint release as described by Barbari and Brevig, [9] thus relocating the proximal phalanx to its anatomical position. With this approach there is no need for plantar capsulotomies of the interphalangeal joints.

If there is difficulty in transferring the distal stumps of the longitudinally split FDL tendon to the dorsal aspect of the proximal phalanx of any digit, the clinician must cut the proximal flexor tendon sheath longitudinally for better FDL tendon exposure. We were able to transfer the FDL tendon via dorsal approach between the FDB hemitendons in100% of second and third digits via a unique single longitudinal incision. We did find it difficult, however, to transfer the FDL "around" the lateral aspects of the FDB hemitendons. This transfer was unsuccessful in 83 (69,16%; N = 120) digits, including 45 (37,5%) second digits and 38 (31,66%) of the third digits. We believe this was a consequence of inadequate proximal tendon sheath dissection. When attempting transfer of the split FDL tendon lateral to the FDB hemitendons, it is difficult to obtain adequate proximal exposure secondary to the depth of the anatomical structures. A mini-osteotome may be used to release the FDL tendon from the plantar aspect of the distal middle phalanx to obtain more tendon and facilitate the transfer.

While passing the split FDL tendons between the hemitendons of the FDB is necessary to cut the flexor tendon sheath.

We also encountered difficulty in transposing the FDL tendon as a consequence of the transverse aponeurotic fibers originating from the EDL tendon. These fibers surround the MTP joint capsule and join in the plantar area with the glenoid plate, the deep MTP ligament, and the sheath of the flexor tendons to insert distally into the plantar base of the proximal phalanx. These aponeurotic fibers and the sheath of the flexor tendons must be cut to allow the split FDL tendon to be repositioned and sutured to the dorsal aspect of the proximal phalanx.

A final challenge associated with this novel surgical approach is ankle positioning while suturing FDL tendon stumps. If the ankle is in plantarflexion the tendon has adequate length to permit suturing to the dorsal aspect of the proximal phalanx without difficulty. When the patient is weight-bearing or walking, however, the ankle is in dorsiflexion, which shortens the FDL tendon and forces the MTP joint into plantarflexion. The FDL tendon should therefore be sutured in its anatomical position to avoid inappropriate flexion or extension positioning of any involved joint.

5. Conclusions

Transfer of the FDL tendon to the dorsum of the proximal phalanx can be performed for the correction of claw and hammer toe deformities in the second and third digits. The meticulous longitudinal incision of the flexor tendon sheath to expose the FDB tendon and its longitudinal incision are essential to the success of the procedure. Furthermore, this approach preserves the integrity of the primary plantar blood supply to the digits of interest.

Author details

Ricardo Becerro de Bengoa Vallejo[1*], Marta Elena Losa Iglesias[2] and Miguel Fuentes Rodriguez[1]

*Address all correspondence to: ibebeva@enf.ucm.es

1 Escuela Universitaria de Enfermería, Fisioterapia y Podología, Universidad Complutense de Madrid, Madrid, Spain

2 Facultad de Ciencias de la Salud, Universidad Rey Juan Carlos, Madrid, Spain

References

[1] Coughlin, M. J. Lesser-toe abnormalities. J Bone Joint Surg Am (2002). , 84, 1446-1469.

[2] Sandeman, J. C. The role of soft tissue correction of claw toes. Br J Clin Pract (1967). , 21, 489-93.

[3] Coughlin, M. J, & Mann, R. A. Lesser Toe Deformities. In: MJ Coughlin, RA Mann *Surgery of the Foot and Ankle,* 7th ed. Mosby, St Louis; (1999). , 328.

[4] Richardson, E. G. Lesser Toe Abnormalities. In: AH Crenshaw. *Campbell's Operative Orthopaedics,* 8th ed. Mosby-Year Book, St Louis; (1992). , 99.

[5] Scheck, M. Etiology of acquired hammertoe deformity. Clin Orthop. (1977). , 123, 63-9.

[6] Engle, E. T, & Morton, D. J. Notes on foot disorders among natives of the Belgian Congo. J Bone Joint Surg. (1931).

[7] Lutter, L. D. Toe Deformities. In: *Atlas of Adult Foot and Ankle Surgery,* Mosby-Year Book, St Louis; (1997). , 74.

[8] Cyphers, S. M, & Feiwell, E. Review of the Girdlestone-Taylor procedure for clawtoes in myelodysplasia. Foot Ankle. (1988). , 8, 229-33.

[9] Barbari, S. G, & Brevig, K. Correction of clawtoes by the Girdlestone-Taylor flexor-extensor transfer procedure. Foot Ankle. (1984). , 5, 67-73.

[10] Newman, R. J, & Fitton, J. M. An evaluation of operative procedures in the treatment of hammertoe. Acta Orthop Scand. (1979). , 50, 709-12.

[11] Parrish TF: Dynamic correction of clawtoesOrthop Clin North Am. (1973). , 4, 97-102.

[12] Pyper, J. B. The flexor-extensor transplant operation for claw toes. J Bone Joint Surg Br. (1958). , 40, 528-33.

[13] Taylor, R. G. The treatment of claw toes by multiple transfers of flexor into extensor tendons. J Bone Joint Surg Br. (1951). , 33, 539-42.

[14] Becerro de Bengoa Vallejo RViejo Tirado F, Prados Frutos JC, Losa Iglesias ME, Jules KT. Transfer of the flexor digitorum brevis tendon. JAPMA. (2008). , 98, 27-35.

[15] Sarrafian, S. K. *Anatomy of the Foot and Ankle*. JB Lippincott, Philadelphia, (1983). , 243.

[16] Sgarlato, T. E. Transplantation of the flexor digitorum longus muscle tendon in hammertoes. JAPA. (1970). , 60, 383-8.

[17] Marcinko, D. E, Lazerson, A, Dollard, M. D, et al. Flexor digitorum longus tendon transfer: a simplified technique. JAPA. (1984). , 74, 380-5.

[18] Coughlin, M. J. Crossover second toe deformity. Foot Ankle. (1987). , 8, 29-39.

[19] Coughlin, M. J. Subluxation and dislocation of the second metatarsophalangeal joint. Orthop Clin North Am. (1989). , 20, 535-51.

[20] Kuwada, G. T. A retrospective analysis of modification of the flexor tendon transfer for correction of hammer toe. J Foot Surg. (1988). , 27, 57-9.

[21] Thompson, F. M, & Deland, J. T. Flexor tendon transfer for metatarsophalangeal instability of the second toe. Foot Ankle. (1993). , 14, 385-8.

[22] Gazdag, A, & Cracchiolo, A. Surgical treatment of patients with painful instability of the second metatarsophalangeal joint. Foot Ankle Int. (1998). , 19, 137-43.

[23] Boyer, M. L, & Deorio, J. K. Transfer of the flexor digitorum longus for the correction of lesser-toe deformities. Foot Ankle Int. (2007). , 28, 422-30.

[24] LeDouble AF*Traité des variations du systéme musculaire del l´homme et de leur signification au point de vue de l´anthropologie et zoologique,* Schleicher Fréres, Paris, (1897). , 2, 327.

[25] Nathan, H, & Gloobe, H. Flexor digitorum brevis: anatomical variations. Anat Anz. (1974). , 135, 295-301.

[26] Testut, L. *Les anomalies musculaires chez l´homme expliqueés par l´anatomie comparée: Leur importance en anthropologie.* Masson, Paris, (1884). , 588.

[27] Testut, L. *Les anomalies musculaires considérées du point de vue de la ligature des artéres.* Doin, Paris, (1892). , 38-40.

[28] Thompson, F. M, & Deland, J. T. Flexor tendon transfer for metatarsophalangeal instability of the second toe. Foot Ankle. (1993).

[29] Gazdag, A, & Cracchiolo, A. Surgical treatment of patients with painful instability of the second metatarsophalangeal joint. Foot Ankle Int. (1998).

[30] Coughlin, M. J. Second metatarsophalangeal joint instability in the athlete. Foot Ankle Int. (1993).

[31] Kuwada, G. T. A retrospective analysis of modification of the flexor tendon transfer for correction of hammertoe. J Foot Surg. (1988).

[32] Coughlin, M. J. Subluxation and dislocation of the second metatarsophalangeal joint. Orthop Clin North Am. (1989).

[33] Thompson, F. M, & Deland, J. T. Flexor tendon transfer for metatarsophalangeal instability of the second toe. Foot Ankle Int. (1993). , 14, 385-8.

[34] Mendocino, R. W, Statler, T. K, Saltrick, K. R, & Catanzariti, A. R. Predislocation syndrome: a review and analysis of eight patients. J Foot Ankle Surg. (2001). , 40, 214-24.

[35] Myerson, M. S, & Jung, H. G. The role of toe flexor-to-extensor transfer in correcting metatarsophalangeal joint instability of the second toe. Foot Ankle Int. (2005). , 29, 675-9.

[36] Bouché, R. T, & Heit, E. J. Combined plantar plate and hammertoe repair with flexor digitorum longus tendon transfer for chronic, severe sagittal plane instability of the lesser metatarsophalangeal joints: preliminary observations. J Foot Ankle Surg. (2008). , 47, 125-37.

[37] Chen, Y. G, Cook, P. A, Mcclinton, M. A, et al. Microarterial anatomy of the lesser toe proximal interphalangeal joints. J Hand Surg [Am]. (1998). , 23, 256-60.

[38] May JW JrChait LA, Cohen BE, O'Brien BM. Free neurovascular flap from the first web space of the foot in hand reconstruction. J Hand Surg. (1977). , 2, 387-93.

[39] Murakami T: On the position and course of the deep plantar arterieswith special reference to the so-called plantar metatarsal arteries. Okajimas Folia Anat Jpn. (1971). , 48, 295-322.